Clinical Ophthalmology, 7/e
A Systematic Approach, International Edition
Expert Consult Online and Print

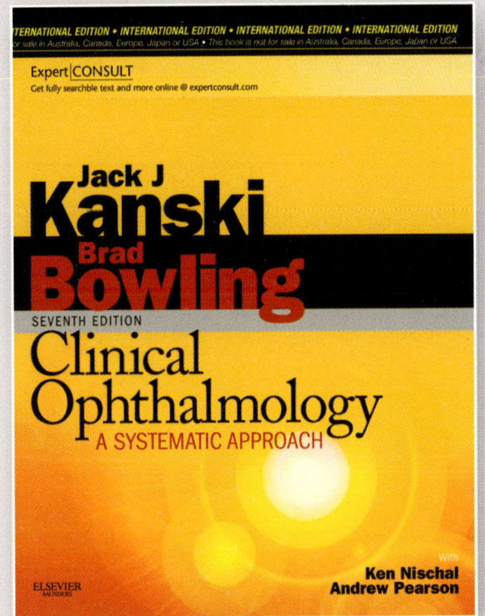

*By **Jack J. Kanski**, MD, MS, FRCS, FRCOphth, Honorary Consultant Ophthalmic Surgeon, Prince Charles Eye Unit, King Edward VII Hospital, Windsor, UK*

***Brad Bowling**, FRCSEd(Ophth), FRCOphth, Consultant Ophthalmic Surgeon, Blackpool Victoria Hospital, Blackpool, United Kingdom, UK*

Ideally suited for rapid reference and efficient, effective recall, this state-of-the-art multimedia resource will keep you up to date with current and evolving practice in the diagnosis and management of ophthalmic disorders, using a visually rich, succinct format that facilitates comprehension for trainees and practitioners. Online and in print, you'll have access to the latest advances in the field.

Features

- Grasp key information and effectively prepare for examinations with a pictorial, bulleted approach – both highly visual and concise, for more efficient study.
- Move rapidly throughout the text to find the information you need, with color coding and at-a-glance key points.
- Approx. 2,743 illustrations (2,436 in full color).
- Access the complete contents online at www.expertconsult.com, with a downloadable image gallery.
- Learn from two renowned experts in the field.
- Includes over 2,700 high-quality images, 1,000 of which appear for the first time in this edition.

ISBN: 9780702040955

www.elsevier.co.in

Spectral-domain
Optical Coherence Tomography
Imaging of the Eye

Spectral-domain Optical Coherence Tomography Imaging of the Eye

ANAND VINEKAR, MD, FRCS

Head, Pediatric Retina Service and Program Director,
KIDROP (Tele-ROP Services),
Narayana Nethralaya Postgraduate Institute of Ophthalmology,
Bangalore, India

KAVITHA AVADHANI, MD

Consultant, Uveitis and Ocular Immunology Service,
Narayana Nethralaya Postgraduate Institute of Ophthalmology,
Bangalore, India

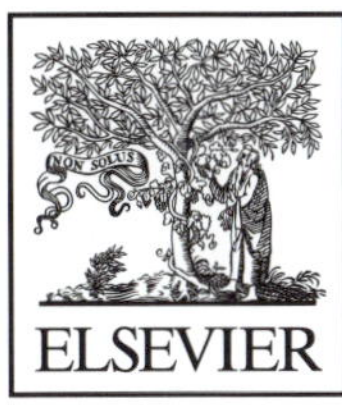

ELSEVIER

A division of
Reed Elsevier India Private Limited

Spectral-domain Optical Coherence Tomography Imaging of the Eye
Anand Vinekar and Kavitha Avadhani

ELSEVIER
A division of
Reed Elsevier India Private Limited

*Mosby, Saunders, Churchill Livingstone, Butterworth-Heinemann and
Hanley & Belfus are the Health Science imprints of Elsevier.*

© 2013 Elsevier

ISBN: 978-81-312-3052-7

Medical knowledge is constantly changing. As new information becomes available, changes in treatment, procedures, equipment and the use of drugs become necessary. The authors, editors, contributors and the publisher have, as far as it is possible, taken care to ensure that the information given in this text is accurate and up-to-date. However, readers are strongly advised to confirm that the information, especially with regard to drug dose/usage, complies with current legislation and standards of practice. ***Please consult full prescribing information before issuing prescriptions for any product mentioned in the publication.***

Published by Elsevier, a division of Reed Elsevier India Private Limited.

Registered Office: 305, Rohit House, 3, Tolstoy Marg, New Delhi – 110 001.
Corporate Office: 14th Floor, Building No. 10B, DLF Cyber City, Phase-II, Gurgaon, Haryana – 122 002, India.

Managing Editor: Shabina Nasim
Development Editor: Goldy Bhatnagar
Copy Editor: Richa Srivastava
Manager – Publishing Operations: Sunil Kumar
Manager – Production: NC Pant
Production Executive: Ravinder Sharma
Cover Designer: Raman Kumar

Typeset by Olympus Premedia Pvt. Ltd. (*formerly* Olympus Infotech Pvt. Ltd.), Chennai, India (www.olympus.co.in).

Printed and bound at Sanat Printers, Kundli (Harayana)

Foreword

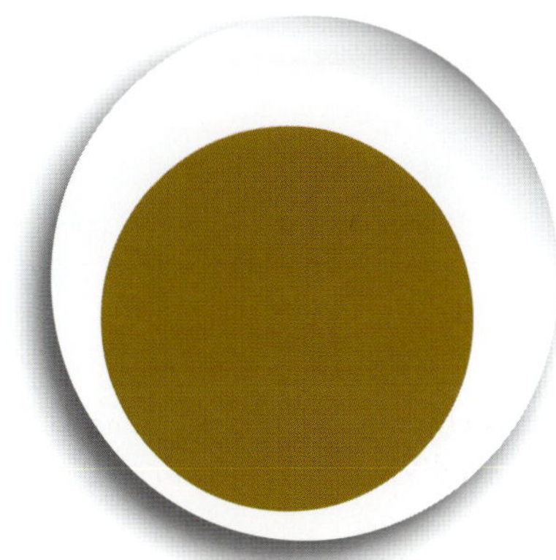

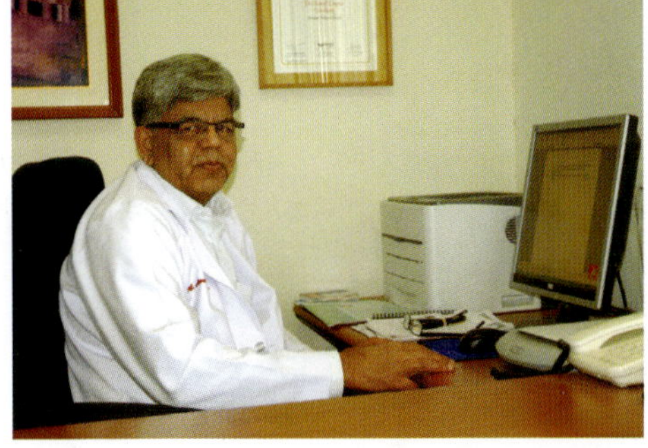

This book is an excellent method of illustrating to the reader, the use of a relatively new ophthalmic imaging technique—Spectral-domain Optical Coherence Tomography (SD-OCT).

What is unique about its style is its ability to present the clinical and SD-OCT images of a disease along with other relevant investigations in an easy-to-read case study style. This helps in emphasizing clinically relevant information to the reader—be it a resident, or fellow, or a specialist consultant who are likely to encounter such cases in routine practice.

Significantly, this book fills a void in available literature by comprehensively dealing with SD-OCT imaging in both anterior and posterior segment diseases between its covers. Optical coherence tomography (OCT) imaging of the cornea and lens, and sections on glaucoma and pediatric retina add new value to the book, making it appealing to general ophthalmologists as well as a large section of subspecialists. International contributors in many sections have added disease entities that are not commonly seen in our part of the world, giving the book an international appeal.

It is also a matter of pride for me as both the chief editors of the book—Dr Anand Vinekar and Dr Kavitha Avadhani—have passed through our portals at the PGI, Chandigarh and have done a wonderful job in putting together this text atlas.

I have no doubt that this book would become an essential requirement on the bookshelves of all those in ophthalmic practice who wish to better understand SD-OCT imaging in eye diseases. I wish the book all success and many more editions in the future.

Professor Amod Gupta, MD
Professor and Head of Department,
Advanced Eye Centre and
Dean, Postgraduate Institute of Medical
Education and Research,
Chandigarh, India

Preface

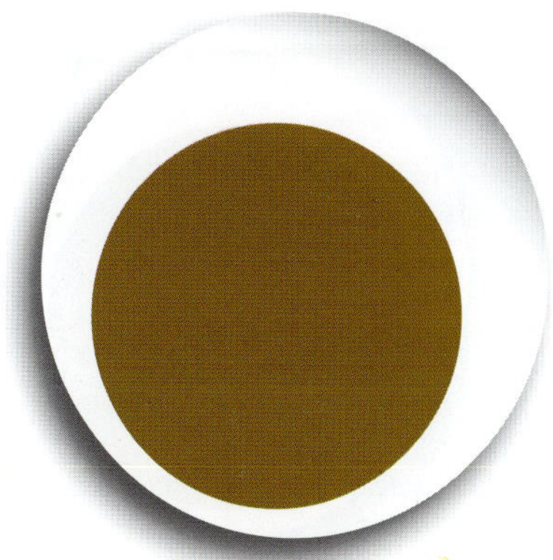

The idea of bringing out this book was not deliberate. It evolved over several weekly "imaging case rounds" with our residents and fellows, each discussing a specific clinical entity and the role of spectral-domain optical coherence tomography (SD-OCT), known more popularly as "SD-OCT", in defining either the diagnosis or influencing the course of their cases. When our institute joined the elite league by possessing a hand-held SD-OCT device, the repertoire of cases only got more diverse and more interesting. Thus, began the serendipitous evolution of the compilation of these cases, which has eventually led to this case atlas.

In this First Edition of **"Spectral-domain OCT Imaging of the Eye"**, we have attempted to maintain the "Case Study" feel of the disorders being discussed. This includes, in most cases, seeking contributors internationally that have either described the disease for the first time or groups who have significant research advancements in that topic. We feel proud that out of the 102 contributors, more than two-thirds are invited faculty.

Again, keeping in with the theme, there has been no attempt to homogenize the content with respect to the form and structure. Each contributor has been allowed to present the case in his or her own style, intonation, and scientific tenor. We hope that in doing so, it would appear as if the authors were "presenting their case" to the reader, rather than a more formal, pedagogic style.

Every attempt has been made to bring to print, common and rare conditions that could be imaged on SD-OCT. Some entities in this book have not been published elsewhere. We thank the untiring efforts of the section editors, who have sought the contributions of renowned faculty in their subspecialty across the globe.

However, we realize that this is neither a compendium nor an exhaustive text, and cannot replace formal textbooks in this field. Our attempt is merely to bring between its covers, what the reader may not have experienced before, i.e., all major subspecialties of eye diseases in an easy-to-read "image heavy" format that tells a story. With this wide spectrum of cases, we hope that the resident, the fellow, the specialist and the academic will find something to hold their interest in this book.

This text atlas strives to visually educate the potential of SD-OCT, which has revolutionized our practice of ophthalmology in the past few decades. Improving technology, better resolution, and faster scans provide newer insights into "old" and "new" diseases which continue to improve our understanding, eventually allowing us to provide better care to our patients.

We hope this book not only answers some of those questions, but also gives rise to several more, to continue to advance this wonderful science we passionately profess—Ophthalmology.

Anand Vinekar and Kavitha Avadhani
Editors-in-Chief

Acknowledgments

This book – *Spectral-domain Optical Coherence Tomography Imaging of the Eye* would not have been possible of course without our imaging teams! Sivakumar Munusamy, Krishnan Narashimha, and Deekshith Suvarna—our posterior segment experts who multitask between several devices, and Nagaraj MC and Dharshan RR for handling the anterior segment. Special thanks to Muhammad Naizal for helping design the cover, Dr Anupama Kiran Kumar during the final stages of editing, and Praveen Sharma who provided the logistic assistance during the evolution of this book.

Editorial Board

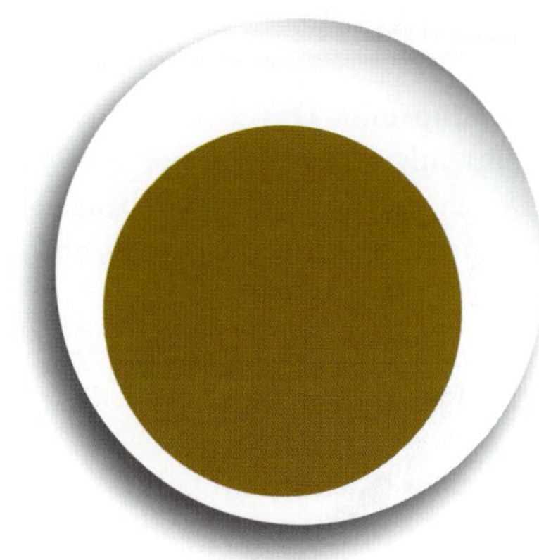

Editor-in-Chief and Subeditor
PEDIATRIC RETINA

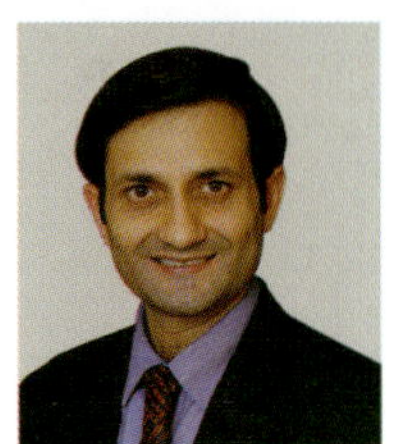

Anand Vinekar, MD, FRCS, is a pediatric retinal specialist, trained at the Postgraduate Institute of Medical Education and Research, Chandigarh, India and Royal Oak, Michigan, USA. He currently serves as the Head of the Pediatric Retina service at Narayana Nethralaya Postgraduate Institute of Ophthalmology, Bangalore. Dr Vinekar has pioneered KIDROP, a unique Tele-ROP program that provides infant eye screening in rural areas. The program is now under the National Rural Health Mission, Ministry of Health and Family Welfare, Government of India. He is the recipient of several awards including the Kataria Gold Medal by the Prime Minister of India, "Young Researcher Award", Positive Health Award, Rajiv Gandhi Excellence Award and finds mention in the Marquis Who's Who of the World. His research interests include pediatric retinal vascular diseases, pediatric OCT imaging, retinal imaging analysis, and community pediatric eye diseases.

Editor-in-Chief and Subeditor
UVEA

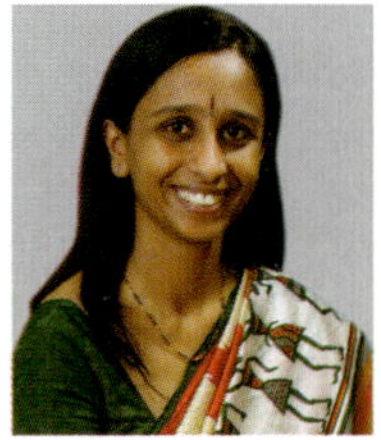

Kavitha Avadhani, MD, trained at Postgraduate Institute of Medical Education and Research, Chandigarh, where she topped her batch. She has subsequently held several teaching positions including serving on the faculty of Kasturba Medical College, Manipal, India. She currently serves as a Senior Consultant in the Department of Uveitis and Immunology at Narayana Nethralaya Postgraduate Institute of Ophthalmology, Bangalore, India. Dr Avadhani has several publications to her credit and has served on the editorial boards of several publications including the All India Ophthalmology Association's Ready Reckoner and several ophthalmic newsletters. Her research interests include posterior segment imaging, retinal imaging analysis and spectral-domain OCT.

CORNEA

Madhusmita Das, MD, trained at L.V. Prasad Eye Institute, Hyderabad, India and currently serves as a senior consultant in the cornea, cataract and refractive service at Vasan Eye Care Hospital, Bangalore, India. Her areas of interest include endothelial keratoplasty, refractive surgery, and keratoprosthesis.

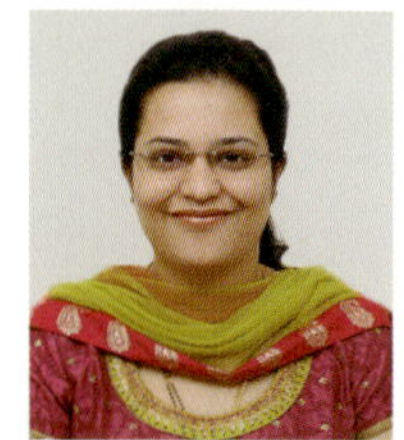

LENS

Mathew Kurien, MD, MBA, is a refractive lens surgeon, with special interest in biostatistics, health care management and surgical training. With an executive MBA from the Indian Institute of Management, he also serves as Medical Superintendent at Narayana Nethralaya, Bangalore, India.

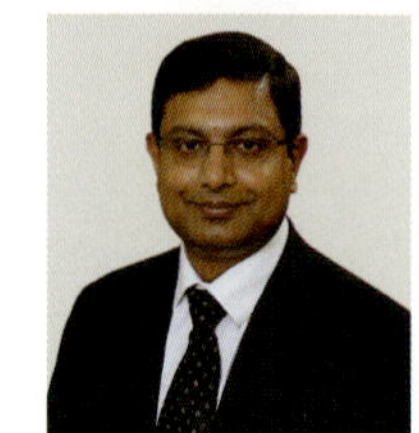

Sudeep Das, MD, is a senior consultant in the Department of Cataract and Refractive Lens Surgery, Narayana Nethralaya, Bangalore, India. He is actively involved in surgical training and evinces special interest in refractive lens surgery and ocular trauma.

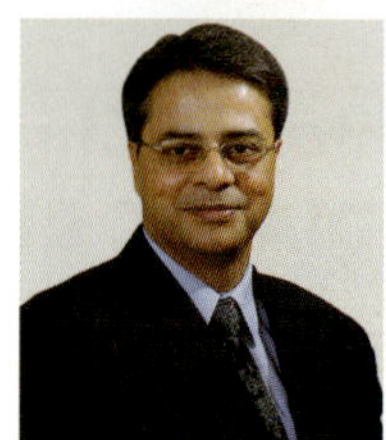

GLAUCOMA

Rajesh S Kumar, MD, is the Deputy Director of Clinical Research. He has been involved in extensive glaucoma research at Sydney Eye Hospital and Singapore Eye Research Institute prior to joining as Senior Consultant at Narayana Nethralaya, Bangalore, India. His special interests include angle closure disease and imaging.

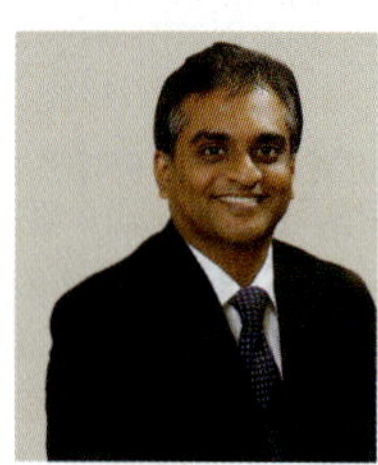

RETINA

Rajani Battu, MD, FRCS, serves as a Senior Consultant at the Department of Vitreo Retina, Narayana Nethralaya, Bangalore, India. Her research interests include inherited retinal dystrophies and genetic eye disorders. She has completed her training from St. John's Medical College, Bangalore and Sankara Nethralaya, Chennai, and Moorfields Eye Hospital, UK.

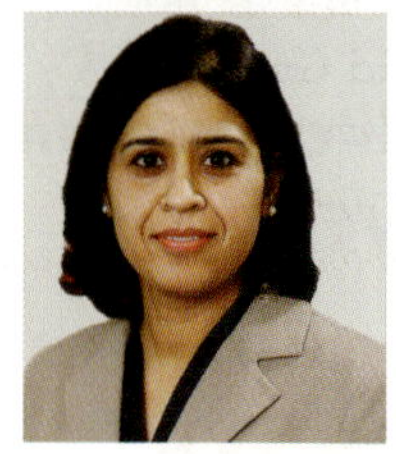

List of Contributors

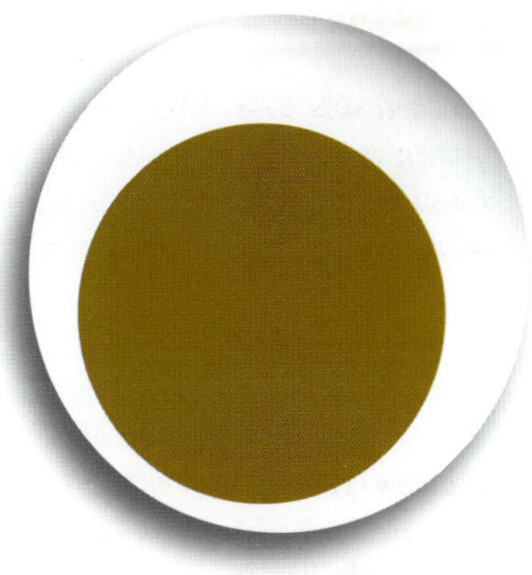

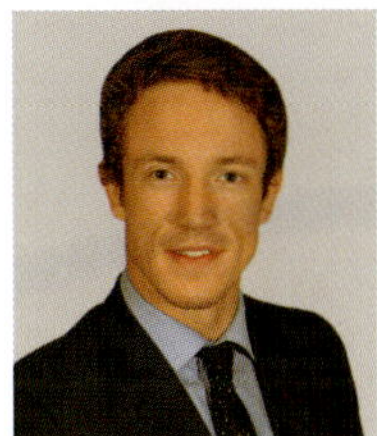

Adam Muzychuk, MD
Department of Surgery, Division of Ophthalmology,
University of Calgary, Canada

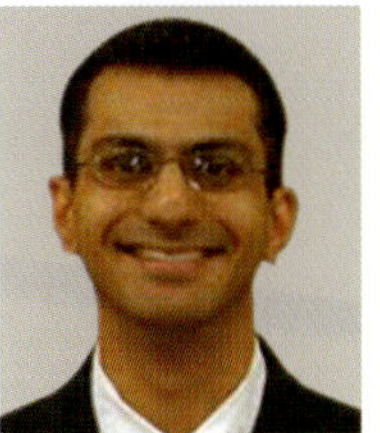

Ajay Shalwala, MD
Vanderbilt Eye Institute,
Vanderbilt University Medical Center,
Nashville, Tennessee,
USA

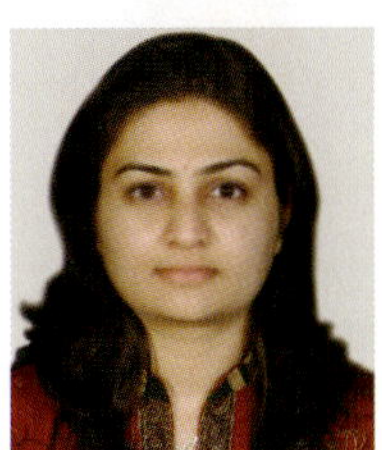

Aditi Ghodke, MD
Fellow, Cataract and Refractive Lens Service,
Narayana Nethralaya Postgraduate Institute of
Ophthalmology, Bangalore, India

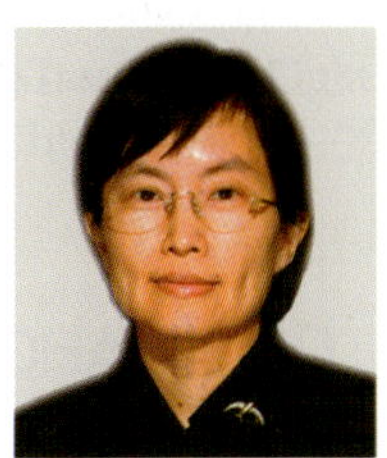

Aliza Jap
Singapore National Eye Centre,
Changi General Hospital,
Singapore

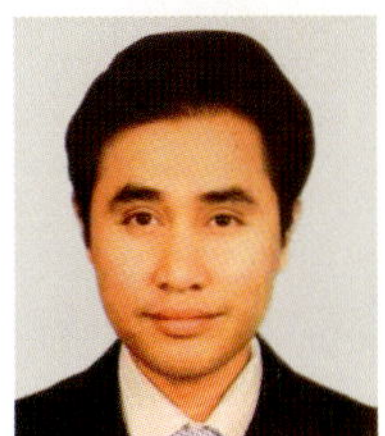

Ainur Rahman Bin Anuar, MD
Singapore Eye Research Institute,
Singapore National Eye Centre, Singapore;
Department of Ophthalmology, Faculty of Medicine,
University of Malaya, Kuala Lumpur, Malaysia;
University of Malaya Eye Research Centre, Faculty of
Medicine, University of Malaya, Kuala Lumpur, Malaysia

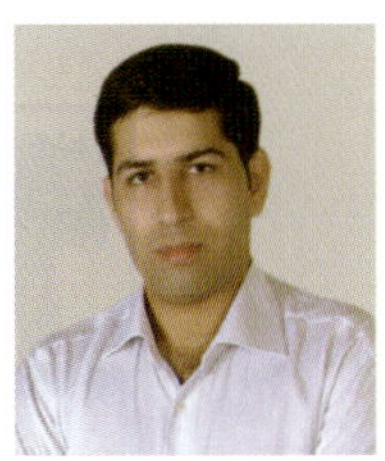

Amit Sobti, MD
Senior Registrar,
Dr Rajendra Prasad Centre for Ophthalmic Sciences,
All India Institute of Medical Sciences,
New Delhi, India

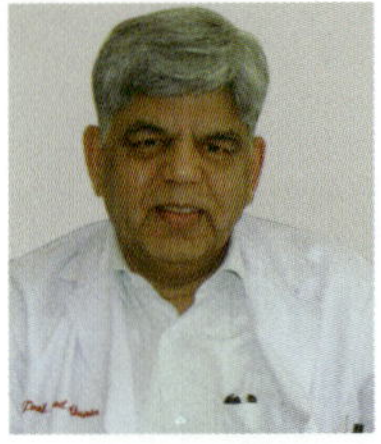

Amod Gupta, MD
*Professor and Head of Department, Advanced Eye Centre,
Dean, Postgraduate Institute of Medical Education and
Research, Chandigarh, India*

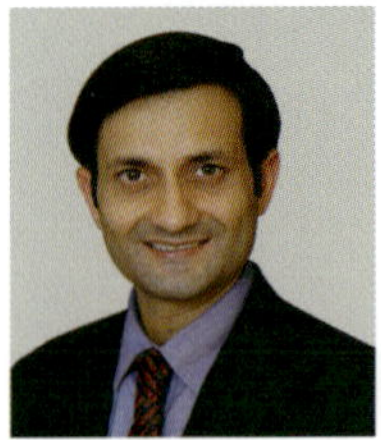

Anand Vinekar, MD, FRCS
*Head, Pediatric Retina Service and Program Director,
KIDROP (Tele-ROP Services),
Narayana Nethralaya Postgraduate Institute of
Ophthalmology,
Bangalore, India*

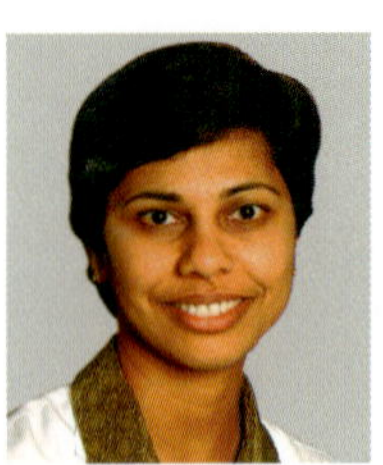

Anita Agarwal, MD
*Associate Professor, Retina and
Vitreous Vanderbilt Eye Institute,
Vanderbilt University Medical Center,
Nashville, Tennessee, USA*

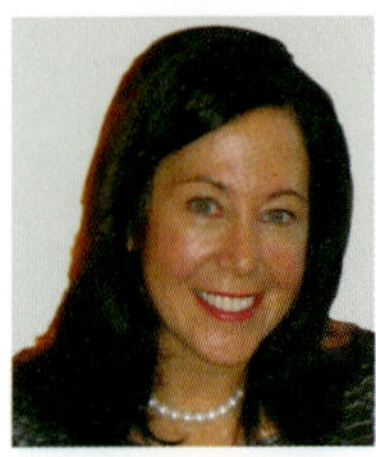

Anna Ells, MD, FRCS (C)
*Ells Retina Centre and University of Calgary,
Calgary, Canada*

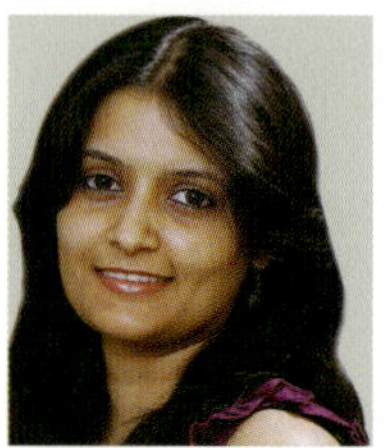

Anupama Kiran Kumar, MD
*Fellow, Department of Vitreo-Retina,
Narayana Nethralaya Postgraduate Institute of
Ophthalmology, Bangalore, India*

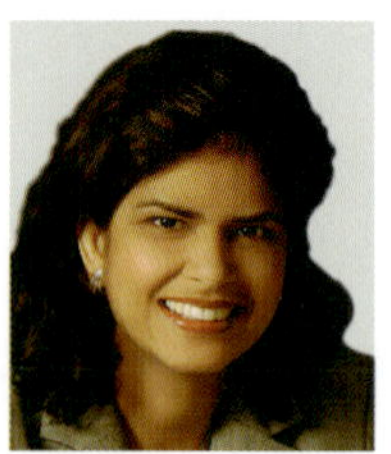

Arundhati Anshu, MD, FRCS (Ed)
*Singapore National Eye Center,
Singapore*

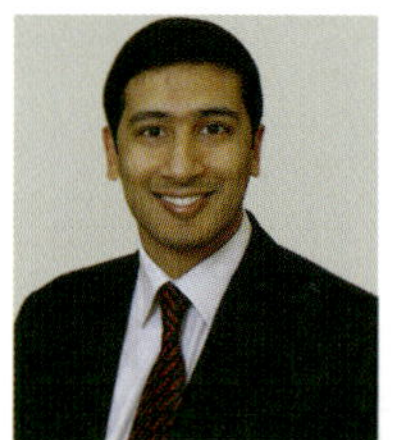

Ashwin Mallipatna, MD
*Consultant, Pediatric Ophthalmology and
Strabismus Service and In-charge,
Retinoblastoma Service,
Narayana Nethralaya Postgraduate Institute of
Ophthalmology, Bangalore, India*

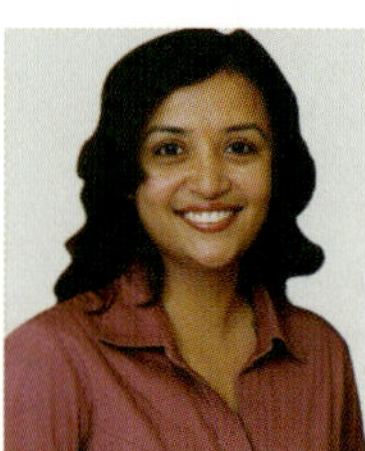

Ashwini Ranganath, MD
*Fellow, Cornea and Refractive Service,
Narayana Nethralaya Postgraduate Institute of
Ophthalmology, Bangalore,
India*

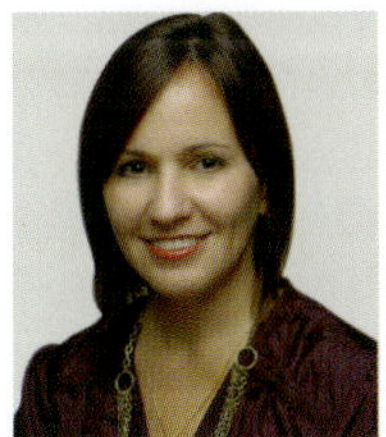

Audina Berrocal, MD
Bascom Palmer Eye Institute, University of Miami,
Miami, Florida, USA

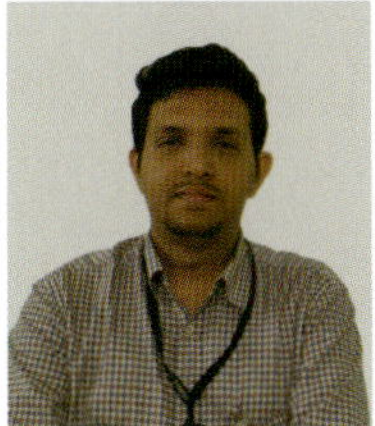

Bhaskar Srinivasan, MD
Senior Consultant,
Dr G Sitalakshmi Memorial Clinic for
Ocular Surface Disorders, Sankara Nethralaya,
Medical Research Foundation, Chennai, India

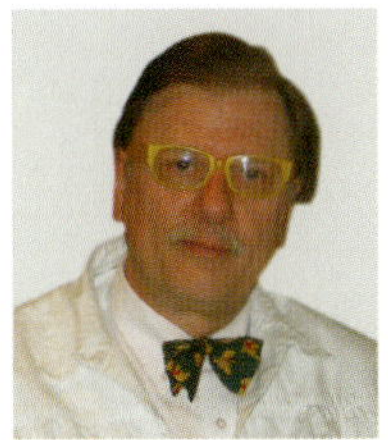

Carl P Herbort, MD, PD
Inflammatory and Retinal Eye Diseases,
Centre for Ophthalmic Specialized Care,
Lausanne, Switzerland, University of Lausanne,
Lausanne, Switzerland

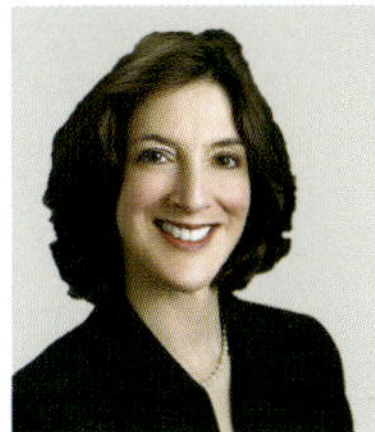

Carol L Karp, MD
Professor of Ophthalmology,
Bascom Palmer Eye Institute,
University of Miami School of Medicine,
Miami, Florida, USA

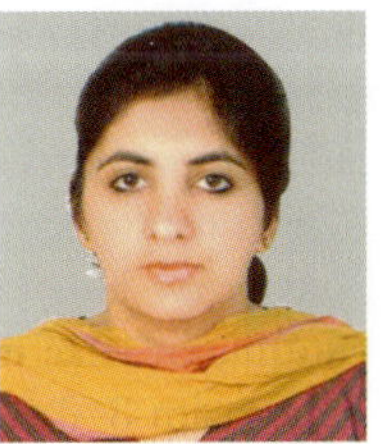

Chintan Malhotra, MD
Assistant Professor, Department of Ophthalmology,
Postgraduate Institute of Medical Education and Research,
Chandigarh, India

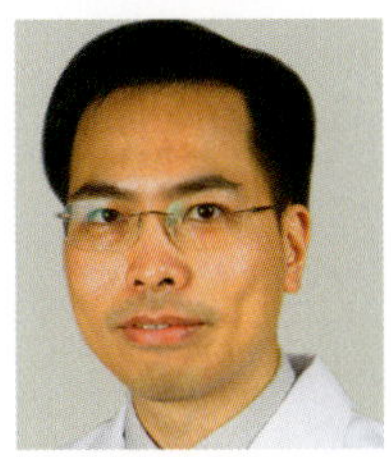

Christopher KS Leung, MD
Professor, Department of Ophthalmology and Visual
Sciences,
The Chinese University of Hong Kong,
Hong Kong, PRC

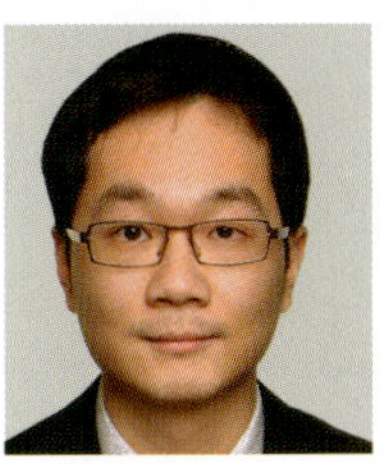

Cong Ye
Imaging Laboratory Manager,
Department of Ophthalmology and Visual Sciences,
The Chinese University of
Hong Kong,
Hong Kong, PRC

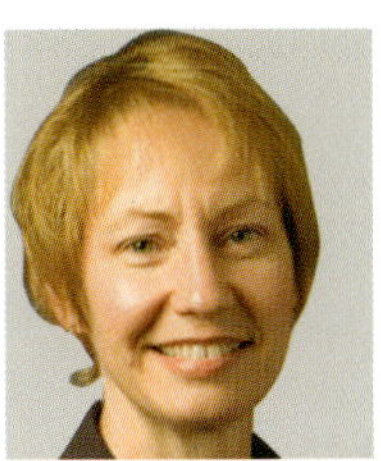

Cynthia Toth, MD
Professor of Ophthalmology and Biomedical Engineering,
Duke University Eye Center, North Carolina, USA

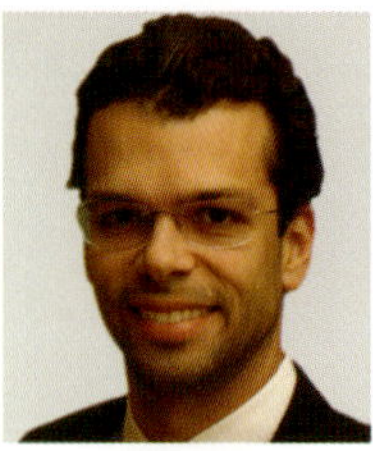

Daniel Vitor Vasconcelos-Santos, MD, PhD
Associate Professor of Ophthalmology,
Universidade Federal de Minas Gerais,
Belo Horizonte, Brazil

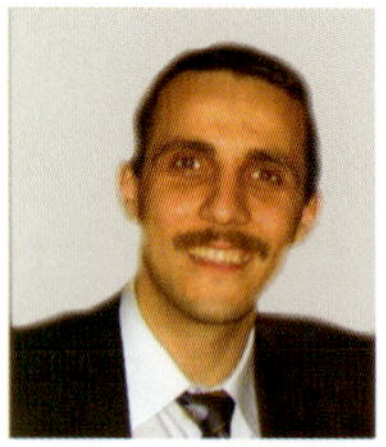

Demetrios G Vavvas, MD, PhD
Department of Ophthalmology,
Massachusetts Eye and Ear Infirmary,
Harvard Medical School, Boston, MA

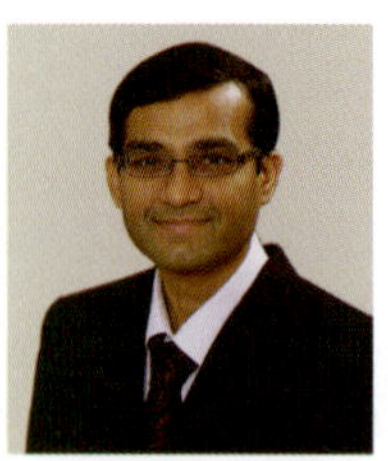

Dhanraj Rao AS, MD
Consultant, Glaucoma Service,
Narayana Nethralaya Postgraduate Institute of
Ophthalmology,
Bangalore, India

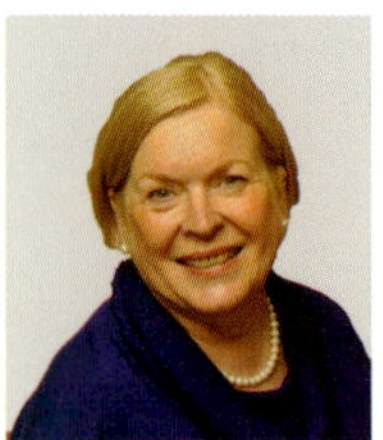

Ditte Hess
Bascom Palmer Eye Institute, University of Miami,
Miami, Florida, USA

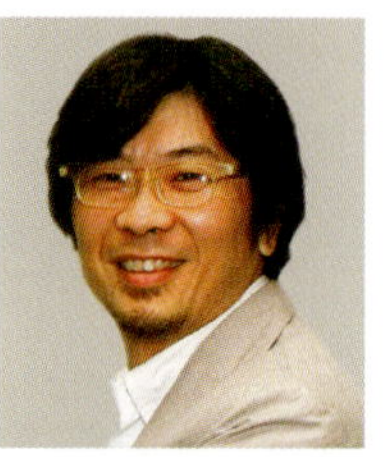

Donald Tan, MD
Singapore National Eye Center,
Singapore

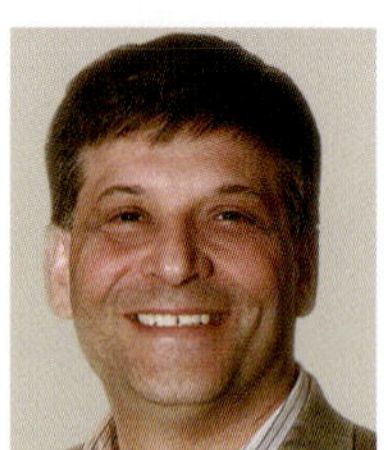

Eric L Buckland, PhD
President and CEO, Bioptigen, Inc.
USA

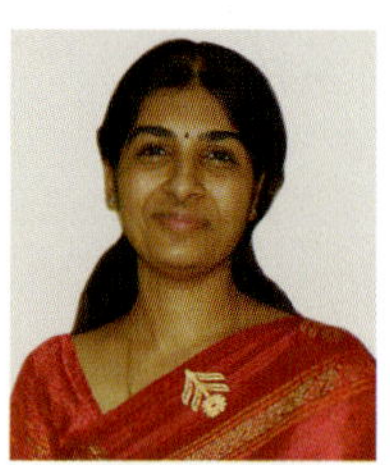

Geetha Iyer, MD
Senior Consultant,
Dr G Sitalakshmi Memorial Clinic for
Ocular Surface Disorders, Sankara Nethralaya,
Medical Research Foundation,
Chennai, India

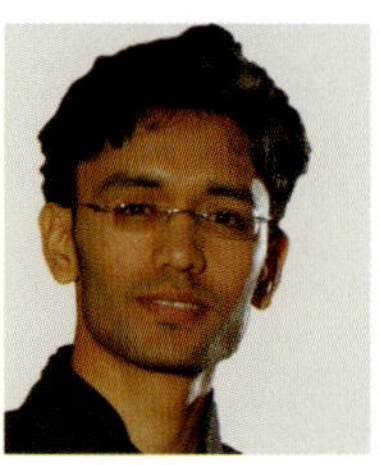

Harsh Yadav, MD
Retina Foundation,
Ahmedabad,
India

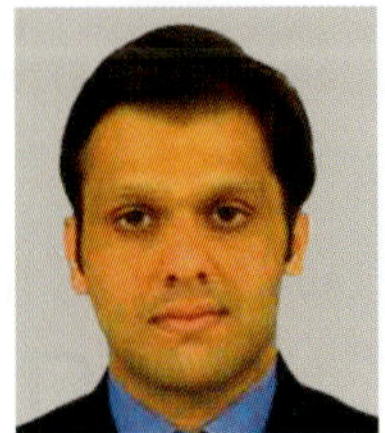

Harsha Pai, MD
Alpha Eye Centre, Mangalore,
India

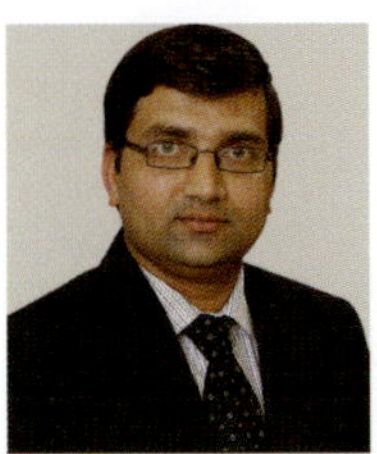

Hemanth Anaspure, MD
Consultant, Pediatric Ophthalmology and
Strabismus Service, Narayana Nethralaya
Postgraduate Institute of Ophthalmology,
Bangalore, India

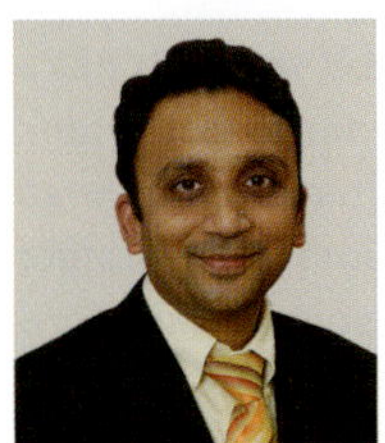

Himanshu Matalia, MD
Medical Superintendent and Head of
Cornea and Refractive Service (NN2)
Narayana Nethralaya Postgraduate Institute of
Ophthalmology, Bangalore, India

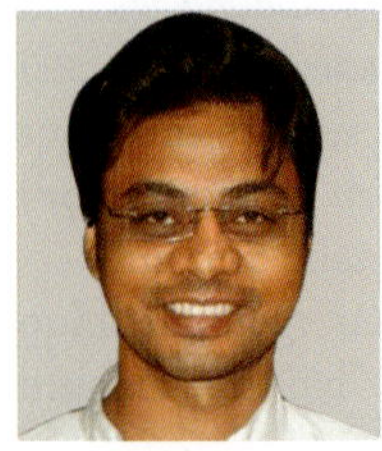

Jainendra Rahud, MD
Retina Foundation,
Ahmedabad, India

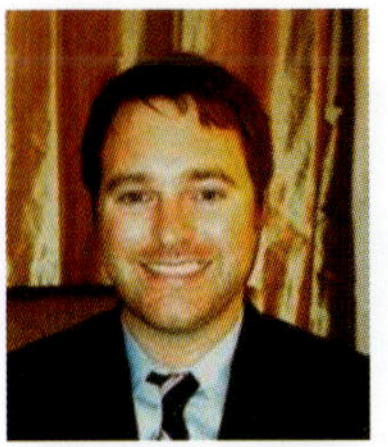

Jared L Matthews, MD
The Florida Lions Ocular Pathology Laboratory,
Bascom Palmer Eye Institute,
University of Miami Miller School of Medicine,
Miami, Florida,
USA

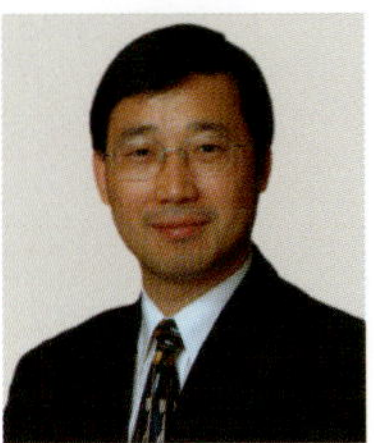

Jianhua Wang, MD, PhD
Associate Professor of Ophthalmology,
Bascom Palmer Eye Institute,
University of Miami School of Medicine,
Miami, Florida,
USA

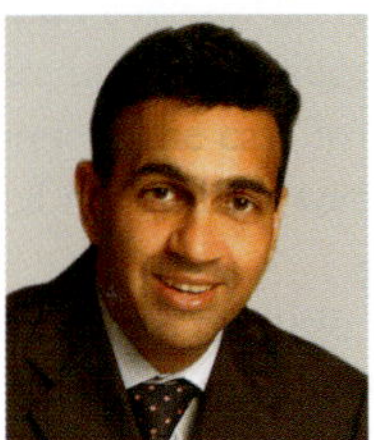

Jodhbir Mehta, BSc (Hons), MBBS,
MRC Ophth, FRCOphth, FRCS (Ed)
Head Corneal and External Eye Disease Service,
Senior Consultant Refractive Service,
Singapore National Eye Centre,
Head, Tissue Engineering and
Stem Cells Group,
Singapore Eye Research Institute,
Associate Professor,
Department of Ophthalmology,
Duke-NUS Graduate Medical School,
Singapore

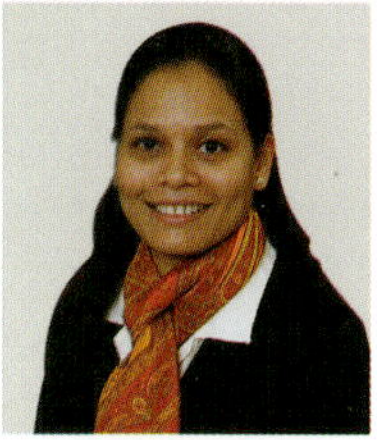

Jyoti Matalia, MD
Consultant, Pediatric Ophthalmology and Strabismus Service, Narayana Nethralaya Postgraduate Institute of Ophthalmology, Bangalore, India

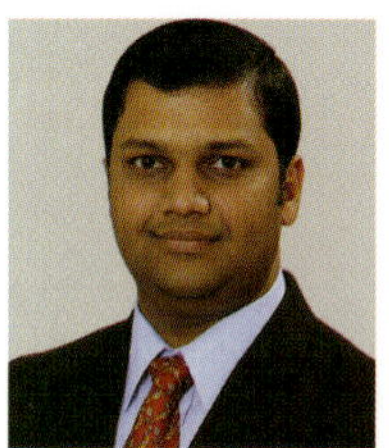

Kanav Gupta, MD
Fellow, Vitreo-Retina Service, Narayana Nethralaya Postgraduate Institute of Ophthalmology, Bangalore, India

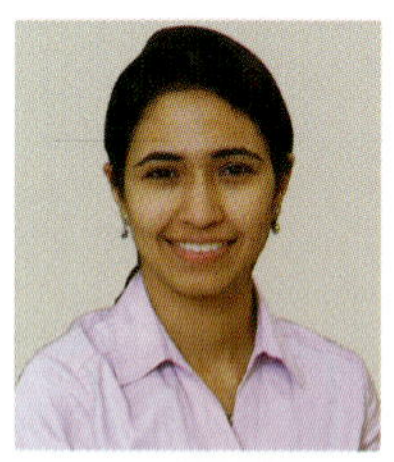

Kareeshma Wadia–Havewala, MD
Fellow, Cornea and Refractive Services, Narayana Nethralaya Postgraduate Institute of Ophthalmology, Bangalore, India

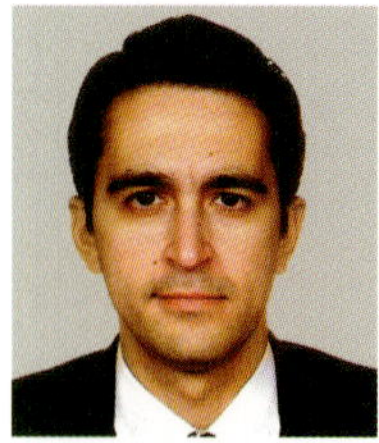

Karim Mohamed–Noriega, MD
Singapore National Eye Centre, Singapore. Tissue Engineering and Stem Cell Group, Singapore Eye Research Institute, Singapore; Dept of Ophthalmology, Faculty of Medicine and University Hospital "Jose Eleuterio Gonzalez", Autonomous University of Nuevo Leon (UANL), Monterrey, Mexico;

Professor, Department of Ophthalmology, Clinics of Cornea and External Diseases, Refractive Surgery and Cataract, Faculty of Medicine and University Hospital "Jose Eleuterio Gonzalez", Autonomous University of Nuevo Leon (UANL), Monterrey, Mexico

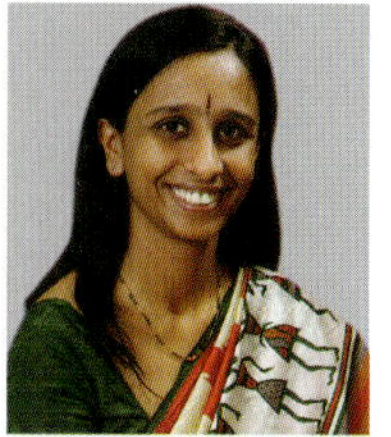

Kavitha Avadhani, MD
Consultant, Uveitis and Ocular Immunology Service, Narayana Nethralaya Postgraduate Institute of Ophthalmology, Bangalore, India

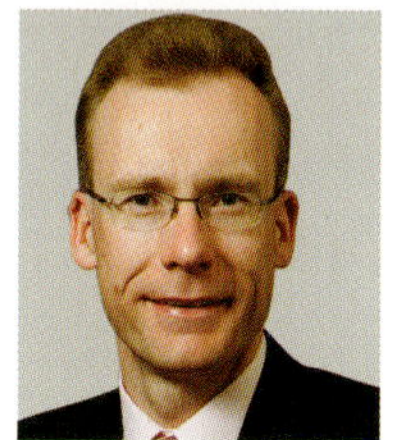

Kester Nahen, PhD
Heidelberg, Germany

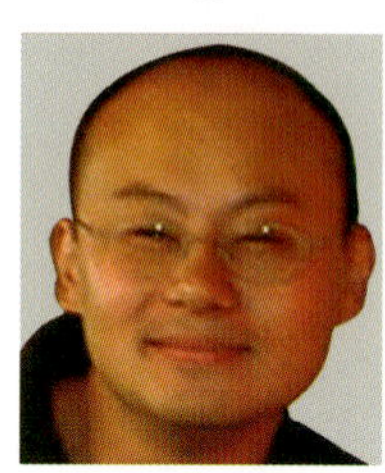

Lisandro M Sakata, MD, PhD
Glaucoma Consultant Department of Ophthalmology, Universidade Federal de São Paulo, Brazil Clinica Sakata Ophthalmology, Curitiba, PR, Brazil

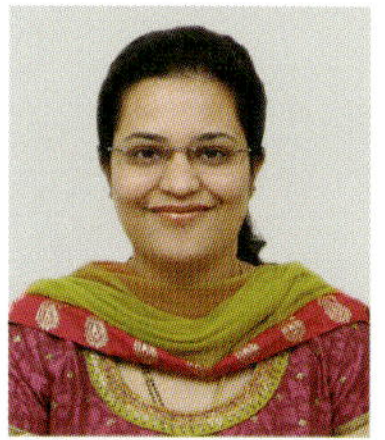

Madhusmita Das, MD
Senior Consultant, Cornea, Cataract and Refractive Services, and Uvea and Ocular Immunology Services, Vasan Eye Care Hospital, Bangalore, India

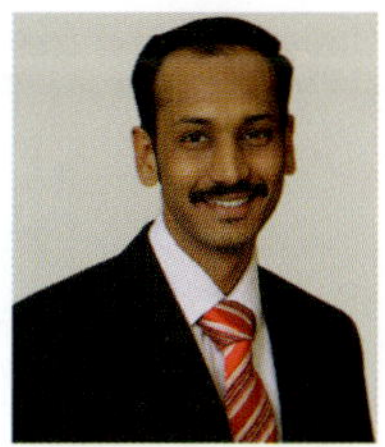

Mahesh Chandargi, MD
Consultant, Vitreo-Retina Service,
Narayana Nethralaya Postgraduate Institute of
Ophthalmology, Bangalore,
India

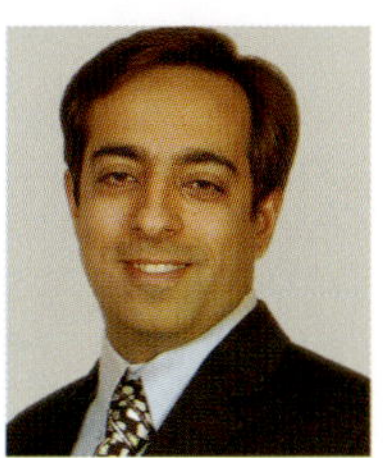

Manish Nagpal, MD, FRCS
Vitreo-Retina Consultant,
Retina Foundation,
Ahmedabad, India

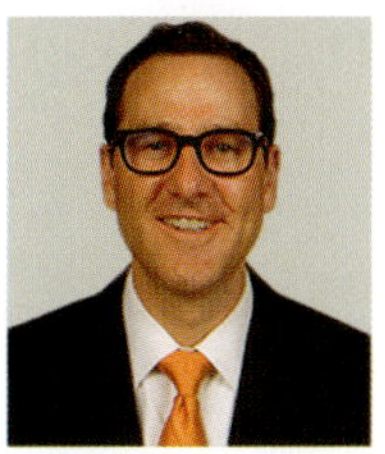

Mark A Greiner, MD
Assistant Professor, Cornea and External Diseases,
University of Iowa Hospitals and Clinics,
Department of Ophthalmology and
Visual Sciences, Iowa City, USA

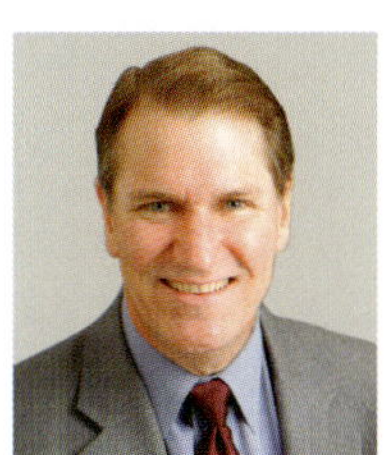

Mark A Terry, MD
Director Corneal Services,
Devers Eye Institute, Professor,
Clinical Ophthalmology,
Oregon Health Sciences University,
Portland, Oregon, USA

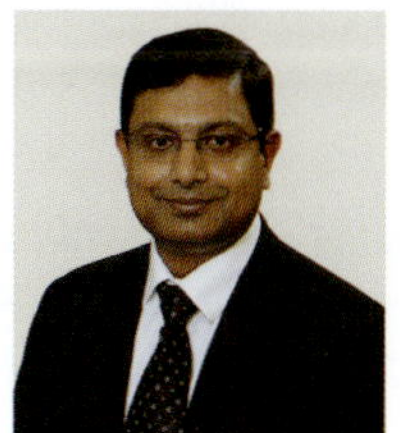

Mathew Kurien, MD
Medical Superintendent (NN1) and
Head Cataract and Refractive Lens Service,
Narayana Nethralaya Postgraduate Institute of
Ophthalmology, Bangalore,
India

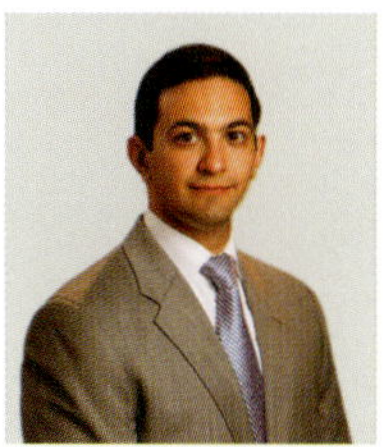

Maziar Lalezary, MD
Southern California Desert Retina Consultants,
Palm Desert,
California, USA

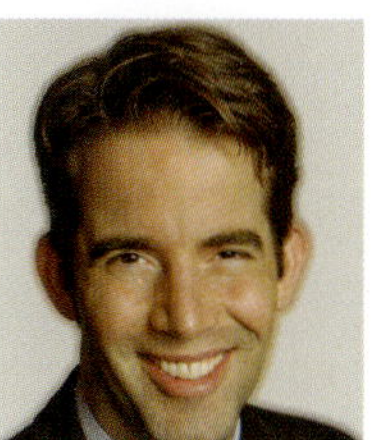

Michael D Straiko, MD
Associate Director, Corneal Services,
Devers Eye Institute,
Portland, Oregon,
USA

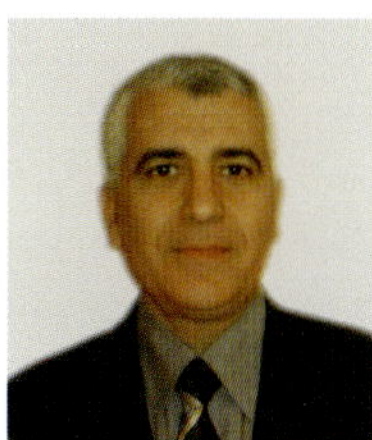

Moncef Khairallah, MD
Department of Ophthalmology,
Fattouma Bourguiba University Hospital,
Faculty of Medicine, University of Monastir,
Monastir, Tunisia

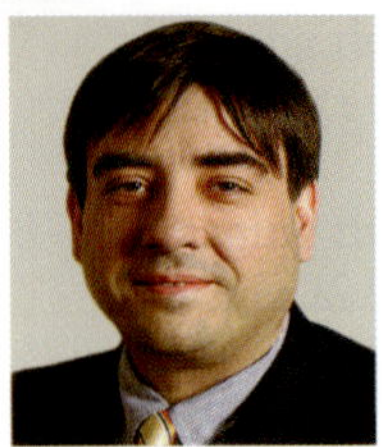

Murat Dogru, MD
Department of Ophthalmology,
Tokyo Dental College School of Medicine,
Chiba, Japan

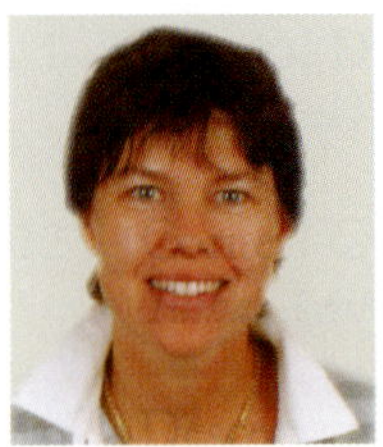

Nadia Bouchenaki, MD
Centre for Ophthalmic Specialized Care,
Lausanne, Switzerland

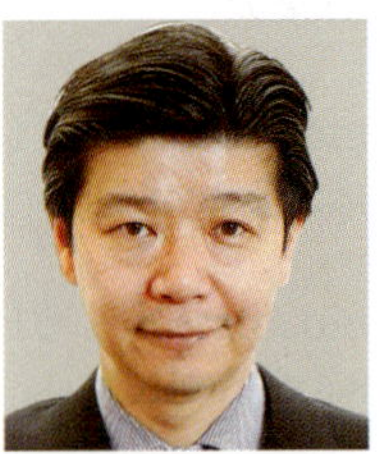

Naoyuki Maeda, MD
Department of Ophthalmology,
Osaka University Graduate School of Medicine,
Suita, Japan

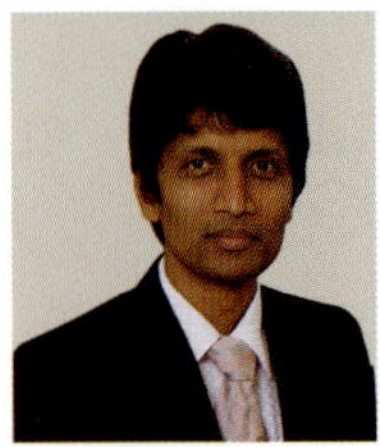

Narendra KP, MD
Consultant, Glaucoma Service,
Narayana Nethralaya Postgraduate Institute of
Ophthalmology,
Bangalore, India

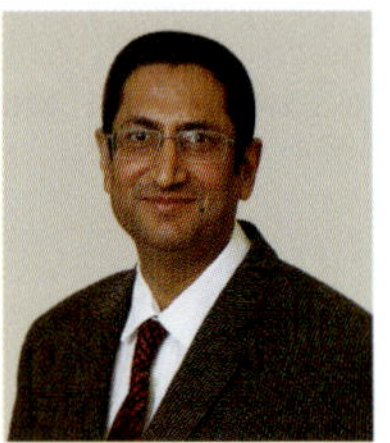

Naresh Kumar Yadav, MD
Head, Vitreo-Retina Service,
Narayana Nethralaya Postgraduate Institute of
Ophthalmology, Bangalore, India

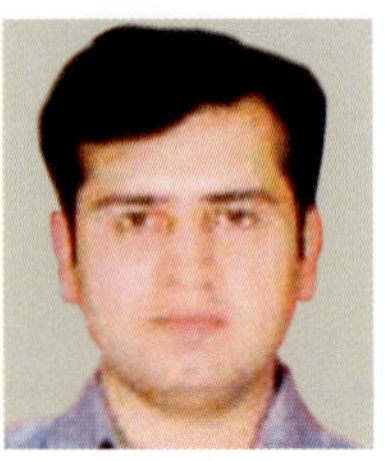

Navneet Mehrotra, MD
Vitreo-Retina Consultant,
Retina Foundation,
Ahmedabad, India

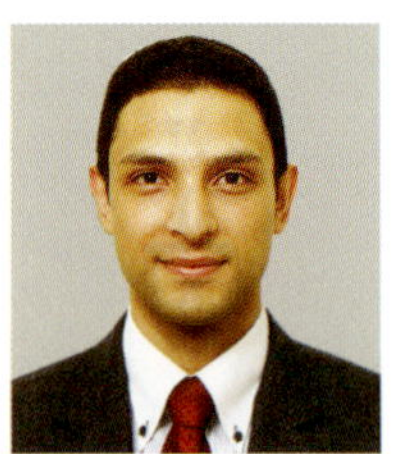

Osama MA Ibrahim, MD
Department of Ophthalmology,
Keio University School of Medicine,
Tokyo, Japan

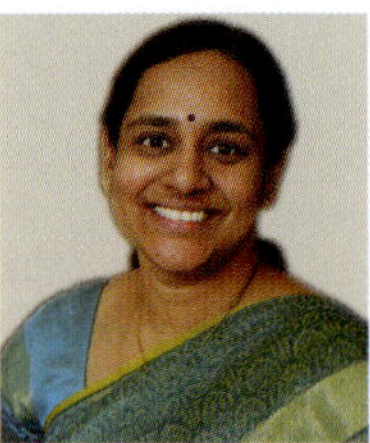

Padmamalini Mahendradas, MD
Head, Uveitis and Ocular Immunology Service,
Narayana Nethralaya Postgraduate Institute of
Ophthalmology, Bangalore, India

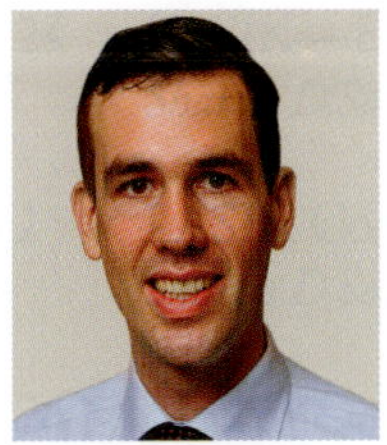

Patrick Oellers, MD
Bascom Palmer Eye Institute,
University of Miami School of Medicine, Miami,
Florida, USA

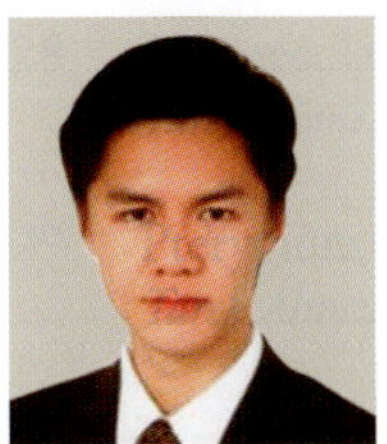

Poemen PM Chan, MD
Glaucoma Specialist,
Hong Kong Eye Hospital,
Hong Kong, PRC

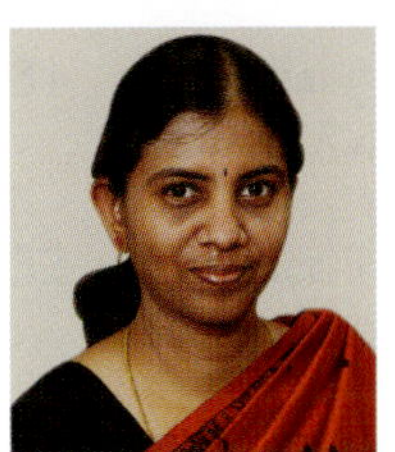

Priya BV, MD
Consultant, Vitreo-Retina Service,
Narayana Nethralaya Postgraduate Institute of
Ophthalmology, Bangalore, India

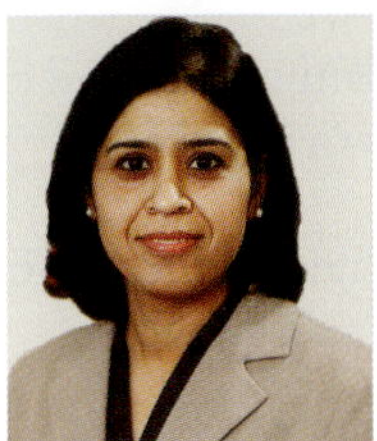

Rajani Battu, MD
Consultant, Vitreo-Retina Service,
Narayana Nethralaya Postgraduate Institute of
Ophthalmology, Bangalore, India

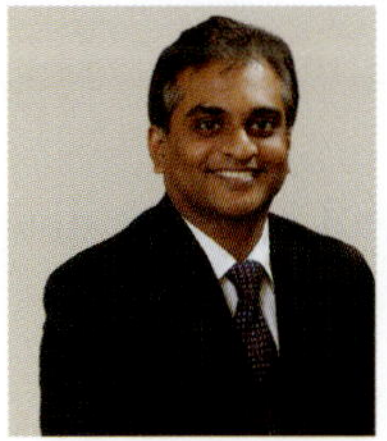

Rajesh S Kumar, MD
Deputy Director Research and Consultant,
Glaucoma Service, Narayana Nethralaya
Postgraduate Institute of Ophthalmology,
Bangalore, India

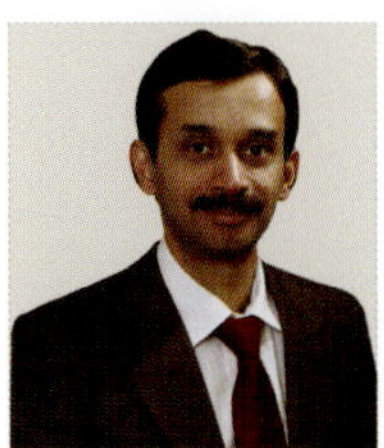

Ramgopal Balu, MD
Consultant, Glaucoma Service,
Narayana Nethralaya Postgraduate Institute of
Ophthalmology, Bangalore, India

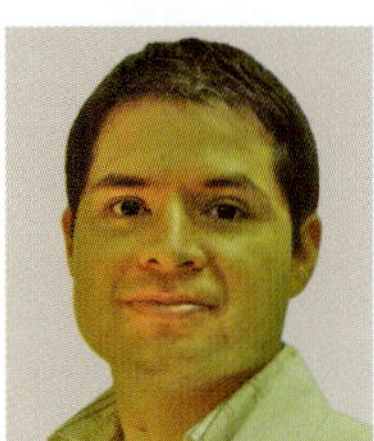

Ramiro Maldonado, MD
Postdoctoral Fellow, Duke University Eye Center,
North Carolina, USA

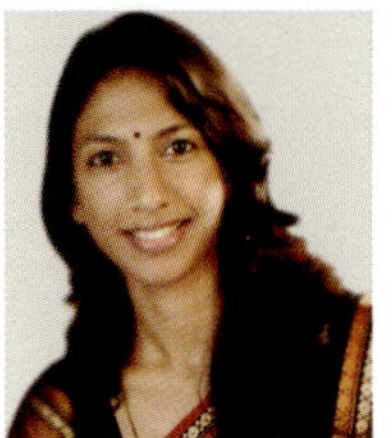

Rashmi Shetty, MD
Fellow, Cataract and Refractive Lens Service,
Narayana Nethralaya Postgraduate Institute of
Ophthalmology, Bangalore, India

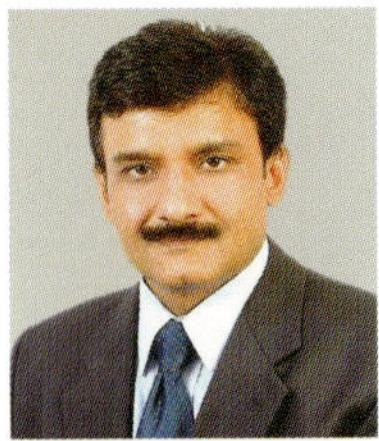

Rasik B Vajpayee, MD
*Professor, Dr Rajendra Prasad Centre for
Ophthalmic Sciences,
All India Institute of Medical Sciences,
New Delhi, India*

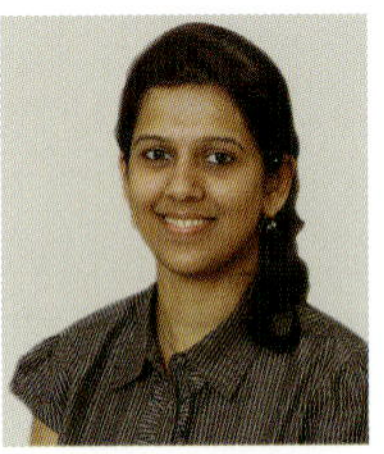

Ridhima Bhagali, MD
*Consultant, Cataract and Refractive Lens Service,
Narayana Nethralaya Postgraduate Institute of
Ophthalmology, Bangalore, India*

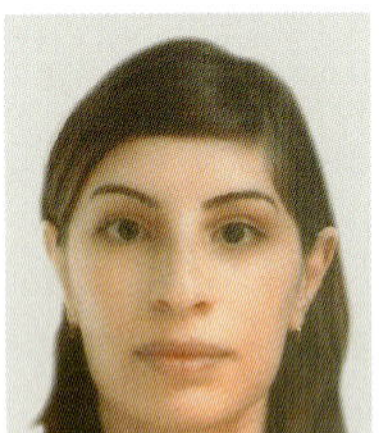

Rim Kahloun, MD
*Department of Ophthalmology,
Fattouma Bourguiba University Hospital,
Faculty of Medicine, University of Monastir,
Monastir, Tunisia*

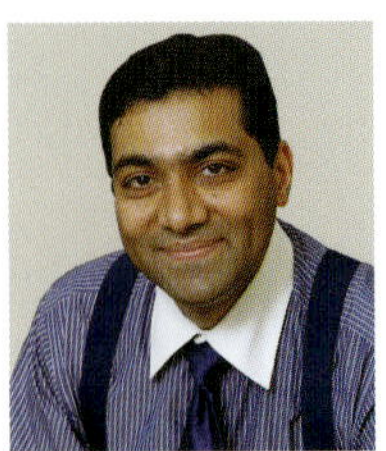

Rohit Shetty, MD, FRCS
*Vice Chairman and Consultant,
Refractive Services, Narayana Nethralaya
Postgraduate Institute of Ophthalmology,
Bangalore, India*

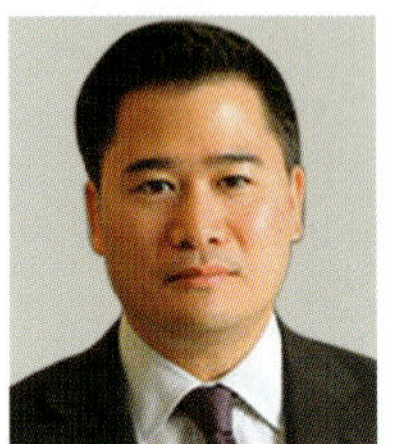

RV Paul Chan, MD, MSc, FACS
*Associate Professor of Ophthalmolgy,
St. Giles, Associate Professor of Pediatric Retina,
Weill Cornell Medical College,
New York, USA*

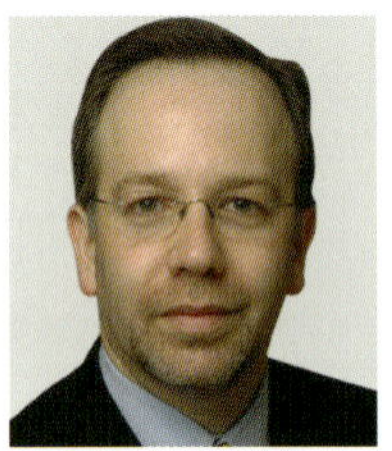

Sander R Dubovy, MD
*Associate Professor of Ophthalmology,
The Florida Lions Ocular Pathology Laboratory,
Bascom Palmer Eye Institute,
University of Miami Miller School of Medicine,
Miami, Florida, USA*

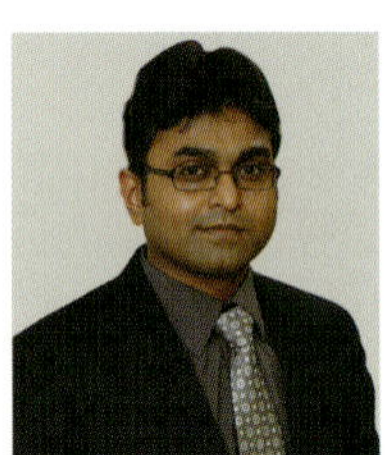

Santosh Gopi Krishna, MD
*Consultant, Vitreo-Retina Service,
Narayana Nethralaya Postgraduate Institute of
Ophthalmology, Bangalore, India*

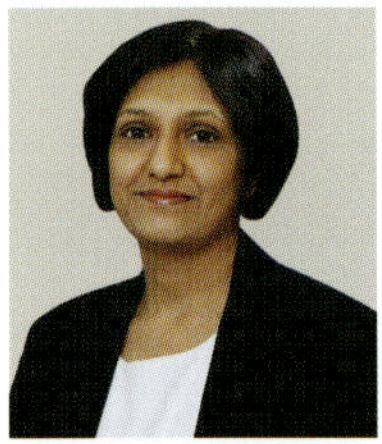

Sathi Devi AV, MD
*Head, Glaucoma Service,
Narayana Nethralaya Postgraduate Institute of
Ophthalmology, Bangalore, India*

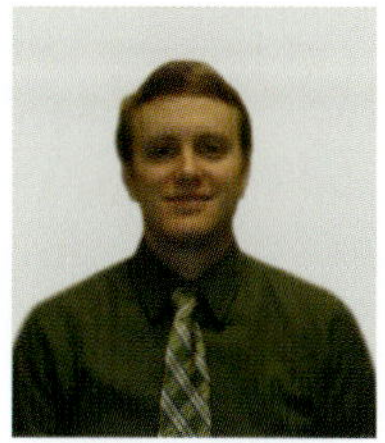

Scott Schoenberger, MD
Vanderbilt Eye Institute,
Vanderbilt University Medical Center,
Nashville, Tennessee,
USA

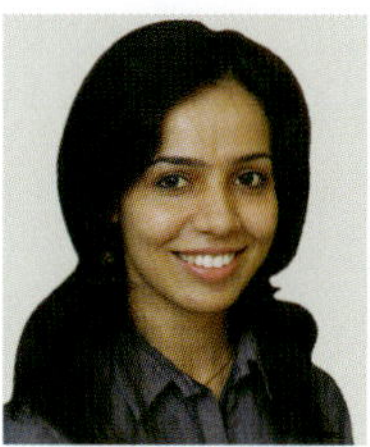

Sharon D'Souza, MD
Consultant, Cornea and Refractive Service,
Narayana Nethralaya Postgraduate Institute of
Ophthalmology,
Bangalore, India

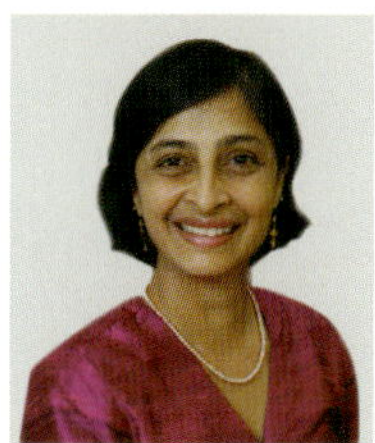

Sherine Braganza, MD
Consultant, Vitreoretinal Service,
Narayana Nethralaya Postgraduate Institute of
Ophthalmology, Bangalore, India

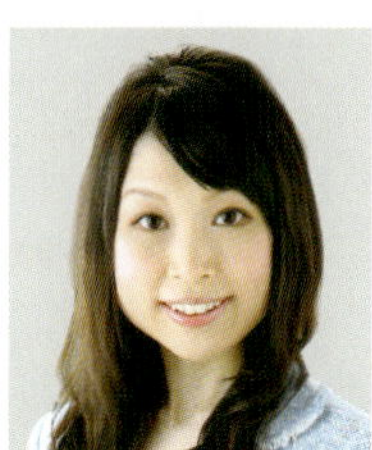

Shizuka Koh, MD
Assistant Professor of
Department of Ophthalmology,
Osaka University Graduate School of Medicine,
Osaka, Japan

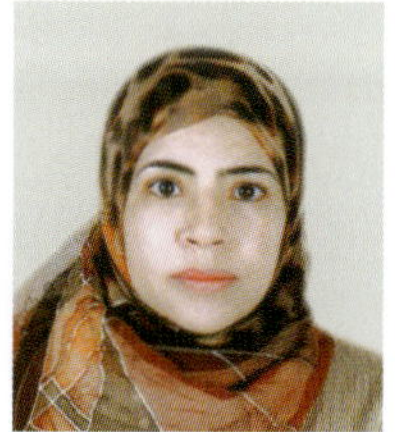

Sonia Attia, MD
Department of Ophthalmology,
Fattouma Bourguiba University Hospital,
Faculty of Medicine, University of Monastir,
Monastir, Tunisia

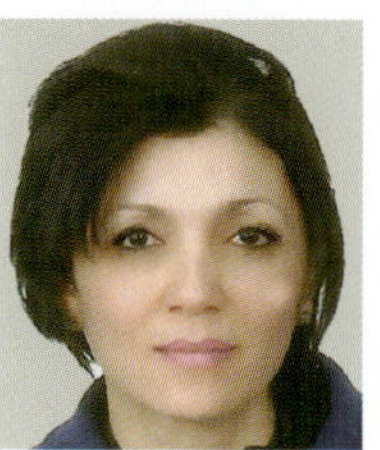

Sonia Zaouali, MD
Department of Ophthalmology,
Fattouma Bourguiba University Hospital,
Faculty of Medicine, University of Monastir,
Monastir, Tunisia

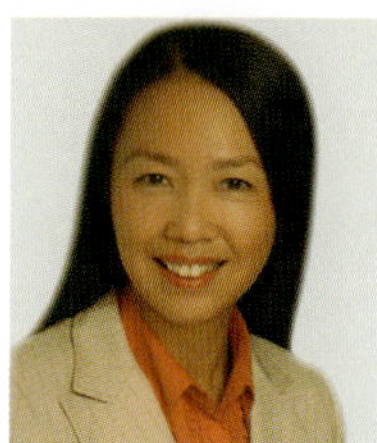

Soon-Phaik CHEE, MD
Singapore National Eye Centre,
Singapore Eye Research Institute,
National University of Singapore,
Duke NUS PGMS, Singapore

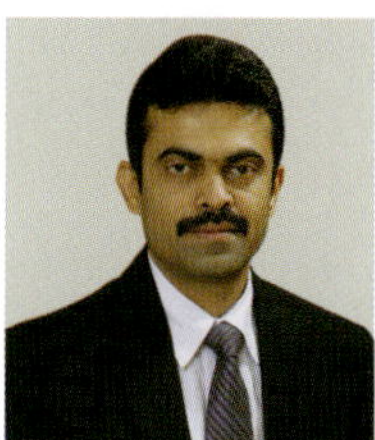

Subhashchandra HD
Consultant, Vitreo-Retina Service,
Narayana Nethralaya Postgraduate Institute of
Ophthalmology, Bangalore, India

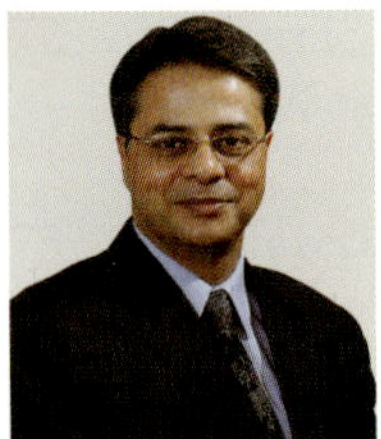

Sudeep Das, MD
Senior Consultant, Cataract and Refractive Lens Service,
Narayana Nethralaya Postgraduate Institute of
Ophthalmology, Bangalore, India

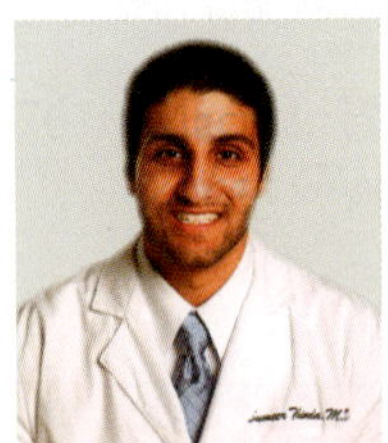

Sumeer Thinda, MD
Vanderbilt Eye Institute, Vanderbilt University Medical
Center, Nashville, Tennessee, USA

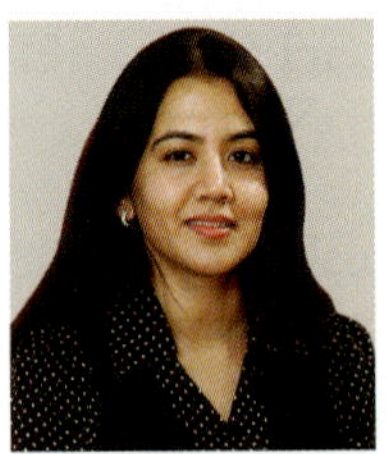

Supriya Dabir, MD
Consultant, Vitreoretinal Service,
Narayana Nethralaya Postgraduate Institute of
Ophthalmology, Bangalore, India

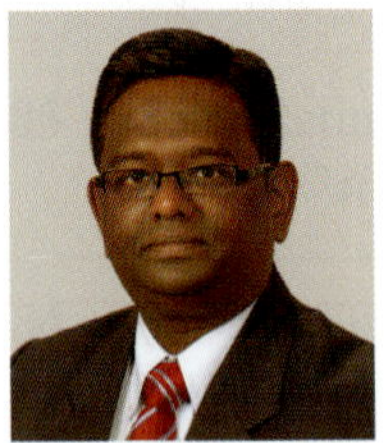

Syril Dorairaj, MD
Glaucoma, Anterior Segment Surgery,
Mayo Clinic, Department of Ophthalmology,
Jacksonville, Florida, USA

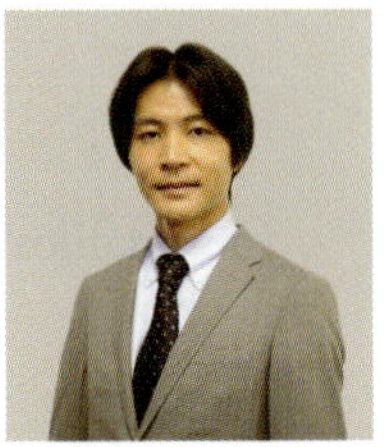

Takashi Kojima, MD
Department of Ophthalmology,
Gifu Red Cross Hospital,
Gifu, Japan

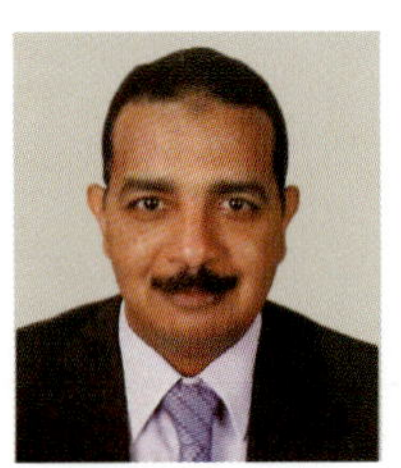

Tarek Ahmed Mohamed, MD
Assistant Professor,
Ophthalmology Department,
Faculty of Medicine,
Assiut University, Assiut,
Egypt

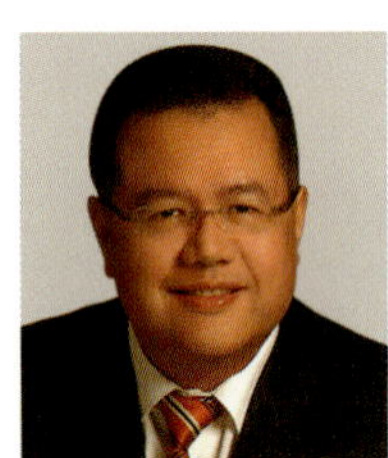

Tin Aung, MBBS, MMed (Ophth),
FRCS (Ed), FRCOphth, FAMS, PhD (Lond)
Senior Consultant and Head,
Glaucoma Service,
Singapore National Eye Centre,
Deputy Director,
Singapore Eye Research Institute;
Professor,
Department of Ophthalmology,
Yong Loo Lin School of Medicine,
National University of Singapore,
Singapore

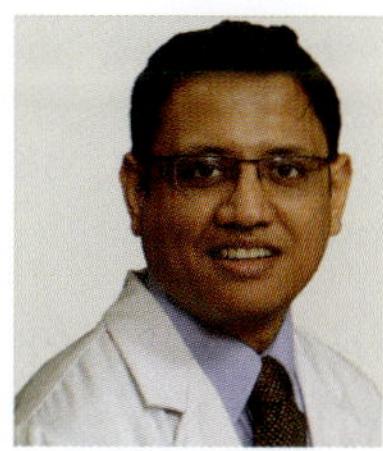

Tushar Agarwal, MD
*Associate Professor of Ophthalmology, Cornea, Lens and
Refractive Surgery Service, Dr Rajendra Prasad Centre for
Ophthalmic Sciences, All India Institute of Medical Sciences,
New Delhi, India*

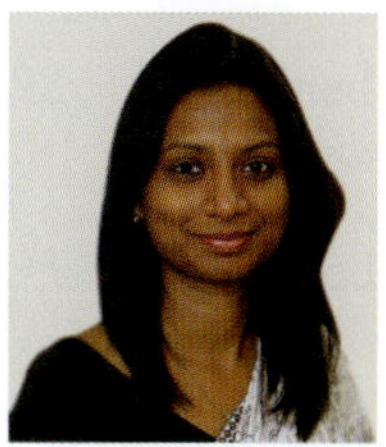

Vandhana Suren, MD
*Resident, Ophthamology, Narayana Nethralaya
Postgraduate Institute of Ophthalmology, Bangalore, India*

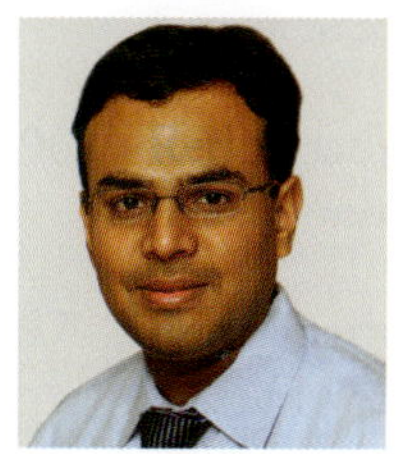

Vishak John, MD
*Bascom Palmer Eye Institute, University of Miami,
Miami, Florida, USA*

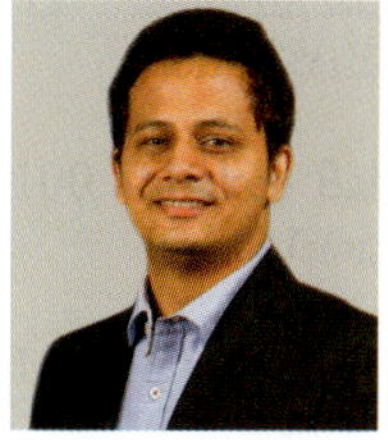

Vishal Jhanji, MD
*Department of Ophthalmology and Visual Sciences,
The Chinese University of Hong Kong,
Hong Kong*

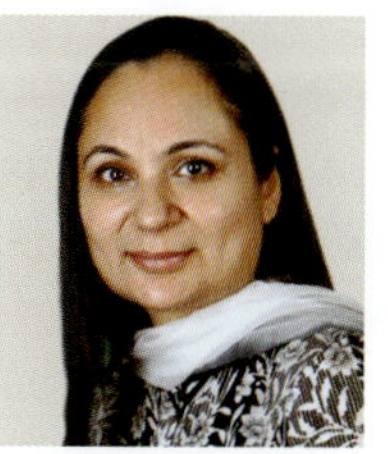

Vishali Gupta, MD
*Senior Consultant, Vitreo-Retina Division,
King Khaled Eye Specialist Hospital, Riyadh, KSA
Adjunct Additional Professor, Advanced Eye Centre,
Postgraduate Institute of Medical Education and Research,
Chandigarh, India*

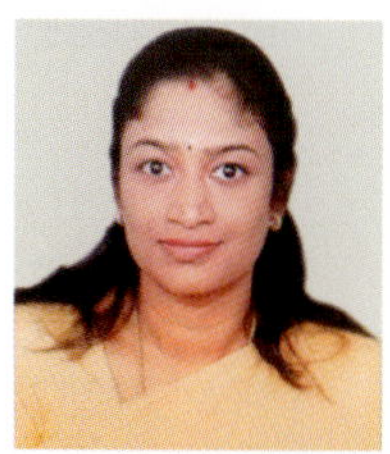

VP Poonkodi, MD
*Consultant Medical Retina, Vasan Eye Care Hospitals,
Bangalore, India*

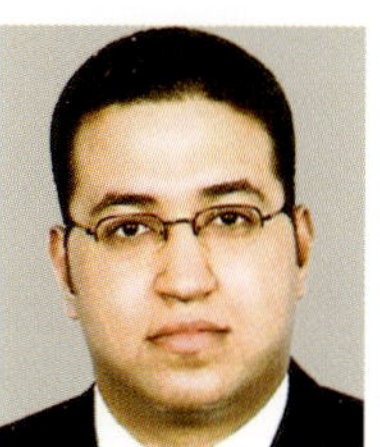

Wael Soliman, MD
*Lecturer, Ophthalmology Department,
Faculty Of Medicine, Assiut University, Assiut, Egypt*

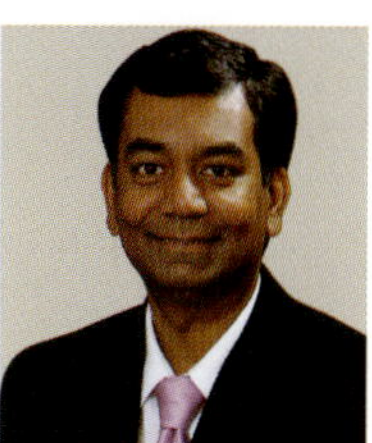

Yathish Shivanna, MD
*Consultant, Cornea Service, Narayana Nethralaya
Postgraduate Institute of Ophthalmology, Bangalore, India*

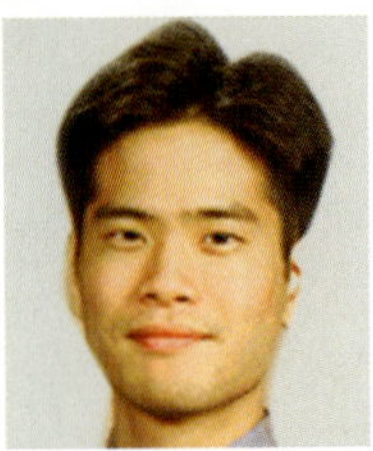

Yoshihiro Yonekawa, MD
Department of Ophthalmology, Massachusetts Eye and Ear Infirmary, Harvard Medical School, Boston, MA, USA

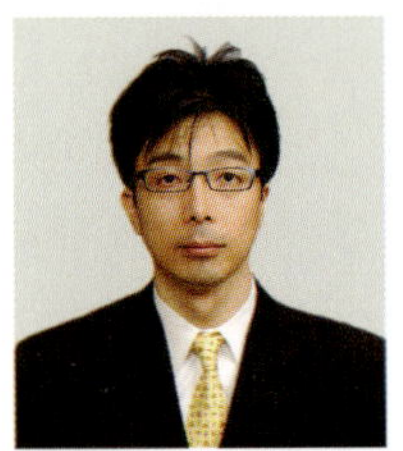

Yukihiro Matsumoto, MD
Department of Ophthalmology, Keio University School of Medicine, Tokyo, Japan

Contents

SECTION VII   PEDIATRIC RETINA

SECTION VIII   UVEA

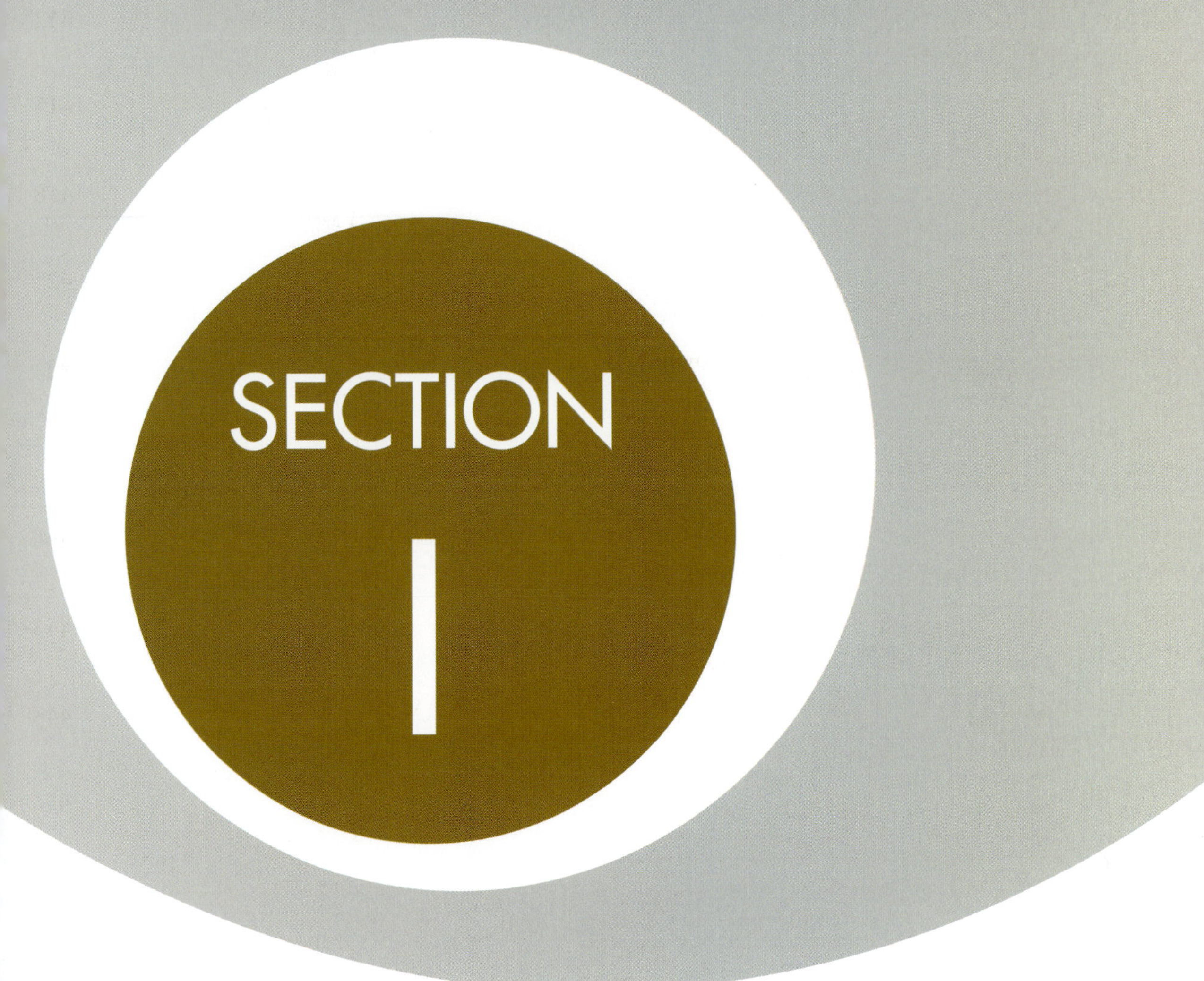

Introduction

Principles of Optical Coherence Tomography

Supriya Dabir

Optical coherence tomography (OCT) is a noncontact, noninvasive, in vivo, high-resolution, cross-sectional imaging of the eye that measures backscattered light. It works on the same principle as ultrasound B-mode imaging, but uses light instead of sound.

In OCT, a beam of light from a light source is scanned across tissue being studied. The OCT system collects reflected light and measures time delay. Light reflected from deeper tissues has longer propagation delays than that reflected from more anterior structures. The amplitude of reflected light can be plotted against delay to demonstrate tissue reflectivity at successively deeper levels of tissue penetration along axis of light propagation. This is called an axial scan (A-scan). Many scans are required to make an image. The OCT is based on principle of low-coherence Michelson interferometer. It uses the technique for high-resolution time and distance measurement using light. Interferometry is a result of combining amplitude of two light waves. This may be constructive (when the two waves are in phase) or destructive (when the waves are out of phase).

The meaning of low coherence is the usage of a wide range of wavelengths. The interferometer has a source of light [superluminescent diode (SLD)], a sample arm, a reference arm fiber, and a detector arm, all centered on a 50/50 fiber optic coupler (Fig. 1.1). The light from the source is directed into a partially reflecting mirror, and is split as a reference beam and a sample beam. The sample beam is reflected from the tissue specimen at different time delays according to internal microstructure. In the reference beam, the light is reflected from a reference mirror at variable distances, which produce variable time delays. The sample beam from the tissue will contain multiple reflections, and the beam from the reference mirror contains a single reflection at a known delay. These beams are then combined at the coupler and produce interference. As the mirror is scanned, each sample reflection gives rise to a single pulse when reference delay matches it. The distance between beam splitter and reference mirror is continuously varied. When the distance between the light source and sample tissue is equal to the distance between the light source and the reference mirror, the reflected light from retinal tissue and the reference mirror interacts to produce an interference pattern. Interferometric signal is converted from light to electric current by a photo detector, processed electronically, and transferred to computer memory. Plot of the signal is an A-scan, which represents amplitude of the reflection versus depth.

In spectral-domain optical coherence tomography (SD-OCT), instead of the reference mirror moving back and forth, there is a spectrometer and a high-speed charge coupled device (CCD) camera to measure interference spectrum (Fig. 1.2). The A-scan measurements can be obtained by calculating Fourier transform. (A Fourier transform is a mathematical operation that extracts frequency content of a signal.)

The image can be thought of as a series of stacked and aligned A-scans to produce a two-dimensional cross-sectional retinal image that resembles that of a histological section.

Digital processing aligns the A-scans to correct for eye motion. Digital smoothing techniques are used to further improve signal-to-noise ratio.

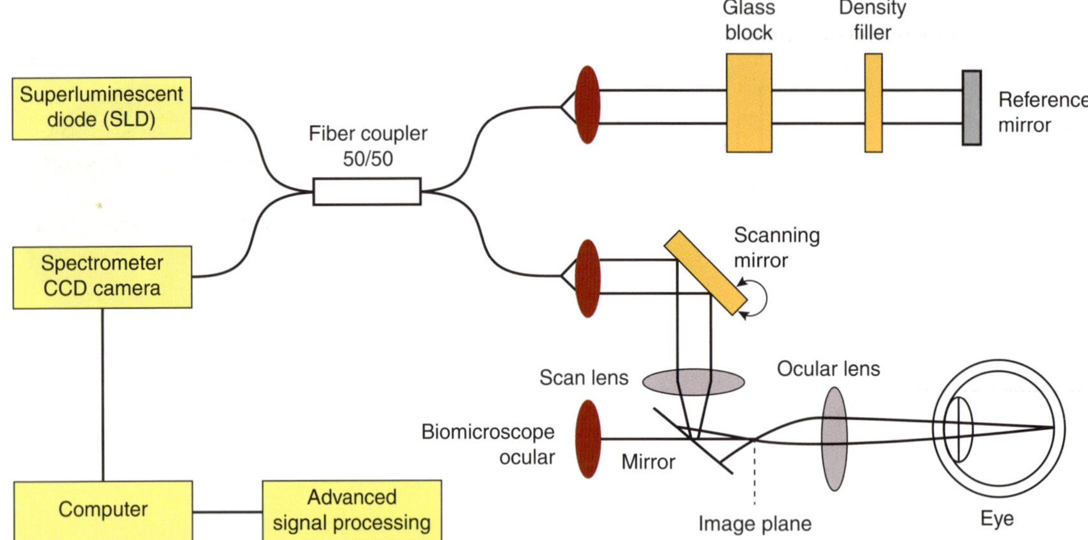

Fig. 1.1 Schematic diagram of time-domain optical coherence tomography (OCT) imaging system: The light source in most time-domain OCT systems is a low-coherence superluminescent diode (SLD) that is coupled to an optical fiber. The reference mirror is mechanically scanned to produce different time delays. (Adapted from Retinal Angiography and Optical Coherence Tomography by J Fernando Arévalo, published by Springer, 2009.)

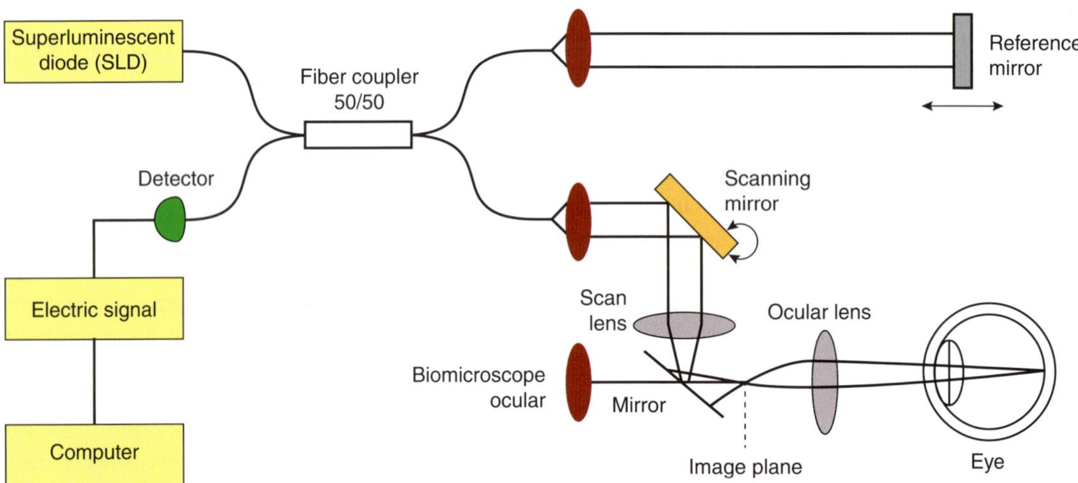

Fig. 1.2 Schematic diagram of spectral/Fourier-domain OCT imaging system: In contrast to time-domain OCT systems, a spectrometer coupled to a charge-coupled device (CCD) camera detects entire interference spectrum from which the Fourier transform is calculated. The position of reference arm does not need to be adjusted. (Adapted from Retinal Angiography and Optical Coherence Tomography by J Fernando Arévalo, published by Springer, 2009.)

The older versions of the OCT required dilation with at least a 5-mm pupil. The newer OCT systems can be used in absence of dilation in many individuals and usually require a 3-mm pupil for adequate visualization.

The OCT image can be displayed on a gray scale, where more reflected light is brighter than less reflected light. Alternatively, it can be displayed in color, whereby different colors correspond to different degrees of reflectivity. On the OCT scanners, currently that are commercially available, highly reflective structures are shown with bright colors (red and white), while those with low reflectivity are represented by darker colors (black and blue). Those with intermediate reflectivity appear green.

In OCT, the image resolution can be considered axial and transverse. The axial (along the incident light beam) resolution is determined by coherence length of the light source, which is inversely proportional to bandwidth. The commercial OCT systems use SLD light sources at near-infrared wavelengths of ~820 nm with a bandwidth of about 20–50 μ. Earlier time-domain OCT could achieve an axial resolution of 8–10 microns in tissue. However, recently the spectral/Fourier-domain OCT systems can achieve 5–8-micron axial resolution.

The transverse (perpendicular to the incident light beam) resolution is determined by the size of focused light beam incident on retina and independent of the bandwidth. The transversal resolution by optics of the eye, number of A-scans used to reconstruct a B-scan, and image depth by the penetration of the laser light into the retinal tissue is limited.

The commercial OCT systems use light sources between 800- and 900-nm wavelength, allowing good imaging of the retina but limited visualization of choroid. For imaging choroid, wavelengths above 1000 nm have been used. Since depth of focus and spot size are dependent, most OCT systems use a 20-micron resolution.

FURTHER READING

1. Fernando AJ: Retinal Angiography and Optical Coherence Tomography. Springer, 2008.
2. Friedrich AF: Optical coherence tomography – development, principles, applications. *Z Med Phys* 20:251–276, 2010.
3. Puliafito CA, Hee MR, Schuman JS, et al.: Optical Coherence Tomography of Ocular Diseases. Thorofare, NJ: Slack Inc, 1996.
4. Stanga PE, Bird AC: Optical coherence tomography (OCT): principles of operation, technology, indications in vitreoretinal imaging and interpretation of results. *Int Ophthalmol* 23:191–197, 2001.
5. Costa RA, Skaf M, Melo LA Jr, et al.: Retinal assessment using optical coherence tomography. *Prog Retin Eye Res* 25:325–353, 2006.

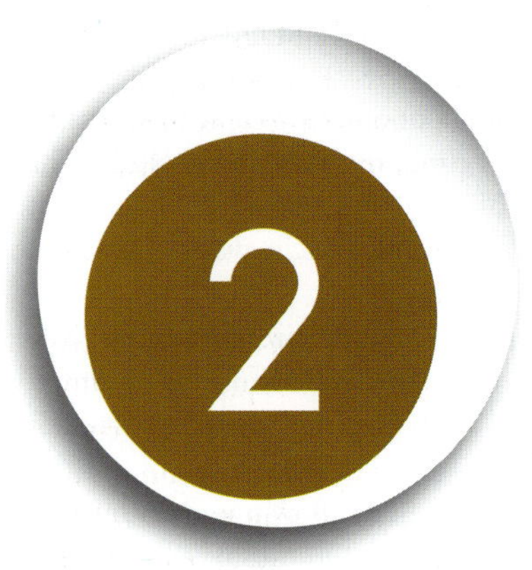

Spectral-domain Optical Coherence Tomography Imaging of the Eye: Limitations and Advances

Sherine Braganza

Spectral-domain optical coherence tomography (SD-OCT) imaging provides high-definition visualization of retinal layers and clear discrimination of interfaces between different reflectance structures. Stratified retinal structures are seen on time-domain optical coherence tomography (TD-OCT).

Noise reduction provides a marked increase in contrast with improved discrimination of fine structures. The stratified retinal structures can be seen on the TD-OCT, but margins of layers with different reflectance characteristics are not clearly delineated; and it is difficult to identify interfaces between these elements.

The SPECTRALIS™ images provide clear visualization and differentiation of each single layer, with sharper definition. Starting from surface these images show:

- Hyperreflective points at the margins of the fovea and at the surface of the avascular pit correspond to adherence of vitreous to internal limiting membrane. This hyperreflectivity is because the A-scans are perpendicular to the vitreous. This advantage is seen with the SPECTRALIS™ OCT.
- Following five layers are easily visualized, namely: nerve fiber layer, ganglion cell layer, inner plexiform layer, inner nuclear layer, and outer plexiform layer. In particular, the margins of the nerve fiber layer are sharper and more clearly characteristic.

In the ganglion cell layer, individual cells are almost visible, whereas time-domain OCT is unable to identify single hyperreflective spots as corresponding to cells. With the SPECTRALIS™, intraretinal vessels are identified not merely as hyper reflective structures, but as clear, tubular, linear structures comprising of the vessel wall with the lumen.

The outer nuclear layer is visible as a hyporeflective structure very similar in the TD and SD-OCT.

The external limiting membrane can almost always be identified by SD-OCT, while this is often difficult to assess with the TD-OCT.

The first hyperreflective band beneath the outer nuclear layer corresponds to inner–outer interface of photoreceptors. With the SPECTRALIS™, this inner segment (IS)–outer segment (OS) junction can be assessed in detail which is useful in dystrophies and degenerative pathologies such as dry and wet age-related macular degeneration (AMD). In these cases, the photoreceptor layer appears homogenous with hyperreflective fine deposits and is often possible to identify a jagged and irregular pattern.

The retinal pigment epithelium (RPE) layer is composed of two distinct hyperreflective bands separated by a fine hyporeflective strip. In TD-OCT, the RPE layer appears only as a hyperreflective band.

Optical coherence tomography (OCT) images obtained with spectral-domain OCT technology, provide good visualization of the main vessels of choroid, possibly due to longer wavelength and decreased absorption by the RPE. In addition, real-time averaging results in a sharper image with fewer artifacts derived from structures beneath the pigment epithelium. Bruch's membrane is not clearly visualized as an independent structure, as it is included in the highly reflective RPE–Bruch's complex.

Finally, the outermost layer visible on SPECTRALIS™ OCT is a moderately reflective structure that corresponds to the sclera not detected by the TD-OCT.

The greatest improvement provided by the spectral domain technology is high acquisition speed and consequently greater number of A-scans for each B-scan; and therefore a very large volume of information is acquired in a single examination. The acquisition speed of SPECTRALIS™ is a hundred times faster than that of STRATUS™. The current software allows OCT acquisition in three different modes. The first mode consists of taking five consecutive raster horizontal scan lines in high-resolution. The operator can move the position of the five lines during examination by analyzing SLO-red free fundus images. Each raster scan line is constructed with a single A-scan, which considerably increases horizontal resolution. In the other two modes, retinal cube sections are acquired. This cube is formed by 512 vertical × 128 horizontal A-scans for macular studies and 200 × 200 A-scans for optic nerve head studies. The acquisition time in each mode is 1 second or a little more. This reduces the possibility of motion artifacts, and is specially useful in patients with poor fixation. SD-OCT has a powerful autoregulation system for polarization and Z-axis position, which facilitates acquisition. Therefore, one can get very high image quality, even in cases with media opacity as in cataracts and also in myopic patients who are difficult to examine.

The spectral (or Fourier) domain OCT (SD-OCT) replaces the moving mirror with a stationary one and performs the Fourier transformation of interference pattern. Therefore, SD-OCT provides a wealth of anatomical information giving the retinologists better information of hitherto unknown features of retinal diseases and thus allowing greater precision in diagnosis and analysis of disease progression.

HOW TO TAKE A GOOD SD-OCT IMAGE?

Experience with the SD-OCT shows that cooperation between ophthalmic technicians and the patient is both essential. Patients must keep still and fixate optimally. Photographers must ensure that the tear film is of good quality, either by having the patient blink at timely intervals or by administering ocular lubricants when the tear film is insufficient. The lens of the OCT machine must be kept at an optimal distance from the patient's eye, and must be kept clean. Technician should try to find the clearest optical media through which imaging is possible and must also bear in mind that deviating too far from visual axis may cause tilting of the image.

It is essential to correlate the OCT with clinical examination and other imaging results. OCT is poor at differentiating between subretinal hemorrhage and neovascular membrane. This distinction is better made on clinical examination. Thus, clinical examination and fluorescein angiography are better able to determine the presence of inactive scarring than OCT. It is important to examine the entire set of the OCT images of any lesion. It is important to understand all the OCT features of the lesion, e.g., outer retinal tubulation in neovascular AMD is a finding not appreciated before the advent of the SD-OCT. These tubules appear as round or ovoid hyporeflective spaces with hyperreflective borders. These represent degenerating photoreceptors. It is, therefore, important to differentiate between tubulation and intraretinal cysts when making re-treatment decisions. The SD-OCT now has a role in the management of many diseases that were previously managed on the basis of clinical examination, visual acuity, and fluorescein angiography. Thus, a quantitative assessment of disease response that was previously impossible has now become possible.

FURTHER READING

1. de Boer JF, Cense B, Park BH, et al.: Improved signal-noise ratio in spectral domain compared with time-domain optical coherence tomography. *Opt Lett* 38:2067–2069, 2003.

2. Coscas G, Coscas F, Vismara S: Optical coherence tomography in age-related macular degeneration. Springer Medizen Verlag Heidelberg, 2009.
3. Cirrus HD OCT 4000. User Manual Carl Zeiss Meditec Inc, 2008.
4. Leitgeb RA, Schmetterer L, Hitzenberger CK, et al.: Real-time measurement of *in vitro* flow by Fourier-domain color Doppler optical coherence tomography. *Opt Lett* 29(2):171–173, 2004.
5. Wolf S, Wolf-Schnurrbusch U: Spectral-domain optical coherence tomography use in macular diseases: a review. *Ophthalmologica* 224(6):333–340, 2010.
6. Kiernan DF, Mieler WF, Hariprasad SM: Spectral-domain optical coherence tomography: a comparison of modern high-resolution retinal imaging systems. *Am J Ophthalmol* 149(1):18–31, 2010.
7. van Velthoven ME, Faber DJ, Verbraak FD, et al.: Recent developments in optical coherence tomography for imaging the retina. *Prog Retin Eye Res* 26(1):57–77, 2007.

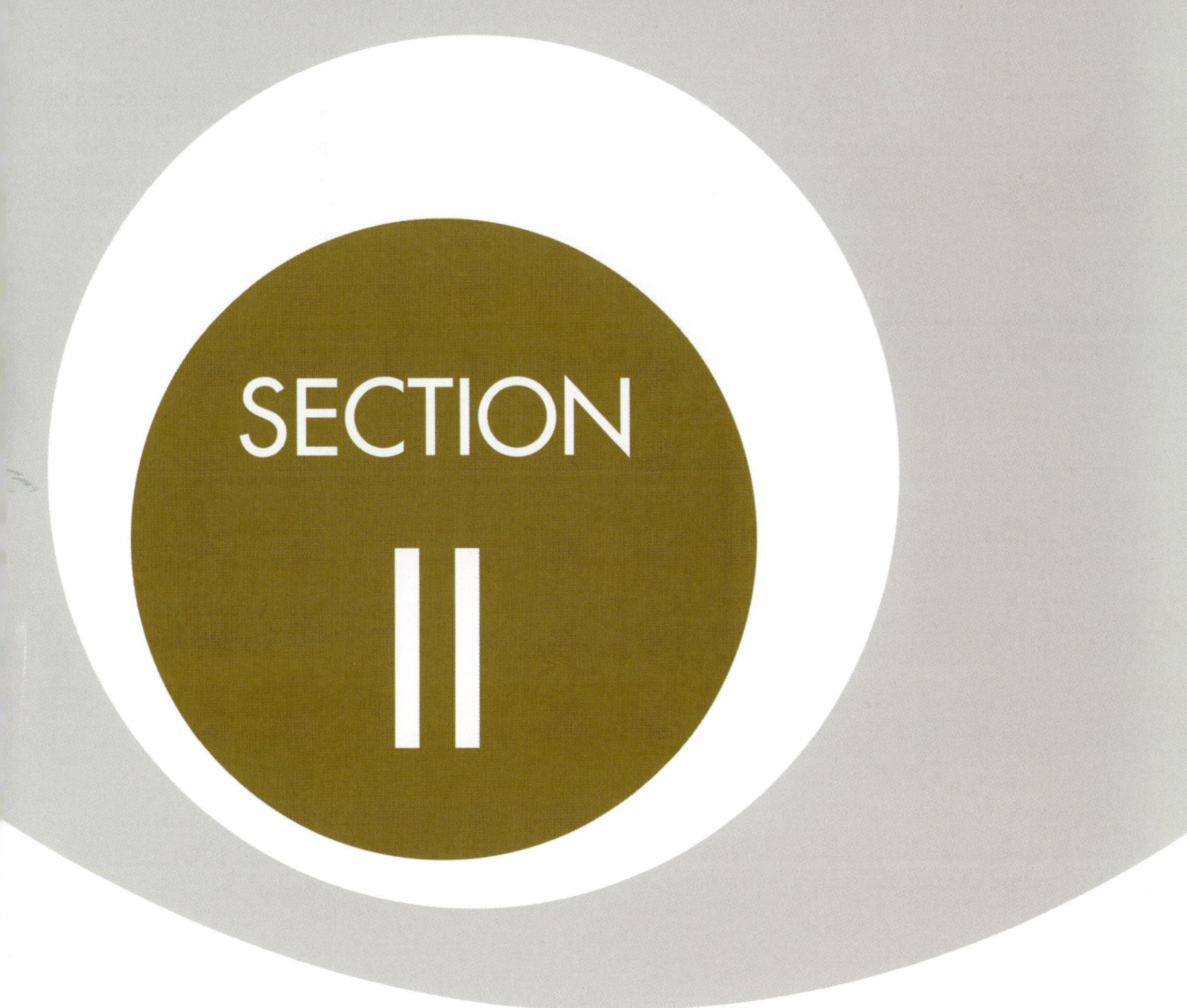

Technology: What's in the Box?

SPECTRALIS™— Heidelberg Engineering

Kester Nahen

The SPECTRALIS™ product family combines confocal scanning laser ophthalmoscopy (cSLO) and spectral-domain optical coherence tomography (SD-OCT) in a single multimodal imaging platform. With the combination of up to six cSLO modes with SD-OCT and enhanced depth imaging (EDI), optical coherence tomography (OCT) provides unique insights in retinal diseases, glaucoma, anterior segment, and neurologic disorders. A variety of SPECTRALIS™ models with different combinations of cSLO and SD-OCT modalities is available, which offers attractive solutions to specialists, general ophthalmologists, and optometrists (**Fig. 3.1**).

SPECTRALIS™ combines SD-OCT with up to six fundus-imaging modalities (**Fig. 3.2**):

- MultiColor
- Red-free imaging (RF)
- Infrared imaging (IR)
- BluePeak™ blue laser autofluorescence (AF) imaging
- Fluorescein angiography (FA)
- Indocyanine green angiography (ICGA)

Diseases are better studied comprehensively with the use of multimodality imaging. Combining insights into function and structure together, with metabolic activity of the retina, would benefit patient's management as well as improve the patient flow in the hospital.

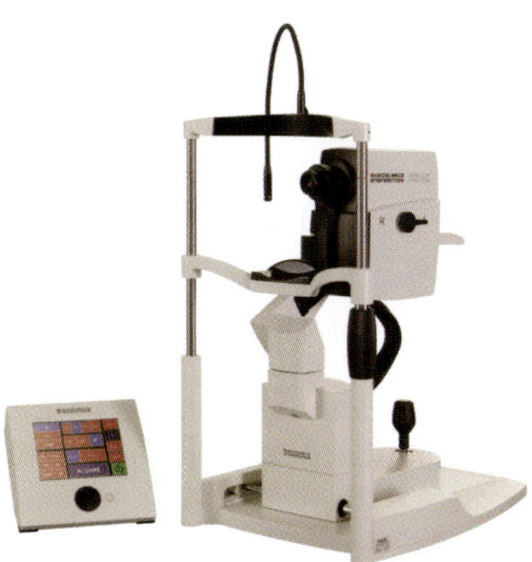

Fig. 3.1 SPECTRALIS™ device.

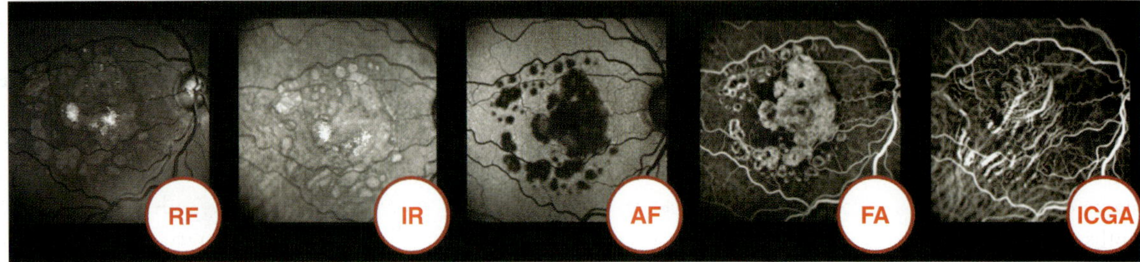

Fig. 3.2 Different acquisition modes of retinal pigment epithelial (RPE) atrophy.

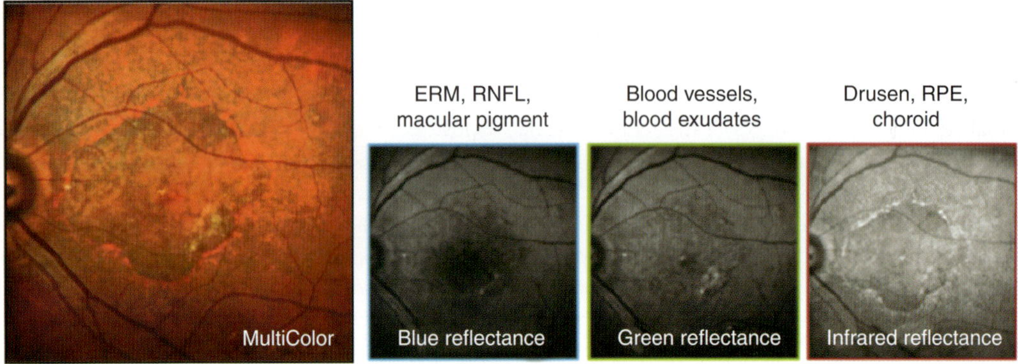

Fig. 3.3 MultiColor and selective depth reflectance images.

CONFOCAL LASER SCANNING

For acquiring digital confocal images, a laser beam is focused on the retina. The laser beam is deflected periodically by means of oscillating mirrors to sequentially scan a two-dimensional section of the retina. The intensity of reflected light or of emitted fluorescent light at each point is measured with a light-sensitive detector. In a confocal optical system, light reflected or emitted outside of the adjusted focal plane is suppressed, resulting in high-contrast images. Furthermore, especially during indocyanine green angiographies (ICGA), the confocal optical system acquires a layer-by-layer three-dimensional (3-D) image. This system allows clinicians to image patients with poorly or nondilated pupils, which is especially important for diabetic patients who do not dilate well and make up a large proportion of patients in a retina clinic.

Since fluorescein dyes require excitation at a narrow band of wavelengths, it is better to use laser to do this. Lasers offer specific wavelengths that can be concentrated for this purpose. This is infinitely better than using an ordinary flash, as used in standard photography. The SPECTRALIS™ requires considerably less retinal light exposure than photographic systems; thus allowing for safer and more patient-friendly examination. Dependent on the SPECTRALIS™ model, the laser sources of the device emit laser light with up to three different wavelengths (Fig. 3.3):

- A blue all-solid-state laser, with a wavelength of 488 nm ± 2 nm, or a blue laser diode with wavelength of 486 ± 3 nm is used to excite fluorescein or intrinsic AF. A barrier filter at 500 nm separates excitation and fluorescence light. Same wavelength without the barrier filter is used to create red-free images, also called blue reflectance images. The SPECTRALIS™ is also capable of high-quality BluePeak™ blue-laser autofluorescence imaging.
- A diode laser at 518-nm wavelength produces green reflectance images.
- A diode laser at 786-nm wavelength is used with a barrier filter at 830 nm to separate excitation from fluorescence in the retina using indocyanine green dye.
- A diode laser at 820-nm wavelength produces infrared (IR) reflectance images.

When using simultaneous imaging modes, each image line is scanned individually by each laser. For example, during simultaneous FA and ICGA, only the 488-/486-nm laser is switched on for first scan of a line, while during second scan only 786-nm laser is switched on. In every acquisition mode, individual images, temporal image sequences, or a focal series of images (layered 3-D images) can be acquired.

MultiColor images are composed of three simultaneously acquired reflectance images taken with 488-nm, 518-nm, and 820-nm wavelengths. An automatic color balance matches the fundus appearance of photographs. View of images of individual laser colors helps gain a better understanding of anatomic and pathologic detail at different depths within the retina. The continuous laser scanning system delivers live MultiColor images, making camera alignment easy. The OCT scan position can be selected on a stabilized MultiColor image.

OPTICAL COHERENCE TOMOGRAPHY (OCT)

SPECTRALIS™ uses SD-OCT technology, also referred to as Fourier-domain OCT (FD-OCT). The beam of a super luminescent diode (SLD) scans across the retina to produce a cross-sectional B-scan image. In order to create high-spatial-resolution–3-D images of the retina, B-scans as close as 11 microns to each other can be acquired. The infrared beam of the SLD has a central wavelength of 870 nm.

TRUTRACK™ ACTIVE EYE TRACKING

By using two separate beams, SPECTRALIS™ captures two images simultaneously. First beam images the fundus and tracks any eye movement. This is the reference or guiding beam. The second beam acquires the OCT image. "Active eye tracking" is the ability to "lock" the OCT scan location to the fundus even if eye movement occurs. Active eye tracking ensures that structures, for example blood vessels, seen on fundus and OCT image match up at the same location. Its biggest advantage is in 3-D volume scans, where motion artifact is a big hurdle because the scan time is longer then the time between microsaccades (**Figs 3.4 and 3.5**).

Red dot indicates the OCT scan and blue dot indicates IR laser. All SPECTRALIS™ SD-OCT devices operate with patented TruTrack active eye tracking technology with dual beam scanning to produce:

- OCT scans free-of-motion artifact.
- Precise registrations of OCT scan to fundus image.
- Precise follow-up examinations with a smallest measurable change of retinal thickness of 1 μm.

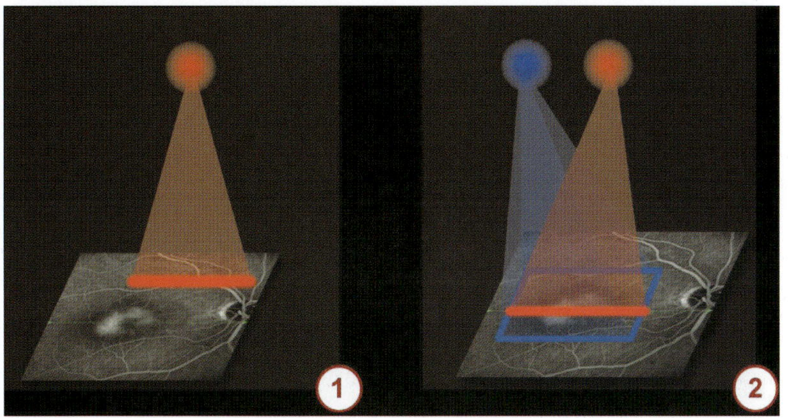

Fig. 3.4 Image without (1) and with (2) active eye tracking.

ENHANCED DEPTH IMAGING (EDI)

Enhanced depth imaging (EDI) is an imaging modality for enhanced visualization of deeper tissue structures in OCT images. Reference plane of the OCT system is shifted such that deeper structures are imaged with maximum sensitivity (Fig. 3.6).

HEIDELBERG NOISE REDUCTION TECHNOLOGY

TruTrack™ active eye tracking enables capture of multiple images in exactly the same location. The automatic real time (ART) function combines these images, helping clinicians to discriminate between image "noise" and true signals from real tissue structures. Noise is effectively eliminated and the results are the images of high contrast with finer detail.

AUTORESCAN™

AutoRescan™ allows clinicians to track change over time. Locating the initial scan is important; locating follow-up scan is critical (Fig. 3.7). By using the fundus image like a fingerprint, SPECTRALIS™ automatically places follow-up OCT scans at precisely the same location as the initial scan. Eliminating subjective placement of follow-up scans is important for confidently identifying small change and for optimizing patient flow.

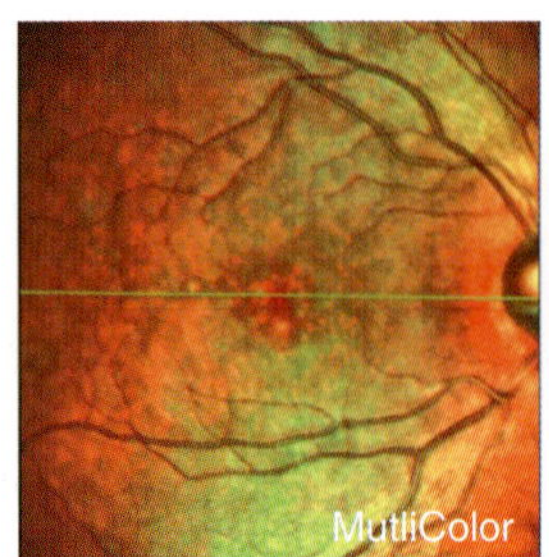
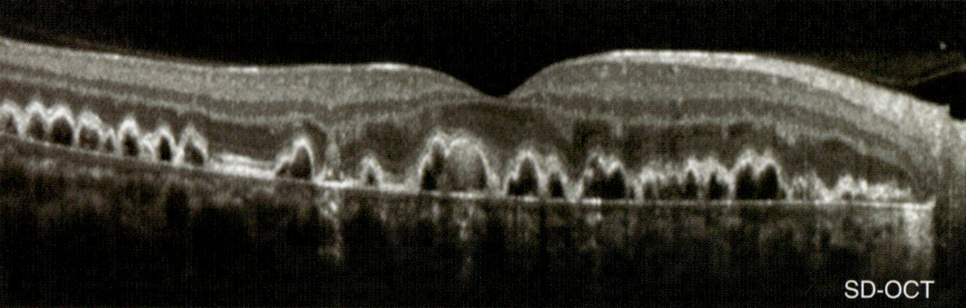

Fig. 3.5 Simultaneous MultiColor and SD-OCT image with active eye tracker-enabled image registration.

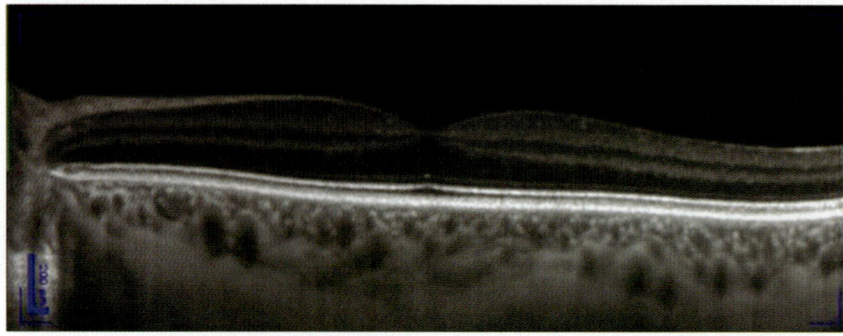

Fig. 3.6 EDI–OCT image showing choroidal structures at high image contrast.

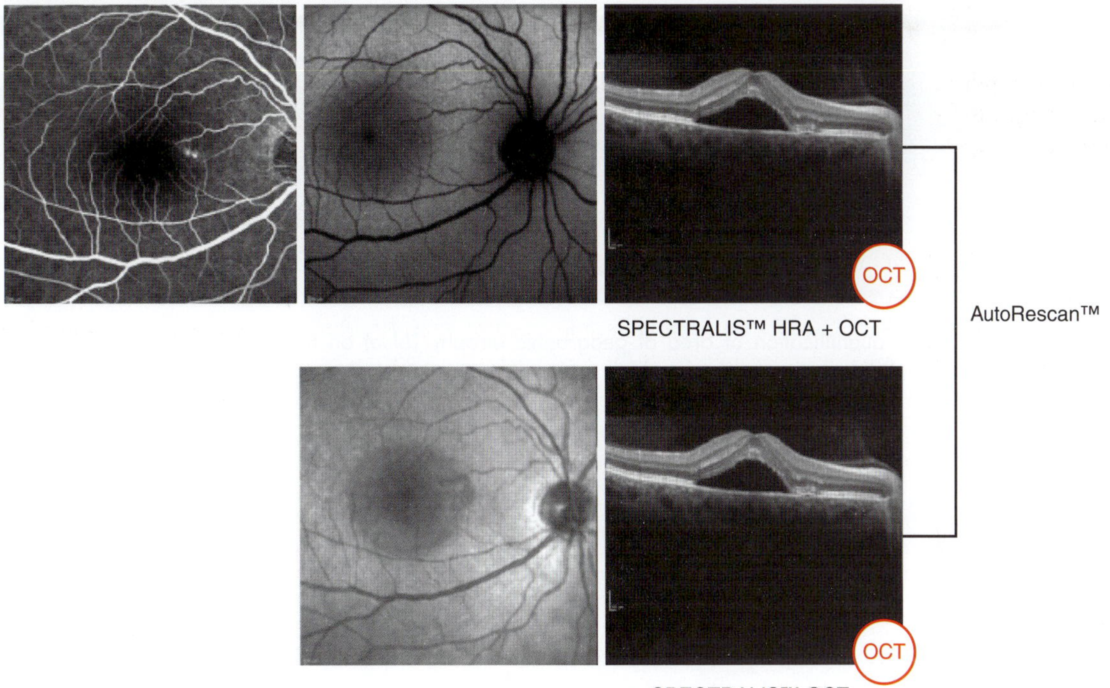

Fig. 3.7 Initial and follow-up examination of a patient: The registration of OCT image to cSLO image allows re-scan simultaneously at exactly same location on the retina.

REGISTRATION LINK

Patients imaged on one SPECTRALIS™ type device can later be followed on any other SPECTRALIS™ device using a common database. The cSLO image acquired simulteous to the OCT image serves as a registration link. The AutoRescan function ensures that all OCT scans are automatically taken at the exact same retinal location. The type of simultaneously acquired cSLO fundus image can vary from one device to the other which supports efficient multimodality imaging.

ANTERIOR SEGMENT MODULE

The anterior segment module offers multimodal imaging of the anterior segment. It captures simultaneous SD-OCT scans, IR, RF, FA, or ICGA images of cornea, sclera, or anterior chamber angle. RF, FA, and ICGA are the cSLO modes at anterior segment imaging, only available for SPECTRALIS™ HRA + OCT. The anterior segment module allows OCT scan widths of 8 mm, 11 mm, and 16 mm. Available OCT scan patterns are single-line scans and volume scans.

REGIONFINDER

The RegionFinder software provides a semi-automatic quantification of well-demarcated regions with significantly decreased AF signal intensity. BluePeak blue laser AF images are digital images taken with a confocal laser scanning

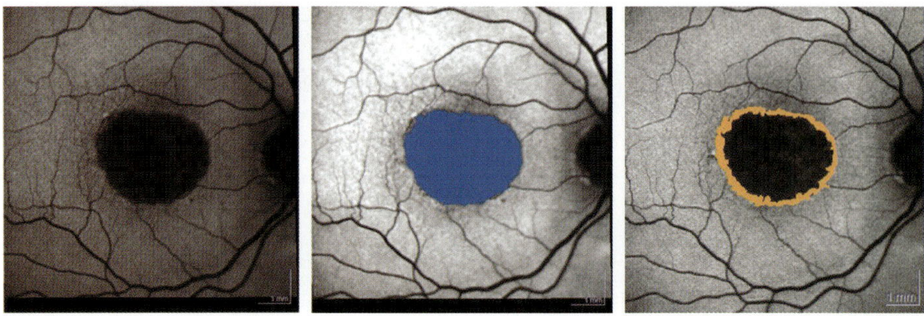

Fig. 3.8 RegionFinder quantification of area of geographic atrophy (*blue*) on BluePeak image and change map (*brown*) of a follow-up exam.

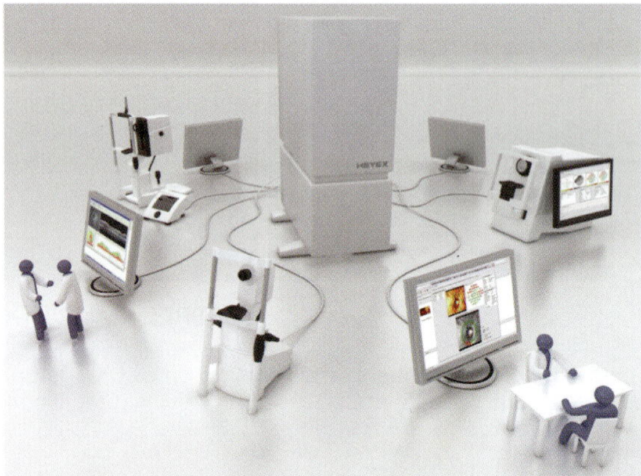

Fig. 3.9 Heidelberg Eye Explorer (HEYEX™) network integration of all Heidelberg Engineering products.

ophthalmoscope, using a blue wavelength. For every picture element (Pixel), there is a well-defined value of AF signal intensity. This value shows a decrease in cases with atrophy due to loss of RPE, e.g., in geographic atrophy (Fig. 3.8). In order to measure these areas of atrophy, the RegionFinder software uses a so-called region-growing algorithm. If the user has defined a seed point inside a region, the algorithm tends to grow towards the border of this region. All pixels with a signal intensity below a certain threshold are included in the region. The parameter "growth power" defines this threshold. The higher the growth power, the larger is the enclosed area. If this parameter is well adjusted, the areas of atrophy can be measured precisely.

HEIDELBERG EYE EXPLORER (HEYEX) SOFTWARE PLATFORM

All Heidelberg Engineering devices operate on the Heidelberg Eye Explorer (HEYEX™) platform. HEYEX™ hosts the patient database, from which the user manages patient files and performs examinations. HEYEX™ also hosts image acquisition and analysis applications for different Heidelberg Engineering devices.

All Heidelberg Engineering devices can be used within a network environment. This allows users to review images from networked PCs, often referred to as viewing stations, using the same analysis software that is used on instrument PC. In a network environment, the common HEYEX™ database containing all patient data is located on a network server. Images acquired with the device are saved to this database. Viewing and analyzing these images are possible at any computer that meets the viewing-station requirements. A viewing station receives access to the database through a network license. The network license can be fixed, permanently assigned to a computer, or floating where many viewing stations share a defined number of licenses. A DICOM interface is available to link HEYEX™ to PACS systems (Fig. 3.9).

FURTHER READING

1. Coscas G: Optical Coherence Tomography in Age-Related Macular Degeneration, Springer, Second Edition, 2010.
2. Wolf-Schnurrbusch, Swanson EA, Lin CP, et al.: Macular thickness measurements in healthy eyes using six different optical coherence tomography instruments. *Invest Ophthalmol Vis Sci* 50(7):3432–3437, 2009.
3. Menke, et al.: Reproducibility of retinal thickness measurements in healthy subjects using Spectralis optical coherence tomography. *Am J Ophthalmol* 147:467–472, 2009.

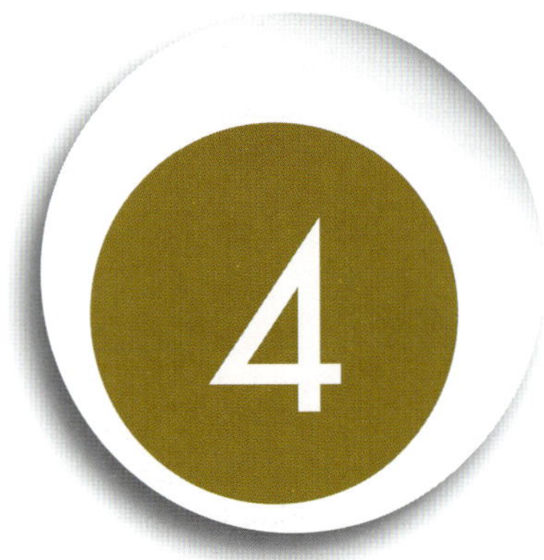

Bioptigen Envisu SD-OCT Primer

Eric L Buckland

INTRODUCTION

Images matter. Bioptigen is committed to developing highest quality ophthalmic imaging systems to meet diverse and growing demands of the ophthalmic translational research community and underserved patient sectors of the ophthalmic and optometric clinical communities. Bioptigen introduced the first commercial ultra-high-resolution spectral-domain optical coherence tomography (SD-OCT) imaging system, the first SD-OCT system convertible for both posterior and anterior imaging, and the first hand-held SD-OCT imaging system for ophthalmology. Bioptigen is a leader in providing benefits of ultra-high-resolution imaging to small animal models for research, developing custom lenses tailored to the specifics of animal eyes from zebra fish to mouse, chick, rabbit to monkey, horse, and elephant, and applicable to cornea, crystalline lens, and retina. Expertise developed in the imaging, the diversity of eyes in the natural world is now being applied to pediatric imaging from a premature neonate to a developing adolescent. At Bioptigen, we believe that an understanding of the natural history of human eye development is still in its infancy and that high-performance SD-OCT is a critical tool both for advancing research related to the developing eye and for improving care of the pediatric patient.

SD-OCT THEORY

Envisu is a SD-OCT system tailored for high resolution imaging. The key image attributes of any SD-OCT system—axial resolution, maximum image depth, and lateral resolution—are nominally independent and provide design choices that are subject to application objectives and technical constraints.

The axial resolution and lateral resolution are independent attributes. The axial resolution is determined by the bandwidth of optical light source—a broader bandwidth yields finer axial resolution. The theoretical resolution for a Gaussian-shaped spectrum is:

$$\Delta z = \frac{2\ln(2)}{\pi} = \frac{\lambda_0^2}{\Delta\lambda}$$

1. Axial resolution

Where, Δz is optical axial resolution, λ_0 is the center wavelength of the source, and $\Delta\lambda$ is the bandwidth (full width at half maximum) of the source.

The numerical aperture (NA) or, equivalently, the f-number (f) of the objective optics determines the lateral resolution. A higher NA (lower f) yields finer lateral resolution. The diffraction-limited resolution for traditional optics is given by:

$$\Delta r = 0.61 \frac{\lambda_0}{N.A.} = 1.22 \lambda_0 f l$$

2. Lateral resolution

These concepts of axial and lateral resolution are symmetrical. Achieving theoretical performance is not generally possible in practice. For example, chromatic dispersion limits ability to realize optimum axial resolution. Envisu uses a combination of hardware and software techniques to minimize axial resolution. Lateral resolution is limited by aberrations of the imaging lens and the eye. Envisu optics is designed to provide fine lateral resolution for both non-mydriatic imaging and mydriatic imaging.

The image depth in SD-OCT is more complex. In contrast to time-domain OCT (TD-OCT), where the image depth is dependent on the range of a scanning reference mirror, the available image depth z_{max} in SD-OCT is constrained by the design of the system's spectrometer. The frequency sampling interval $\delta_s k$, where k is optical wave number sampling interval (or alternatively $\delta_s \lambda$, the wavelength sampling interval) of the spectrometer sets maximum image depth. The narrower the frequency spacing between sampled pixel elements, the deeper the SD-OCT imaging window, as per the following equation:

$$Z_{max} = \frac{\pi}{2 \cdot \delta_s k} = \frac{\lambda_0^2}{4 \cdot \delta_s k}$$

3. Image depth

For a particular camera incorporated in different spectrometers, the spectrometer with narrower total spectral bandwidth will have finer spectral interval ($\delta_s k$) between pixels and greater imaging depth.

As with the axial and lateral resolutions, the maximum imaging window does not necessarily translate into the usable imaging depth in practice. Signal fall-off describes how signal-to-noise ratio decreases with depth. Signal fall-off arises because each pixel has its own finite detection bandwidth. This finite detection bandwidth limits coherence length of each individual spectral element, imposing a depth-dependent interference fringe visibility. For a perfect spectrometer imaging system and square detection pixels, 6-dB depth z_{6dB} is predicted to be:

$$Z_{6dB} = \frac{2 \ln(2)}{\delta_r k} = \frac{\ln(2)}{\pi} \frac{\lambda_0^2}{\delta_r \lambda}$$

4. Fall-off

While the axial resolution and the lateral resolution are strongly decoupled, the axial resolution and maximum image depth are mutually constrained. Image depth improves with a narrower spectrometer bandwidth. Therefore, the image depth and the axial resolution are inversely related.

The 2300 system is designed to have approximately 30% greater imaging depth than the 2200, and is the system recommended for hand-held clinical applications. The increased depth range makes imaging less sensitive to the precise working distance and improves visualization of choroid and cornea. Both 2200 and 2300 systems accept the Bioptigen VHR light source, and optical resolution is virtually indistinguishable. The 2200, however, will have commensurately better digital or pixel resolution in-depth direction.

EXTENDED DEPTH IMAGING

It is more difficult to visualize even translucent structures further from the zero-depth point of the image because of signal fall-off. In SD-OCT, it is possible to play a trick that improves imaging of deeper structures by placing the zero point behind the structure of interest. This extended depth imaging mode places the more highly attenuated deep structures in the SD-OCT window where the fall-off is less. This technique is simply implemented in the Envisu system and can be useful for accentuating the choroid or for imaging posterior lens capsule.

BIOPTIGEN ENVISU PRODUCT LINE

The Bioptigen Envisu™ spectral-domain ophthalmic imaging system (SD-OIS) with hand-held imaging probe is a versatile tool for exploring ocular pathology and physiology of patients from neonatal to adult, ambulatory or supine, awake or under anesthesia, or from cornea to retina (Fig. 4.1).

The Envisu™ product line includes implementations for research (R-series) and clinic (C-series). The R-series systems offer increased flexibility for use in a nonregulated environment, specifically intended for noninvasive pre-clinical research. The C-series systems are fully validated systems approved by one or more major regulatory agencies and will be cleared for clinical use in the country in which they are sold. Technically, there are no significant differences between R-series and C-series systems, except that the C-series system will provide new features to the research market through R-series introductions. Clinical users can be confident that C-series systems meet safety and efficacy guidelines demanded for the clinic. Both product lines are designed with patient safety in mind and operate as Class 1 LEDs,* safe under all operating conditions.

Two Envisu™ models are available, allowing user to select systems optimized for either resolution or imaging depth. The Envisu™ 2200 is designed for finest resolution and is very well suited to research imaging of small animal models. The Envisu™ 2300 is optimized for imaging depth and recommended for clinical applications. Specifications for the two models are compared in Table 4.1.

The Envisu R2200 accepts an external ultra-high-resolution source for finest resolution imaging. This source is not available on the C2200.

The Envisu SD-OIS features a hand-held OCT scanning probe. The probe is lightweight and compact, and is convenient for imaging patients in a seated or supine position. The probe may also be mounted for tabletop imaging with a chin rest for more traditional application with ambulatory patients. The hand-held probe accepts a catalog of imaging lenses for different imaging applications. The general retina lens is suitable for posterior imaging of all patients

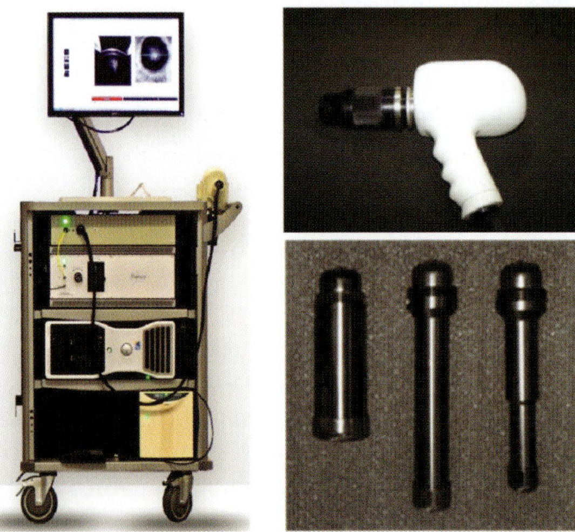

Fig. 4.1 Envisu™ System, left; hand-held imaging probe with retina lens, top right; and telecentric anterior segment lenses, lower right. Lateral resolution of anterior segment lenses, from left to right: 20 μm, 12 μm, and 8 μm, respectively.

*IEC 60825.

Table 4.1 Specifications for Envisu 2200 and Envisu 2300

Imaging speed	C2200 VHR	C2300 VHR
Maximum camera line rate	36 kHz	
Typical imaging line rate	32 kHz	
Axial resolution (measured, in air)	<6.0 μm	
Axial resolution (measured, in tissue)	<4.0 μm	
Maximum imaging depth (in air)	2.3 mm	3.4 mm
Maximum imaging depth (in tissue)	1.7 mm	2.5 mm
Digital resolution, axial (in air)	2.2 μm/pix	3.3 μm/pix
Digital resolution, axial (in tissue)	1.6 μm/pix	2.4 μm/pix
Coherence length oversampling	2.7	1.8
Hand-held scanner weight	<1.6 kg	
System weight	125 kg	
Electrical	110°/220 V	

Table 4.2 Attributes of imaging lenses

Bores	Retina (1)	18 mm Telecentric (2)	12 mm Telecentric (3)
Field of view	70 deg	14 mm	8 mm
Working distance	13.0 mm	20.0 mm	15.0 mm
Lateral resolution	11.0 μm	12.0 μm	8.5 μm
Depth of focus	0.9 mm	1.15 mm	0.54 mm

with a focal range of −12D to +10D and a 70° scan range. Three fixed focus telecentric lenses are available for anterior segment imaging. These lenses offer the photographer a choice in optimizing images for highest lateral resolution or maximum depth of field. High resolution is preferred for imaging microstructure of the cornea, for example, and high depth of field improves imaging of the iridocorneal angle. The attributes of each lens are listed in Table 4.2.

Envisu™ is managed through Bioptigen's InVivoVue™ Clinic (IVVC) software interface. IVVC is a feature-rich platform that provides researcher and the clinician with flexibility to design exam protocols to meet unique needs of any study or diagnostic challenge. IVVC allows real-time imaging and displays at high frames rates without display lag for true ("what you see is what you get" WYSIWYG) visualization. IVVC has both an aiming mode and a free-run mode. In aiming mode, orthogonal cross-sectional B-scans are displayed to assist the photographer with centering of the scan. When set, a foot-pedal-mediated snapshot acquires a single volume of data. In free-run mode, volumetric data is acquired, repetitively, allowing extended exploration of the eye. When stopped, last full volume of data is saved.

IVVC allows complete flexibility of scan settings with a variety of scan patterns, including raster scans, radial scans, and annular scans. The length and width of scans are continuously variable, as are the scan densities. This flexibility allows the photographer to set the scan pattern most relevant to physiology or pathology and the scan density to be chosen to optimize the trade-off between image speed and image quality. At low density, full volume scans of 60 frames and 600 lines per frame are acquired in 1 second. For a 6 mm × 6 mm scan, the spacing between frames is 100 μm. At high density, a full-volume scan of 100 frames and 1000 lines per frame is acquired in 3 seconds. An isotropic scan up to 400 frames + 400 lines is acquired in 5 seconds (Table 4.3).

The IVVC display shows the depth-resolved cross-sectional B-scans (Fig. 4.2) next to enface image or volume intensity projection (VIP), derived directly from the OCT data. This VIP image is an OCT fundus image that provides direct registration between the depth-resolved OCT data and the fundus view, assuring that OCT-resolved

Table 4.3 Comparative benefits of scan-sampling densities

Volume type	Lines per B-scan	B-scans per volume	Frames per B-scan	Imaging time (seconds)	A-scan spacing (μm) 6 mm × 6 mm	B-scan spacing (μm) 6 mm × 6 mm	Benefit/ appli- cation	Speed	B-scan quality	En face quality
"Standard"	1000	100	1	28	6	60	General purpose imaging; high quality B-scans	Better	Better	Better
High speed volume	600	60	1	1	10	100	Superior acquisition speed, screening of active subjects	Best	Good	Average
Averaged	1000	25	4	28	6	240	High quality B-scans with better SNR	Better	Better	Ok
Isotropic volume	350	350	1	3.4	17	17	Optimal 3D sampling, still subjects	Average	Average	Best

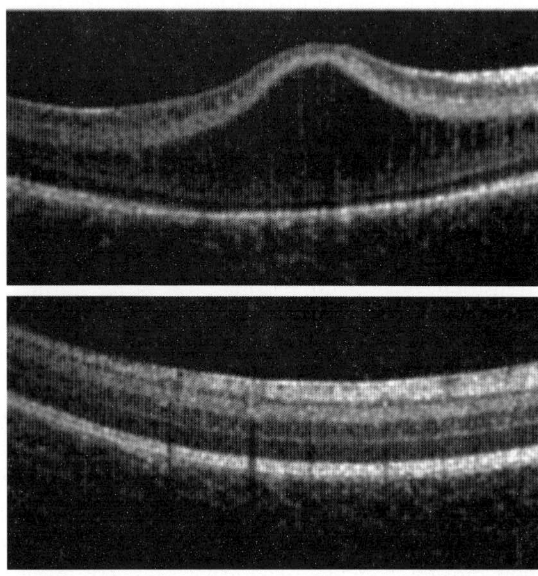

Fig. 4.2 B-scans acquired at 600 lines.

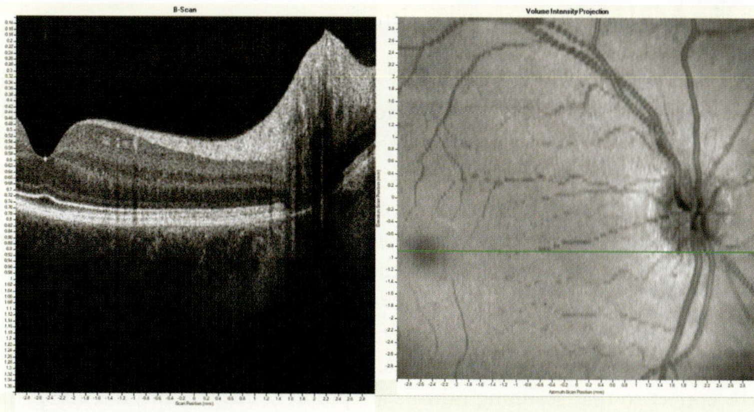

Fig. 4.3 B-scan and associated VIP of 6 mm × 6 mm scan acquired at 1000 lines × 100 frames. The green line on the VIP shows the location of the displayed B-scan.

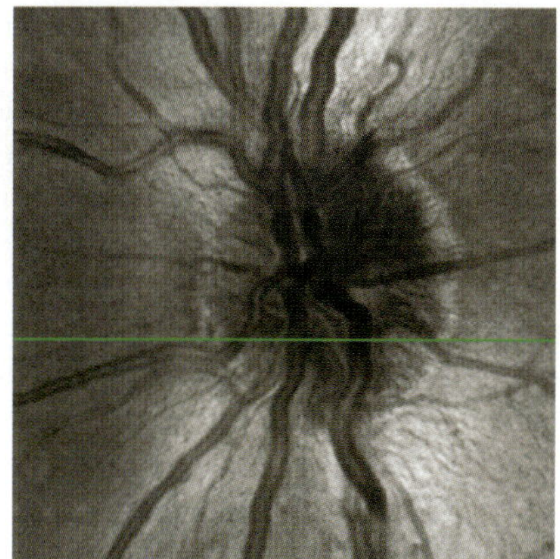

Fig. 4.4 VIP of 3 mm × 3 mm scan acquired at 350 lines by 300 frames.

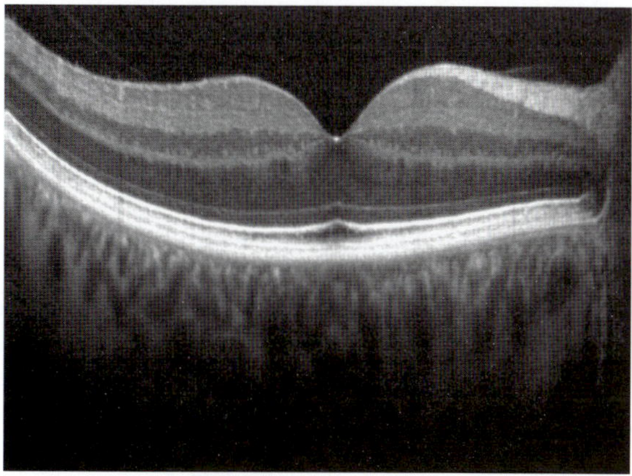

Fig. 4.5 Hand-held image of adult macula of 6-mm scan length, 1000 lines and averaging 4×.

pathologies can be identified against the landscape of the fundus. This is a useful feature for longitudinal comparisons. The absolute precision in alignment is not required to compare pathology changes over time. High sampling density and automatic registration to a fundus view both assure the photographer that pathologies are unlikely to be missed during a scan, and position of the scan is always evidenced by the VIP image (horizontal green line in **Figures 4.3 and 4.4**).

While IVVC allows complete customization of scan settings, ease of use features include custom scans and custom protocols. The user can save frequently used scan settings named custom scans. Additionally, IVVC enables the user to save a collection of scans used in exam as a custom protocol. These protocols may be attached to studies, allowing for efficient and accurate recreation of scan settings for clinical trials.

In addition to these basic features, IVVC allows user-settable averaging for the highest image quality. Generally, averaging levels of three-to-five times results in quality images, as shown in **Figure 4.5**. IVVC has a caliper function for manual measurement of any features observed on B-scans or VIP images. These measurements are saved in a single step into a spreadsheet file for ease of analysis. IVVC includes a feature-rich–3D-visualization tool. Also included are Doppler imaging for the qualitative visualization of blood flow, and an extended depth imaging mode provides some improvement in the imaging of posterior features of an imaged structure, for example, to highlight the choroid or to visualize posterior lens capsule.

HAND-HELD IMAGING

Hand-held imaging is a new technique enabled by the Envisu SD-OIS system, allowing the photographer to bring the instrument to the patient, instead of the patient to the instrument. This is very useful for nonambulatory patients, pediatric patients, and any other class of patient or imaging environment where tabletop imaging is not indicated. With hand-held imaging, the clinician is free to explore the eye unconstrained by the mechanics of the tabletop system. The Envisu system has a number of attributes that lend the system to hand-held imaging, including lightweight and fast real-time imaging. As the Envisu system is noncontact and uses very low levels of near-infrared illumination, the imaging experience is comfortable for the patient.

It is useful to understand imaging optics for successful retinal imaging with a noncontact hand-held SD-OCT system. In contrast to taking photos with fundus cameras, acquiring images with OCT systems requires a higher level of precision in obtaining a correct working distance. There are two reasons for this. First, the distance to pupil of the patient must be correct so that scanning mirrors are properly imaged into the eye of the patient. Without a proper working distance, the scanned OCT image will exhibit significant vignetting, particularly in nonmydriatic patients. Second, the reference arm setting of the OCT system must match total path length to region of interest, for example, the retina. For mature eyes, these conditions are not dramatically different from patient to patient. For imaging of patients from newborn to adult, these conditions require extra attention.

With tabletop imaging, control of various geometric relationships are simplified with a patient positioned in a chin rest and the imaging probe secured in a mount. Hand-held imaging requires more dexterity and attention to visual cues. The Envisu optics are designed for nonmydriatic imaging—an accurately aligned probe at correct working distance to the cornea will provide the same image quality for patients with dilated or undilated pupils. The proper alignment requires that the scanned beam waist is directed through the center of the pupil, as shown in **Figure 4.6**. Image distortions will occur if the working distance is not correct, as shown in **Figure 4.7**. If the retina appears convex, as shown in the rightmost image (**Fig. 4.7**, *left panel*), the reference arm is likely to be too short, and the lens held is too close to the patient's eye. Conversely, if the retina appears overly concave (**Fig. 4.7**, *right panel*) the lens is too far from the patient's eye and reference arm is set too long. **Figure 4.8** provides visual cues for lateral misalignment (lens held off-center of the pupil). Of course, vignetting will be more sensitive to misalignment with nonmydriatic patients. The lens rotates around the nodal point—the pupil center—in order to image away from

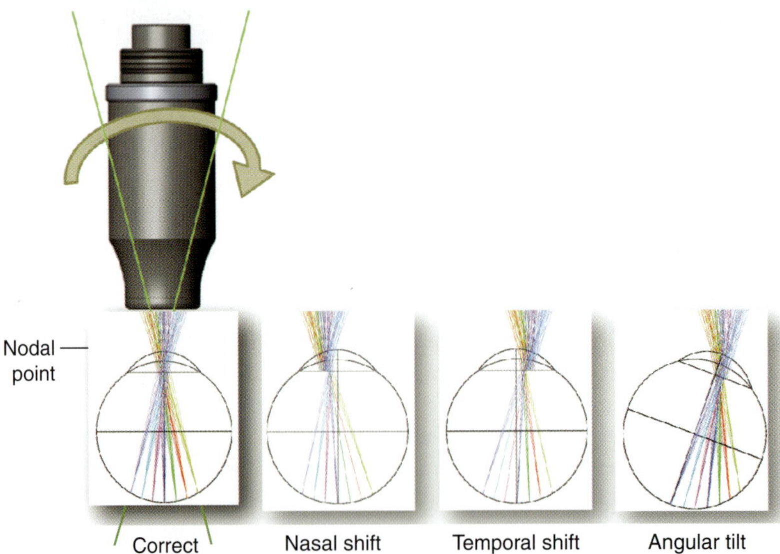

Fig. 4.6 Proper alignment of scanning OCT beam. Proper working distance and alignment for imaging fovea centralis, left to right. Vignetting due to nasal and temporal shifts from center (OD), proper alignment and rotation for imaging peripheral to fovea centralis (OD) or imaging optic nerve head (OS).

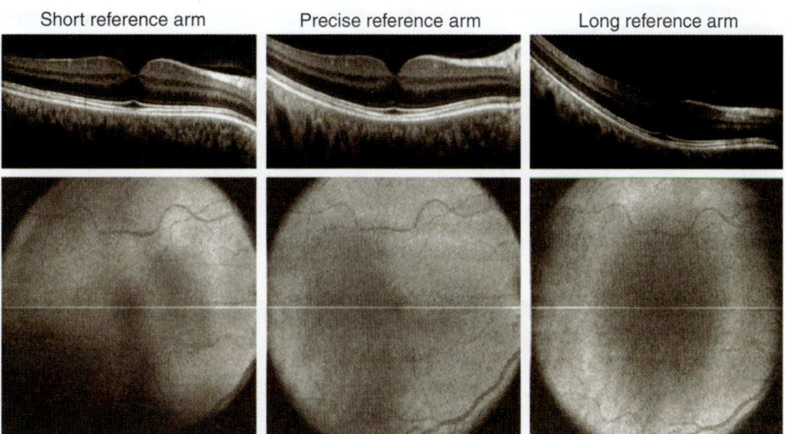

Fig. 4.7 Visual cues when imaging with improper working distance and reference arm setting. Top images are unaveraged B-scans. Bottom images are corresponding en face views. Note convex appearance of retina when reference arm is too short (and working distance too close), and concave appearance when reference arm is too long (and working distance too far).

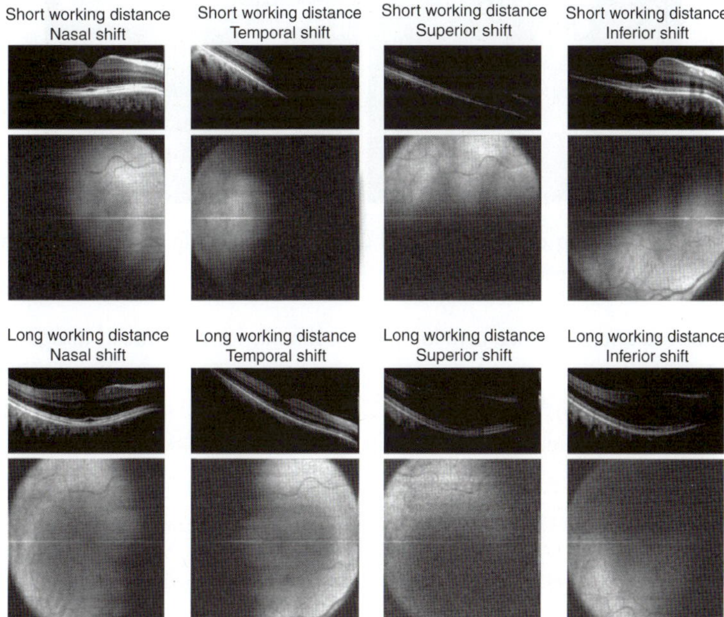

Fig. 4.8 Visual cues associated with lateral shifts of the imaging probe relative to the pupil, right (OD) eye. At precise working distance, vignetting associated with lateral shifts will be more uniform across the image plane.

fovea centralis. In practice, it is recommended that the photographer develops confidence with alignment to the fovea before rotating the lens to observe peripheral features of the retina. With practice, the photographer can adjust to visual cues and obtain high-quality hand-held images for a wide range of patient physiology and pathology.

PEDIATRIC IMAGING

Imaging very young children presents a unique challenge to the ophthalmic photographer. Clearly, neonates and preadolescent children cannot cooperate to verbal instructions from the photographer. Frequently, children will be in a neonatal unit, held by nervous parents, or imaged under anesthesia. Tabletop imaging is not appropriate for these circumstances. Additionally, the eye continues to develop after birth. The eye length and cellular structure continues to develop after birth. There are also pathologies unique to childhood eye and visual development, including retinopathy of prematurity, retinoblastoma, and shaken baby syndrome. Hand-held imaging systems are desirable to support clinical evaluation and treatment of the child.

The Envisu SD-OIS system is the first OCT system dedicated to imaging the pediatric eye. As a noncontact imaging system with very low radiant optical powers, the imaging experience is less traumatic to patient than other modalities such as contact fundus photography or ultrasound biomicroscopy. The Envisu system power output is

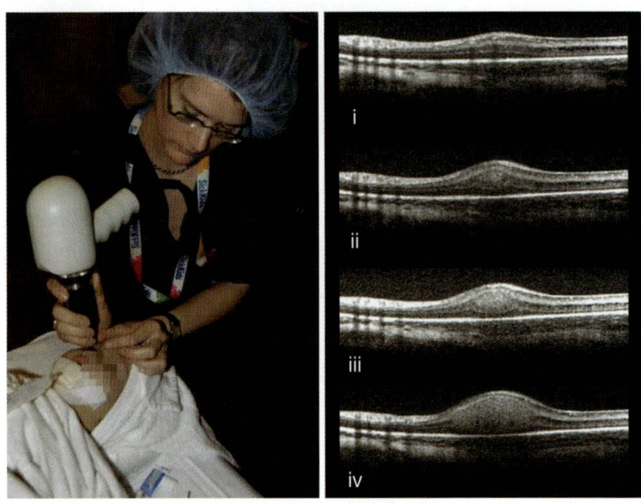

Fig. 4.9 Hand-held SD-OCT imaging of a young child under anesthesia. Images on the right are cross-sections of pathology assessed by clinician to be retinoblastoma.

Table 4.4 Refractive errors and reference arm length adjustments for age-based imaging

Age (Gestational)	Reference error (D)	Axial length (mm)	Change in reference arm settings (Envisu units)
30–35 wk	−1	15.1	97
35–39 wk	0.3	16.1	86
39–41 wk	0.4	16.8	79
0–1 mo	0.9	17.4	72
1–2 mo	0.3	18.6	59
2–6 mo	0.5	18.9	56
6–12 mo	0.6	19.2	52
12–18 mo	0.7	20.1	43
18 mo–2 yr	0.9	21.3	30
2–3 yr	1	21.8	24
3–4 yr	0.6	22.2	20
4–5 yr	−0.8	22.3	19
5–9 yr	−0.6	22.7	14
10 yr–Adult	−0.5	24	0

limited to 750 µW of optical energy in the 800–900 nm wavelength range; the system is certified as a nonhazardous class 1 LED. The system is designed to image eye lengths from < 14 mm to > 25 mm, accommodating neonates to adults. The scan head weighs only 3 lbs and is comfortable to hold in multiple positions for the photographer.

The use of the Envisu system for imaging a young child with evident retinoblastoma under anesthesia [exam under anesthesia (EUA)] is shown in **Figure 4.9**.

Maldonado et al. studied refractive error and eye length of children as a function of gestational age, establishing settings for imaging with the hand-held Envisu SD-OIS. The Envisu system has a manual system for the reference arm length adjustment; larger units on the reference arm counter are associated with shorter reference arm length and eye length. **Table 4.4** provides guidelines for adjusting refractive error (Diopter) and eye length of the patients according to age. These are starting points; fine adjustment for individual cases may be desired for the best images.

CONCLUSION

The Envisu Hand-held Spectral-Domain Ophthalmic Imaging System is a unique platform for depth-resolved imaging of nonambulatory patients. High resolution and high signal-to-noise ratio with real-time feedback during image acquisition enables the photographer to obtain high-density volumetric images for patients from neonate to adult with a wide range of pathologies. The Envisu SD-OIS should prove to be a valuable diagnostic adjunct for pediatric and perioperative ophthalmology.

FURTHER READING

1. Gerth C, Zawadzki RJ, Elise Héon, et al.: High-resolution retinal imaging in young children using a handheld scanner and Fourier-domain optical coherence tomography. *AAPOS* 13(1):72–74, 2009.
2. Chong GT, Farsiu S, Freedman SF, et al.: Abnormal foveal morphology in ocular albinism imaged with spectral-domain optical coherence tomography. *Arch Ophthalmol* 127(1):37–44, 2009.
3. Scott AW, Farsiu S, Enyedi LB, et al.: Imaging the infant retina with a hand-held spectral-domain optical coherence tomography device. *Am J Ophthalmol* 147(2):364–373, 2009.
4. VandenHoven C, Kelly MP: An introduction to the first commercially available hand-held spectral domain optical coherence tomography unit. *Journal of Ophthalmic Photography* 31(SD OCT Supplement):80–85, 2009.
5. Bremner R: Retinoblastoma, an Inside Job. *Cell* 137(6):992–994, 2009.
6. Chavala SH, Farsiu S, Maldonado R, et al.: Insights into advanced retinopathy of prematurity using handheld spectral domain optical coherence tomography imaging. *Ophthalmology* 116(12):2448–2456, 2009.
7. Maldonado RS, Freedman SF, Cotten CM, et al.: Reversible retinal edema in an infant with neonatal hemochromatosis and liver failure. *AAPOS* 15(1):91–93, 2010.
8. Muni RH, Kohly RP, Charonis AC, et al.: Retinoschisis detected with handheld spectral-domain optical coherence tomography in neonates with advanced retinopathy of prematurity. *Arch Ophthalmol* 128(1):57–62, 2010.
9. Muni RH, Kohly RP, Sohn EH, et al.: Hand-held spectral domain optical coherence tomography finding in shaken-baby syndrome. *Retina* 30(4):S45–S50, 2010.
10. Day S, Maldonado RS, Toth CA, et al.: Preretinal and intraretinal exudates in familial exudative vitreoretinopathy. *Retina* 31(1):193–194, 2011.
11. Vajzovic L, Toth CA, Hendrickson AE, et al.: Maturation of the human fovea: correlation of spectral-domain optical coherence tomography findings with histology. *Am J Ophthalmol* 154(5):779–789, 2012.
12. Maldonado RS, Toth CA, Rachelle O'Connell, et al.: Spectral-domain optical coherence tomographic assessment of severity of cystoids macular edema in retinopathy of prematurity. *Arch Ophthalmol* 130(5):569–578, 2012.
13. Dubis AM, Carroll J, Costakos DM, et al.: Evaluation of normal human foveal development using optical coherence tomography and histologic evaluation. *Arch Ophthalmol* 130(10):1291–1300, 2012.

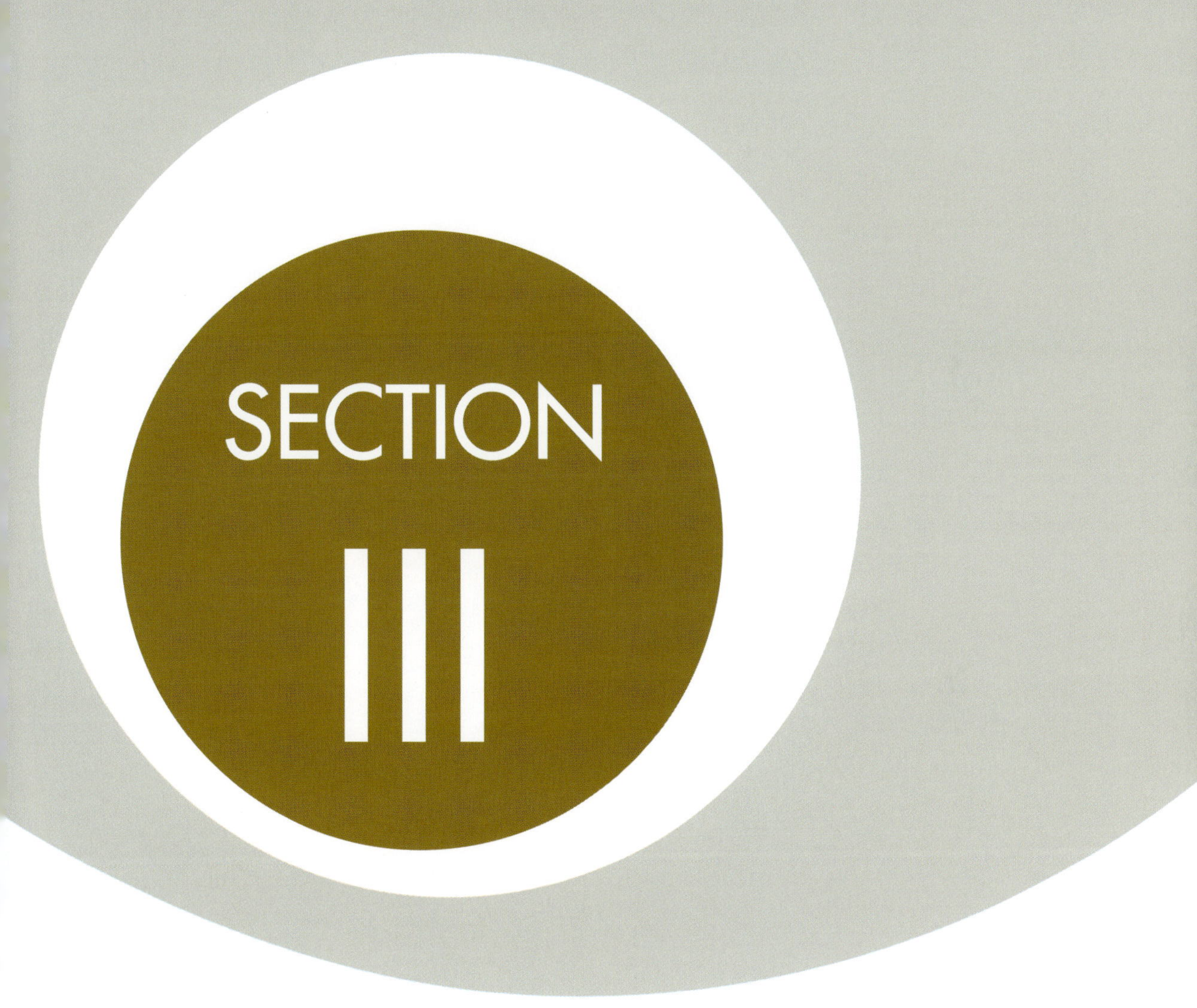

Cornea

Interpreting Corneal Images with Spectral-domain Optical Coherence Tomography

Naoyuki Maeda

INTRODUCTION

Optical coherence tomography (OCT) imaging of the anterior segment of the eye was first published in 1994. Ever since, anterior-segment optical coherence tomography (AS-OCT) is frequently used not only for diagnosing pathology of the anterior segment, but also for planning and evaluating anterior segment surgeries. This is because one can visualize and quantify cross-sectional images of the cornea, anatomic structures of angle, and anterior chamber biometry using the AS-OCT in a noninvasive fashion in the clinic.

Currently, AS-OCTs are classified into three categories based on the principle: time-domain (TD) OCT, spectral-domain (SD) OCT, and swept-source (SS) OCT.

Time-domain (TD) OCT

The time-domain optical coherence tomography (OCT) at 1310 nm is a first-generation OCT. The resolution in vertical direction is 18 μm and the speed of A-scan is 2000 scan/second. The wavelength of 1310 nm is generally used for OCT that is exclusively for anterior segment instead of 840 nm that is common in OCTs for the posterior segment of the eye. This is because deeper penetrance in opaque tissue can be obtained with 1310 nm than with 840 nm. Therefore, second-generation OCT only for the anterior-segment SS-OCT also employs 1310 nm. Its vertical resolution is 10 μm with 30,000 A-scan/second for 16-mm diameter. The 1310 nm AS-OCT finds use in investigating distribution of corneal thickness, graft–host junction in keratoplasty, interface following lamellar corneal surgery, dimensions of the anterior chamber, and lesions of various corneal pathologies.

Spectral-domain (SD) OCT

Opposite to the AS-OCT that covers wider area with low magnification and low resolution, higher resolution (5 μm) and faster speed of A-scan (26000 scan/second) can be obtained with the 840-nm spectral-domain OCT such as RTVue-100 (Optovue Inc., Fremont, CA).

As the SD-OCT was designed to image the posterior segment of the eye, working distance and magnification should be modified during measurement of the anterior segment of the eye. **Figures 5.1 and 5.2** show cornea/anterior

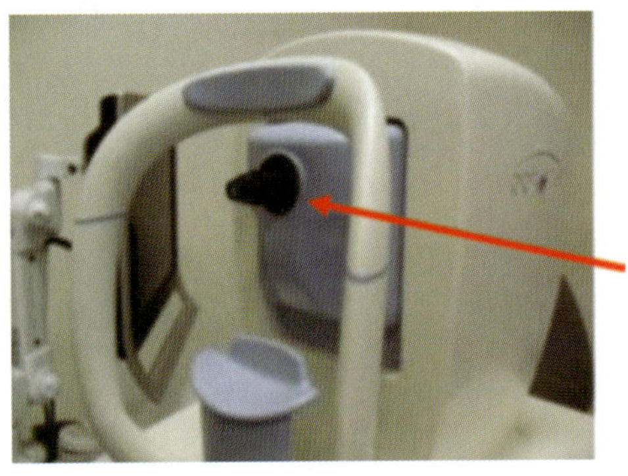

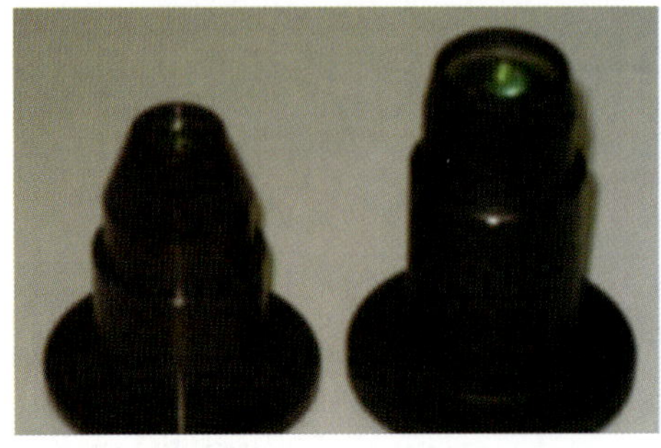

Fig. 5.1 Cornea/anterior measurement (CAM) modules in RTVue.

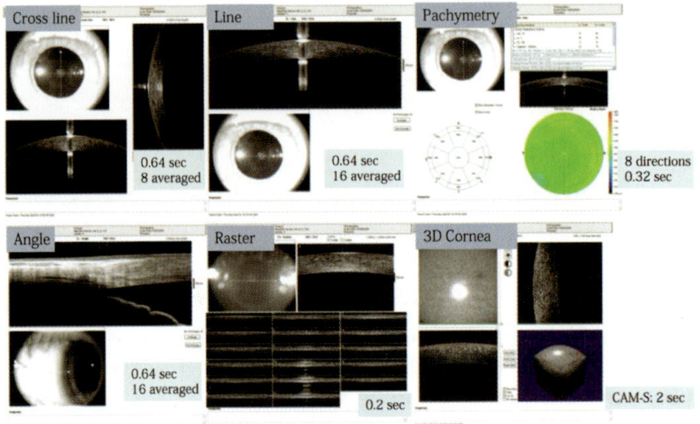

Fig. 5.2 Images obtained with eight modes in normal cornea.

measurement (CAM) modules in RTVue. With line mode, Bowman's layer can be seen as parallel lines. One of the biggest advantages of the SD-OCT over the TD- or SS-OCT is that thickness profile of the epithelium and stroma of the cornea can be analyzed separately.

SELECTIVE LAMELLAR KERATOPLASTY

Recently, we are in the middle of a paradigm shift in keratoplasty. Selective lamellar keratoplasty including DSAEK (Descemet's stripping automated endothelial keratoplasty) and DALK (deep anterior lamellar keratoplasty) have their advantages and disadvantages over penetrating keratoplasty (PKP). With the use of SD-OCT, thickness profiles of the host and the graft can be easily evaluated separately.

CASE STUDY 1

A 72-year-old female patient had necrotizing keratitis due to herpes simplex virus (HSV) in her left eye. The DALK was performed and slit lamp examination following the DALK showed clear graft, as shown in **Figure 5.3**. Although it gave us the impression that the whole cornea was replaced by donor graft except Descemet's membrane and endothelium, images obtained with cross-line mode by the SD-OCT indicated residual stromal bed. The central thickness of the stromal bed and graft were 73 μm and 538 μm, respectively. We need to look out for corneal

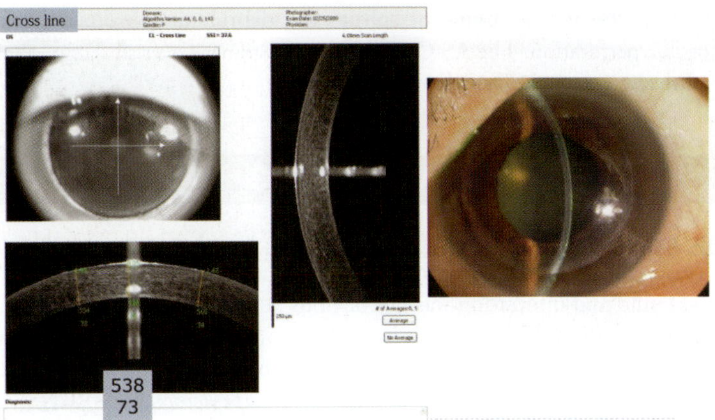

Fig. 5.3 DALK for HSV keratitis.

neovascularization at this interface and monitoring stromal thickness will be helpful for following up this patient in terms of recurrence of herpetic stromal keratitis.

CASE STUDY 2

Descemet's stripping automated endothelial keratoplasty (DSAEK) was done in an 84-year-old man for pseudophakic bullous keratopathy (PBK; Fig. 5.4). Slit lamp examination revealed the clear-graft and clear-host cornea. The SD-OCT images, however, indicated high intensity at subepithelial stroma and inhomogeneous distribution of intensity at the posterior part of the host's stroma. These findings suggested that the subepithelial and pre-Descemet's stromal scars existed probably due to longstanding bullous keratopathy before surgery. In addition, measurements of the thicknesses in the host and the graft are helpful for checking rejection reaction that is generally milder than that in PKP and is difficult to diagnose.

INFECTIOUS KERATITIS

Although it is not difficult to diagnose infectious keratitis with conventional ophthalmic examinations, it is not easy to estimate the depth of the focus and residual stromal thickness with slit lamp examination because of abscess

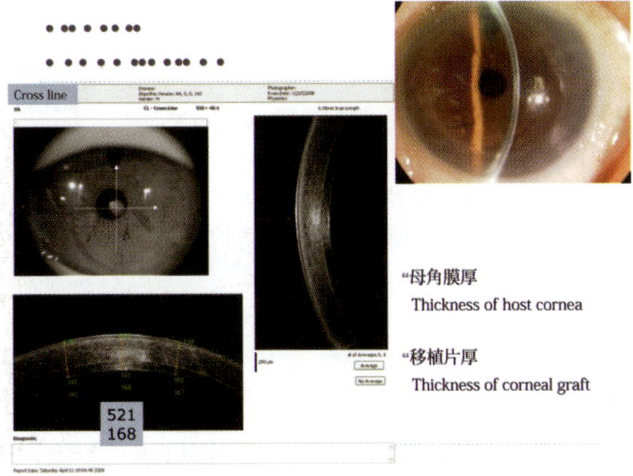

Fig. 5.4 DSAEK for PBK.

and edema at the focus. In such cases, scraping for culture and debridement around the focus might be deferred because of the fear of possible perforation. The AS-OCT has big advantages over slit lamp examination for observation inside opaque tissues and measuring corneal thickness at the lesion.

A 29-year-old female was referred to our clinic because of neurotrophic ulcer with a combination of trigeminal nerve palsy and facial nerve palsy. Slit lamp examination showed irregular and dirty surface on the neurotrophic ulcer. Conjunctival injection was mild and infiltration was not obvious beneath the ulcer.

The cross-sectional images by the OCT, as shown in **Figure 5.5**, revealed that the high-intensity area was limited to the anterior corneal surface and posterior stroma appeared to be intact. Therefore, the lesion was scraped. The culture was positive for methicillin-resistant coagulase-negative *staphylococcus* (MRCNS). Topical application of arbekacin and minocycline ointment was effective as a treatment.

After scarring of the lesion and epithelization of the neurotrophic ulcer, therapeutic soft contact lens was worn to prevent recurrence of neurotrophic ulcer due to lagophthalmos for a while. The OCT images indicated disappearance of the high-intensity area at the corneal surface and soft contact lens on the cornea.

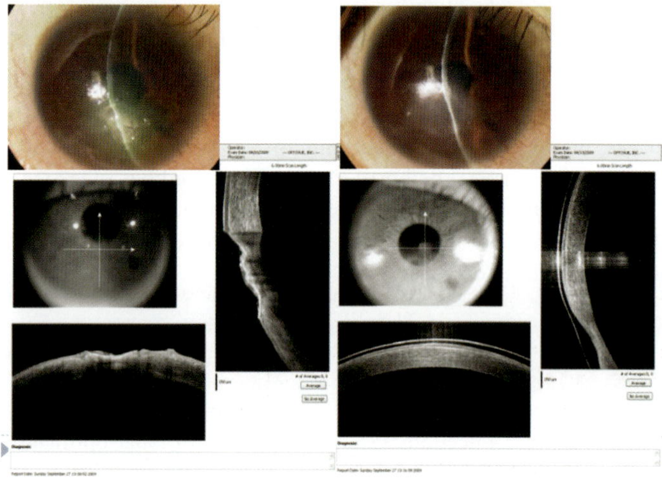

Fig. 5.5 Bacterial keratitis due to MRCNS.

PSEUDOPHAKIC BULLOUS KERATOPATHY

The presence of the stromal scar will induce scattering and corneal deformation; thus giving rise to irregular astigmatism. This, in turn, will lead to deterioration of quality of vision following the DSAEK. The corneal stroma should be checked carefully preoperatively, and AS-OCT is a valuable tool for the same.

A 69-year-old male visited the hospital complaining of pain in his left eye. As shown in **Figure 5.6**, bulla formation associated with pseudophakic bullous keratopathy was noted. The images of SD-OCT showed remarkable bulla formation as obvious space between the epithelium and the stroma. There were a couple of intraepithelial spaces or clefts.

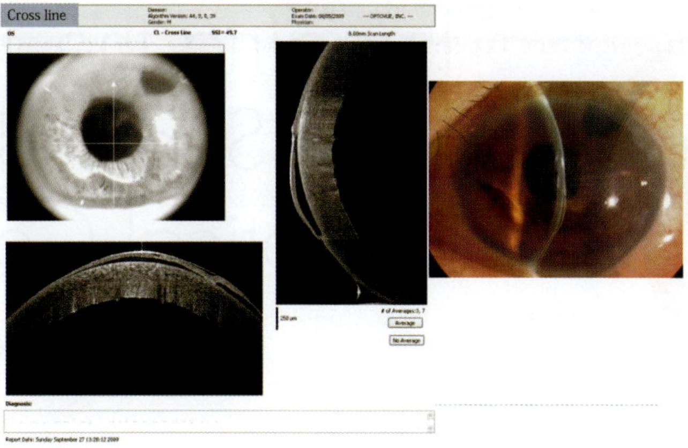

Fig. 5.6 Pseudophakic bullous keratopathy.

In addition, folds in the Descemet's membrane, stromal edema, and irregular pattern in the anterior stroma were also visible.

In addition to the examples shown here, wound healing process at the stroma, compensational thickening of corneal epithelium, thickness distribution of LASIK flap, or epithelial ingrowth between LASIK flap and stromal bed can be evaluated precisely with the SD-OCT. The OCT technology, being a noninvasive and quantitative modality for examining anterior pathology of the eye, is gaining a crucial role in planning and evaluating anterior segment surgeries.

FURTHER READING

1. Izatt JA, Hee MR, Swanson EA, et al.: Micrometer-scale resolution imaging of the anterior eye *in vivo* with optical coherence tomography. *Arch Ophthalmol* 112:1584–1589, 1994.
2. Konstantopoulos A, Hossain P, Anderson DF: Recent advances in ophthalmic anterior segment imaging: a new era for ophthalmic diagnosis? *Br J Ophthalmol* 91:551–557, 2007.
3. Chen J, Lee L: Clinical applications and new developments of optical coherence tomography: an evidence-based review. *Clin Exp Optom* 90:317–335, 2007.
4. Simpson T, Fonn D: Optical coherence tomography of the anterior segment. *Ocul Surf* 6:117–127, 2008.
5. Ramos JL, Li Y, Huang D: Clinical and research applications of anterior segment optical coherence tomography – a review. *Clin Experiment Ophthalmol* 37:81–89, 2009.
6. Maeda N: Optical coherence tomography for corneal diseases. *Eye Contact Lens* 36:254–259, 2010.

6

Imaging the Tear Film on Spectral-domain Optical Coherence Tomography

Shizuka Koh

Recent development in anterior-segment imaging technique with anterior-segment optical coherence tomography (AS-OCT) enables noninvasive observation of the tear film. On the ocular surface, tears are distributed in the upper and lower tear menisci, precorneal tear film, and cul-de-sac. Cross-sectional images of the tear meniscus can be directly visualized with the AS-OCT (Figs 6.1 and 6.2). Also, imaging with the AS-OCT allows us to quantify the

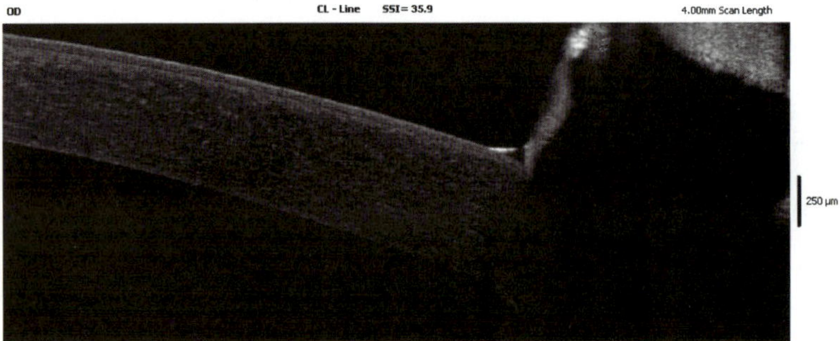

Fig. 6.1 Upper tear meniscus.

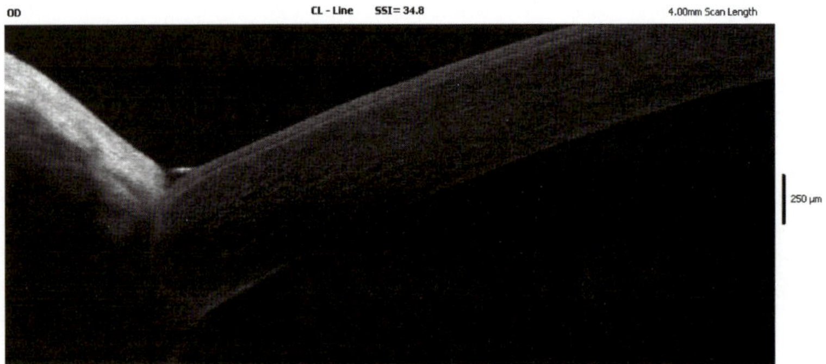

Fig. 6.2 Lower tear meniscus.

tear meniscus dimensions. It is believed that the tear meniscus reflects total tear volume and noninvasive quantitative assessment of the tear meniscus with the AS-OCT can be a useful tool in the diagnosis of dry eye. It is also useful in the examination of other tear-film related cases such as contact lens fitting. Moreover, spectral-domain optical coherence tomography (SD-OCT) can allow acquisition of better quality cross-sectional images of the tear meniscus in a much shorter time than time-domain optical coherence tomography (TD-OCT).

Shown here are cross-sectional images of the upper and lower tear menisci of a normal eye without dry eye with the SD-OCT (RTVue-100; Optovue, Inc., Fremont, CA). Although both the upper and lower tear menisci cannot be imaged in a single image because of the limitation in the scan length of the RTVue-100, the tear boundary can be identified clearly for both the tear menisci (**Figs 6.3 and 6.4**).

The RTVue-100 and other frequency-domain optical coherence tomography (FD-OCT) systems have a caliper software, and quantification of the tear meniscus dimensions can be performed easily.

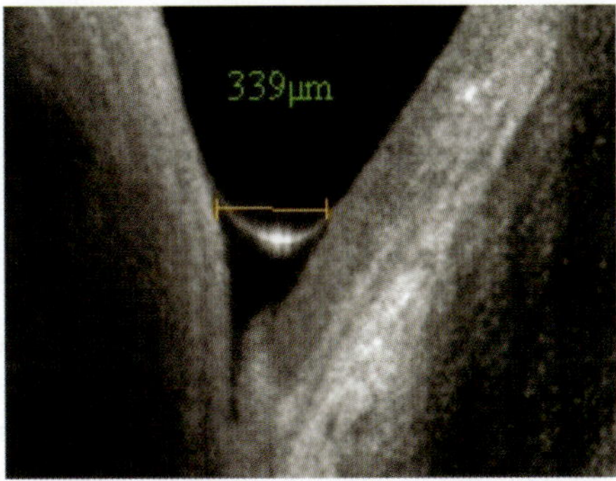

Fig. 6.3 Lower tear meniscus of normal eye, lower-tear-meniscus height = 339 µm.

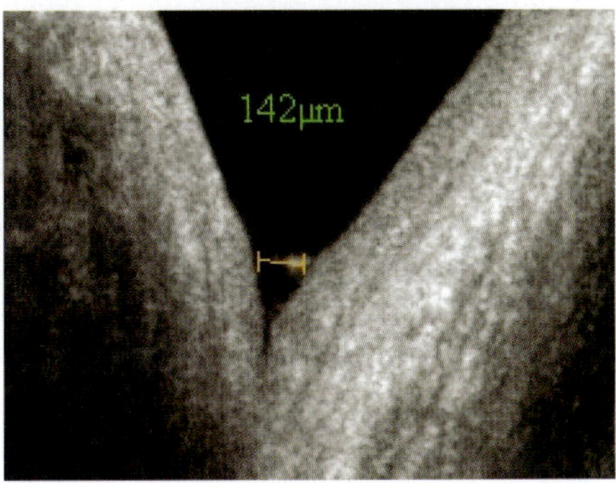

Fig. 6.4 Lower tear meniscus of aqueous-tear-deficient dry eye, lower-tear-meniscus height = 142 µm.

FURTHER READING

1. Radhakrishnan S, Rollins AM, Roth JE, et al. Real-time optical coherence tomography of the anterior segment at 1310 nm. *Arch Ophthalmol* 119:1179–1185, 2001.
2. Wang J, Aquavella J, Palakuru J, Chung S, Feng C. Relationships between central tear film thickness and tear menisci of the upper and lower eyelids. *Invest Ophthalmol Vis Sci* 47:4349–4355, 2006.

Imaging the Tear Film in Normal and Dry Eyes

Osama MA Ibrahim,

Takashi Kojima,

Yukihiro Matsumoto, and

Murat Dogru

Dry eye is a multifactorial disease of tears and ocular surface that results in symptoms of discomfort, visual disturbance, and tear film instability with a potential damage to the ocular surface, which may be associated with tear deficiency. Several methods have been used for diagnosis and assessment of dry eye disease including Schirmer test, Rose Bengal, and fluorescein staining. However, these tests are criticized for their invasive nature and low repeatability. Optical coherence tomography (OCT) tear meniscus height measurement has been reported to be a quick, noninvasive method for assessing the tear meniscus height with acceptable sensitivity, specificity, and repeatability.

Visante OCT shows reduced heights of upper and lower tear menisci (0.17 mm and 0.17 mm, respectively) in the dry eye patient compared to those (0.29 mm and 0.37 mm, respectively) in the normal subject, respectively (Fig. 7.1).

CASE STUDY 1

A 67-year-old female patient with a history of eye dryness and foreign body sensation in both eyes for 2 years was diagnosed to have dry eye disease based on tear film break-up time measurement, vital staining assessment, and Schirmer's test.

The patient was advised to receive artificial tear supplementation. However, the patient's symptoms and signs did not improve after 2 months of treatment. Upper and lower punctal occlusion with silicone plugs (SUPERFLEX® plugs) (Eagle Vision, Memphis, Tennessee, USA) was used for retention of the tears on the ocular surface. After 1 month of punctal occlusion, the patient underwent the examinations performed before insertion of punctal plugs. The increase in upper and lower tear meniscus heights measured by Visante OCT, as shown in Figure 7.2, was accompanied with an improvement of the patient's ocular surface tests.

CASE STUDY 2

A 69-year-old female patient was diagnosed with primary Sjögren syndrome, according to the Japanese diagnostic criteria of Sjögren syndrome. The patient had a history of using nonpreserved 0.1% hyaluronic acid eye drops for 12 weeks without improvement in her ocular symptoms and signs. The patient was given pilocarpine 5-mg tablets (Salagen, Kissei pharmaceutical Co., Ltd, Nagano, Japan) two times/day (morning and evening) for 3 months. The data was analyzed for 1 week, 1 month, and 3 months after treatment. The OCT tear meniscus height measurement showed low upper and lower tear meniscus heights, as shown in Figure 7.3.

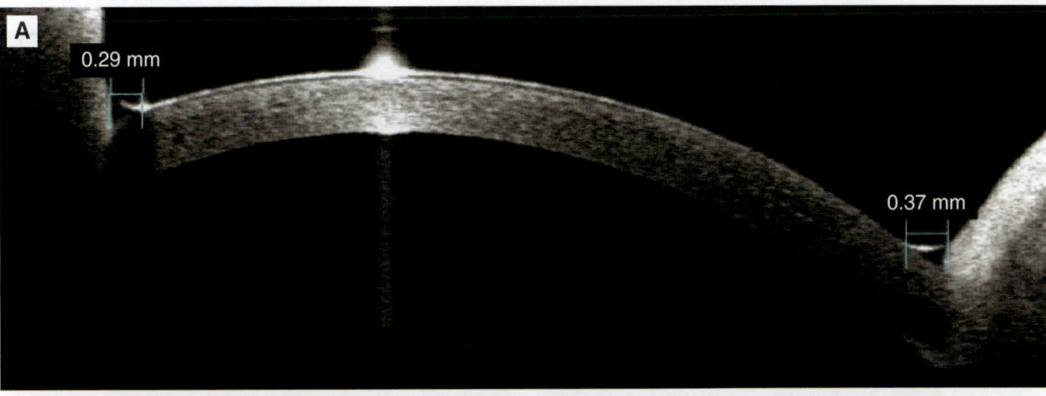

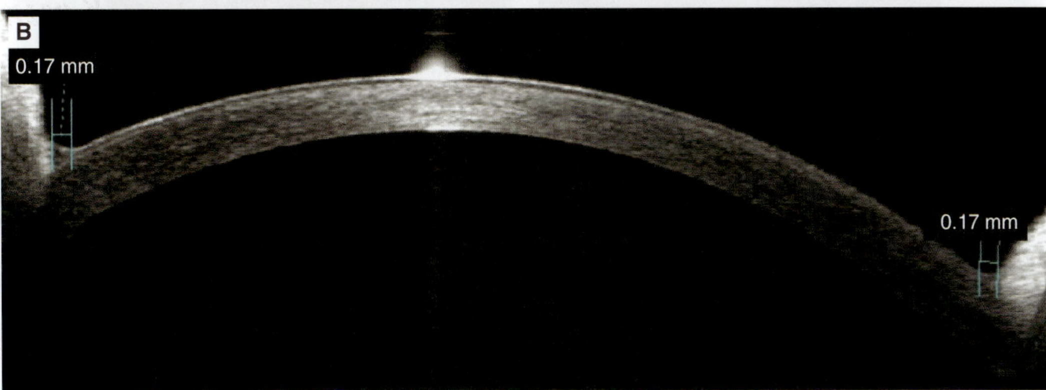

Fig. 7.1 Visante OCT images of the left eye of a female normal subject aged 64 years (A) and a female dry eye patient aged 67 years (B).

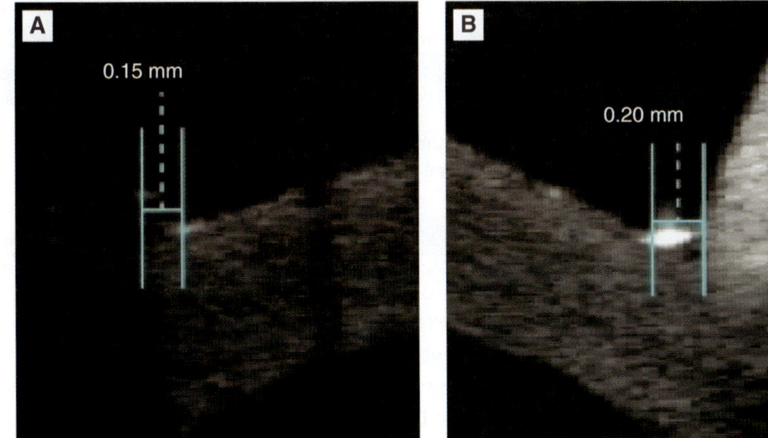

Fig. 7.2 OCT upper- and (A) lower-tear-meniscus (B) height measurement performed before punctal occlusion.

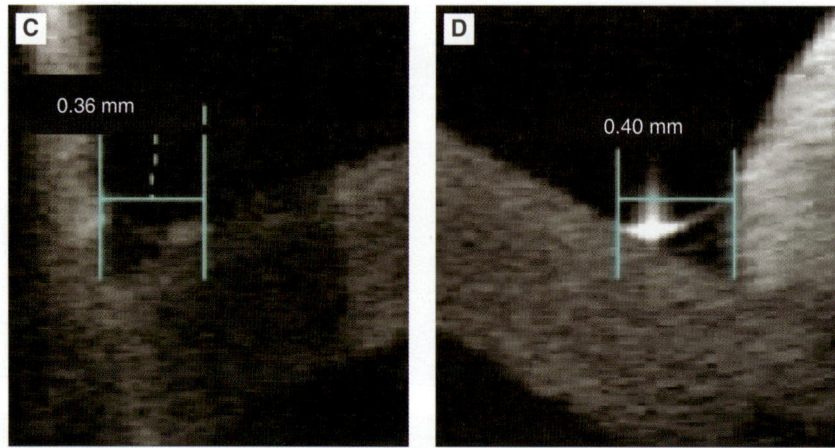

Fig. 7.2 (*Continued*) OCT upper **(C)** and lower tear meniscus **(D)** heights measurement performed after 1 month. Note the increase in tear meniscus height after punctal occlusion.

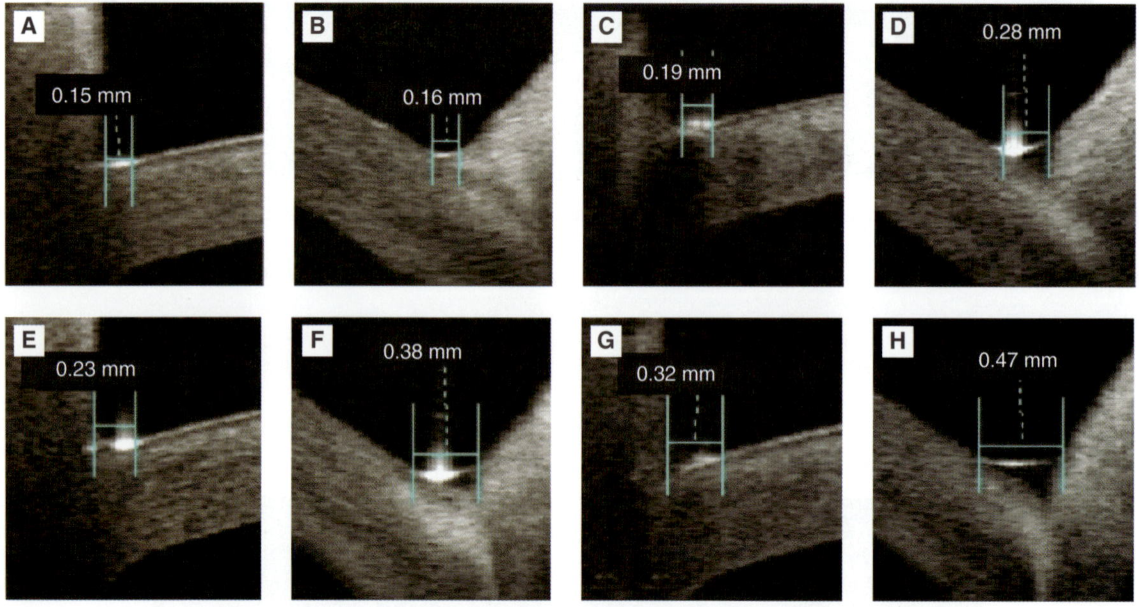

Fig. 7.3 Upper and lower tear meniscus heights measured with Visante OCT before **(A, B)**, after 1 week **(C, D)**, 1 month **(E, F)**, and 3 months of pilocarpine treatment **(G, H)**, respectively.

Improvements in the tear meniscus heights were observed after 1 week, further improved after 1 month, and reached its highest values after 3 months of pilocarpine treatment (**Fig. 7.3**). The patient's ocular surface examinations maintained at normal range and reduction of the dry eye symptoms was observed throughout the follow-up.

The tear meniscus height has been reported to reduce in tear-deficient dry eye and its measurement is of great value in diagnosis of the disease. Recently, new technologic developments such as the OCT has revealed great potential to evaluate the tear meniscus and ocular surface status more precisely. The OCT system allows high-resolution view of the tear meniscus with an ability to compare data during the follow-up of a patient providing a more objective follow-up. Clinically, the OCT is of value in analyzing tear dynamics and assessment of the tear meniscus after application of the dry eye treatment, including the punctal plugs and oral sialogogue. The ability of the OCT to monitor improvement of the tear meniscus height recommends this new methodology to be a useful clinical tool in evaluating ocular surface response to different treatment protocols.

FURTHER READING

1. DEWS Definition and Classification committee. Report of the Definition and Classification Subcommittee of the International Dry Eye Work Shop. *Ocul Surf* 5:75–92, 2007.
2. Ibrahim OM, Dogru M, Satake Y, et al.: Application of visante optical coherence tomography tear meniscus height measurement in the diagnosis of dry eye disease. *Ophthalmology* 117:1923–1929, 2010.
3. Mainstone JC, Bruce AS, Golding TR: Tear meniscus measurement in the diagnosis of dry eye. *Curr Eye Res* 15:653–661, 1996.
4. Oguz H, Yokoi N, Kinoshita S: The height and radius of the tear meniscus and methods for examining these parameters. *Cornea* 19:497–500, 2000.
5. Ibrahim OM, Dogru M, Kojima T, et al.: Optical coherence tomography assessment of tear meniscus after punctal occlusion in dry eye disease. *Optom Vis Sci* 89:770–776, 2012.

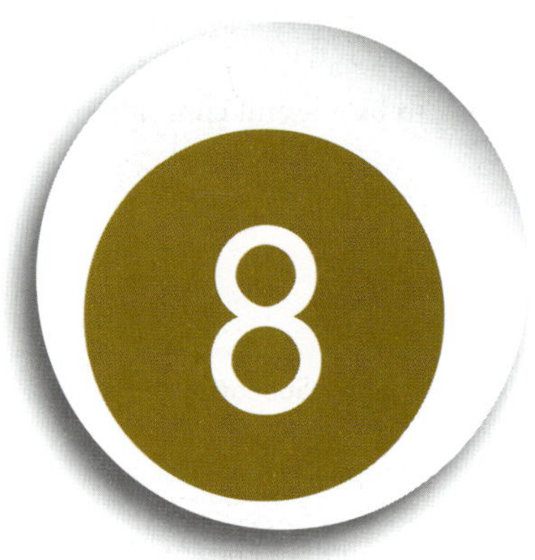

Imaging the Tear Film in Contact Lens Users

Shizuka Koh and Madhusmita Das

The tear film is important for maintaining the health of the cornea and the conjunctiva. In addition, because the tear film is the first and most powerful ocular refractive surface, it is an important optical element. This is also true for eyes that are corrected by contact lenses. In the latter, a contact lens divides the tear film into two layers—the pre- and postlens tear-film layers, and the lens itself might affect dynamics of the tear film. Edge of the lens especially plays an important role in tear fluid exchange beneath the lens and in the mobility of the lens over the conjunctiva and cornea. The lens edge has a considerable effect on objective compatibility and wearing comfort, especially for patients who wear rigid gas-permeable (RGP) lenses. Spectral-domain optical coherence tomography (SD-OCT), one of the Fourier-domain OCTs, can image fit of the edge of the lens and will add to understanding of interaction between the lens and the ocular surface (including the tear film) during contact lens wear.

The thicknesses of the pre- and postlens tear-film layers are of great interest, and some researchers have succeeded in quantifying the prelens and postlens tear-film layers using a custom-built anterior segment optical coherence tomography (AS-OCT). However, with the currently commercially available AS-OCT, it has been difficult to quantify the prelens and postlens tear-film thicknesses.

RIGID GAS-PERMEABLE LENS

The images of nasal and temporal sides of the lens (Fig. 8.1A–D) were obtained for each eye by rotating the OCT probe to target the limbus. The tear film beneath the edge of the lens is visualized clearly.

Figures 8.2A and B shows the same eye as in the previous figure (Fig. 8.1) with three-dimensional AS-OCT (SS-1000, Tomey Corporation, Inc., Nagoya, Japan) based on swept source OCT technology, which is a variation of Fourier-domain OCT.

Soft Contact Lens

Images of upper, lower, and temporal sides of the lens in the right eye are shown (Fig. 8.3). In the images of the upper and lower sides, both the upper and lower tear menisci are seen.

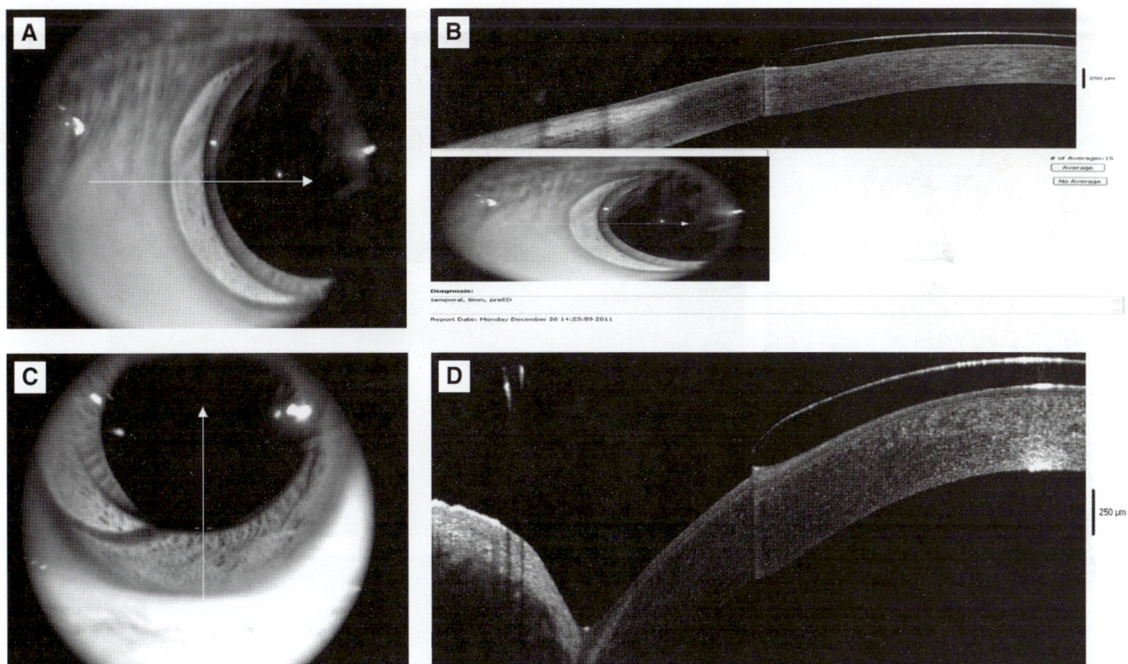

Fig. 8.1 (A–D) SD-OCT images (RTVue-100; Optovue Inc., Fremont, CA) of RGP lens after instillation of artificial tears.

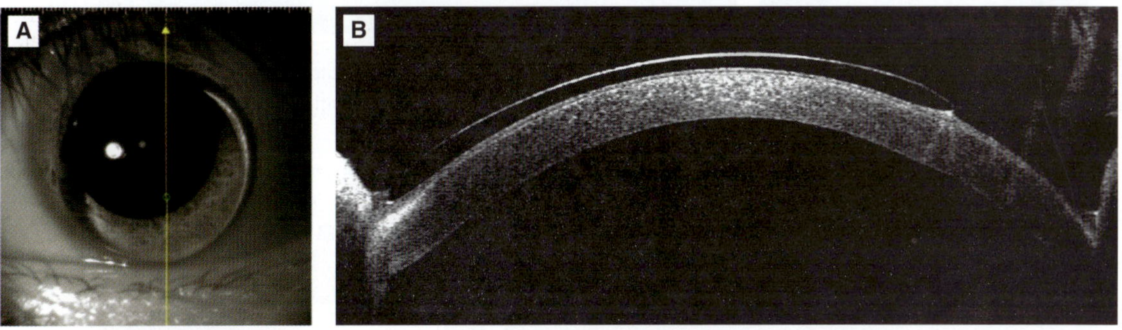

Fig. 8.2 (A and B) AS-OCT images obtained in three-dimensional swept source technology.

KERATOCONUS WITH CONTACT LENSES

Keratoconus is a corneal disorder characterized by progressive thinning of the central stroma and anterior corneal protrusion. To correct irregular astigmatism induced by asymmetric corneal protrusion, RGP contact lenses are prescribed most often.

CASE STUDY 1

A 28-year-old man with keratoconus was fitted with customized RGP lens (MZ lens, Sun Contact Lens Co. Ltd., Kyoto, Japan). The edge of the RGP lens and the postlens tear-film layer in the left eye are seen clearly. Gaps in the tear film between the lens and cornea seen in the slit photograph are seen in the OCT image. The peripheral groove on the customized lens surface is also seen (**Figs 8.4A and B**).

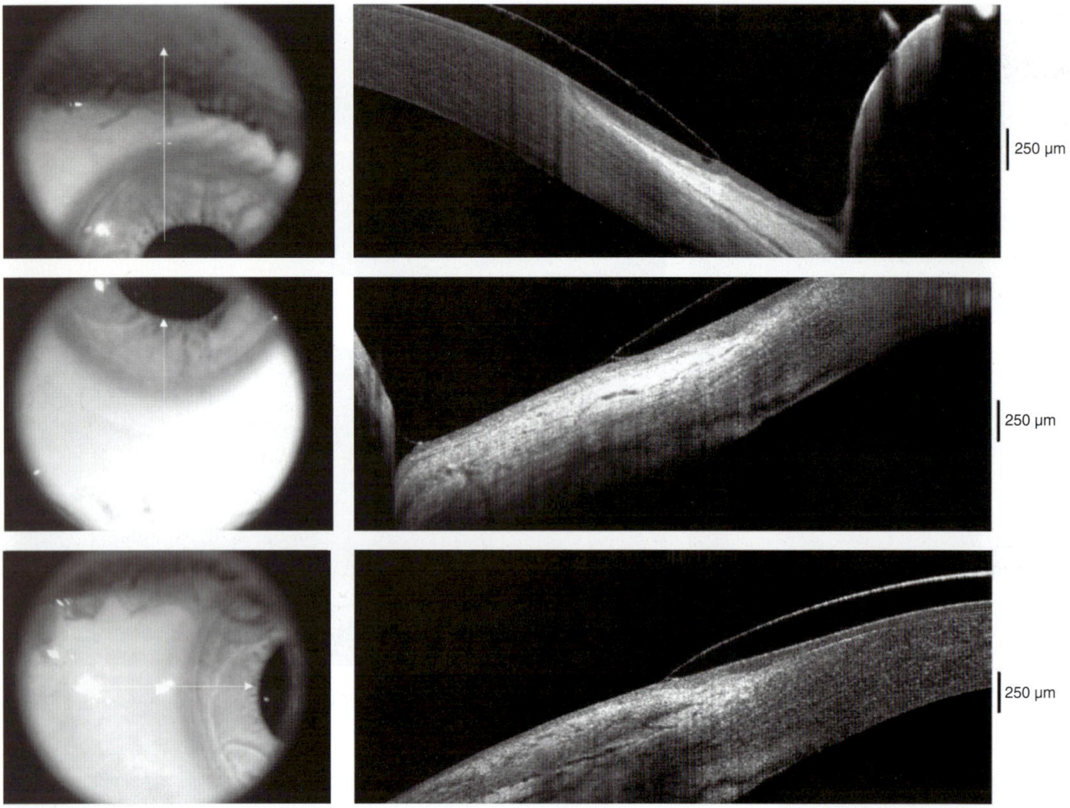

Fig. 8.3 SD-OCT images (RTVue-100) of a 37-year-old woman wearing an Etalfilcon A lens (1-Day ACUVUE®; Johnson & Johnson KK Vision Care Company, Tokyo, Japan) after instillation of artificial tears.

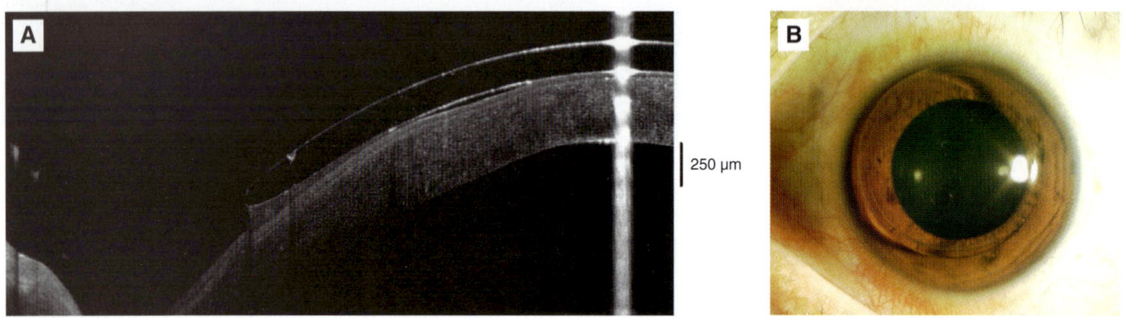

Fig. 8.4 **(A)** SD-OCT image (RTVue 100) of RGP lens in keratoconus. **(B)** The slit photograph of the left eye showing RGP contact lens.

CASE STUDY 2

A 26-year-old man diagnosed with keratoconus having a history of acute hydrops in his right eye was fitted with a RGP lens. In addition to the RGP contact lens and postlens gaps in the tear film, apical scarring due to resolved hydrops is seen clearly in the SD-OCT image (**Figs 8.5A and B**).

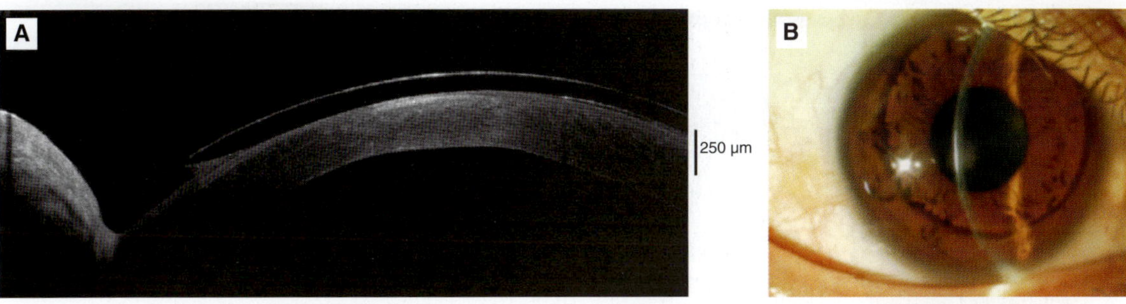

Fig. 8.5 **(A)** SD-OCT image (RTVue-100) of RGP contact lens in keratoconus with resolved hydrops. **(B)** The slit lamp photograph demonstrating apical scarring in keratoconus with RGP contact lens.

FURTHER READING

1. Chen Qi, Wang J, Tao A, et al.: Ultrahigh-resolution measurement by optical coherence tomography of dynamic tear film changes on contact lenses. *Invest Ophthal Vis Sci* 51:1988–1993, 2010.
2. Shen M, Cui L, Wang J, et al.: Characterization of soft contact lens edge fitting using ultra-high resolution and ultra-long scan depth optical coherence tomography. *Invest Ophthal Vis Sci* 52(7):4091–4097, 2011.
3. Cui L, Shen M, Wang J, et al.: Micrometer-scale contact lens movements imaged by ultrahigh-resolution optical coherence tomography. *Am J Ophthalmol* 153(2):275–283, 2012.

Bee Stinger

Madhusmita Das, Yathish Shivanna,
and Chintan Malhotra

Ocular bee sting injuries are rarely reported and have a potential to cause severe vision-threatening complications. Ocular bee stings can present in an immunologic, penetrating, or toxic form, or as a combination of all three forms. Apamin, a phospholipase A2-related mast cell degranulating peptide, and melittin are the major active peptidergic components that result in inflammation and pain. Corneal edema with striate and toxic keratopathy, uveitis, and glaucoma caused by toxic trabeculitis are the complications encountered most often. Lens subluxation and cataracts may result in a subacute stage. Catarrhal conjunctivitis, conjunctival nodules, keratoconjunctivitis, keratitis, iris hypochromia, iris atrophy, internal ophthalmoplegia, iridoplegia, iris nodules, vitritis, papillitis, or chorioretinopathy have also been reported.

The treatment of corneal bee stings essentially consists of stinger removal from stroma followed by treatment with antibiotics and/or topical steroids. In case of barbed stingers, attempts to manually remove the stinger may result in retention of stinger fragments within the cornea. Corneal incision along the injured plane or keratectomy is at times needed to remove the stinger intact from the corneal layers. The stingers should be removed as soon as possible because they may release venom.

CASE STUDY 1

A 19-year-old Indian male presented to our cornea clinic with chief complaints of pain, diminished vision for far and near and watering since 2 days following a honey bee hitting his left eye 2 days back. His visual acuity was 20/20 in the right eye and counting fingers close to face, perception of light (PL) present, projection of rays (PR) accurate in the left eye (oculus sinister-OS). Intraocular pressure (IOP) oculus uterque [both eyes (OU)] was within normal limits (WNL) with noncontact tonometry. Slit lamp examination (SLE) of OS revealed corneal edema and a bee stinger embedded in the superior part of the cornea at a paracentral location (**Figs 9.1 and 9.2**). Bioptigen images (**Fig. 9.3**) demonstrated deep intrastromal location of the stinger, adjacent tissue edema, and that the stinger had not gone into the anterior chamber. The stinger was removed using a 30-G needle under aseptic precautions and bandage contact lens (BCL) was applied (**Fig. 9.4**). The patient was administered topical steroids and antibiotics. Fundus OU was WNL. Specular microscopy of the oculus sinister (OS) done after 2 weeks did not reveal good endothelial architecture and a cell density (CD) of 1514 cells/mm^2. Oculus dexter (OD) cell density by specular was 3006 cells/mm^2.

He was followed-up on a regular basis in our cornea clinic, and at his last visit was 4 months postinjury; he had OS visual acuity of 20/200 improving to 20/40 with pin hole and with polymethylmethacrylate (PMMA) contact lens (CL) vision improved to 20/25.

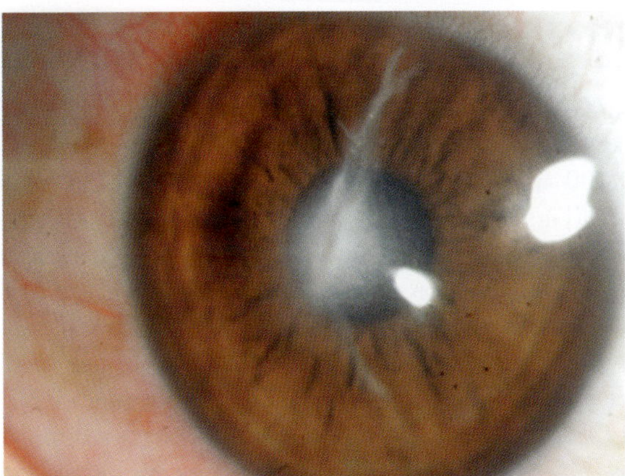

Fig. 9.1 Slit lamp photograph diffuse illumination post-bee sting injury.

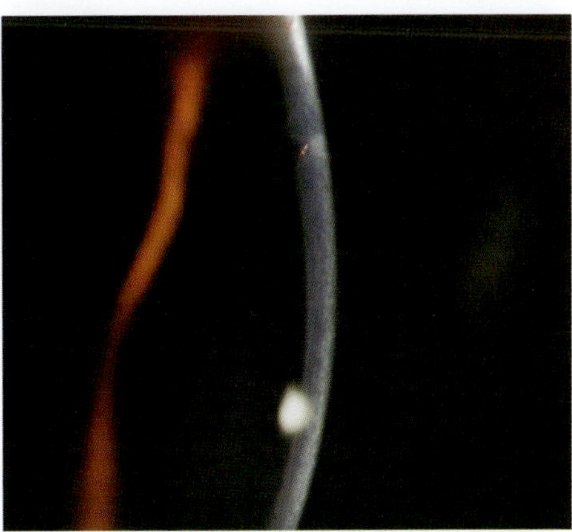

Fig. 9.2 Optical section showing bee stinger at mid-stromal level.

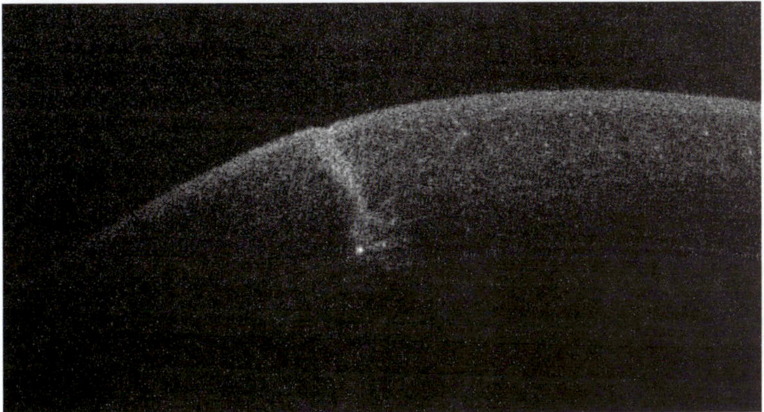

Fig. 9.3 Bioptigen image (6 mm × 6 mm, rectangular volume scan) demonstrating the intrastromal bee stinger, adjacent tissue edema, and that the stinger has not entered the anterior chamber.

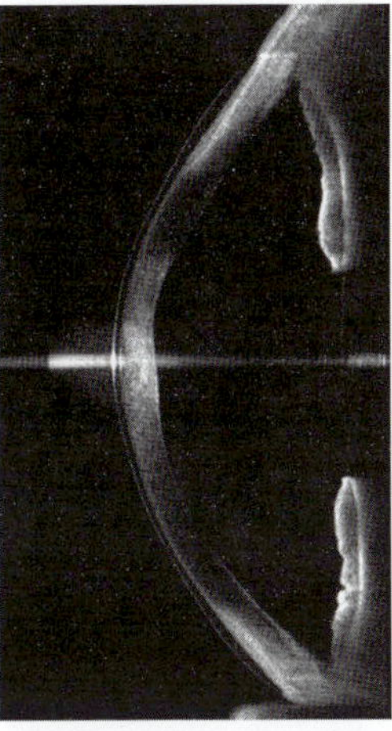

Fig. 9.4 Tomey AS-OCT image taken 2 days post-stinger removal and BCL placement demonstrating minimal corneal edema at the area of stinger removal.

A 37-year-old male presented to our cornea clinic with complaints of diminished vision and pain OS following honey bee sting 2 months back. He had consulted a local doctor and was on topical antiglaucoma drops and topical NSAID drops. Visual acuity at presentation was OD 20/100 and OS counting finger close to face. Slit lamp examination (SLE) of OD revealed superficial corneal abrasions (**Fig. 9.5**), retained stinger on the upper tarsal conjunctiva (**Fig. 9.6**), deep and quiet anterior chamber (AC), and atrophic patches on the iris. SLE of OS revealed corneal edema, focal midstromal scar, diffuse superficial punctate keratitis, atrophic patches on the iris, peripheral anterior synechiae (PAS) extending from 3 o'clock to 7 o'clock, and anterior polar cataract (**Fig. 9.7**). Intraocular pressure (IOP) with Tono-Pen was 18 mmHg in OD and 50 mmHg in OS. Gonioscopy showed open angles in all quadrants in OD, PAS at the inferior angle, and hazy view of the other angles in OS. Fundus examination of OD showed a cup:disc (C:D) ratio of 0.5:1 and OS C:D ratio of 0.8:1. The retained stinger (OD) was removed under sterile aseptic precautions at the slit lamp with a sterile forceps. The patient was administered topical antibiotics and lubricants in OD, and oral antiglaucoma medication, topical antiglaucoma drops, topical cycloplegics, topical steroids, and hypertonic (5% Sodium Chloride eye drops) for OS and was followed-up on a regular basis at our Cornea, Glaucoma, and Uvea clinics. Spectral-domain optical coherence tomography (SD-OCT) (Bioptigen) of OS revealed anterior polar cataract (**Fig. 9.8**) and corneal edema, bullae, keratic precipitates in OS, and showed no retained stinger in the corneal layers, angle, and lens (**Fig. 9.9**). The IOP was consistently high even after maximum medical therapy,

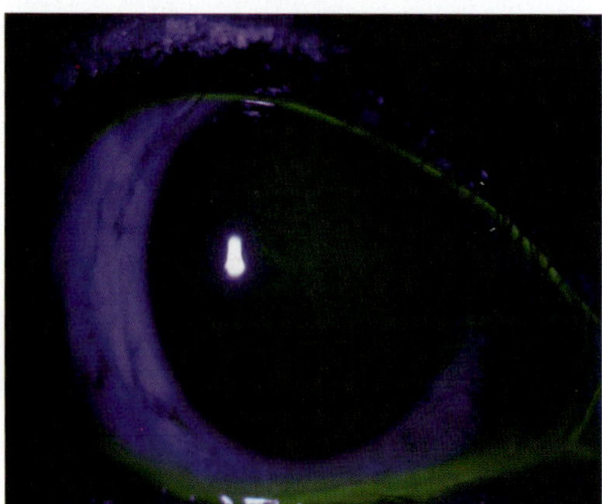

Fig. 9.5 Slit lamp photo OD under cobalt blue filter with Fluorescein staining demonstrating corneal abrasions.

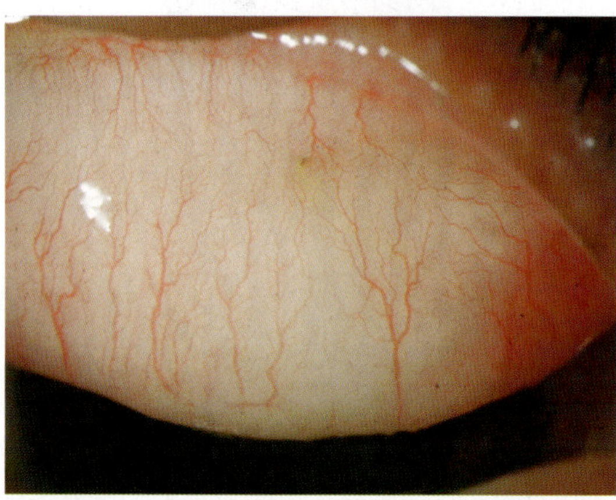

Fig. 9.6 Slit lamp photo diffuse illumination showing stinger in the upper tarsal conjunctiva (OD).

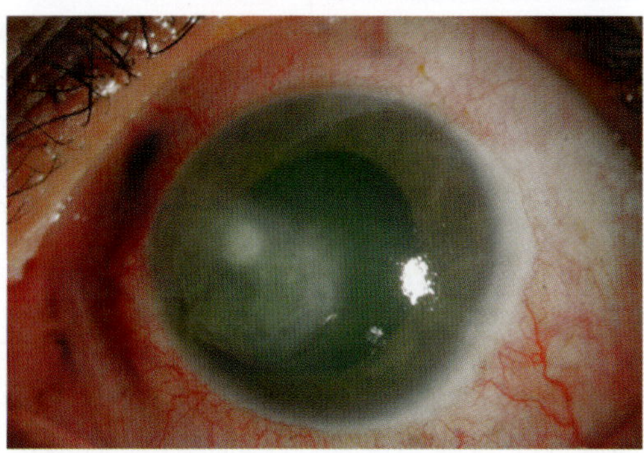

Fig. 9.7 Slit lamp photo demonstrating area of corneal decompensation, corneal scarring, anterior polar cataract, and atrophic patches on the iris (OS).

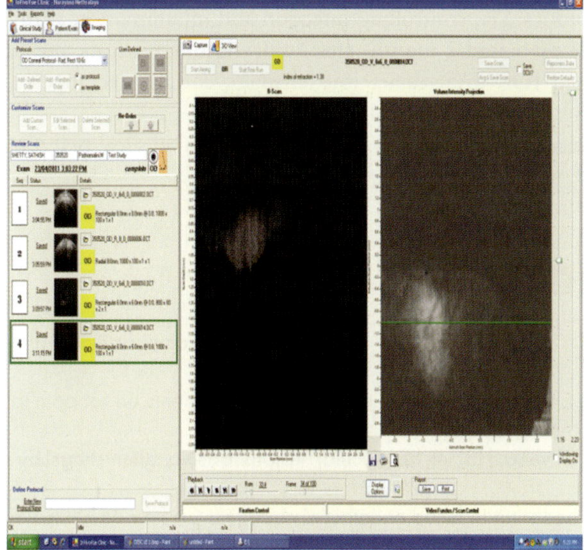

Fig. 9.8 Bioptigen 6 mm × 6 mm rectangular volumes scan demonstrating anterior polar cataract (OS).

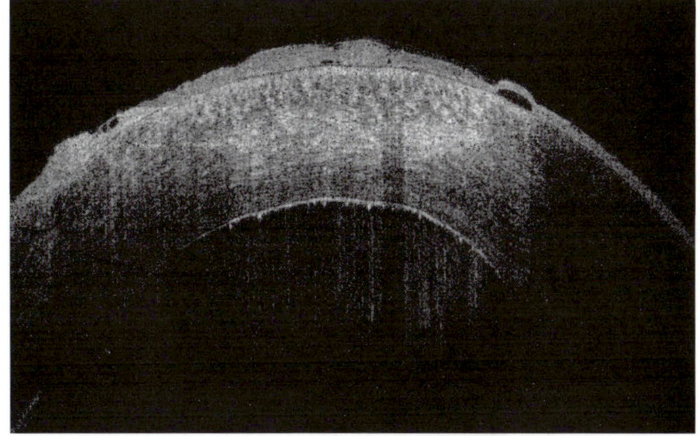

Fig. 9.9 Bioptigen 8 mm × 8 mm rectangular volume scan showing bullae, stromal edema, and keratic precipitates stuck to endothelium due to intense inflammation post bee sting injury and no retained stinger (OS).

and patient underwent OS trabeculectomy under highly guarded visual prognosis, as a measure to control IOP and cataract extraction with or without penetrating keratoplasty was planned to give him some visual rehabilitation. Post-trabeculectomy, IOP in OS was controlled and cataract surgery with posterior-chamber intraocular lens (PCIOL) was planned.

Anterior-segment imaging may prove extremely useful in localizing bee stingers, if any, within the layers of cornea or in anterior chamber, in cases of intense corneal edema limiting visibility on SLE. The role of specular microscopy and confocal microscopy in demonstrating endothelial damage post-bee sting injury has been illustrated in our cases. Bioptigen imaging could beautifully demonstrate keratic precipitates stuck to the endothelium in Case 2, in spite of the intense corneal edema, illustrating severe inflammation due to bee sting. The clarity in viewing the keratic precipitates and anterior polar cataract by Bioptigen in spite of the intense corneal edema in Case 2 prompts us to believe that this imaging modality might be of immense use in localizing bee stingers if any in the corneal layers (not visible on SLE due to edema) and in angles or in other parts of the anterior chamber; thus aiding in planning immediate appropriate surgical management.

A potential triad of penetrating, immunologic, and toxic injury must be taken into consideration while addressing bee sting injuries. Vision can be restored by early removal of the stinger and prompt administration of topical and/or oral steroids and topical antibiotics, i.e., controlling infection and inflammation at first presentation to the ophthalmologist (Case 1). Case 2 had presented 2 months after injury to our Institute and had already developed sequelae of intense inflammation (raised IOP, PAS, cataractous changes, corneal decompensation, and scarring), therefore making the management at this stage more difficult.

Detailed history and a meticulous examination, along with proper surgical planning ensures satisfactory management of these cases.

FURTHER READING

1. Lin PH, Wang NK, Hwang YS, et al.: Bee sting of the cornea and conjunctiva: management and outcomes. *Cornea* 30:392–394, 2011.
2. Chen YN, Li KC, Li Z, et al.: Effects of bee venom peptidergic components on rat pain-related behaviours and inflammation. *Neuroscience* 138:631–640, 2006.
3. Arcieri ES, França ET, de Oliveria HB, et al.: Ocular lesions arising after stings by hymenopteran insects. *Cornea* 21:328–330, 2002.
4. Gürlü VP, Erda N: Corneal bee sting-induced endothelial changes. *Cornea* 25:981–983, 2006.
5. Chuah G, Law E, Chan WK, et al.: Case reports and mini review of bees stings of the cornea. *Singapore Med J* 37:389–391, 1996.
6. Choi MY, Cho SH: Optic neuritis after bee sting. *Korean J Ophthalmol* 14:49–52, 2000.
7. Yuen KSC, Lai JSM, Law RWK, et al.: Confocal microscopy in bee sting corneal injury. *Eye* 17:845–847, 2003.
8. Jain V, Shome D, Natarajan S: Corneal bee sting misdiagnosed as viral keratitis. *Cornea* 26:1277–1278, 2007.

Collagen Cross-linking with Riboflavin

Rohit Shetty

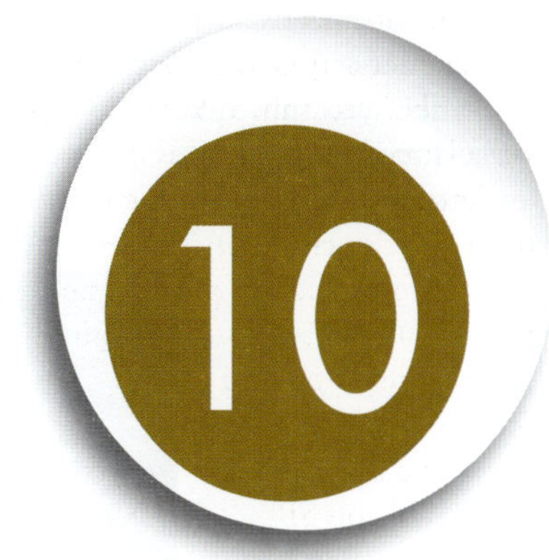

Corneal ectasia is a weakening of corneal integrity and can occur due to acquired and congenital conditions such as keratoconus. There are various modalities to treat ectasia; however none address the inherent pathology—an increased laxity of corneal stroma. The basic priniciple in collagen cross-linking is to strengthen the stroma by inducing cross-links between neighboring collagen fibers; thereby resulting in an increase in corneal tensile strength. Clinically, treated patients display stabilization of the condition and improvement in both visual acuity and keratometric readings.

CASE STUDY

A 25-year-old male patient with a history of progressive diminution of vision in both the eyes since past 3 years was diagnosed to have keratoconus based on slit lamp examination and corneal topography. On serial follow-up, topography showed progressive keratoconus, as shown below in **Figure 10.1**.

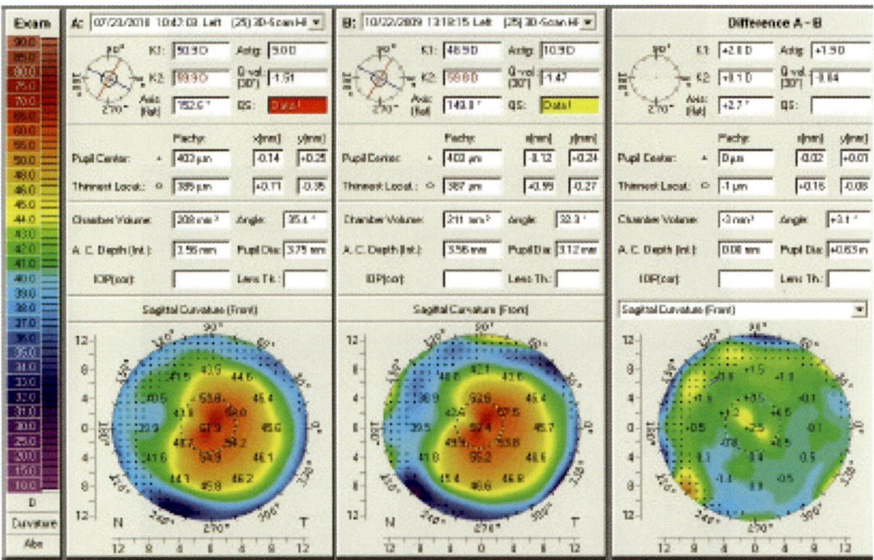

Fig. 10.1 Pentacam images of left eye of the patient shows a progression of 2.5 D over 9 months on difference map.

The patient was advised cross-linking in the left eye. Spectral-domain optical coherence tomography (SD-OCT) of the anterior corneal stroma, performed on the hand-held Bioptigen, was done 30 minutes after cross-linking (**Fig. 10.2**).

Patient was subsequently followed-up at 1 week, 1 month, and 3 months after procedure. At 1 month post-op visit, demarcation line was noticed on slit lamp examination, which was again imaged on the Bioptigen and confocal microscopy (**Figs 10.3 and 10.4**).

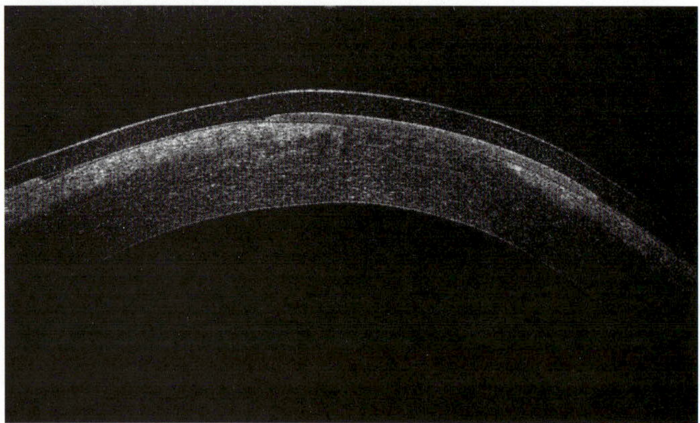

Fig. 10.2 Scan shows percolation of riboflavin drops into anterior stroma only in areas where epithelium was removed.

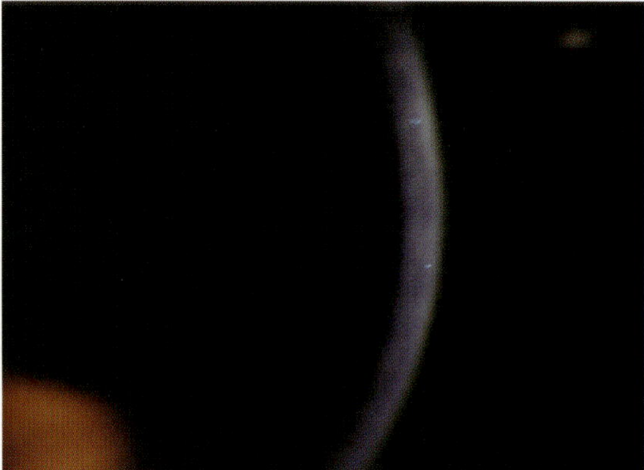

Fig. 10.3 Slit lamp photograph showing demarcation line in midstroma.

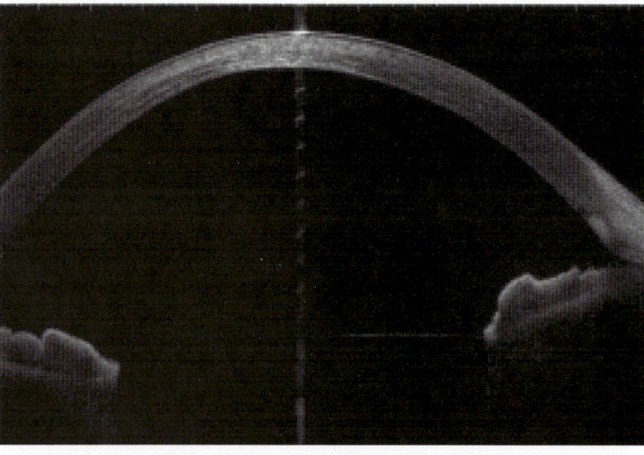

Fig. 10.4 AS-OCT showing demarcation line at a depth of 320 microns.

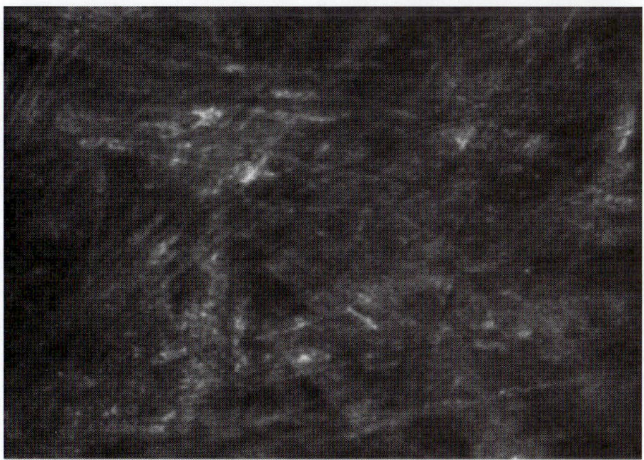

Fig. 10.5 Confocal microscopy images showing cross-linking at a depth of 330 microns, which correlates with depth of demarcation line as measured on AS-OCT.

The patient has since been on routine follow-up and is showing a stabilization of keratoconus.

Until recently, corneal surgeons did not have methods available to directly monitor the effect of corneal cross-linking on the anterior corneal stroma. After cross-linking treatment, one should be able to differentiate between treated anterior corneal stroma and untreated posterior corneal stroma. This can be done by recognizing the demarcation line clinically and by imaging it on the AS-OCT and confocal microscopy (**Fig. 10.5**).

This line, usually seen at around 60% depth of corneal thickness, denotes effectiveness of the cross-linking, and also helps us identify the depth of the stroma at which cross-linking has occurred.

FURTHER READING

1. Cannon DJ, Foster CS: Collagen cross-linking in keratoconus. *Invest Ophthalmol Vis Sci* 17:63–65, 1978.
2. Spoerl E, Seiler T: Techniques for stiffening the cornea. *J Refract Surg* 15:711–713, 1999.
3. Spoerl E, Huhle M, Seiler T: Induction of cross-links in corneal tissue. *Exp Eye Res* 66:97–103, 1998.
4. Wollensak G, Spoerl E, Wilsch M, et al.: Keratocyte apoptosis after corneal collagen cross-linking using riboflavin/UVA treatment. *Cornea* 23:43–49, 2004.
5. Wollensak G, Spoerl E, Reber F, et al.: Corneal endothelial cytotoxicity of riboflavin/UVA treatment *in vitro*. *Ophthalmic Res* 35:324–328, 2003.
6. Seiler T, Hafezi F: Corneal Cross-Linking–Induced Stromal Demarcation Line. *Cornea* 25:1057–1059, 2006.

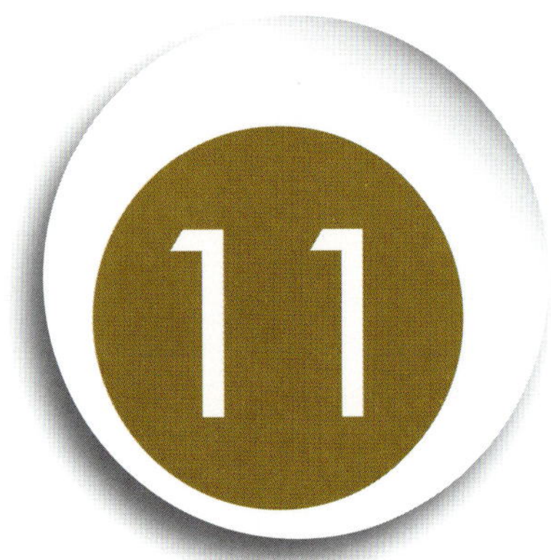

Corneal Dystrophies

Arundhati Anshu, Donald Tan, and Madhusmita Das

INTRODUCTION

Traditionally, "corneal dystrophy" has been referred to a group of inherited corneal diseases that are typically bilateral, symmetric, slowly progressive, and have no relationship to environmental or systemic factors. Several exceptions to this definition have been noted and therefore an International Committee for Classification of Corneal Dystrophies (IC3D) was created that proposed a classification that was anatomically based. Dystrophies were classified according to the layer chiefly affected—epithelial and subepithelial, Bowman layer, stromal, and those affecting Descemet's membrane and endothelium (Table 11.1).

Table 11.1 IC3D classification of corneal dystrophies

Epithelial and Subepithelial Dystrophies
1. Epithelial basement membrane dystrophy (EBMD)
2. Epithelial recurrent erosion dystrophy (ERED) (Smolandiensi variant)
3. Subepithelial mucinous corneal dystrophy (SMCD)
4. Mutation in keratin genes: Meesmann corneal dystrophy (MECD)
5. Lisch epithelial corneal dystrophy (LECD)
6. Gelatinous drop-like corneal dystrophy (GDLD)

Bowman's Layer Dystrophies
1. Reis–Bücklers' corneal dystrophy (RBCD)—Granular corneal dystrophy type 3
2. Thiel–Behnke corneal dystrophy (TBCD)
3. Grayson–Wilbrandt corneal dystrophy (GWCD)

Stromal Dystrophies
1. TGFBI corneal dystrophies
   A. Lattice corneal dystrophy
      a. Lattice corneal dystrophy, TGFBI type (LCD)
      b. Lattice corneal dystrophy, gelsolin type (LCD2) (This is not a true corneal dystrophy but is included here for ease of differential diagnosis.)
   B. Granular corneal dystrophy
      a. Granular corneal dystrophy, type 1 (classic) (GCDl)
      b. Granular corneal dystrophy, type 2 (granular lattice) (GCD2)
      c. Granular corneal dystrophy, type 3 (GCD3) = Reis–Bücklers'
2. Macular corneal dystrophy (MCD)
3. Schnyder corneal dystrophy (SCD)
4. Congenital stromal corneal dystrophy (CSCD)
5. Fleck corneal dystrophy (FCD)
6. Posterior amorphous corneal dystrophy (PACD)
7. Central cloudy dystrophy of Francois (CCDF)
8. Pre-Descemet's corneal dystrophy (PDCD)

(Continued)

Table 11.1 (*Continued*)

Descemet's Membrane and Endothelial Dystrophies
1. Fuchs' endothelial corneal dystrophy (FECD)
2. Posterior polymorphous corneal dystrophy (PPCD)
3. Congenital hereditary endothelial dystrophy 1 (CHED1)
4. Congenital hereditary endothelial dystrophy 2 (CHED2)

PTK IN MANAGEMENT OF EPITHELIAL BASEMENT MEMBRANE DYSTROPHY

Epithelial basement membrane dystrophy (EBMD) usually presents in adult life with recurrent corneal erosions resulting from poor adhesion of basal epithelial cells to abnormal basal laminar material. On-axis lesions may also cause blurring of vision due to irregular astigmatism. Asymptomatic patients may have varying signs consisting of maps, dots, fingerprints, or bleb-like pattern. Most cases have no documented inheritance pattern, and many are considered degenerative or secondary to trauma.

CASE STUDY 1

A 23-year-old man presented with chief complaints of watering and mild blurring of vision oculus uterque (OU) for the last 3 months. Slit lamp examination revealed OU vesicle-like lesions (**Fig. 11.1**) in cornea, principally in the epithelial and basement membrane zone. Spectral-domain optical coherence tomography (SD-OCT) (Bioptigen) imaging (**Fig. 11.2**) revealed irregularities in the epithelial–basement membrane complex region and exact depth of involvement. The patient was initially treated with ocular lubricants for 3 months; however, he had a repeat episode of watering and pricking sensation, and was not getting much comfort with only tear substitutes. He was given the option of phototherapeutic keratectomy (PTK), which he underwent subsequently. Post-PTK (**Figs 11.3 and 11.4**), he has been followed-up in our clinic for 1 year, has had no recurrences, and is doing well.

Although PTK is an effective method of alleviating clinical symptoms of EBMD, the dystrophy can recur with time. The relationship between postoperative development of clinical symptoms and corneal morphologic features is complex, and requires further investigation. Diamond burr polishing of Bowman's membrane in the treatment of recurrent corneal erosions associated with the anterior basement membrane dystrophy is also a safe and less expensive alternative.

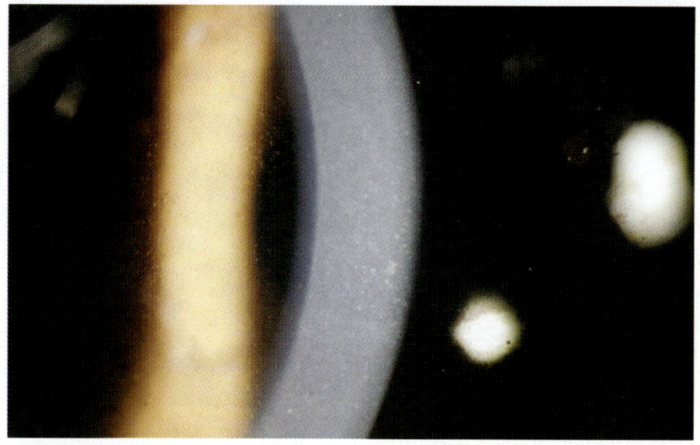

Fig. 11.1 Slit lamp photograph demonstrating EBMD.

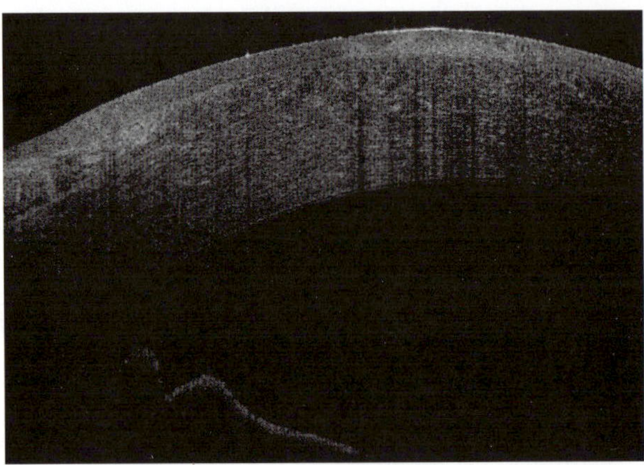

Fig. 11.2 SD-OCT (Bioptigen) images demonstrating irregular contour of epithelial basement membrane complex due to EBMD.

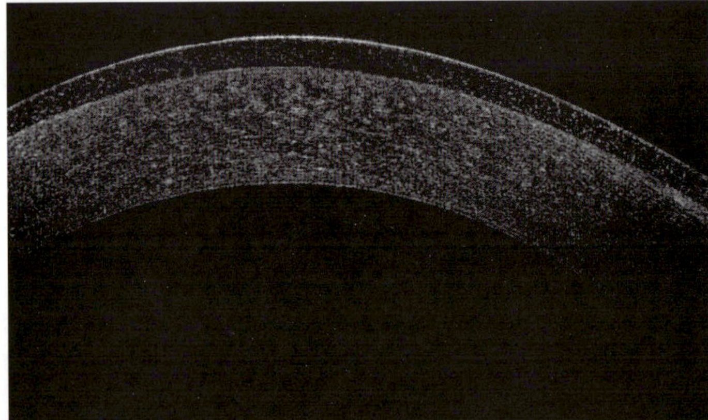

Fig. 11.3 First postoperative day following PTK in EBMD–BCL on.

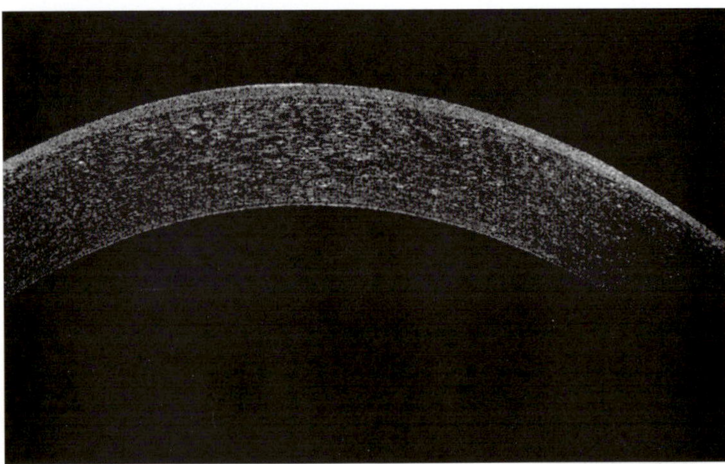

Fig. 11.4 SD-OCT (Bioptigen images) 1 month post-PTK demonstrating a smooth epithelial–basement membrane complex.

AUTOMATED LAMELLAR THERAPEUTIC KERATOPLASTY (ALTK)—AN OPTION IN GRANULAR DYSTROPHY

Granular dystrophy is a slowly progressive stromal disorder characterized by the presence of white granular lesions that spare the limbus and are usually localized to superficial cornea. It has an autosomal dominant pattern of inheritance and presents with decreased vision or recurrent corneal erosions as the condition progresses.

Automated lamellar therapeutic keratoplasty (ALTK) is a surgical procedure for the treatment of pathology affecting anterior corneal stroma. It has been employed for anterior stromal dystrophies, scars resulting from complicated refractive surgery procedures like PRK, and other anterior stromal scars that have a regular and smooth contour. It allows the surgeon to tailor the surgery to the needs of each patient, transplanting only minimal amount of corneal tissue necessary to improve vision.

CASE STUDY 2

A 58-year-old man presented with progressive blurring of vision in both the eyes. He was diagnosed to have bilateral granular dystrophy (Fig. 11.5) as well as bilateral cataracts based on slit lamp examination. SD-OCT was performed to assess the depth of opacities to determine the type of anterior lamellar keratoplasty needed for visual rehabilitation. Scan showed granular opacities largely localized to the anterior corneal stroma (Fig. 11.6).

The patient was offered ALTK that was performed in two stages. In stage 1, a microkeratome was used to perform lamellar dissection of a large diameter (exceeding intended graft diameter) in the recipient cornea, which was then replaced and left to heal. In stage 2, performed 2 months later, a conventional corneal graft vacuum trephine was used to trephine through the previous flap, followed by removal of the central lamellar flap. A large-diameter lamellar dissection was then performed on the donor using the ALTK unit and the donor was trephined within the large-diameter flap. The donor was then sutured into position on the recipient bed.

SD-OCT showed smooth interface between the donor and recipient stromal bed with a clear lamellar graft, 1 week postoperatively. ALTK is useful in the management of superficial corneal pathology, and SD-OCT is a useful tool in assessment of the depth of the lesions in planning for surgery.

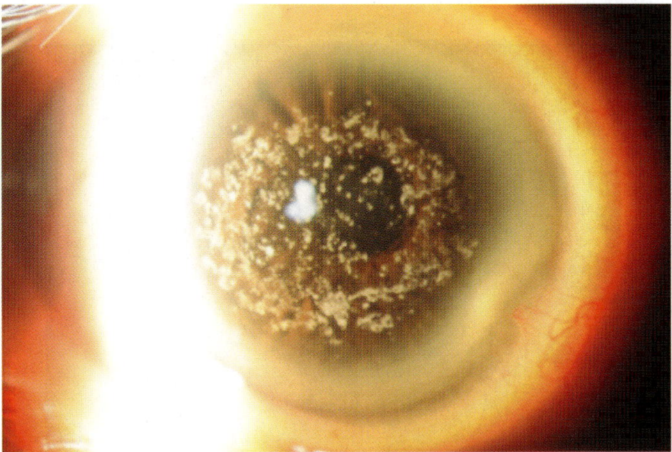

Fig. 11.5 Slit lamp photograph—Granular dystrophy.

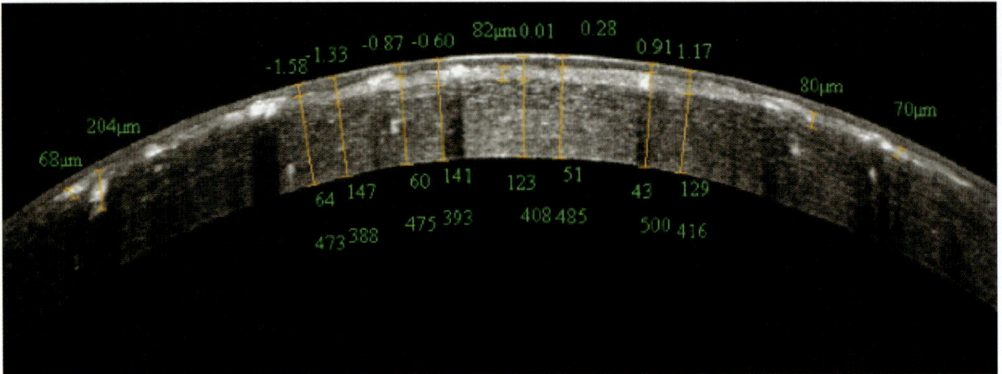

Fig. 11.6 AS-OCT granular dystrophy.

BIG BUBBLE DEEP ANTERIOR LAMELLAR KERATOPLASTY (DALK) IN LATTICE DYSTROPHY

Lattice corneal dystrophy is a bilateral inherited stromal dystrophy with an onset in the first decade of life. The lesions start centrally and superficially, and spread deeper, but spare the limbus, Descemet's membrane, and endothelium. The patients may present with recurrent corneal erosions and/or decreased visual acuity. If visual acuity is impaired lamellar or penetrating keratoplasty (PK) can be performed. Anterior lamellar keratoplasty in the form of manual deep anterior lamellar keratoplasty (DALK) or big-bubble DALK is the preferred surgical modality since endothelium is spared.

CASE STUDY 3

A 35-year-old lady presented with progressive blurring of vision secondary to bilateral lattice dystrophy (Fig. 11.7). She underwent DALK using modified-big-bubble technique in her right eye (OD) (Fig. 11.8). She had an uneventful postoperative recovery and 2 years after surgery achieved a best-corrected visual acuity of 6/6, with no recurrence of the lattice dystrophy. In patients undergoing lamellar surgery, AS-OCT is a useful preoperative tool in assessing the depth of the lesions and determining the appropriate form of surgical technique needed. AS-OCT is also useful postoperatively to look for DM detachment and double anterior chambers as well as monitoring over time for resolution of the detachment.

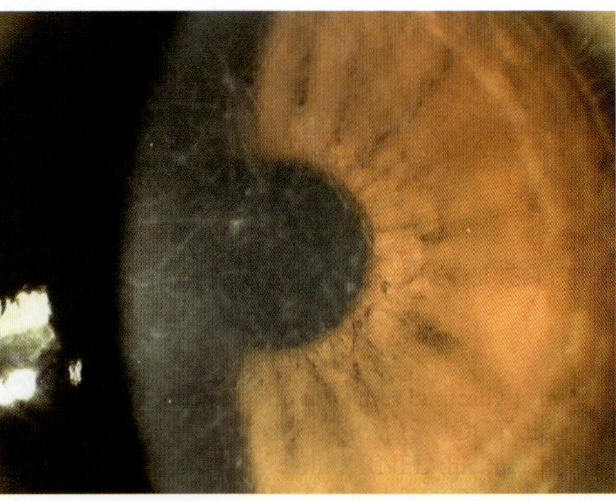

Fig. 11.7 Slit lamp photograph—lattice dystrophy.

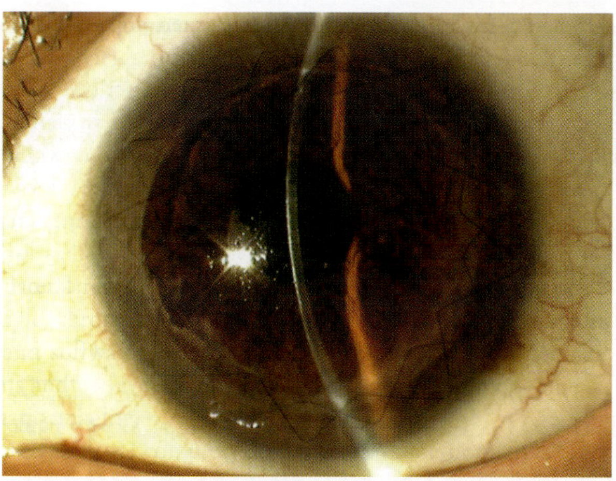

Fig. 11.8 Slit lamp photograph—DALK in lattice dystrophy.

MACULAR DYSTROPHY

Macular dystrophy is an autosomal recessive form of stromal dystrophy with onset in childhood. The lesions are elevated, irregular, and whitish, and unlike granular dystrophy, they have no clear space in between. With progression of disease, the opacities extend to the limbus and can also affect corneal endothelium with stromal thickening secondary to endothelial decompensation. It causes severe visual impairment early in life and requires keratoplasty for visual rehabilitation.

CASE STUDY 4

A 16-year-old man presented to our clinic with chief complaints of blurred vision for far and difficulty in opening eyes in sunlight. He was accompanied by his elder brother (18 years of age) who also had the same complaints. Slit lamp examination revealed the presence of whitish opacities in the cornea of both the eyes with intervening haze between the opacities. Deposits were confined to anterior one-fourth to anterior one-third of the cornea. **Figure 11.9** demonstrates

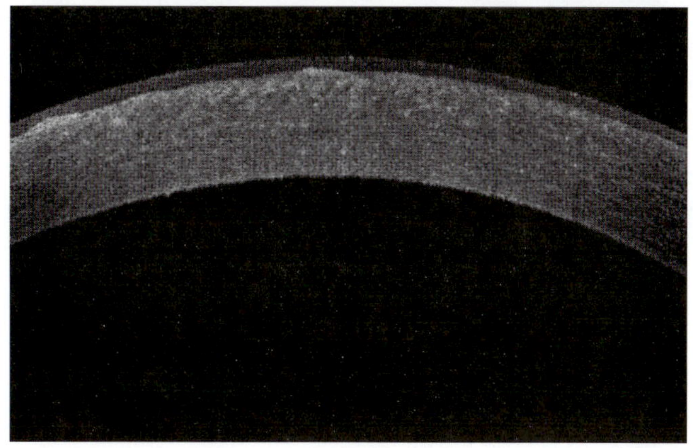

Fig. 11.9 SD-OCT image of macular dystrophy.

hyperlucent opacities in the layers of the cornea, more in the anterior one-third of the cornea, on SD-OCT (Bioptigen) imaging in this patient.

As this patient's best-corrected visual acuity was OU 6/9, he was prescribed tinted glasses with his subjective acceptance values and was asked to come for a review after 1 year. He was also explained about the progressive nature of the disease, need for regular follow-up, and need for keratoplasty in the future when vision is grossly impaired for daily tasks.

Visualization of the exact depth of the opacities in macular dystrophy is at times challenging, particularly in relatively advanced cases, where involvement of deep stromal layers hampers visualization of endothelial involvement. SD-OCT can be a useful tool to assess the exact depth of the deposits in such advanced cases of macular dystrophy and plan DALK in selected cases.

DESCEMET'S STRIPPING AUTOMATED ENDOTHELIAL KERATOPLASTY (DSAEK): THE PROCEDURE OF CHOICE FOR FUCHS' ENDOTHELIAL DYSTROPHY

Fuchs' endothelial dystrophy may have an autosomal dominant pattern of inheritance (although most cases have no known inheritance pattern) with a late onset, progressive visual impairment secondary to stromal and/or epithelial edema. Asymptomatic patients manifest with corneal guttae. Confocal microscopy shows pleomorphism and polymegathism of endothelial cells and is helpful in diagnosis as well as follow-up. In the past, PK was performed for visual rehabilitation. Currently, Descemet's stripping automated endothelial keratoplasty (DSAEK) is considered the procedure of choice for this condition, given the advantages it offers over PK in terms of rapid and predictable visual recovery as well as increased tectonic integrity.

CASE STUDY 5

A 56-year-old man presented with blurring of vision and ocular discomfort in his right eye, and was diagnosed to have bilateral asymmetrical Fuchs' dystrophy with evidence of corneal decompensation in the right eye (Fig. 11.10) and asymptomatic guttae in the left eye. He was initially managed conservatively with hypertonic saline eyedrops but had recurrent erosions caused by epithelial bullae. He underwent uneventful DSAEK surgery and has a clear graft at last follow-up (Fig. 11.11). Postoperatively, anterior-segment optical coherence tomography (AS-OCT) was performed

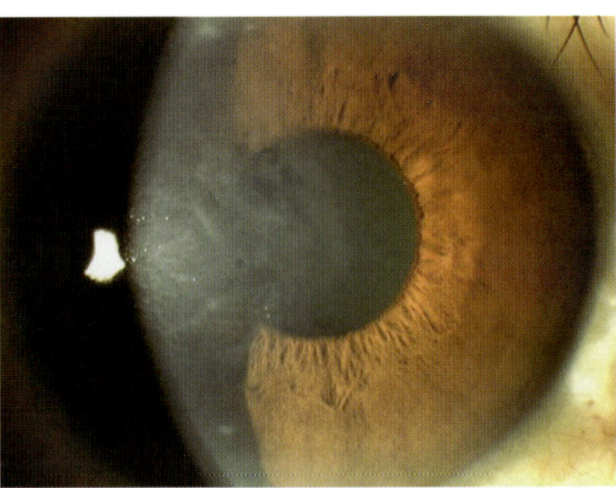

Fig. 11.10 Fuchs' endothelial dystrophy—preoperative slit lamp photo.

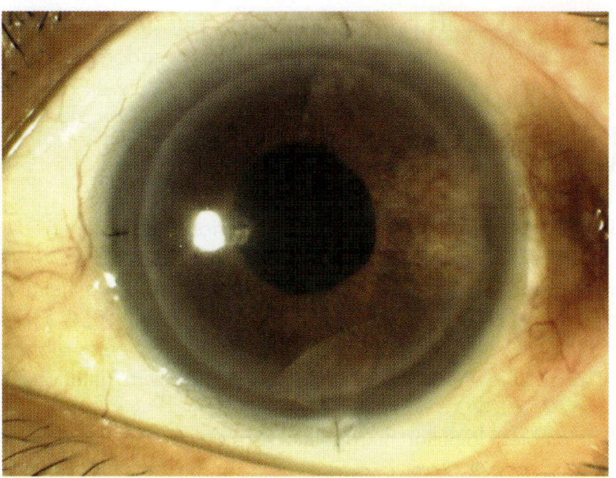

Fig. 11.11 Fuchs' endothelial dystrophy—postoperative (post-DSAEK) slit lamp photo.

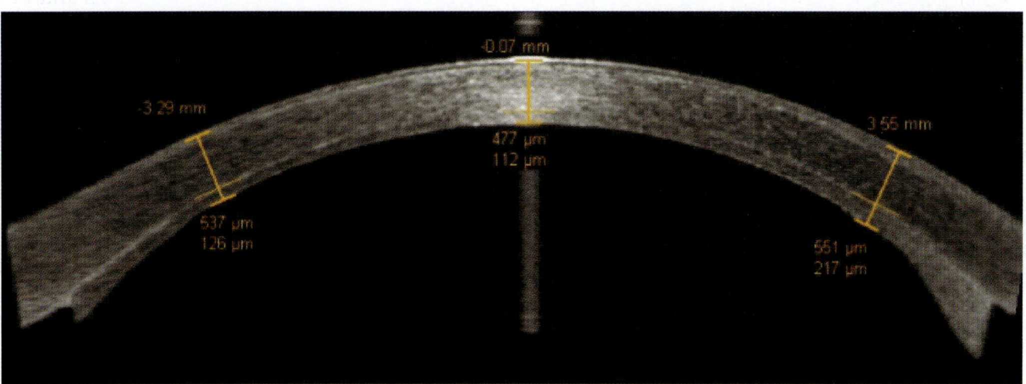

Fig. 11.12 AS-OCT image demonstrating well-attached lenticule and lenticule thickness in the center and periphery.

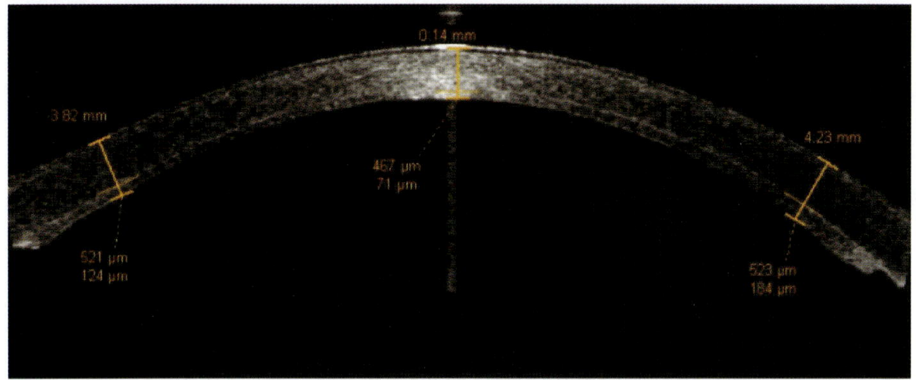

Fig. 11.13 AS-OCT image demonstrating graft deturgescence (reduction of lenticule thickness in the center and periphery) over time.

on follow-up visits and shows DSAEK graft deturgescence over time (**Figs 11.12 and 11.13**). The preoperative endothelial cell density was 2617 cells/mm^2; and 1 year later, he had an endothelial cell density of 1972 cells/mm^2.

FURTHER READING

1. Weiss JS, Rapuano CJ, Klintworth GK, et al.: The IC3D classification of the corneal dystrophies. *Cornea* 27 Suppl 2: S1–S83, 2008.
2. Germundsson J, Fagerholm P, Lagali N: Clinical outcome and recurrence of epithelial basement membrane dystrophy after phototherapeutic keratectomy a cross-sectional study. *Ophthalmology* 118(3):515–522, 2011.
3. Sridhar MS, Rapuano CJ, Cosar CB, et al.: Phototherapeutic keratectomy versus diamond burr polishing of Bowman's membrane in the treatment of recurrent corneal erosions associated with anterior basement membrane dystrophy. *Ophthalmology* 109(4):674–679, 2002.
4. Tan D, Ang LP: Modified automated lamellar therapeutic keratoplasty for keratoconus—a new technique. *Cornea* 25:1217–1219, 2006.
5. Busin M, Zambianchi L, Arffa RC: Microkeratome-assisted lamellar keratoplasty for the surgical treatment of keratoconus. *Ophthalmology* 112:987–997, 2005.
6. Klintworth GK, Smith CF, Bowling BL: CHST6 mutations in North American subjects with macular corneal dystrophy: A comprehensivemolecular genetic review. *Mol Vis* 12:159–176, 2006.
7. Akama TO, Nishida K, Nakayama J, et al.: Macular corneal dystrophy type I and type II are caused by distinct mutations in a new sulphotransferase gene. *Nat Genet* 26:237–241, 2000.

Corneal Cyst

Tushar Agarwal and Amit Sobti

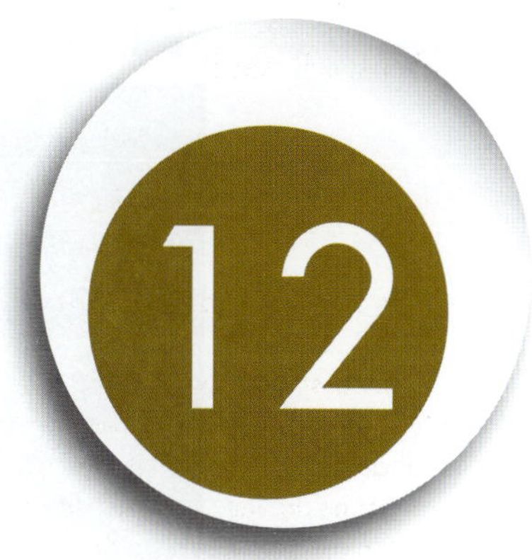

Corneal cyst is a rare clinical entity. These are congenital and progressive in course. However, they can occur following ocular trauma or ocular surgery.

In most cases, history of injury is not found. A trivial, undetected accident can force some epithelial cells into the stroma, where they become isolated due to closure of the surface wound.

CASE STUDY

A 4-year-old male presented with the complaint of progressive diminution of vision in the left eye for the last 2 months. He presented with history of trauma to the right eye sustained with a broom stick 3 months back. Slit lamp examination showed a cystic structure in the cornea with normal epithelium and stroma (Fig. 12.1).

Anterior-segment optical coherence tomography (AS-OCT) (Visante) showed a cyst of homogenous moderate reflectivity originating from the inferior angle with a clear separation from iris, pupil, and lens, which was attached to the endothelium (Fig. 12.2). Corneal epithelium and stroma appeared uninvolved by the cyst. The patient underwent cyst aspiration and excision of the mouth of the cyst.

On follow-up, although some corneal haze persisted (Fig. 12.3), a significant improvement in vision was noted. AS-OCT showed no residual cyst at 1 year of follow-up (Fig. 12.4).

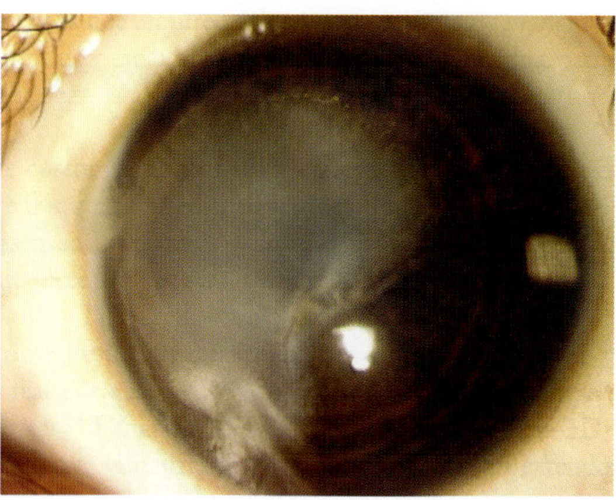

Fig. 12.1 Slit lamp photograph showed a cystic structure in the cornea with normal epithelium and stroma.

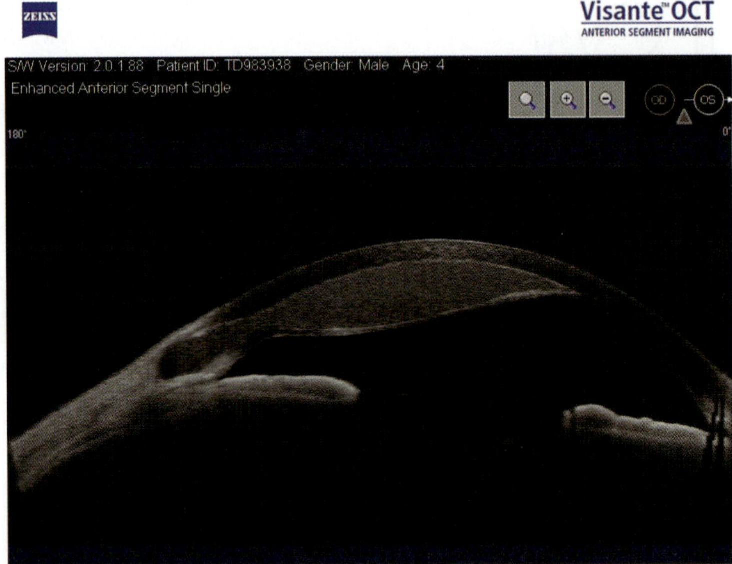

Fig. 12.2 AS-OCT (Visante) showed a cyst of homogenous moderate reflectivity.

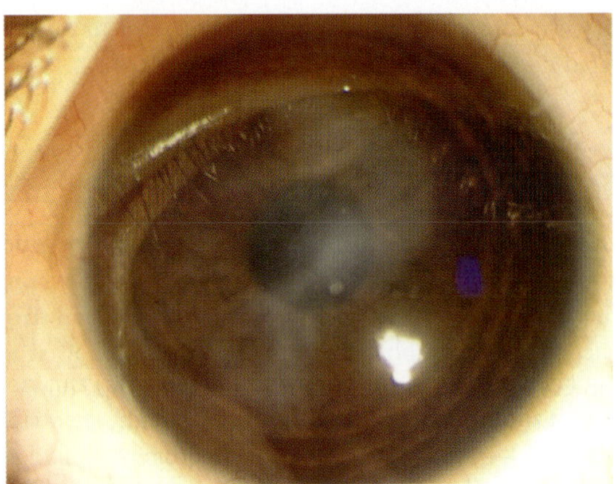

Fig. 12.3 Appearance at 1 month following cyst removal.

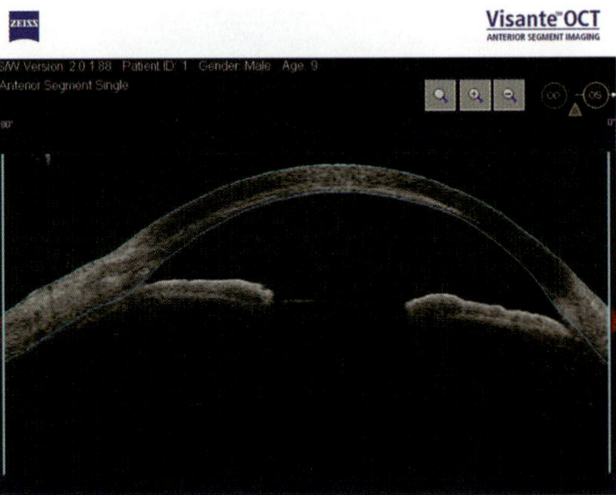

Fig. 12.4 AS-OCT showed no residual cyst at 1 year of follow-up.

Corneal cysts are a rare entity. Documenting the complete extent of the lesion is very important, especially in phakic patients for a sound surgical plan. AS-OCT can be a useful investigative modality that can help to clearly delineate extent of the cyst and can also be used as a monitoring tool postoperatively to ensure complete removal.

FURTHER READING

1. Reed JW, Dohlman CH: Corneal cysts. A report of eight cases. *Arch Ophthalmol* 86(6):648–652, 1971.
2. Sanders N: Corneal intrastromal cyst. *Am J Ophthalmol* 71:1138–1139, 1971.
3. Liakos GM: Intracorneal and sclerocorneal cysts. *Br J Ophthalmol* 62:155–158, 1978.
4. Mifflin MD, Byers TL, Elliot R, et al.: Surgical treatment of an intrastromal epithelial corneal cyst. *Cornea* 20(2):222–225, 2001.

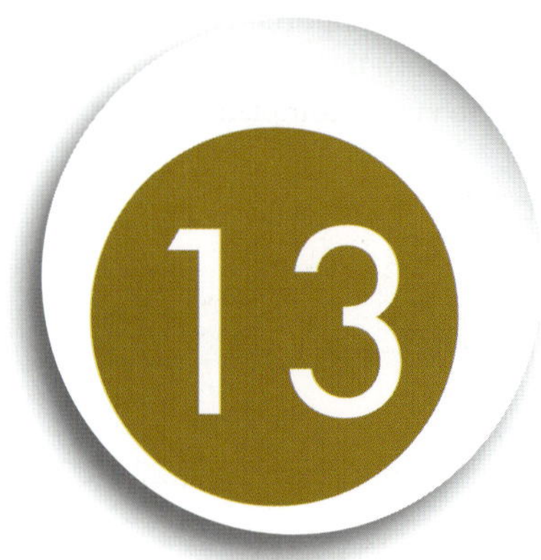

Descemet's Membrane Detachment

Vishal Jhanji and Rasik B Vajpayee

Descemet's membrane detachment (DMD) has been reported to occur following cataract extraction, trabeculectomy, lamellar keratoplasty, and during insertion of intraocular lens. The incidence of DMD is on a rise in the past few years due to a proportional increase in the number of lamellar corneal surgeries. Factors associated with DMD include shallow anterior chamber, use of blunt microkeratomes, shelved incisions, and inadvertent injection of antibiotics into the supra-Descemet's membrane (supra-DM) space. DMD can be classified as planar or nonplanar based on the distance between detached DM from the overlying corneal stroma. Another classification includes description of DMD into "peripheral" and "peripheral with central" type. Although most of these cases resolve spontaneously, a minority would result in persistent double anterior chamber and corneal edema, therefore necessitating surgical intervention.

Surgical management of DMD, if contemplated, includes injection of air or isoexpansile gas into the anterior chamber followed by appropriate positioning of the patient. Imaging devices such as anterior-segment optical coherence tomography (AS-OCT) are extremely useful in the management and follow-up of cases with postoperative DMD, especially when severe corneal edema precludes visualization of detached DM on slit lamp examination. We have used AS-OCT for categorizing the extent and severity of DM detachments in order to decide whether or not surgical intervention is required. It is of paramount importance not to perform surgery unless absolutely indicated, since injection of intracameral air/gas is fraught with risks of inducing cataract and intractable glaucoma. In cases with small, localized, inferior detachments that do not involve the visual axis, it is prudent to observe. In cases with extensive DM detachments, rolled DM, and DMD with a "fish-mouth" tear, an early surgical intervention can potentially prevent endothelial cell damage and salvage useful vision. There have been reports of drainage of fluid from the supra-DM space in cases with extensive nonplanar DM detachments. All such interventions can be performed safely with the help of AS-OCT imaging.

CASE STUDY

A 23-year-old female with bilateral keratoconus underwent deep anterior lamellar keratoplasty in her left eye using the "big-bubble" technique. Surgery was complicated by a small perforation of the DM intraoperatively. However, lamellar keratoplasty was successfully completed. Massive corneal edema was noted on day 1 postoperatively. Topical corticosteroids and antibiotics were continued, but edema failed to resolve after 5 days of observation. An AS-OCT was performed, which showed complete detachment of DM with thickening of overlying corneal stroma (Fig. 13.1). Isoexpansile mixture of C3F8 (14%) was injected into the anterior chamber under local anesthesia. Serial follow-ups showed complete resolution of DM detachment on day 3 postinjection. Complete corneal clarity was achieved over the next 2 weeks.

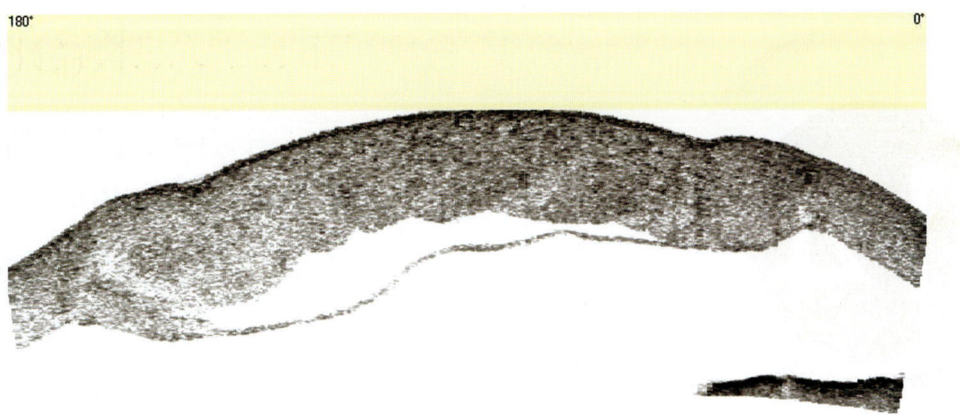

Fig. 13.1 Anterior-segment optical coherence tomography image showing a large Descemet's membrane detachment after deep lamellar keratoplasty.

AS-OCT is a useful tool for management and follow-up of cases with postoperative DM detachment. Appropriate timing of surgical intervention can be decided based on AS-OCT images in such cases.

FURTHER READING

1. Macsai MS: Total detachment of Descemet's membrane after small-incision cataract extraction. *Am J Ophthalmol* 114(3):365–366, 1992.
2. Mulhern M, Barry P, Condon P: A case of Descemet's membrane detachment during phacoemulsification surgery. *Br J Ophthalmol* 80(2):185–186, 1996.
3. Kansal S, Sugar J: Consecutive Descemet's membrane detachment after successive phacoemulsification. *Cornea* 20: 670–671, 2001.
4. Wigginton SA, Jungschaffer DA, Lee DA: Postoperative Descemet's membrane detachment with maintenance of corneal clarity after trabeculectomy. *J Glaucoma* 9:200–202, 2000.
5. Mannan R, Jhanji V, Sharma N, et al.: Intracameral C(3)F(8) injection for descemet membrane detachment after phacoemulsification in deep anterior lamellar keratoplasty. *Cornea* 26(5):636–638, 2007.
6. Mannan R, Pruthi A, Jhanji V, et al.: Descemet membrane detachment during foldable intraocular lens implantation. *Eye Contact Lens* 37(2):106–108, 2011.

Madhusmita Das, Naoyuki Maeda, and Shizuka Koh

KERATITIS-ADENOVIRAL

Epidemic keratoconjunctivitis (EKC) is an adenoviral infection that typically starts with a unilateral foreign body sensation. This gradually develops, within a few hours or days, into bilateral keratoconjunctivitis, manifested as marked chemosis, epiphora, and photophobia. Persistence of subepithelial corneal infiltrates (nummuli) and residual scars leads to irregular astigmatism and visual impairment. Steroids, calcineurin inhibitors, virostatic drugs, and disinfecting agents in the acute phase have not demonstrated any clear benefit in randomized clinical trials. Cyclosporin A eye drops can accelerate regression of subepithelial infiltrates in the chronic phase. Conscientious hand and surface disinfection can reduce spread of the disease. It is caused by adenoviruses that are highly resistant to environmental influences and are transmitted from person-to-person by way of infectious secretions, mainly tear fluid. In the Western world, transmission often occurs in places where a large number of people gather together, such as schools, homes for elderly, and factories, as well as in healthcare institutions such as hospitals and doctors' offices (including ophthalmologists' offices). The 54 types of adenovirus now known to be pathogenic in man are classified in seven groups, which are labeled from A to G.

Adenoviruses are double-stranded DNA viruses, roughly 80–110 nm in size. They are surrounded by an icosahedral capsid-bearing group and type-specific antigens; they have no outer lipid bilayer. They are highly resistant to environmental influences and can survive contact with many of the usual commercially available types of disinfectants.

Slit lamp microscopy reveals conjunctival redness and swelling, sometimes with pseudomembrane formation. Corneal component of the disease can arise from the fourth day onwards, but it can also be entirely lacking. If the cornea is affected, the first sign is usually the development of small epithelial punctate spots that tend to enlarge and then remain visible, once the acute phase is over, as individual or confluent lesions called nummuli. These consist of immune complexes deposited beneath the epithelium in the anterior-third of the corneal stroma. The acute phase heals in 3–6 weeks.

CASE STUDY 1

An 18-year-old woman presented to our Cornea Clinic with chief complaints of redness, watering, and photophobia for the last 3 days. Her father too had the same complaints and red eyes. She denied similar episodes in the past. On examination, her visual acuity oculus uterque (OU) unaided was 6/6P and OU lids showed edema, conjunctiva showed follicles in the upper and lower tarsal conjunctiva, and pseudomembranes oculus dexter (OD). Examination of the cornea OU revealed multiple active subepithelial infiltrates (Fig. 14.1). She was advised OU topical prednisolone acetate 1% eye drops and topical lubricants. On her review visit after 1 week, she was symptomatically

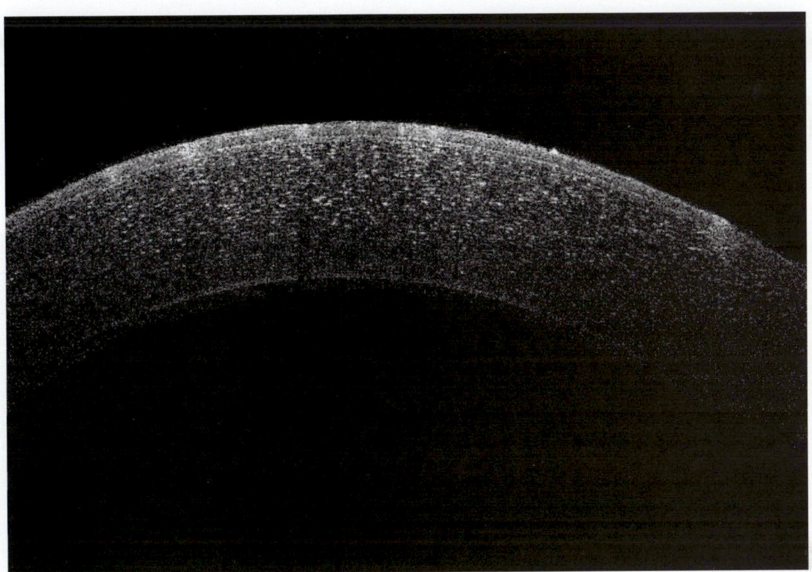

Fig. 14.1 Bioptigen image (rectangular 6-mm scan) demonstrating active subepithelial infiltrates of adenoviral keratoconjunctivitis.

much better and steroid eye drops were tapered over the next few weeks. On last follow-up visit, her cornea OU was clear (Fig. 14.2) and she was comfortable. **Figures 14.3 and 14.4** demonstrate slit lamp photographs of a patient with few active lesions and scars of previous episode of adenoviral keratoconjunctivitis.

Although it is not difficult to diagnose infectious keratitis with conventional ophthalmic examinations, it is not easy to estimate the depth of focus and residual stromal thickness with slit lamp examination because of abscess and edema at the focus. In such cases, scraping for culture and debridement around the focus might be deferred because of possible perforation. Anterior-segment optical coherence tomography (AS-OCT) has a big advantage over slit lamp examination for observing the inside of opaque tissues and measuring corneal thickness at the lesion.

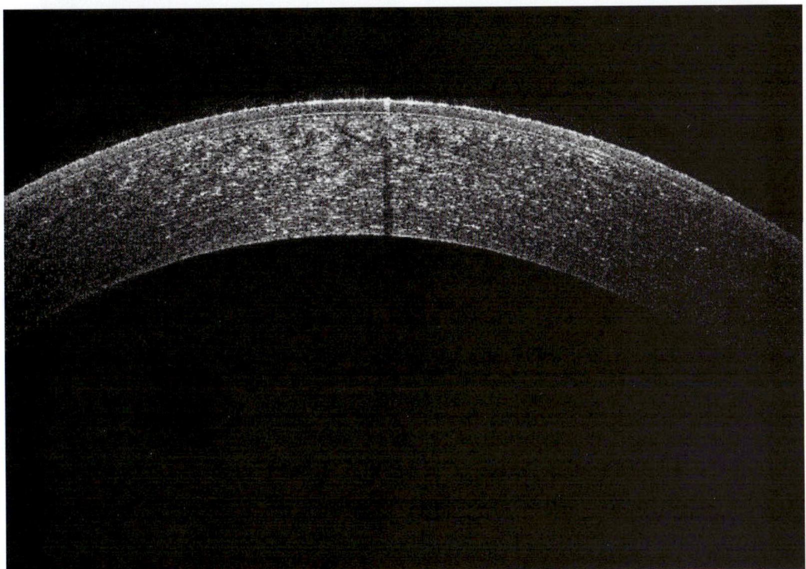

Fig. 14.2 Bioptigen image (rectangular 6-mm scan) demonstrating a clear cornea with total resolution of subepithelial infiltrates post-timely management.

CASE STUDY 2

A 29-year-old woman was referred to our clinic for the treatment of neurotrophic ulcer OD with a combination of trigeminal nerve palsy and facial nerve palsy. Slit lamp examination showed irregular and dirty surface on the neurotrophic ulcer. The conjunctival injection was mild and infiltration was not obvious beneath the ulcer.

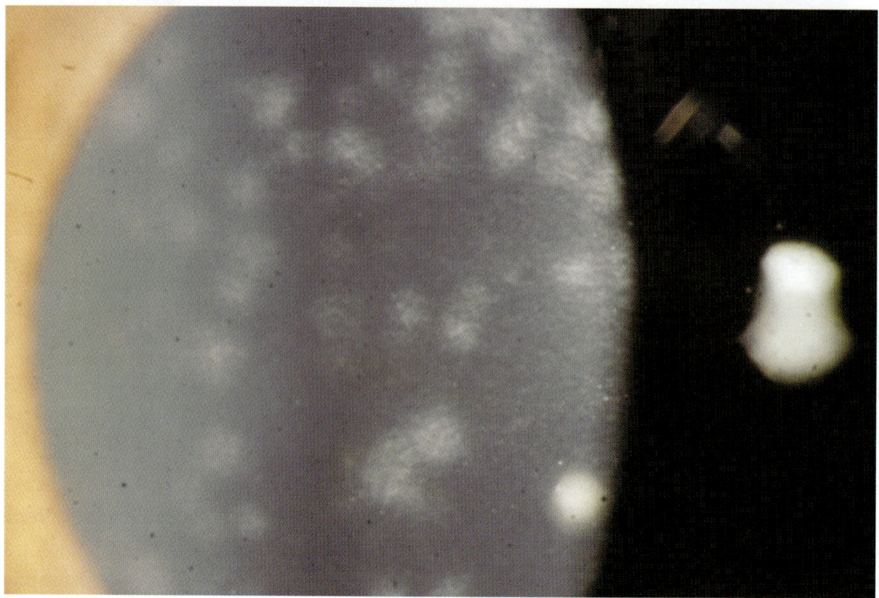

Fig. 14.3 Slit lamp photo of a patient with few active lesions and scars of previous episode of adenoviral keratoconjunctivitis.

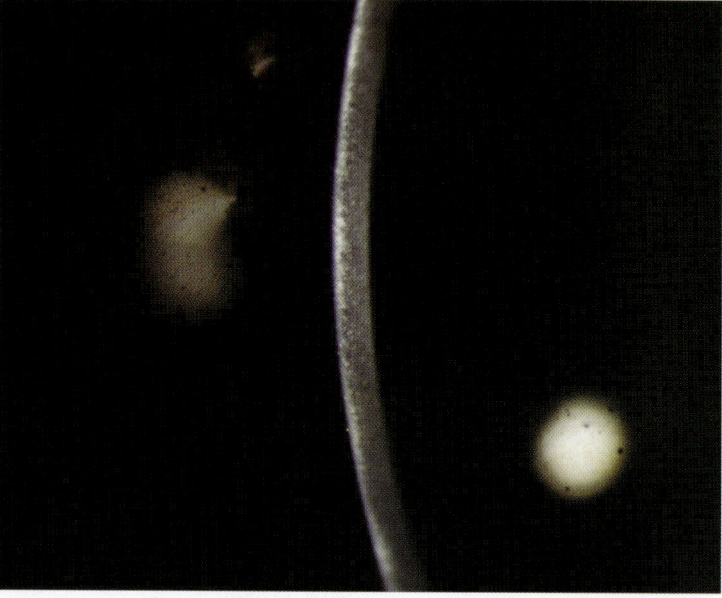

Fig. 14.4 Slit lamp photo (optical section) of a patient with few active lesions and scars of previous episode of adenoviral keratoconjunctivitis.

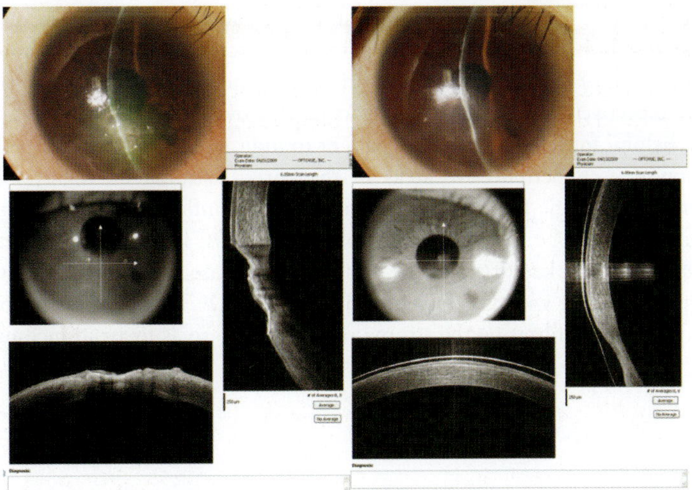

Fig. 14.5 Bacterial keratitis due to MRCNS.

The cross-sectional images by optical coherence tomography (OCT), as shown in **Figure 14.5**, revealed that the high-intensity area was limited to the anterior corneal surface and the posterior stroma appeared to be intact. The lesion was therefore scraped without fear of perforation. The culture was positive for methicillin-resistant coagulase-negative *Staphylococcus*. Topical application of arbekacin and minocycline ointment gave good resolution of the ulcer.

After scarring of the lesion and epithelialization of the ulcer, therapeutic soft contact lens was prescribed to prevent recurrence of the ulcer due to lagophthalmos. OCT images showed disappearance of high-intensity area at the corneal surface and soft contact lens on the cornea.

VIRAL KERATITIS (HERPES SIMPLEX VIRAL KERATITIS)

CASE STUDY 3

A 72-year-old woman presented with necrotizing keratitis due to herpes simplex virus in her left eye. Deep anterior lamellar keratoplasty (DALK) was performed and slit lamp examination following DALK showed clear graft as shown

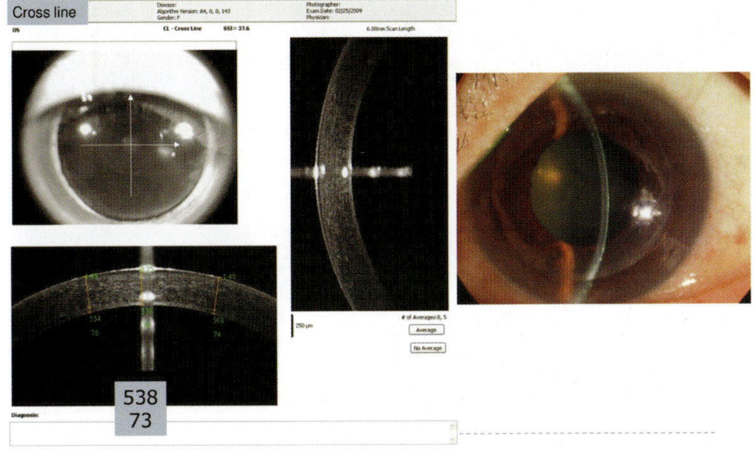

Fig. 14.6 DALK for HSV keratitis.

in **Figure 14.6**. Although it gave us the impression that the whole cornea was replaced by donor graft except Descemet's membrane and endothelium, images obtained with the cross-line mode of the spectral-domain optical coherence tomography (SD-OCT) indicated residual stromal bed. The central thickness of the stromal bed and graft was 73 μm and 538 μm, respectively. We need to look for corneal neovascularization at this interface, and monitoring stromal thickness will be helpful for following-up this patient to indicate recurrence of herpetic stromal keratitis.

Corneal infiltrates appear as hyperreflective areas in the corneal stroma on high-resolution AS-OCT scans. Imaging of the retrocorneal pathologic features and anterior-chamber inflammatory cells can also be accomplished. Thickness of corneal infiltrates can be measured with callipers. AS-OCT imaging provides numerous parameters that can be used to assess microbial keratitis and the treatment response objectively. Sun et al. have demonstrated the role of anterior-segment imaging with OCT in fungal ulcers. AS-OCT helped in assessing the depth of corneal ulcers and the depth of the lesion infiltrating the stroma preoperatively so as to avoid incomplete removal and postoperative recurrence.

FURTHER READING

1. Chintakuntlawar AV, Chodosh J: Cellular and tissue architecture of conjunctival membranes in epidemic keratoconjunctivitis. *Ocul Immunol Inflamm* 18(5):341–345, 2010.
2. Rajaiya J, Chodosh J: New paradigms in infectious eye disease: adenoviral keratoconjunctivitis. *Arch Soc Esp Oftalmol* 81:493–498, 2006.
3. Kaufman HE: Adenovirus advances: new diagnostic and therapeutic options. *Curr Opin Ophthalmol* 22(4):290–293, 2011.
4. Jabbur NS, O'Brien TP: Recurrence of keratitis after excimer laser keratectomy. *J Cataract Refract Surg* 29(1):198–201, 2003.
5. Meyer-Rüsenberg B, Loderstädt U, Richard G, et al.: Epidemic keratoconjunctivitis: the current situation and recommendations for prevention and treatment. *Dtsch Arztebl Int* 108(27):475–480, 2011.
6. Konstantopoulos A, Yadegarfar G, Hossain P, et al.: In vivo quantification of bacterial keratitis with optical coherence tomography. *Invest Ophthalmol Vis Sci* 52:1093–1097, 2011.
7. Sun G, Li S, Shi W, et al.: Clinical observation of removal of the necrotic corneal tissue combined with conjunctival flap covering surgery under the guidance of the AS-OCT in treatment of fungal keratitis. *Int J Ophthalmol* 5(1):88–91, 2012.
8. Konstantopoulos A, Kuo J, Hossain P, et al.: Assessment of the use of anterior segment optical coherence tomography in microbial keratitis. *Am J Ophthalmol* 146(4):534–542, 2008.

Keratoconus

Rohit Shetty and Kareeshma Wadia–Havewala

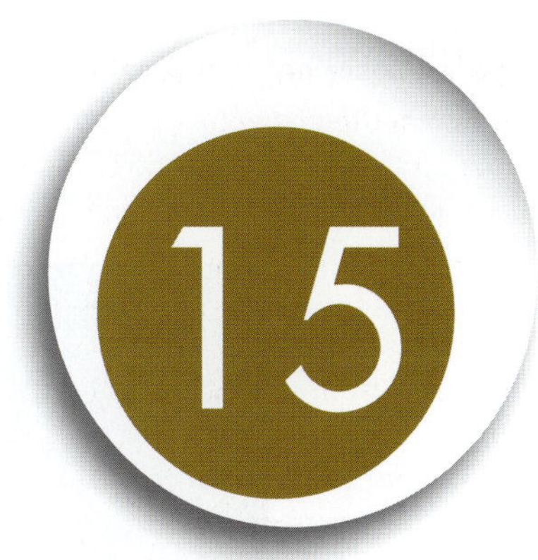

15

Keratoconus (from Greek: *kerato*-horn, cornea; and *konos* cone) is a noninflammatory ectatic disorder of the eye in which there is corneal thinning and the cornea changes to a more conical shape than its normal gradual curve. Keratoconus has its onset at puberty and is progressive up to the third to fourth decade of life, when it usually arrests. Nevertheless, it may commence later in life and progress or arrest at any age. Keratoconus has no male or female preponderance and occurs in all ethnic groups. It may be congenital in rare cases.

Though there are multiple singular reports of coexistence with other disorders, keratoconus is usually an isolated condition. Commonly seen associations include Down's syndrome, Leber's congenital amaurosis, and connective tissue disorders.

The reported incidence of keratoconus varies in literature, with most estimates being between 50 and 230 per 100,000 in the general population (approximately 1 per 2000). Prevalence is 54.5 per 100,000.

CASE STUDY 1

A 17-year-old man presented with complaints of frequent change in spectacles and blurring of vision since the past 8 months. He also had severe itching and redness in both the eyes.

Clinical examination revealed increased curvature of the cornea and stromal thinning. There was also a Fleischer's ring suggestive of keratoconus (**Fig. 15.1**). Anterior-segment optical coherence tomography (AS-OCT) confirmed the stromal thinning and increased corneal curvature (**Fig. 15.2**).

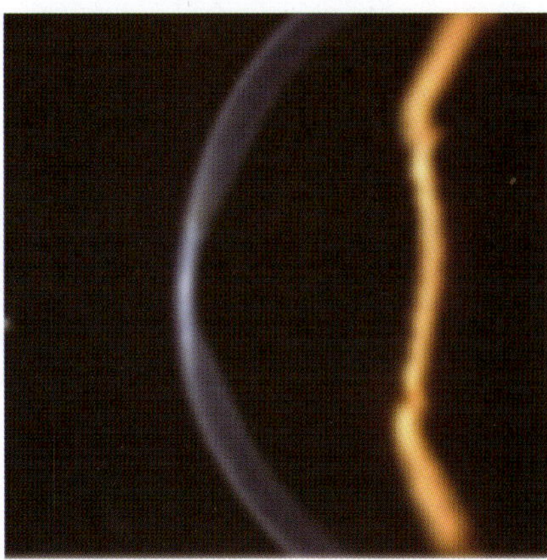

Fig. 15.1 Clinical picture reveals increased curvature of the cornea and stromal thinning. There was also a Fleischer's ring suggestive of keratoconus.

The patient underwent collagen cross-linking with riboflavin 0.1% under UV-A light. The anterior-segment optical coherence tomography (AS-OCT) postprocedure revealed subepithelial haze and a faint demarcation line (Fig. 15.3).

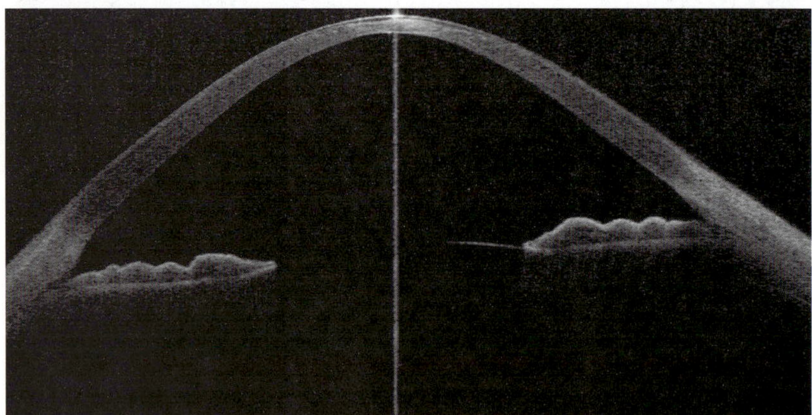

Fig. 15.2 Keratoconus – increased curvature and stromal thinning.

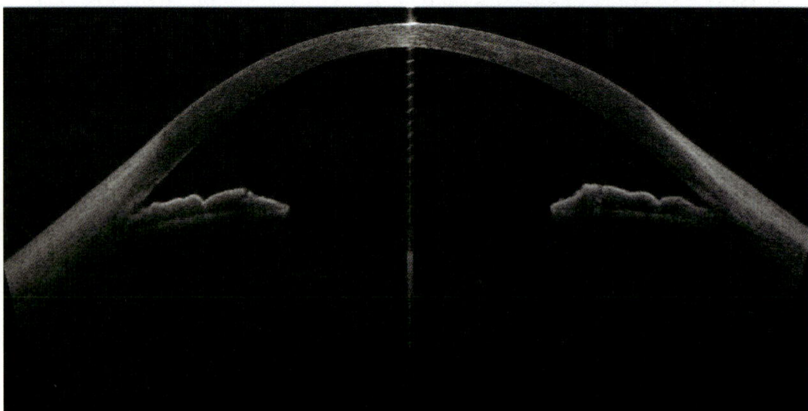

Fig. 15.3 Post cross-linking, AS-OCT demonstrates subepithelial haze, a faint demarcation line and stromal edema in the early postoperative period.

CASE STUDY 2

A 25-year-old woman, wearing glasses since the past 5 years, complained of sudden, painful diminution of vision in the left eye. There was no history of trauma or any systemic illness. A detailed history revealed that her refractive error was fluctuating constantly over the past 1 year, associated with blurring of vision in the eye. She had recurrent episodes of redness and itching in the eyes.

Clinical examination and AS-OCT revealed tears in the Descemet's membrane with overlying stromal edema suggestive of acute hydrops (Fig. 15.4).

Full-thickness compression sutures and intracameral C3F8 (perfluoropropane gas) was injected to treat the condition by apposing the detached Descemet's membrane. A penetrating keratoplasty can be performed at a later date.

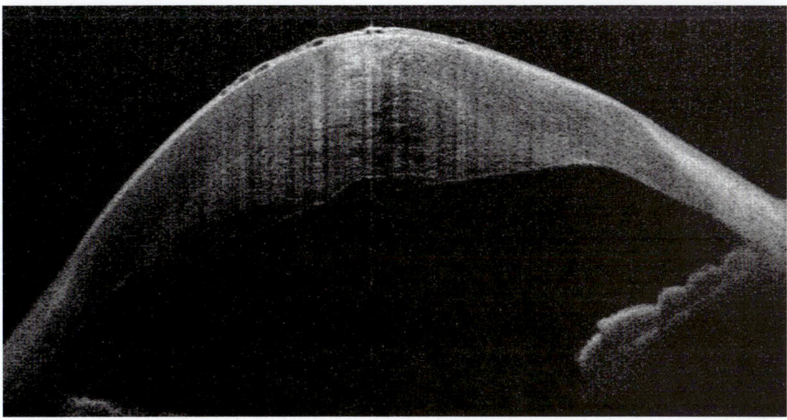

Fig. 15.4 Tears in the Descemet's membrane with overlying stromal edema.

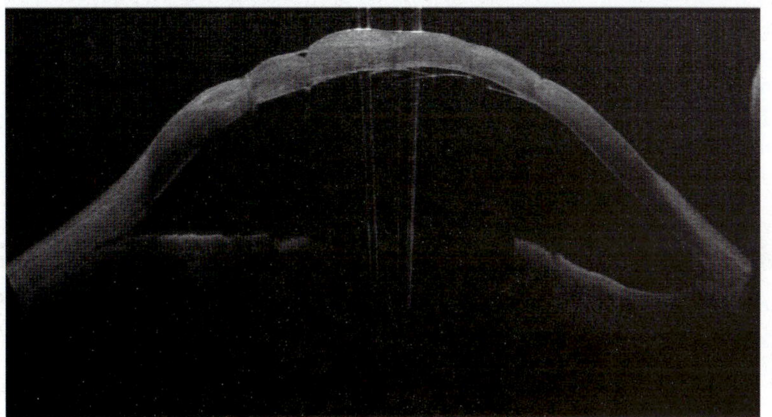

Fig. 15.5 Full-thickness compression sutures seen on AS-OCT.

Full-thickness compression sutures were placed in areas where the Descemet's membrane ruptures due to hydrops, and can be visualized on the AS-OCT (Fig. 15.5).

FURTHER READING

1. Smolin G: Dystrophies and degenerations. In Smolin G, Thoft RA, editors: The Cornea: Scientific Foundations and Clinical Practice, Boston, Little, Brown, ed 2, 448–449, 1987.
2. Duke-Elder S, Leigh AG: System of ophthalmology. Diseases of the outer eye, Vol 8. London, Henry Kimpton, 964–976, 1965.
3. Krachmer JH, Feder RS, Belin MW: Keratoconus and related noninflammatory corneal thinning disorders. *Surv Ophthalmol* 28:293–322, 1984.

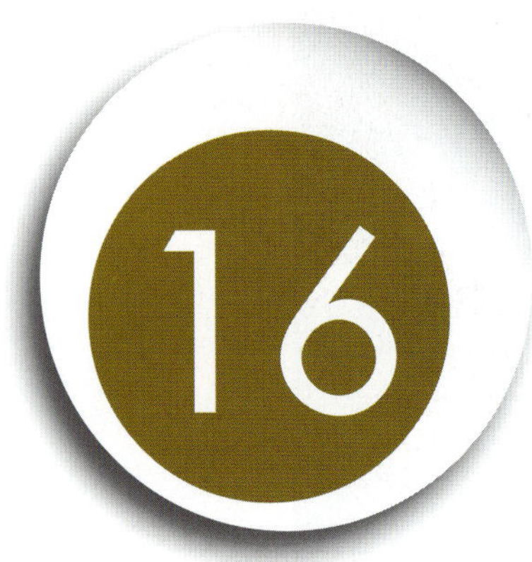

Keratoconus with Proud Nebulae

Ainur Rahman and Jodhbir S Mehta

Proud nebulae or corneal "pip" are usually seen in the context of contact lens use in keratoconic patients, and are rarely seen in normal subjects. It is a focal area of raised corneal tissue, usually located at or near the apex of the keratoconic cone. Thought to have a histologic resemblance to Salzmann degeneration, raised profile of the proud nebula can cause problems in contact lens fitting, rendering its use intolerable or rarely on its own, obscure vision.

CASE STUDY

A 26-year-old woman, a known case of keratoconus, presented with poor vision in both eyes. The patient had no history of eye surgery, trauma, or systemic disease, and was intolerant to contact lenses. At presentation, her best-corrected visual acuity (BCVA) was 6/45[+1] OD (right eye) and 6/15 OS (left eye).

Slit lamp biomicroscopy showed bilateral steepening of the cornea inferiorly, with opacities near the apex of both keratoconic cones. Corneal opacities appeared dense; but in the left eye, they were smaller in size and more superficial in location (Fig. 16.1).

Fourier-domain optical coherence tomography (FD-OCT, RTVue; Optovue, Inc., Fremont, CA) sections of the opacity in the left cornea showed that the plane of the lesion was above the level of Bowman's membrane (corneal "pip" or proud nebula). A similar nebula-like lesion was also seen in the right eye; but it was accompanied by underlying areas of scarring, extending beyond the Bowman's membrane (Fig. 16.1).

The patient underwent a surgical superficial keratectomy to the left eye. Under topical anesthesia, corneal opacity was successfully cleared after excision of overlying corneal epithelium and careful dissection of the plane above Bowman's membrane. Postoperative BCVA of the left eye was 6/7.5[+1].

The right eye underwent deep anterior lamellar keratoplasty (DALK) resulting in a BCVA of 6/18[−2] 1 week postoperatively (Fig. 16.2).

The principle of management of proud nebulae necessitates removal of these subepithelial lesions to improve contact lens tolerance. For more superficial scars, surgical superficial keratectomy and excimer laser phototherapeutic keratectomy (PTK) may be adequate for visual rehabilitation. However, if associated with deeper scarring a DALK or penetrating keratoplasty are indicated to improve vision.

The FD-OCT characteristics of high signal-to-noise ratio coupled with the high depth of resolution and high speed allowed for precise identification and differentiation of key corneal anatomical landmarks, invaluable to the surgeon in deciding on the most-appropriate surgical approach for treatment.

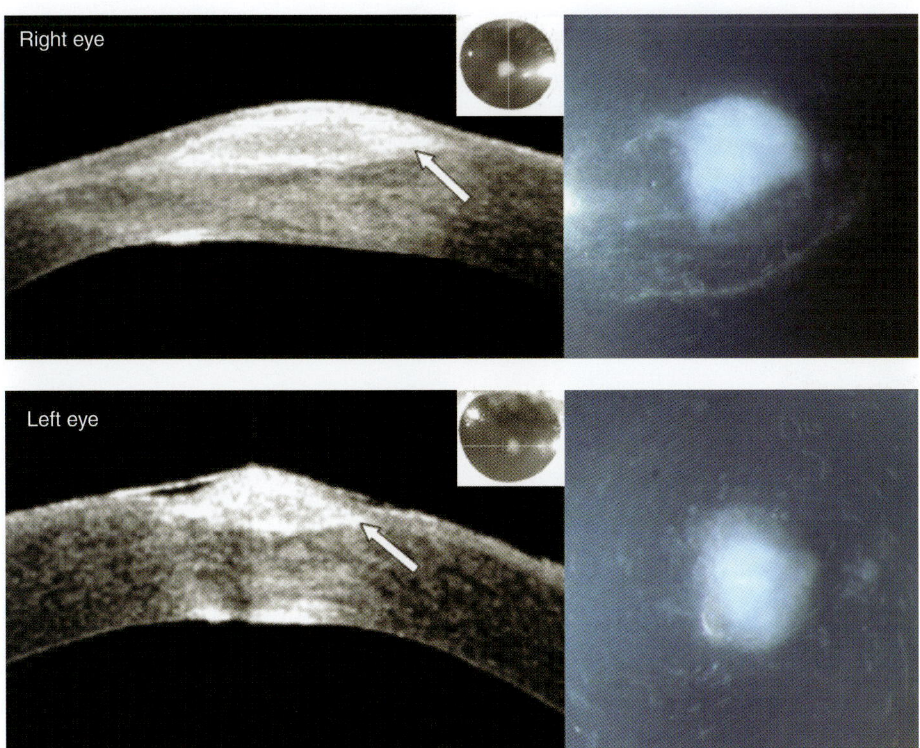

Fig. 16.1 Slit lamp biomicroscopy of right and left cornea with corresponding FD-OCT images (*arrows delineate Bowman's membrane*).

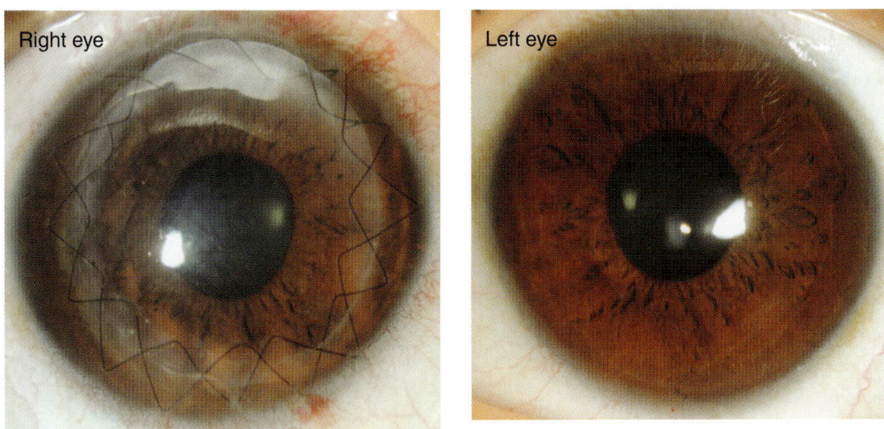

Fig. 16.2 Slit lamp photograph of the right (left panel) and left (right panel) eyes after deep anterior lamellar keratoplasty (DALK) and surgical superficial keratectomy, respectively.

FURTHER READING

1. Moodaley L, Buckley RJ, Woodward EG: Surgery to improve contact lens wear in keratoconus. *CLAO J* 17(2):129–131, 1991.
2. Dasa V, Gangadhar KRK, Michael D: Wagoner Superficial Keratectomy. *Duane's Ophthalmology* 2005–2010–01 Ed: Lippincott Williams & Wilkins; 2006.

3. Moodaley L, Liu C, Woodward EG, et al.: Excimer laser superficial keratectomy for proud nebulae in keratoconus. *Br J Ophthalmol* 78(6):454–457, 1994.
4. Han DC, Han D, Mehta JS, et al.: Comparison of outcomes of lamellar keratoplasty and penetrating keratoplasty in keratoconus. *Am J Ophthal* 148(5):744–751, 2009.
5. Hall RC, Mohamed FK, Htoon HM, et al.: Laser in situ keratomileusis flap measurements: comparison between observers and between spectral-domain and time-domain anterior segment optical coherence tomography. *J Cataract Refract Surg* 37:544–551, 2011.
6. Ramos JL, Li Y, Huang D: Clinical and research applications of anterior segment optical coherence tomography—a review. *Clin Experiment Ophthalmol* 37(1):81–89, 2009.

Keratoconus—INTACS™

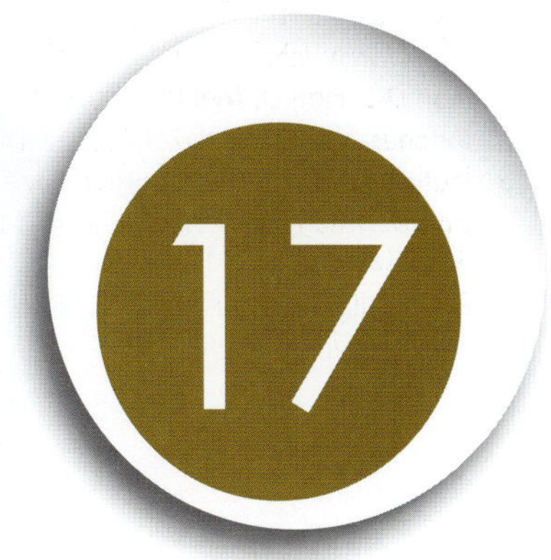

Kareeshma Wadia–Havewala and Rohit Shetty

The category of patients most likely to benefit from implantation of INTACS™ usually are those with lower initial keratometric readings ($K < 53$ D) as opposed to higher ($K > 55$ D). It should ideally be used in patients with relatively clear central corneas who are contact lens intolerant, or for whom keratoplasty is the only remaining option, and have thinnest pachymetry of more than 450 microns at the planned incision site.

Insertion of intrastromal corneal ring segments (ICRS) is being used to defer corneal graft surgery in eyes with keratoconus. The ICRS are inserted in the corneal stroma in an arc fashion, and several studies report successful results. By thickening the peripheral corneal stroma in the area of the ICRS, the central cornea is flattened as a result of the coupling forces exerted on the cornea.

INTACS™ ICRS (Addition Technology, Inc.) have been shown to produce up to 4.00 diopters (D) of corneal flattening, a benefit that decreases markedly when keratometry (K) exceeds 53.00 D. INTACS™ SK (Steep Keratometry) ICRS (Addition Technology, Inc.) were designed to work more effectively in cases of moderate to severe keratoconus (Table 17.1). The segments have an elliptical design and an inner diameter of 6.0 mm. By virtue of its position closer to the visual axis and corneal center, this segment has a greater flattening effect on the central cornea.

Each INTACS™ segment has a hexagonal cross-section that lies along a conic section with a large, clear central optic zone. Each segment has a small positioning hole located at each end of the segment to aid with surgical manipulation. The segments are placed equidistant on each side of the incision.

They are manufactured from polymethylmethacrylate (PMMA) using techniques similar to those employed in intraocular lens (IOL) manufacturing.

Table 17.1 Standard recommendation for sizing of rings

Type of keratoconus	Recommended thickness preoperative spherical equivalent = −3.00 D	Recommended thickness preoperative spherical equivalent > −3.00 D
Asymmetrical cone	0.250 mm/0.300 mm	0.250 mm/0.350 mm
Moderate asymmetry	0.350 mm/0.400 mm	0.400 mm/0.450 mm
High asymmetry	0.250 mm/0.400 mm	0.250 mm/0.450 mm
Global cone/central cone	0.400 mm/0.400 mm	0.450 mm/0.450 mm

(INTACS® Corneal Implants for the Treatment of Keratoconus, *International Surgeon Training Manual*)

CASE STUDY

A 25-year-old man, known case of mild keratoconus, presented to our cornea clinic with the chief complaints of decrease in visual acuity for the last 3–4 months. He had been comfortably using conventional rigid gas permeable

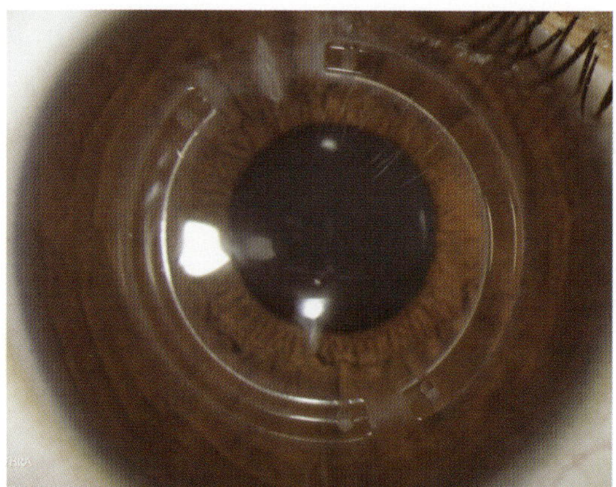

Fig. 17.1 Slit lamp photograph showing INTACS™.

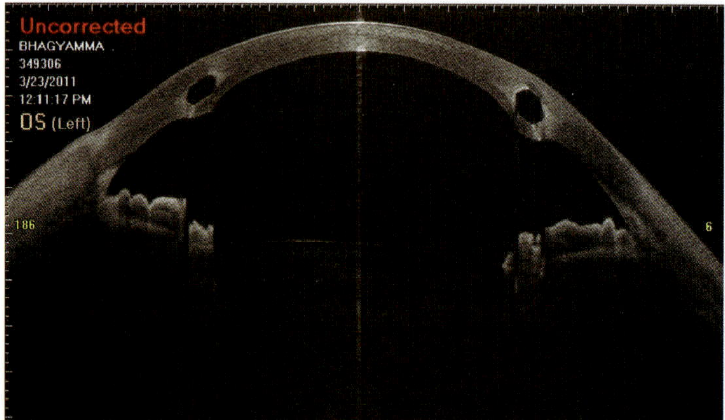

Fig. 17.2 AS-OCT (Tomey) image showing hexagonal cross-section of INTACS™.

(RGP) lenses for the last 2 years. However, for the last 6 months, he was not comfortable with the RGP lenses. Slit lamp examination revealed inferotemporal cone and a central clear cornea (Fig. 17.1). The thinnest pachymetry was 462 microns in the area of the cone. INTACS™ (Intracorneal microthin prescription inserts: Addition Technology Inc., USA) were used for this patient (Fig. 17.2).

FURTHER READING

1. Shetty R, Kannan MN, Shetty KB, et al.: Safety and efficacy of intacs in Indian eyes with keratoconus: an initial report. *Indian J Ophthalmol* 57(2):115–119, 2009.
2. Colin J, Cochener B, Savary G: Correcting keratoconus with intracorneal rings. *J Cataract Refract Surg* 26:1117–1122, 2000.
3. Alio J, Salem T, Artola A, et al.: Intracorneal rings to correct corneal ectasia after laser in situ keratomileusis. *J Cataract Refract Surg* 28:1568–1574, 2002.
4. Zare MA, Hashemi H, Salari MR: Intracorneal ring segment implantation for the management of keratoconus: safety and efficacy. *J Cataract Refract Surg* 33:1886–1891, 2007.
5. INTACS® Corneal Implants for the Treatment of Keratoconus, International Surgeon Training Manual.

Keratoconus— KERAFLEX™ (Microwave Thermoplasty)

Kareeshma Wadia–Havewala and Rohit Shetty

Keraflex™ is the latest procedure for treatment of keratoconus. It is a nonincisional procedure that preserves the biomechanical integrity of the cornea and reshapes it without any tissue removal.

In a Keraflex procedure, the machine delivers a single low-energy microwave pulse for less than a few seconds on the cornea. The single pulse raises the temperature of the selected region of corneal stroma to approximately 65°C, thereby causing shrinkage of collagen and forming a toroidal lesion in the upper 150 microns of the stroma. Subsequently, an in built cooling technique on the surface prevents any thermal effect due to microwaves.

This is followed by collagen cross-linking with riboflavin under UV-A light (CXL/ACXL) after a few days. It is not a refractive procedure and patients will still require glasses or contact lenses after this.

Keraflex is CE marked and is licensed for use in Europe.

Clinical trials to suggest its efficacy are still on-going.

CASE STUDY

A 21-year-old woman, a known case of keratoconus complained of progressive diminution of vision over the past 1 year. She now has advanced keratoconus. The Keraflex procedure was performed for her left eye (Figs 18.1A and 18.1B). Figure 18.2 shows anterior-segment optical coherence tomography (AS-OCT) image of the same eye on first postoperative day, demonstrating the depth to which the microwave pulse energy penetrates.

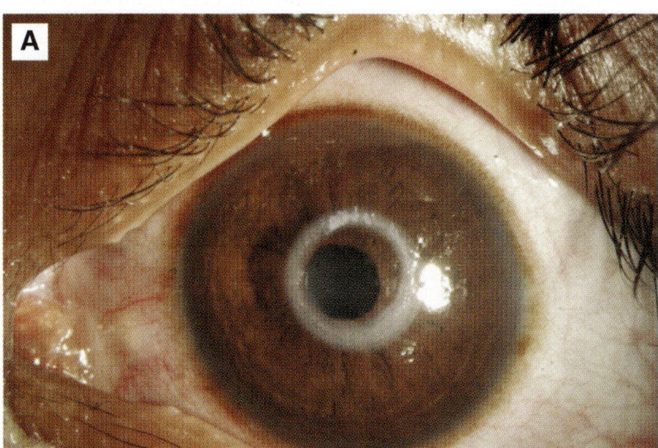
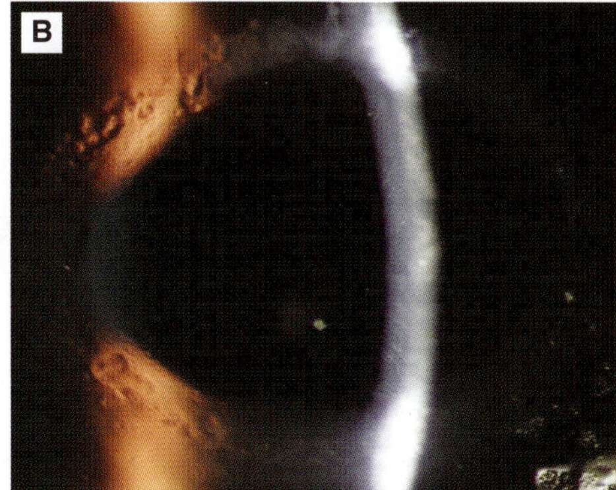

Fig 18.1 (A) and (B) Slit lamp images of the keraflex ring immediately postprocedure.

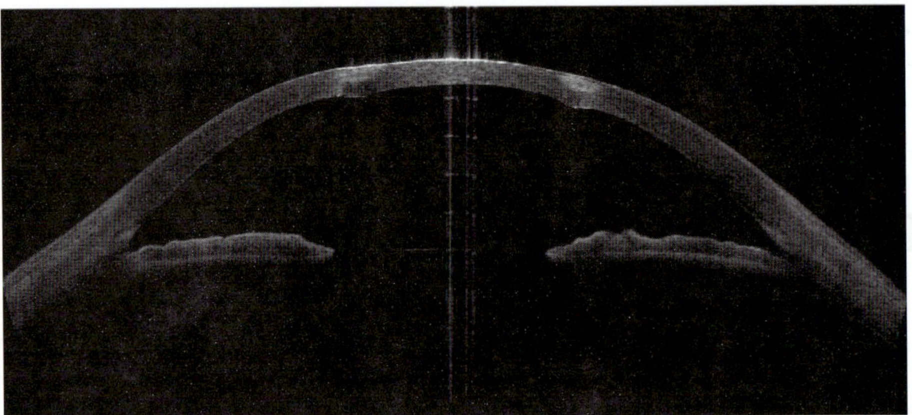

Fig. 18.2 AS-OCT image shows the depth to which the microwave pulse energy penetrates.

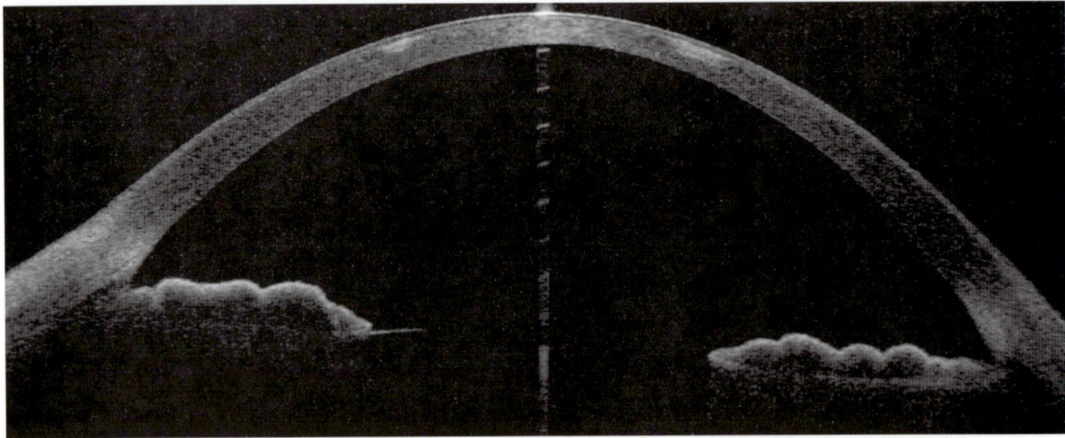

Fig. 18.3 AS-OCT shows a faint scar of the KERAFLEX™ ring at 4 months postprocedure.

The keratometry changed by a mean of 20 Diopters on the first postoperative day. Regression of this effect is seen over the next 48–72 hours, with the KERAFLEX™ ring becoming slightly faint on subsequent visits (Fig. 18.3). On day 3, she underwent accelerated corneal collagen cross-linking (ACXL).

FURTHER READING

Cummings A: Combining Keraflex and Corneal Collagen Crosslinking. Cataract and Refractive Surgery Today: September 2011.

Keratoplasty—Endothelial Keratoplasty

Mark A Greiner, Michael D Straiko, and Mark A Terry

BACKGROUND

Endothelial keratoplasty (EK) is a newer technique of corneal transplantation that selectively replaces endothelium while leaving anterior cornea relatively untouched. EK is a rapidly evolving technique (Fig. 19.1) that has now supplanted penetrating keratoplasty (PK) as a standard of care for endothelial dysfunction. Descemet's stripping-automated endothelial keratoplasty (DSAEK)—where donor endothelium, Descemet's membrane, and a thin layer

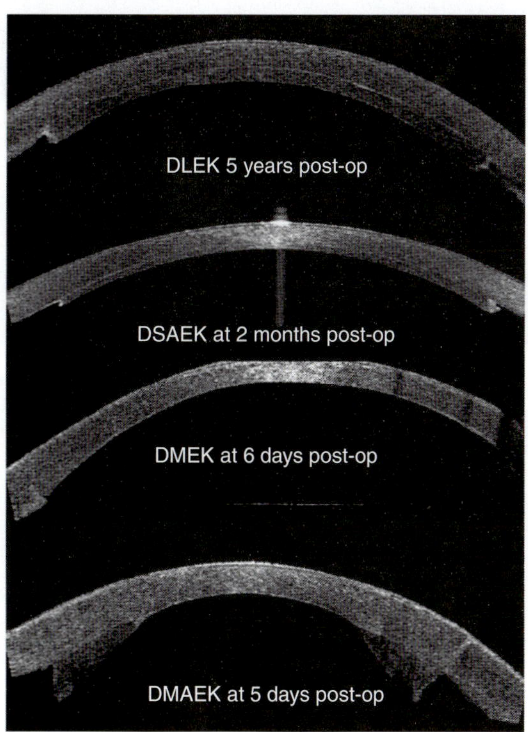

Fig. 19.1 AS-OCT images demonstrating evolution of endothelial keratoplasty.

of stroma are transplanted—is currently the most commonly performed method of EK; although investigation into Descemet's membrane endothelial keratoplasty (DMEK)—where only donor endothelium and Descemet's membrane are transplanted—is burgeoning.

The ascendance of DSAEK and DMEK over PK for the treatment of endothelial dysfunction has occurred for myriad reasons, including a more rapid recovery of vision, no suture-related complications, and minimal alteration of anterior corneal curvature, spherical equivalent, and refractive cylinder. As the donor endothelium clears the edema, mean thickness of the graft decreases over time, with thinning of edges occurring more rapidly than at vertex (Fig. 19.2).

The most common complication following DSAEK and DMEK surgery is dislocation of the transplant requiring reinjection of a second air bubble to reattach tissue. Fluid in the interface between the donor and recipient stroma that is not evacuated adequately at the time of surgery, or that migrates centrally through a peripheral fluid cleft or lifted graft edge, may resolve spontaneously or may lead to detachment of the graft. Careful clinical examination for interface fluid is required in the early postoperative period.

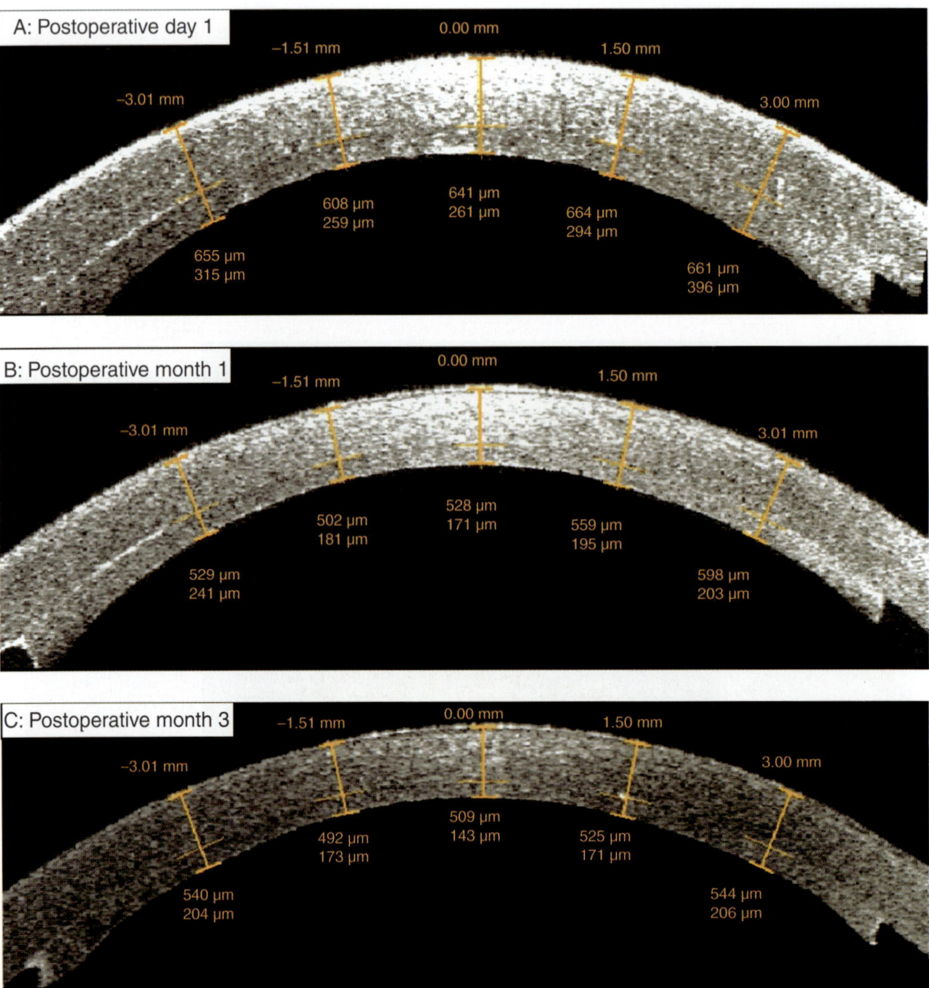

Fig. 19.2 Sequential AS-OCT cornea images after DSAEK surgery with thickness measurements at corneal vertex, ±1.5 mm from the vertex, and ±3 mm from the vertex. **(A)** 1 day after DSAEK. **(B)** 1 month after DSAEK. **(C)** 3 months after DSAEK.

INTERFACE FLUID WITH ATTACHED DSAEK GRAFT

CASE STUDY 1

A 73-year-old pseudophakic woman with Fuchs' endothelial dystrophy experienced a progressive painless visual decline since her cataract surgery and was diagnosed with visually significant endothelial dysfunction and corneal edema in both eyes. She elected to have DSAEK surgery in the right eye.

Uncomplicated DSAEK surgery was performed utilizing a 5-mm scleral tunnel incision, Descemet's membrane stripping with a reverse Terry–Sinskey hook (Bausch & Lomb Surgical, St. Louis, MO), and scraping of peripheral recipient bed with a Terry scraper (Bausch & Lomb Surgical, St. Louis, MO) under Healon (Abbott Medical Optics, Santa Ana, CA). After evacuation of Healon, tissue precut by eye bank staff was inserted using noncoapting Charlie forceps (Bausch & Lomb Surgical, St. Louis, MO). The graft was positioned and interface fluid was removed with gentle external compression using a Cindy sweeper (Bausch & Lomb Surgical, St. Louis, MO). No residual interface fluid was noted. A freely mobile 8-mm air bubble was left in the anterior chamber, and the eye was patched and shielded overnight.

Uncorrected visual acuity (UCVA) 1 day after DSAEK surgery was 20/200. Slit lamp examination revealed a well-centered DSAEK graft attached peripherally but detached centrally with significant central interface fluid and recipient corneal edema. Anterior-segment optical coherence tomography (AS-OCT) imaging was obtained (Fig. 19.3). Decision was made to observe the area of the central interface fluid because the graft was attached peripherally and not dislocated. No further air was injected.

The patient was instructed to spend additional time in supine position, and serial AS-OCT images were obtained postoperatively to supplement slit lamp examination and track the interface fluid. At 5 days postoperatively, UCVA remained 20/200 and examination revealed enlargement of the interface fluid pocket and new central bullous keratopathy (Fig. 19.4). Because the graft remained attached at the superior periphery and was well centered, observation of the interface fluid without intervention was continued.

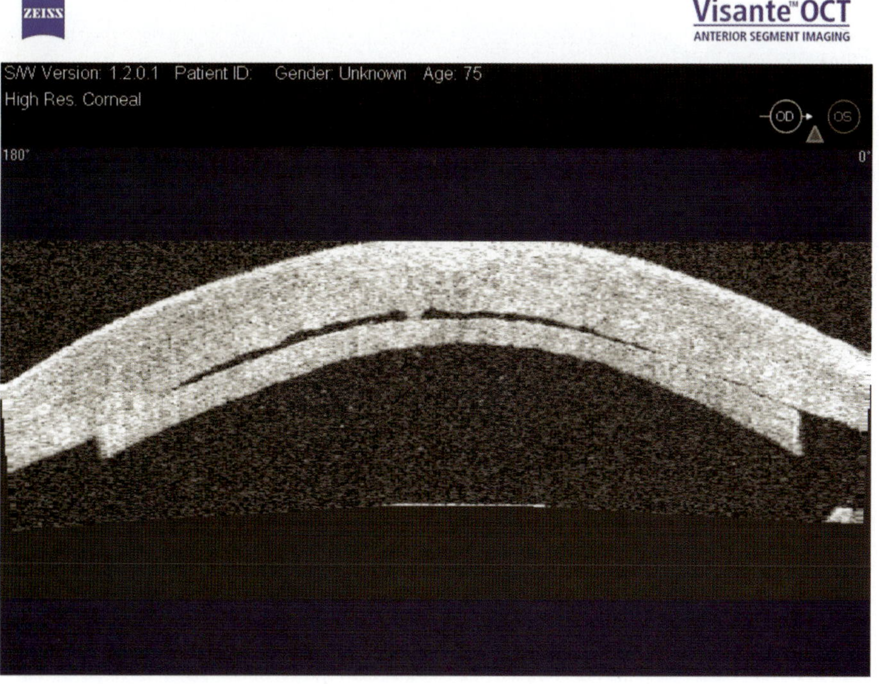

Fig. 19.3 AS-OCT of the right eye, 1 day after uncomplicated DSAEK surgery. Significant interface fluid at the center of the graft is present, but the graft is well-centered due to firm attachment at the periphery where peripheral scraping had been performed as described previously by our group.

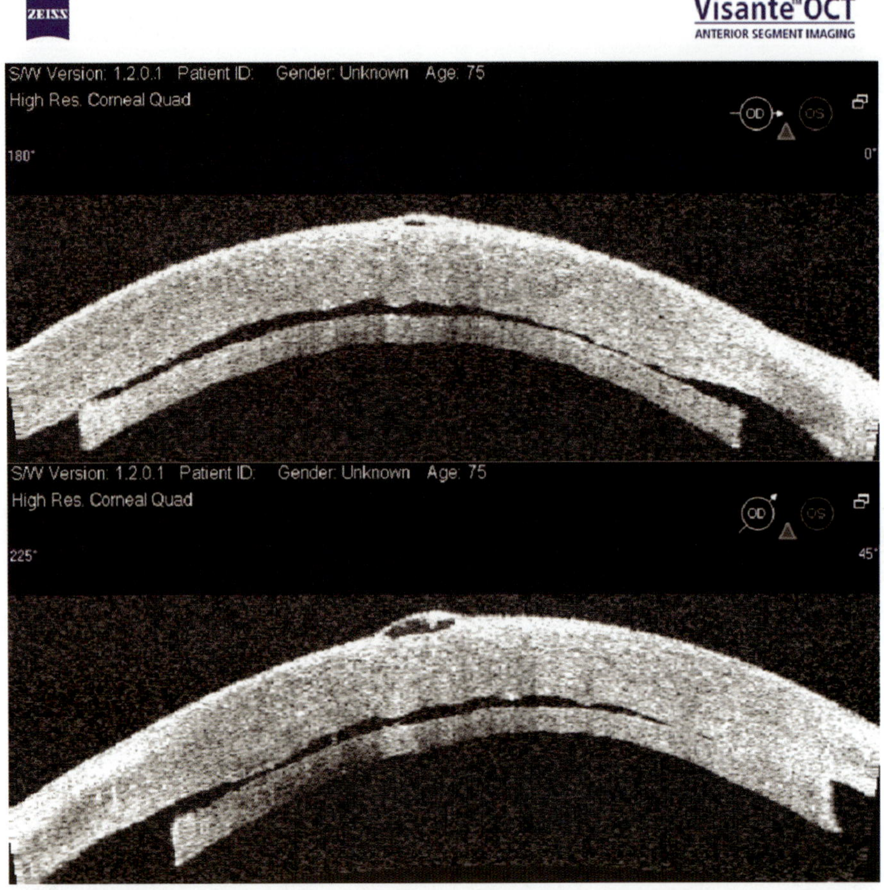

Fig. 19.4 AS-OCT of the right eye, 5 days after uncomplicated DSAEK surgery. Enlargement of the central interface fluid pocket and new epithelial bullae are noted, but observation without intervention was continued because the graft remains attached peripherally and well-centered.

The area of interface fluid and attendant corneal edema stabilized by postoperative day 6 and clear evidence of reduced interface fluid was noted on postoperative day 7 (**Fig. 19.5**). Improvement in UCVA to 20/80 and complete resolution of the interface fluid along with a well-centered compact cornea were notable at postoperative month 1 (**Fig. 19.6**). Best-corrected visual acuity (BCVA) 6 months postoperatively was 20/30, with the vision limited by anterior stromal haze secondary to chronic preoperative corneal edema.

Fluid in the interface between the donor and recipient stroma can occur after uncomplicated DSAEK surgery. As long as the graft is attached, well-centered, and does not incorporate a full-thickness edge from eccentric trephination (**Fig. 19.7**), the tissue will continue to evacuate the interface fluid and a rebubbling procedure generally is not required. Early postoperative AS-OCT imaging supplements slit lamp examination, helps confirm attachment, and provides a baseline for assessing resolution of interface fluid. Serial AS-OCT imaging is an important component in basing clinical decision to observe or rebubble. We rebubble if graft detachment is imminent, especially if an anterior chamber intraocular lens (ACIOL) or glaucoma-drainage tube is present in the anterior chamber, or if the patient's visual needs require more immediate improvement in vision.

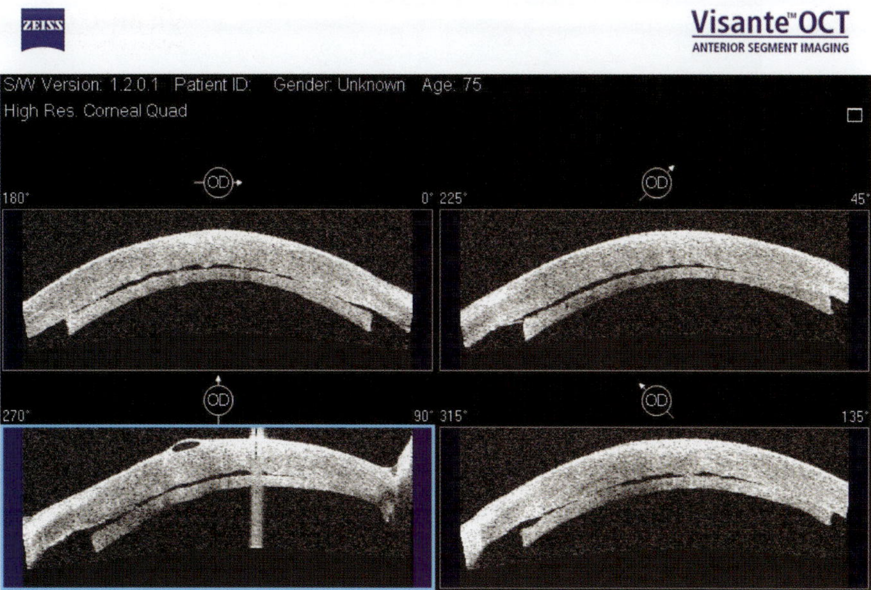

Fig. 19.5 AS-OCT of the right eye, 1 week after uncomplicated DSAEK surgery. The area of interface fluid is improving with observation alone.

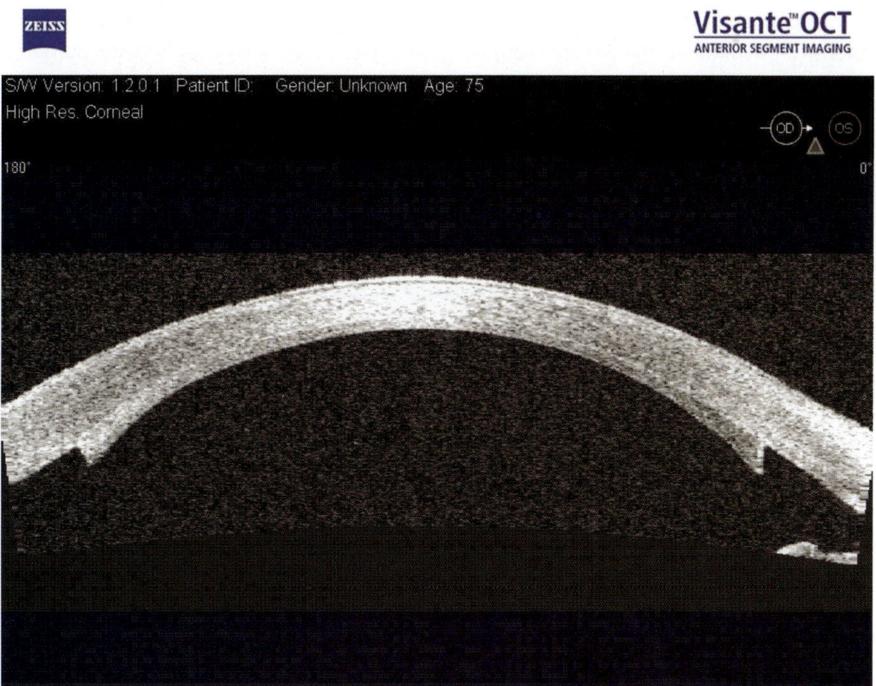

Fig. 19.6 AS-OCT of the right eye, 1 month after uncomplicated DSAEK surgery. Interface fluid and corneal edema resolved completely without intervention.

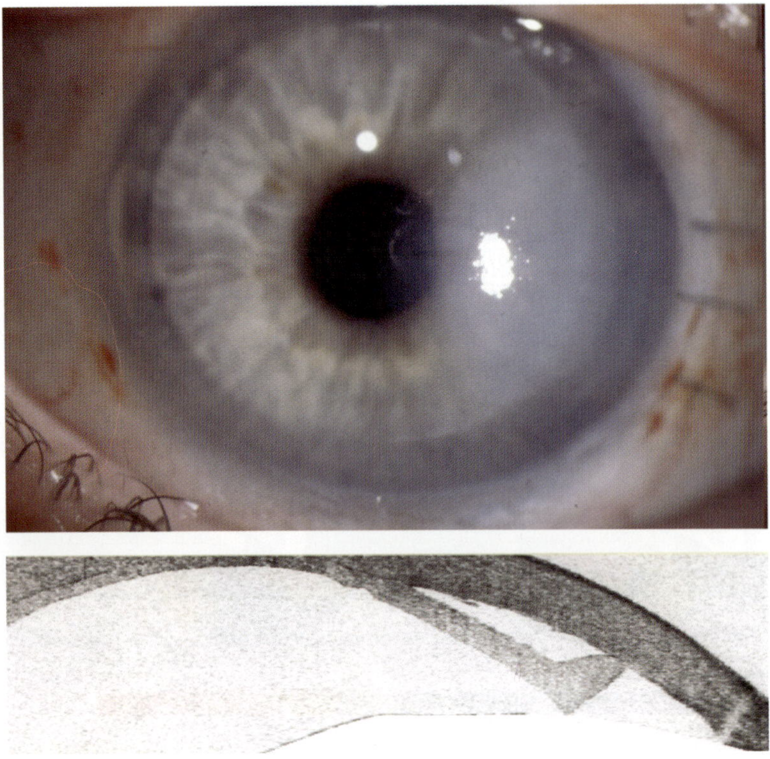

Fig. 19.7 Slit lamp photo (*above*) and corresponding AS-OCT (*below*) of the left eye, 1 month after uncomplicated DSAEK surgery. The patient was referred for non-clearing corneal edema. A full-thickness edge due to eccentric trephination of the donor graft was noted. The patient required graft explantation and repeat DSAEK surgery.

INTERFACE FLUID THREATENING DMEK GRAFT

CASE STUDY 2

A 76-year-old pseudophakic woman with progressive painless visual decline over the past 12 months and a history of Fuchs' endothelial dystrophy was diagnosed with visually significant endothelial dysfunction in both eyes. She elected to have DMEK surgery in the left eye.

Uncomplicated DMEK surgery was performed utilizing a 2.8-mm scleral tunnel incision and stripping of Descemet's membrane with a reverse Terry–Sinskey hook under Healon. After evacuation of Healon, the donor graft was prepared manually from a corneoscleral cap stored in Optisol-GS (Bausch & Lomb, Rochester, NY) and inserted using an injector (STAAR® Surgical, Monrovia, CA). The graft was unfolded under sequential injections of air and balanced salt solution (BSS) and positioned using gentle external compression from a Cindy sweeper. No residual interface fluid was noted. A freely mobile 8-mm air bubble was left in the anterior chamber and the eye was patched and shielded overnight.

UCVA was 20/80 + 1,1 day after DMEK surgery. Slit lamp examination revealed an attached DMEK graft with 2 clock hours of graft edge separation of the inferior graft and stromal edema with bullous keratopathy in the superior nasal cornea. AS-OCT imaging was obtained (**Fig. 19.8**). The decision was made to observe the small sector of edge separation because the graft was attached and well centered, and interface fluid was confined to the graft edges.

At 1 week postoperatively, UCVA was 20/100 and examination revealed progression of the graft edge separation, with enlarged interface fluid collections at the inferior graft quadrant and new interface fluid clefts at the temporal graft quadrant (**Fig. 19.9**). Observation without intervention was continued because over 90% of the graft remained attached, including the central graft, but the frequency of prednisolone acetate 1% topical suspension was increased to every 2 hours and sodium chloride 5% topical solution was added every 2 hours.

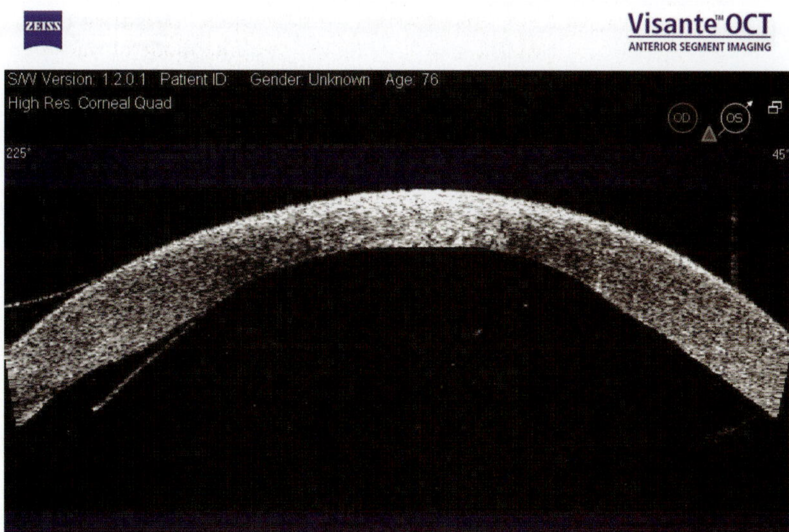

Fig. 19.8 AS-OCT of the left eye, 1 day after uncomplicated DMEK surgery. A limited amount of interface fluid is present due to edge lift of the inferior graft.

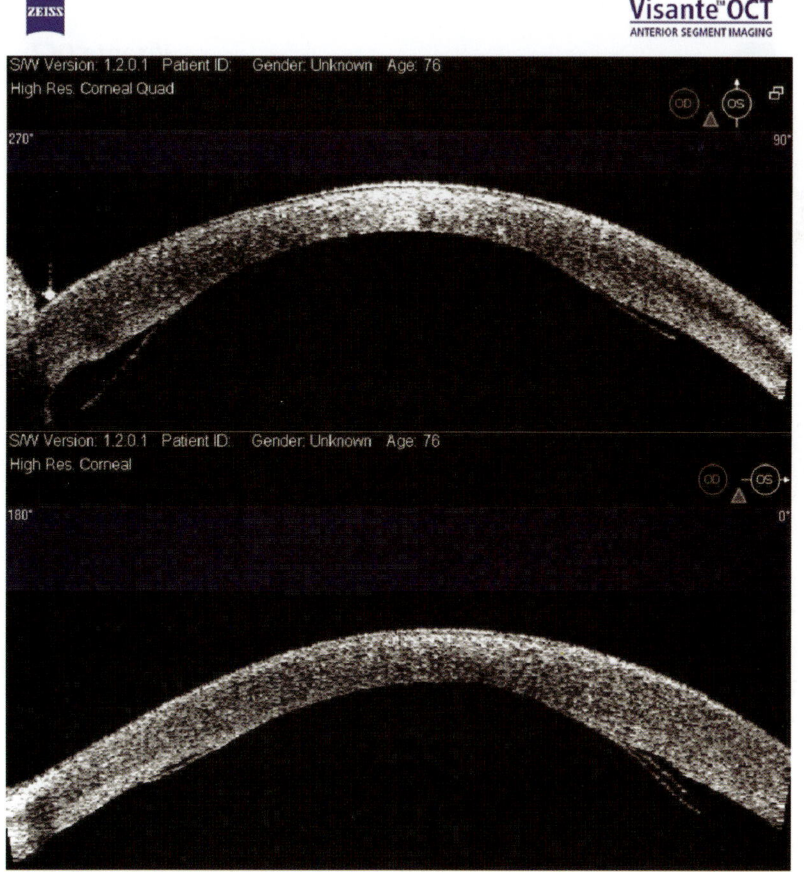

Fig. 19.9 AS-OCT images of the left eye, 1 week after uncomplicated DMEK surgery. An increased amount of peripheral interface fluid is noted inferiorly and temporally, but the graft remains mostly attached.

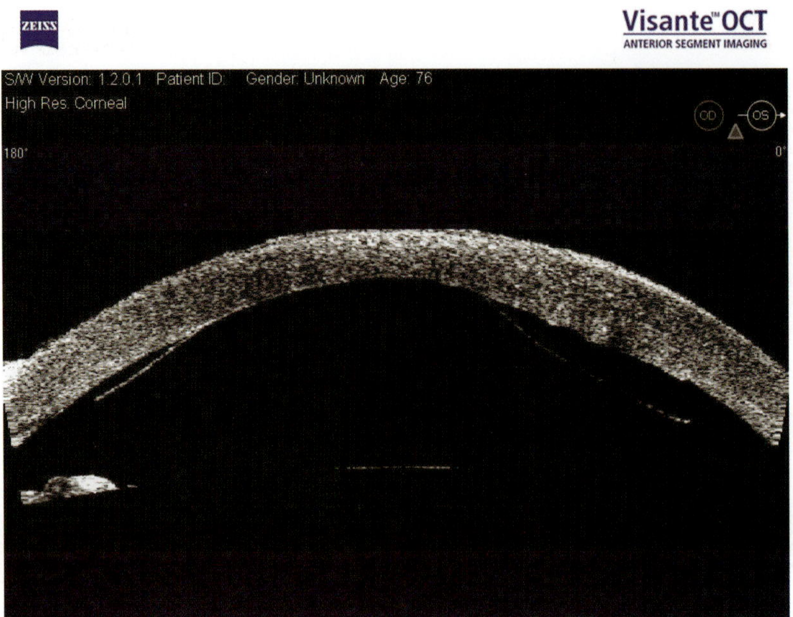

Fig. 19.10 AS-OCT of the left eye, 3 weeks after uncomplicated DMEK surgery. Progressive detachment of the graft is noted, prompting the decision to rebubble.

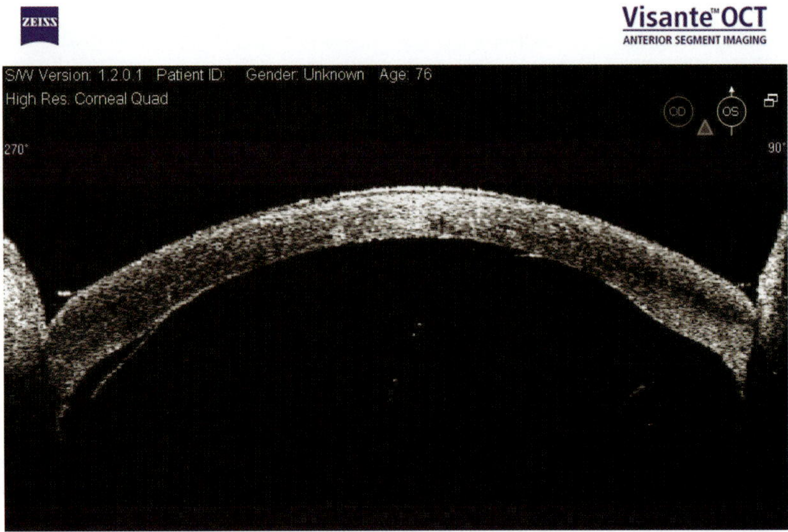

Fig. 19.11 AS-OCT of the left eye, 1 day after rebubbling of the DMEK graft. Firm graft attachment with a persistent small area of edge lift inferiorly and full resolution of the interface fluid are noted.

Serial clinical examinations with AS-OCT imaging continued. Examination 2 weeks after DMEK revealed UCVA of 20/40 with persistent, unchanged peripheral interface fluid collections and associated corneal edema. However, the examination at postoperative week 3 revealed extension of interface fluid clefts temporally, and inferiorly that were found to abut the visual axis in the paracentral cornea (Fig. 19.10). The decision was made to perform a rebubbling procedure because the graft detachment was progressive and threatened the visual axis.

Immediate improvements were noted 1 day after rebubbling of the DMEK graft, with the examination notable for UCVA improving to 20/50 + 1, full resolution of the interface fluid, and firm graft attachment with only a persistent small area of edge lift inferiorly (Fig. 19.11). UCVA of 20/25 + 2 without interface fluid or corneal

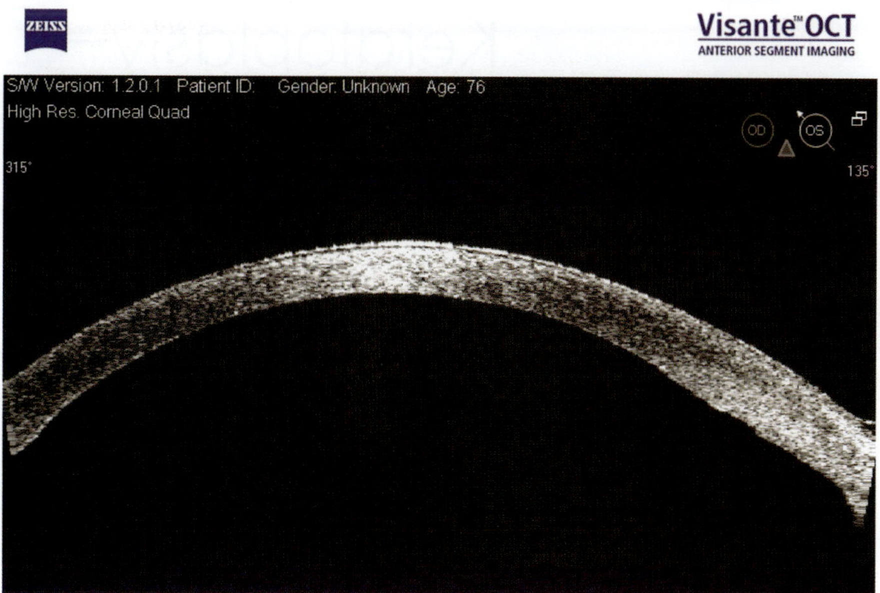

Fig. 19.12 AS-OCT of the left eye, 1 month after DMEK surgery and 1 week after graft rebubbling procedure.

edema were achieved by postoperative month 1 after DMEK and postoperative week 1 after rebubbling of the graft (Fig. 19.12).

At this time, graft detachment occurs more frequently after DMEK surgery than DSAEK surgery, and is one of several significant reasons for the reticence of surgeons to adopt DMEK. Although DMEK complication rates may decline with passage of the steep learning curve, the higher rate of DMEK graft detachment relative to DSAEK surgery makes careful postoperative tracking of any interface fluid essential after DMEK surgery, especially since injection of a second air bubble must be anticipated. DMEK grafts are thinner and more difficult to visualize at the slit lamp, especially in the presence of significant recipient corneal edema, making it of particular importance to follow status of these grafts in the postoperative period with AS-OCT imaging. As with DSAEK surgery, we base the decision to rebubble the DMEK graft if detachment is imminent, progressing, or if the patient's visual needs require more immediate improvement in vision.

FURTHER READING

1. Terry MA: Endothelial keratoplasty (EK): history, current state, and future directions. *Cornea* 25:873–878, 2006.
2. Melles GRJ, Ong TS, Ververs B, et al.: Descemet membrane endothelial keratoplasty (DMEK). *Cornea* 25:987–990, 2006.
3. Price MO, Giebel AW, Fairchild KM, et al.: Descemet's membrane endothelial keratoplasty: prospective multi-center study of visual and refractive outcomes and endothelial survival. *Ophthalmology* 116:2361–2368, 2009.
4. Terry MA, Shamie N, Chen ES, et al.: Pre-cut tissue for Descemet's stripping endothelial keratoplasty: Vision, astigmatism, and endothelial survival. *Ophthalmology* 116:248–256, 2009.
5. Dirisamer M, Ham L, Dapena I, et al.: Efficacy of Descemet membrane endothelial keratoplasty: clinical outcome of 200 consecutive cases after a learning curve of 25 cases. *Arch Ophthalmol* 129:1435–1443, 2011.

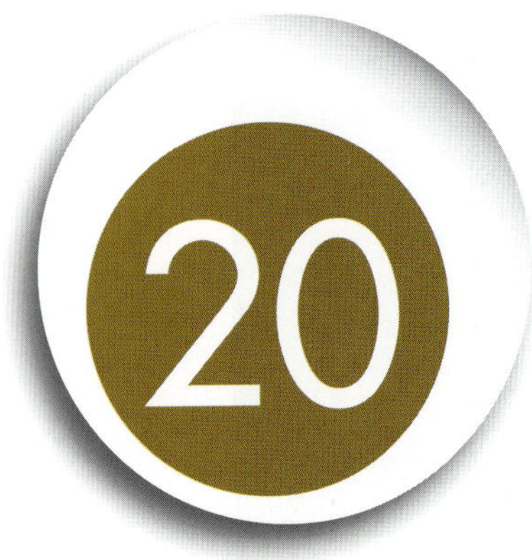

Keratoplasty—Deep Anterior Lamellar Keratoplasty

Karim Mohamed–Noriega, Ainur Rahman, and Jodhbir S Mehta

A descemetocele is characterized by herniation of Descemet's membrane (DM) through an area of eroded corneal stroma. Recognized as one of the end-stage complications of corneal ulcers or melting, imminent perforation with loss of ocular integrity may ensue.

Deep anterior lamellar keratoplasty (DALK) is a selective corneal transplantation procedure indicated for corneal opacities limited to the stroma when DM and endothelium are unaffected. In this case, we describe use of intraoperative anterior-segment optical coherence tomography (AS-OCT) to aid completion of a DALK in management of a patient with a descemetocele.

CASE STUDY

A 73-year-old male with previous history of herpes zoster (VHZ) keratouveitis in his right eye presented with culture-negative corneal ulcer, descemetocele, and anterior chamber reaction and hypopyon. Blood screening for hepatitis B, hepatitis C, human immunodeficiency virus (HIV), and Veneral Disease Research Laboratory (VDRL) were negative. A diagnosis of right eye neurotrophic ulcer with superimposed bacterial infection complicated by a descemetocele was made, and he was empirically treated with intensive topical and systemic antimicrobials. After 7 weeks, the inflammation and probable infection had abated but the epithelized descemetocele remained (**Figs 20.1 and 20.2**).

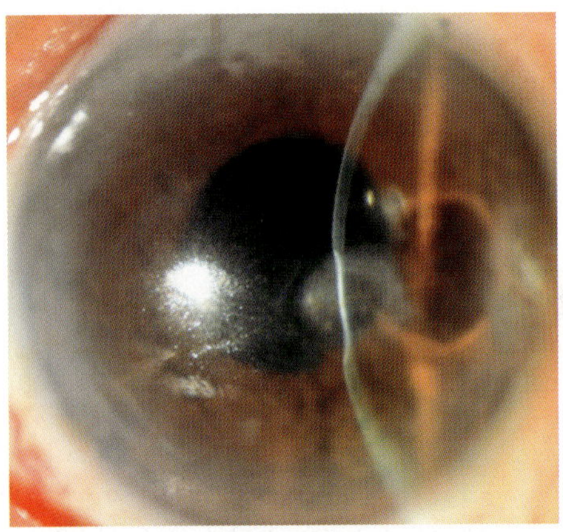

Fig. 20.1 Slit lamp evaluation showing corneal thinning with epithelization of descemetocele.

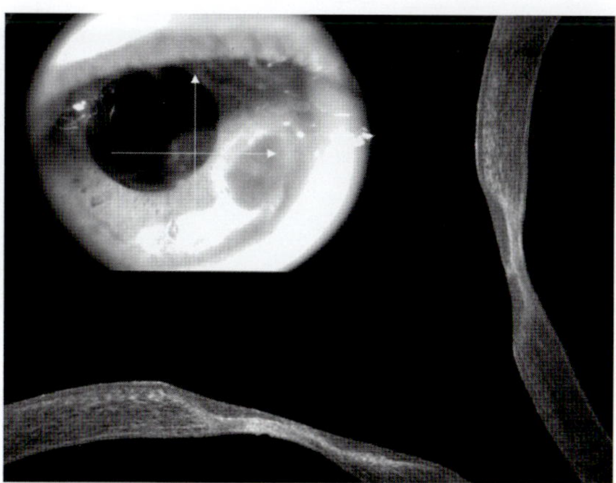

Fig. 20.2 Fourier-domain optical coherence tomography (FD-OCT, RTVue®; Optovue, Inc., Fremont, CA) showed an epithelized descemetocele with some posterior stroma fibers or scar tissue remaining over descemetocele.

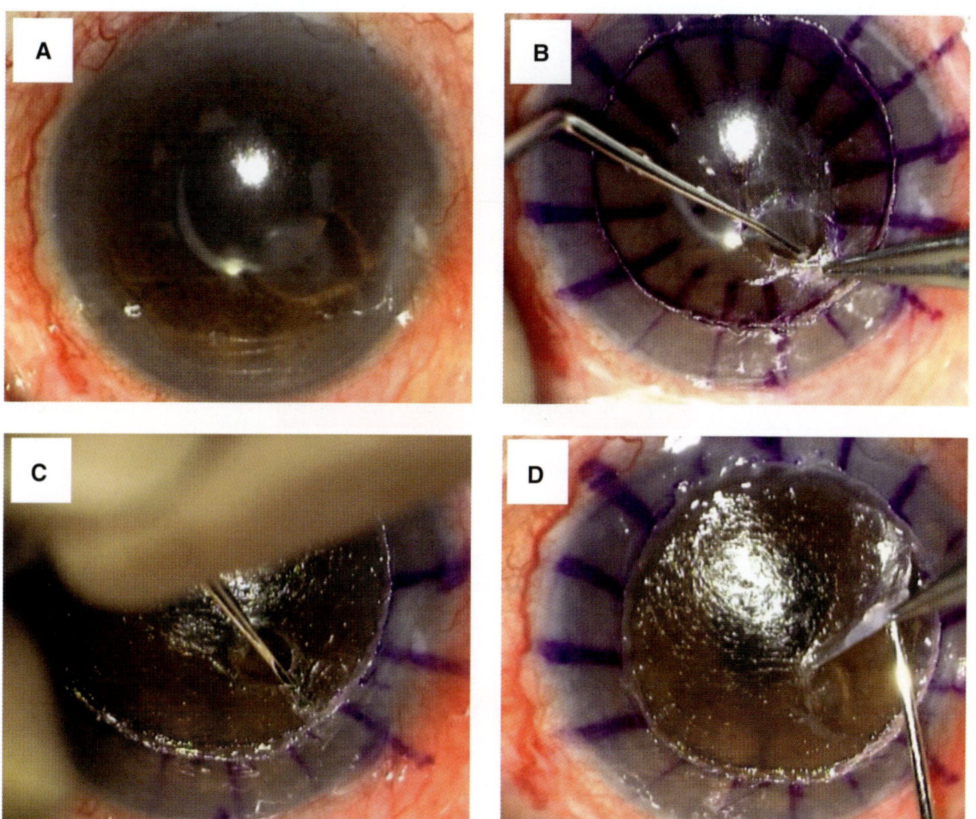

Fig. 20.3 Tectonic manual DALK for a descemetocele and intraoperative FD-OCT in a descemetocele. **(A)** Preoperative image (surgeon view). **(B)** With the aid of a blunt marginal dissector, the dissection was initiated from within the descemetocele. **(C and D)** Deeper surgical planes were further recognized, requiring multiple lamellar dissections.

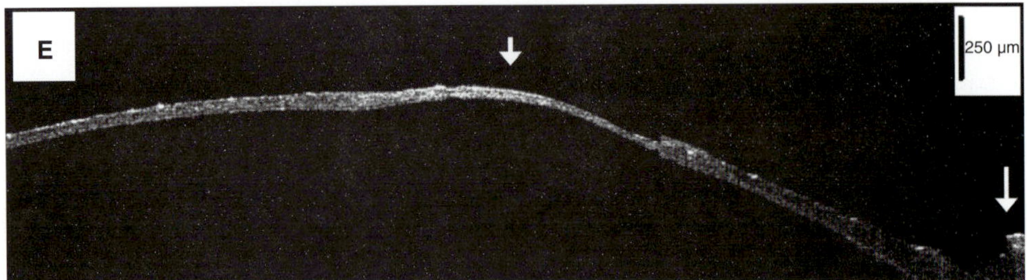

Fig. 20.3 (E) Intraoperative FD-OCT was used to assess thickness of remaining posterior stroma (30–60 μm). The herniated descemetocele (*small arrow*) and the trephination edge (*long arrow*) are also visualized.

Based on these observations the patient underwent a therapeutic manual DALK (**Fig. 20.3**). During the surgery, the FD-OCT (RTVue®; Optovue, Inc., Fremont, CA) was used to assess thickness of remaining posterior stroma (**Fig. 20.3E**). A description of the surgery can be found in **Figure 20.3**.

At day 10 postoperatively the graft was clear, well attached to the remaining posterior stroma, and had completely epithelized (**Figs 20.4 and 20.5**).

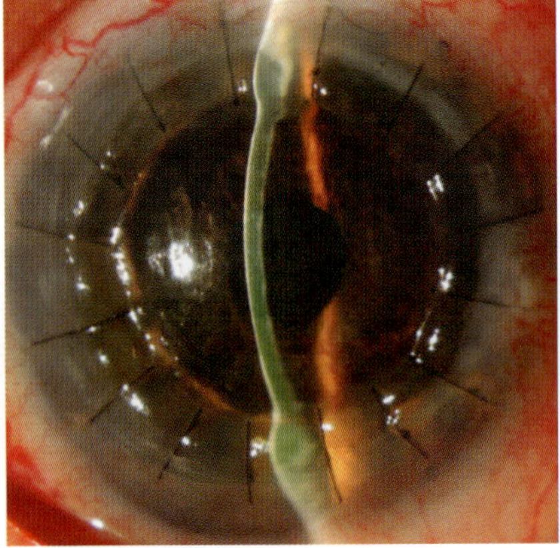

Fig. 20.4 Slit lamp photograph 10 days after DALK.

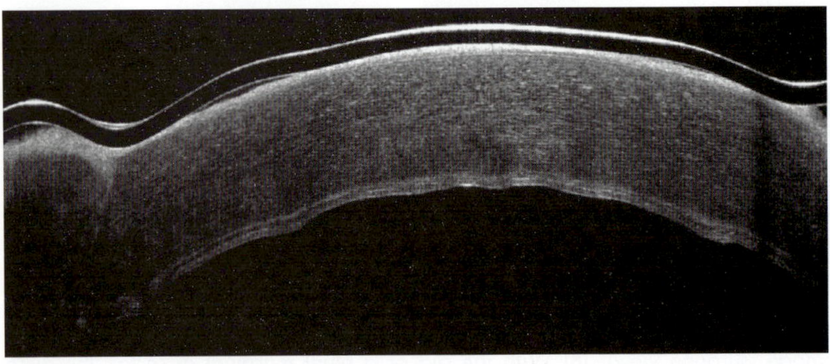

Fig. 20.5 The FD-OCT 10 days after DALK showed no DM detachment. Donor cornea had epithelized and a bandage contact lens is observed prior to removal.

DISCUSSION

DALK is an attractive surgical option in the management of descemetoceles. DALK has many advantages, including reduced risk of graft rejection, lower risk of intraocular infection, and better visual outcomes compared to penetrating keratoplasty (PK). However, the most frequent complication of DALK is inadvertent perforation of DM (Descemet's membrane) during surgery. Ultrasound pachymetry is routinely used to address this problem to assess depth of dissection plane; but it only measures the thickness of a single point on the cornea and is often inaccurate at sub-100-micron thicknesses. The advantage of the intraoperative FD-OCT is that it allows for multiple and simultaneous measurements that are shown as a pachymetric mapping and as a cross-sectional image of the cornea. This helps the surgeon to define whether he needs to dissect deeper or has reached the desired dissection depth. Therefore, it may help to reduce risk of inadvertent perforation. This aids the surgeon in planning the surgical approach, better-delineate anatomical planes, and improves intraoperative and postoperative successful achievement of a lamellar keratoplasty.

FURTHER READING

1. Gabison EE, Doan S, Catanese M, et al.: Modified deep anterior lamellar keratoplasty in the management of small and large epithelialized descemetoceles. *Cornea* 30(10):1179–1182, 2011.
2. Sharma N, Kumar C, Mannan R, et al.: Surgical technique of deep anterior lamellar keratoplasty in descemetoceles. *Cornea* 29(12):1448–1451, 2010.
3. Luengo-Gimeno F, Tan DT, Mehta JS, et al.: Evolution of deep anterior lamellar keratoplasty (DALK). *Ocul Surf* 9(2): 98–110, 2011.
4. Tan DT, Anshu A, Mehta JS: Paradigm shifts in corneal transplantation. *Ann Acad Med Singapore* 38(4):332–338, 2009.
5. Noble BA, Agrawal A, Collins C, et al.: Deep Anterior Lamellar Keratoplasty (DALK): Visual outcome and complications for a heterogeneous group of corneal pathologies. *Cornea* 26(1):59–64, 2007.
6. Anshu A, Parthasarathy A, Mehta JS, et al.:Outcomes of therapeutic deep lamellar keratoplasty and penetrating keratoplasty for advanced infectious keratitis. *Ophthalmology* 116(4):615–623, 2009.
7. Hosny M: Common complications of deep lamellar keratoplasty in the early phase of the learning curve. *Clin Ophthalmol* 5:791–795, 2011.
8. Hall RC, Mohamed FK, Htoon HM, et al.: Laser in situ keratomileusis flap measurements: comparison between observers and between spectral-domain and time-domain anterior segment optical coherence tomography. *J Cataract Refract Surg* 37:544–551, 2011.
9. Lim LSL, Aung HTH, Aung TT, et al.: Corneal imaging with anterior segment optical coherence tomography for lamellar keratoplasty procedures. *Am J Ophthalmol* 145(1):81–90, 2007.

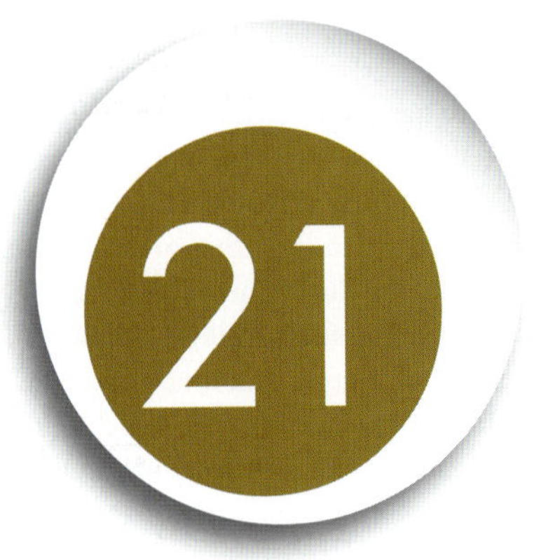

Keratoplasty—Femtosecond Laser-enabled Keratoplasty (FLEK)

Ashwini Ranganath, Himanshu Matalia, and Madhusmita Das

Advances in techniques and instrumentation in corneal transplantation have resulted in improved patient outcomes. With the advent of femtosecond laser, we now have potential for more finite control and precision in corneal surgery with minimal distortion of corneal tissue. Contoured or stepped-wound configurations can be achieved, the advantages of which are that the lamellar rim facilitates healing, keeps the anterior graft edge at a safe distance from the limbus, and gives freedom of transplanting either a relatively large or small diameter of endothelial cells, depending on the corneal pathology for which surgery is being performed. The laser allows for patterns and angles of incisions that are not achievable with conventional trephines.

Femtosecond laser is capable of creating the following patterns of trephination cuts:

1. Straight trephination cuts.
2. Complex-pattern trephination cuts (provides better wound integrity of the graft–host junction)
   a. Top-hat (with a larger diameter cut posteriorly): useful in conditions with diseased host endothelium like pseudophakic or aphakic bullous keratopathy.
   b. Mushroom (with a larger diameter cut anteriorly): useful in conditions with diseased anterior layers of cornea and healthy host endothelium like keratoconus.
   c. Zig-zag.
   d. Christmas tree.

Advantages of femtosecond laser-assisted penetrating keratoplasty (FLAK) over conventional manual penetrating keratoplasty:

- Superior incision integrity compared to traditional penetrating keratoplasty (PK)
  * Enhanced precision of the cuts
  * Highly reproducible dimensions of the cuts made in both host and donor tissues
  * Enhanced fit between donor and recipient cornea.
- Larger area of contact at donor–host junction.
- Rapid and better wound healing as well as less-induced astigmatism, there by promoting faster visual recovery.

CASE STUDY 1

A 31-year-old woman with OU (oculus uterque—both eyes)-advanced keratoconus underwent a mushroom-shaped FLAK in the right eye (Fig. 21.1). Preoperative best-corrected visual acuity was 6/60 in the right eye, with a spherical

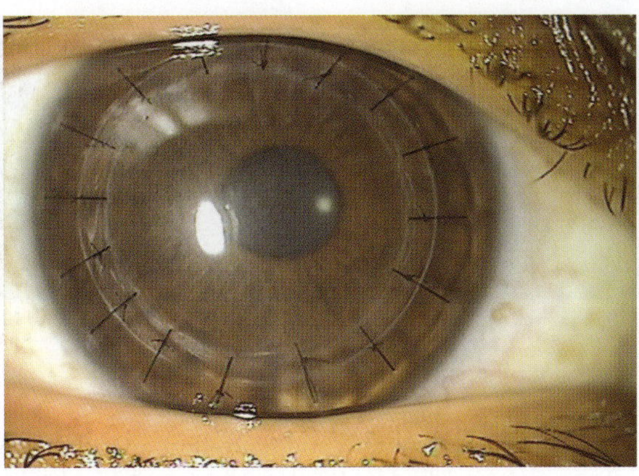

Fig. 21.1 Slit lamp image OD at 6-months follow-up.

equivalent of −10 D. One-month postoperatively, her uncorrected visual acuity was 6/18 improving to 6/9 with a spherical equivalent of −2.5 D. At sixth postoperative month, her uncorrected visual acuity was 6/9 with no refractive correction, which was maintained throughout 2 years of follow-up.

Anterior-segment optical coherence tomography (AS-OCT) was used to evaluate graft–host apposition and wound healing. The graft–host apposition was excellent, with both anterior and posterior corneal surfaces showing good alignment. The wound edge displayed mushroom-pattern cut and a good scar formation with increased signal, even as early as 1 month, with increasing signal intensity over subsequent follow-ups (**Fig. 21.2**). The stability was maintained at all times till the latest follow-up.

CORNEAL WOUND HEALING

Figure 21.3 shows AS-OCT images of a patient who underwent manual straight-cut PK at his first and third month of follow-up.

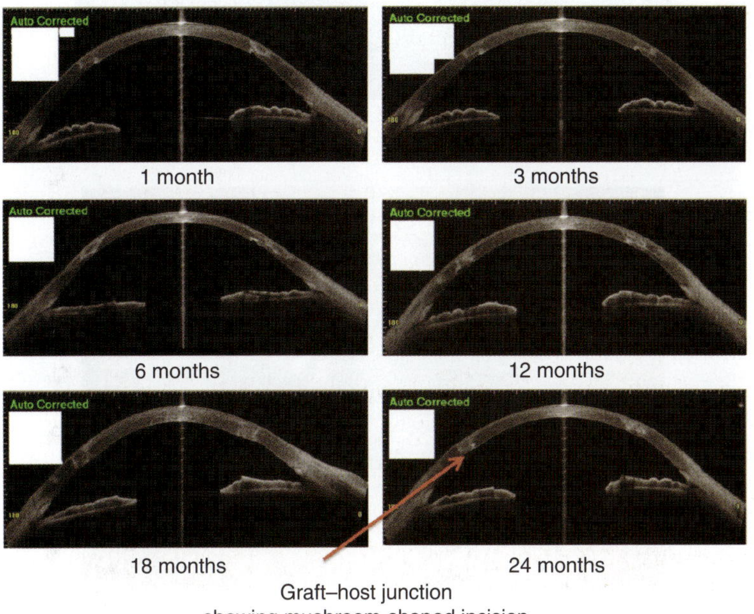

Fig. 21.2 Tomey AS-OCT images post-FLAK.

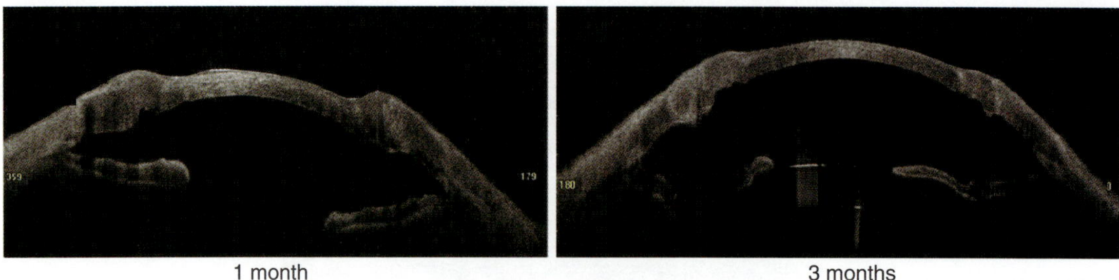

1 month   3 months

Fig. 21.3 AS-OCT images of a patient after penetrating keratoplasty.

We can note the difference in posterior graft contour and graft–host apposition between the AS-OCT images of the straight-cut PK and the mushroom-shaped FLAK. Mushroom-shaped FLAK reveals more-regular wound edges and better wound healing compared to manual PK in the early postoperative period.

CASE STUDY 2

Mushroom-shaped PK with eight sutures only (**Figs 21.4 and 21.5**) was done for a 23-year-old female with advanced keratoconus. She had unaided vision of 6/9, 1-month postoperatively.

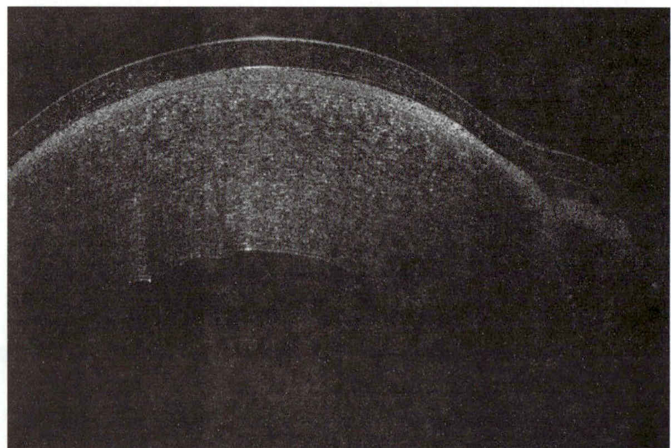

Fig. 21.4 SD-OCT (Bioptigen) images post-FLAK.

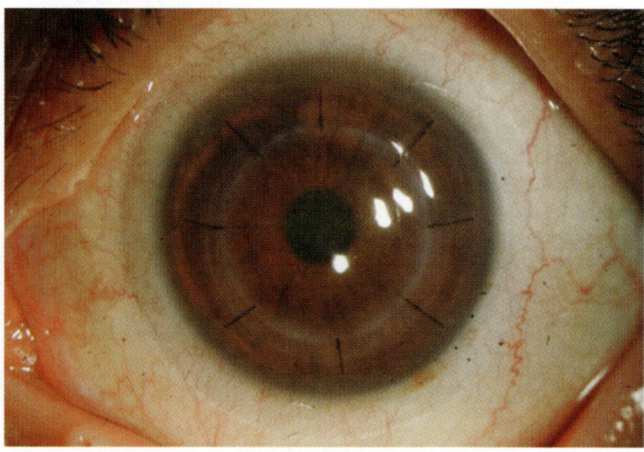

Fig. 21.5 Slit lamp photo 1 day post-FLAK.

FLAK is a feasible option for patients requiring penetrating keratoplasty; and it overcomes major postoperative problems associated with conventional manual PK like prolonged visual rehabilitation, and large and variable refractive errors. FLAK is a safe procedure, and is associated with early visual rehabilitation, faster refractive and topographic stabilization, and rapid and superior wound healing.

Femtosecond lasers are being used now in Descemet's stripping endothelial keratoplasty and deep anterior lamellar keratoplasty too.

FURTHER READING

1. Busin M: A new lamellar wound configuration for penetrating keratoplasty surgery. *Arch Ophthalmol* 121:260–265, 2003.
2. Busin M, Arffa RC: Microkeratome-assisted mushroom keratoplasty with minimal endothelial replacement. *Am J Ophthalmol* 140:138–140, 2005.
3. Farid M, Steinert RF, Gaster RN, et al.: Comparison of penetrating keratoplasty performed with a femtosecond laser zigzag incision versus conventional blade trephination. *Ophthalmology* 116:1638–1643, 2009.
4. Hoffart L, Proust H, Matonti F, et al.: Short term results of penetrating keratoplasty performed with the Femtec femtosecond laser. *Am J Ophthalmol* 146:50–55, 2008.
5. Binder PS: The effect of suture removal on post-keratoplasty astigmatism. *Am J Ophthalmol* 105:637–645, 1988.
6. Price FW, Price MO: Femtosecond laser shaped penetrating keratoplasty: one year results using a top hat configuration. *Am J Ophthalmol* 145:210–214, 2008.
7. Holzer MP, Rabsilber TM, Auffarth GU: Penetrating keratoplasty using femtosecond laser. *Am J Ophthalmol* 143:524–526, 2007.
8. Yoo SH, Hurmeric V: Femtosecond laser-assisted keratoplasty. *Am J Ophthalmol* 151(2):189–191, 2011.
9. Cheng YY, Hendriske F, Pels E, et al.: Preliminary results of femtosecond laser-assisted descemet stripping endothelial keratoplasty. *Arch Ophthalmol* 128(10):1351–1356, 2008.
10. Farid M, Steinert RF: Deep anterior lamellar keratoplasty performed with the femtosecond laser zig-zag incision for the treatment of stromal corneal pathology and ectatic disease. *J Cataract Refract Surg* 35(5):809–813, 2009.

Keratoprosthesis

Bhaskar Srinivasan and Geetha Iyer

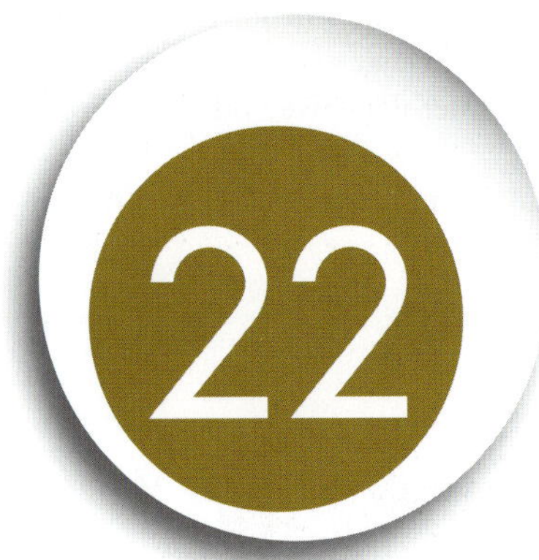

The Boston Keratoprosthesis (KPro) Type 1 is primarily used for those conditions wherein a conventional penetrating keratoplasty is likely to fail. This includes multiple graft failures and conditions with limbal stem cell deficiency without any underlying immunological condition (in a moist eye with adequate blink mechanism and lack of exposure). Recent modifications in design of prosthesis, technique, and postoperative regimen have ensured better results in terms of good retention rates, fewer incidences of melt, and infection.

CASE STUDY 1

A one-eyed–40-year-old male patient with decrease in vision due to multiple graft failures secondary to silicone oil-induced keratopathy underwent Boston Type 1 KPro.

The Visante anterior-segment optical coherence tomography (AS-OCT)(Carl Zeiss) shows normal appearance following the Boston KPro Type 1 in the following scan (**Fig. 22.1**).

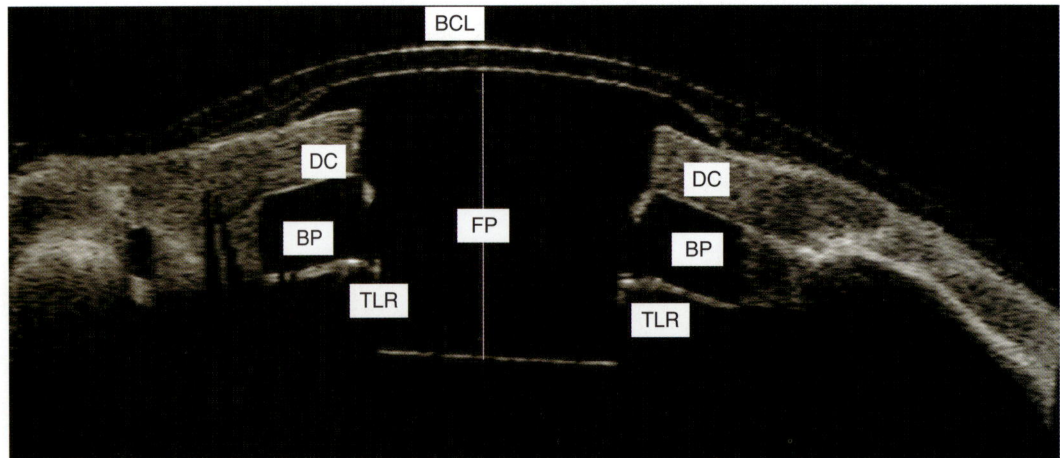

Fig. 22.1 BCL–bandage contact lens; FP–front plate; BP–back plate; DC–donor cornea; TLR–titanium locking ring.

CASE STUDY 2

A one-eyed–50-year-old male patient with decrease in vision due multiple graft failures secondary to silicone oil-induced keratopathy underwent Boston Type 1 Keratoprosthesis. The AS-OCT scan (**Fig. 22.2**) shows the presence of a retrokeratoprosthetic membrane thickening along the posterior surface of the front plate. Also noted in the scan is a hypoechoic area below the optic corresponding to an area of graft melt (**Fig. 22.2**) secondary to loss of bandage contact lens, as also observed in the slit lamp photograph (**Fig. 22.3**).

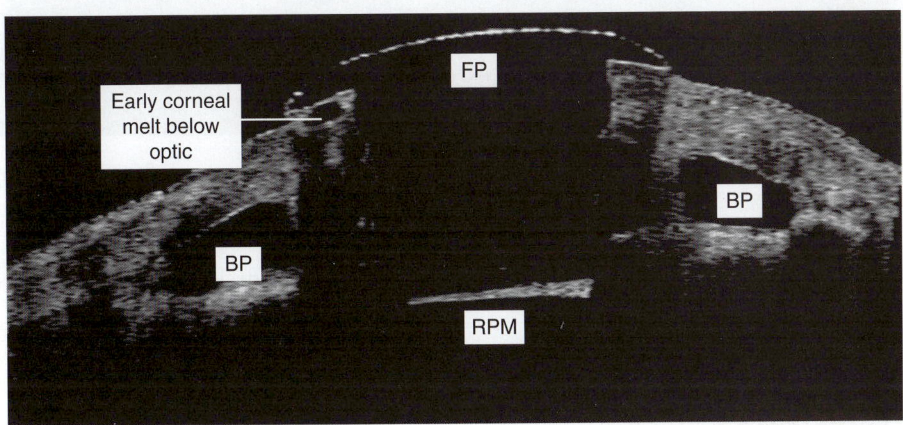

Fig. 22.2 RPM–retroprosthetic membrane. Note absence of bandage contact lens.

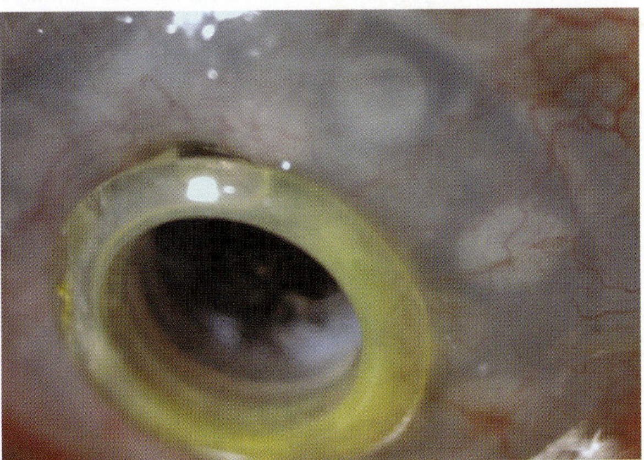

Fig. 22.3 Slit lamp photograph showing Boston Type 1 Keratoprosthesis (KPro) in situ, with melt below the optic superiorly and presence of retroprosthetic membrane.

CASE STUDY 3

A 30-year-old male with bilateral chemical injury underwent Boston KPro Type 1. The AS-OCT scan (**Fig. 22.4**) shows an intact posterior capsule in an aphakic eye with high reflective echoes in the anterior segment, probably corresponding to severe anterior segment inflammation in the immediate postoperative period.

The status of the implanted the Boston Type 1 KPro in terms of KPro–donor cornea interface and structural integrity of the assembled device can be better understood with the AS-OCT. These imaging techniques aid in evaluation of

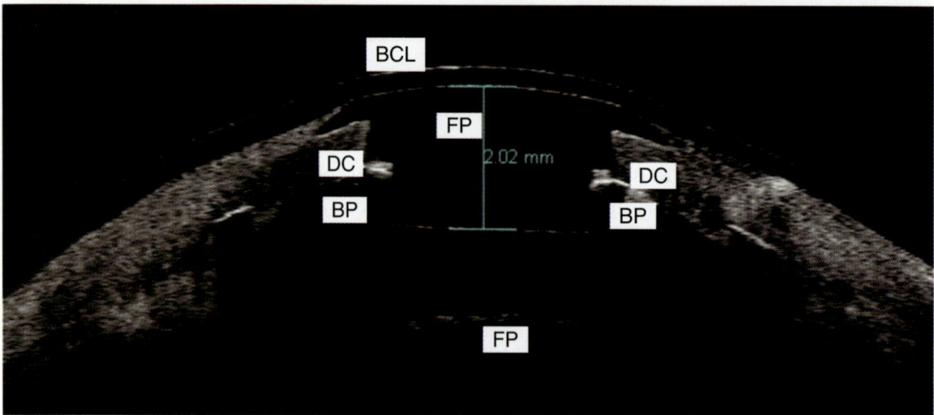

Fig. 22.4 BCL–bandage contact lens; FP–front plate; BP–back plate ; DC–donor cornea; PC–posterior capsule.

placement and position of the KPro, assist in understanding dynamics of the device, and help monitor early adverse developments.

FURTHER READING

1. Garcia JP Jr, Ritterband DC, Buxton DF, et al.: Evaluation of the stability of Boston type I keratoprosthesis-donor cornea interface using anterior segment optical coherence tomography. *Cornea* 29(9):1031–1035, 2010.
2. Garcia JP Jr, de la Cruz J, Rosen RB, et al.: Imaging implanted keratoprostheses with anterior-segment optical coherence tomography and ultrasound biomicroscopy. *Cornea* 27(2):180–188, 2008.

LASIK—Flaps

Sharon D'Souza and Rohit Shetty

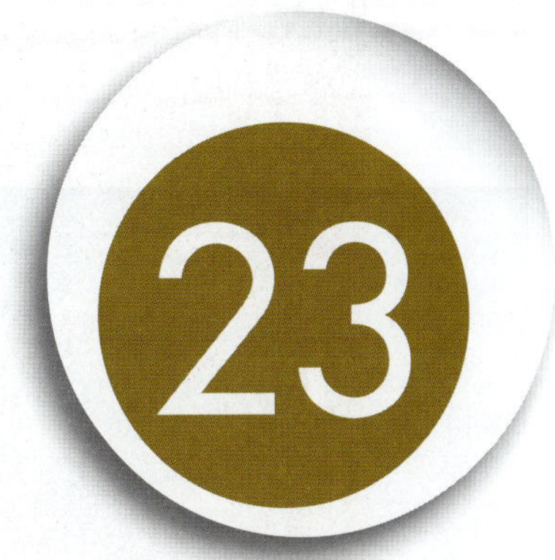

LASIK (laser-assisted in-situ keratomileusis) is a type of refractive surgery for correcting myopia, hyperopia, astigmatism, and even presbyopia. In this procedure a flap is created on the cornea using either a microkeratome or femtosecond laser. A microkeratome is a precise hand-held surgical instrument, with an oscillating metal blade which is used to make a horizontal incision at a particular depth in the corneal stroma to create a corneal flap. The femtosecond laser photo disrupts tissue at a preset depth, producing microcavitation bubbles of water and carbon dioxide. When the bubbles expand, it forms a resection plane by separating corneal lamellae. The flap is then lifted and excimer laser ablation is done on the stromal bed under the flap according to the refractive error to be corrected, after which the flap is replaced into position.

A good corneal flap is critical to ensure a successful outcome for the LASIK surgery and to prevent flap-related complications such as decentered flaps, free flaps, irregular flap edges, and buttonholes. Femtosecond lasers have evolved over the last decade and are becoming increasingly popular for flap creation; but the microkeratome blade is still widely used. In some studies it has been shown that corneal flaps created with the femtosecond laser are more predictable in depth and also have the advantage of customization according to the depth, morphology, and side-cut configuration. The various flap-creation modalities lead to different flap architectures. Femtosecond laser flaps (**Figs 23.1 and 23.2**) have been found to have a planar configuration, while microkeratome flaps are typically meniscus shaped (**Figs 23.3 and 23.4**). Either method of flap creation is acceptable, but femtosecond laser LASIK may induce fewer corneal aberrations, which could make it more suitable for wavefront-guided custom ablation.

CASE STUDY

A 26-year-old female patient presented to the hospital with a history of wearing spectacles since 12 years, with her last change in glass prescription being 3 years back. She was interested in undergoing LASIK for correcting her refractive error.

On examination
- Best-corrected visual acuity: 6/6 for the both eyes.
- Refraction: OD − 4.5 DSph / −1.0 DCyl × 170.
- OS − 4.0 DSph/ − 0.75 DCyl × 180 (same as previous prescription).
- Anterior segment examination was within normal limits.
- Dilated fundoscopy OU was within normal limits.
- Corneal topography done by Orbscan and Pentacam was within normal limits.
- Patient underwent femtosecond LASIK for both the eyes.
- Postoperative unaided visual acuity was 6/6 for both the eyes.

SD-OCT IMAGES

Femtosecond flap

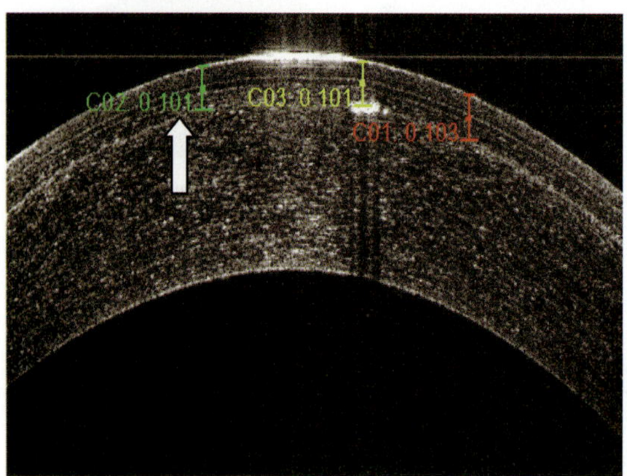

Fig. 23.1 Intraoperative measurement of femtosecond flap showing thickness of the flap at various points. [Photo courtesy: *Journal of Refractive Surgery* Vol. 28, Issue 11:S817 (Fig. 1B), November 2012.]

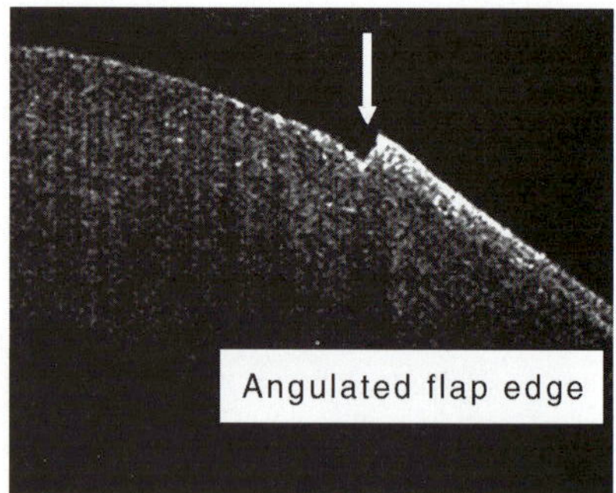

Fig. 23.2 Intraoperative measurement of femtosecond flap showing right-angled configuration of the flap edge. [Photo courtesy: *Journal of Refractive Surgery* Vol. 28, Issue 11:S818 (Fig. 4), November 2012.]

Microkeratome flap

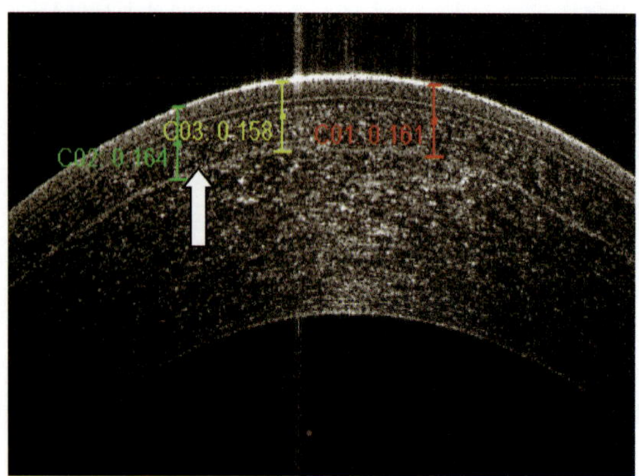

Fig. 23.3 Intraoperative measurement of microkeratome flap showing flap thickness at various points. [Photo courtesy: *Journal of Refractive Surgery* Vol. 28, Issue 11:S817 (Fig. 2B), November 2012.]

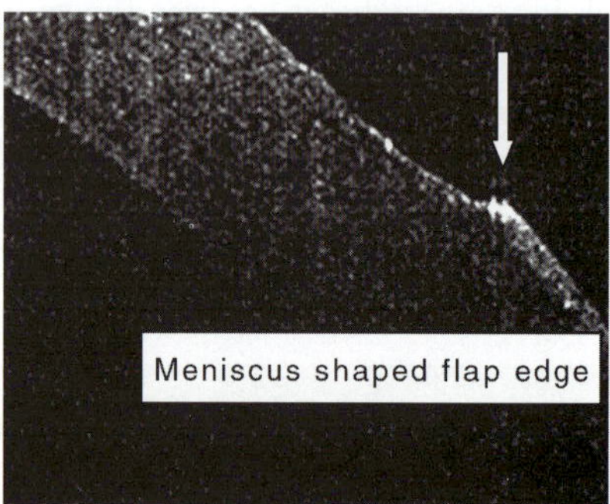

Fig. 23.4 Intraoperative measurement of microkeratome flap showing meniscus-shaped flap edge. [Photo courtesy: *Journal of Refractive Surgery* Vol. 28, Issue 11:S818 (Fig. 5), November 2012.]

FURTHER READING

1. Zhang ZH, Jin HY, Patel SV, et al.: Femtosecond laser versus mechanical microkeratome laser in situ keratomileusis for myopia: meta-analysis of randomized controlled trials. *J Cataract Refract Surg* 37:2151–2159, 2011.
2. Stulting RD, Carr JD, Thompson KP, et al.: Complications of laser in situ keratomileusis for the correction of myopia. *Ophthalmology* 106:13–20, 1999.

3. Gimbel HV, Anderson Penno EE, van Westenbrugge JA, et al.: Incidence and management of intraoperative and early postoperative complications in 1000 consecutive laser in situ keratomileusis cases. *Ophthalmology* 105:1839–1847, 1998.
4. Vaddavalli PK, Yoo SH: Femtosecond laser in-situ keratomileusis flap configurations. *Curr Opin Ophthalmol* 22(4): 245–250, 2011.
5. Holzer MP, Rabsilber TM, Auffarth GU: Femtosecond laser assisted corneal flap cuts: morphology, accuracy, and histopathology. *Invest Ophthalmol Vis Sci* 47:2828–2831, 2006.
6. Krueger RR, Dupps WJ: Biomechanical effects of femtosecond and microkeratome-based flap creation: prospective contralateral examination of two patients. *J Refract Surg* 23:800–807, 2007.
7. Alio JL, Pinero DP: Very high-frequency digital ultrasound measurement of the LASIK flap thickness profile using the IntraLase femtosecond laser and M2 and Carriazo-Pendular microkeratomes. *J Refract Surg* 24:12–23, 2008.
8. vonJagow B, Kohnen T: Corneal architecture of femtosecond laser and microkeratome flaps imaged by anterior segment optical coherence tomography. *J Cataract Refract Surg* 35:35–41, 2009.

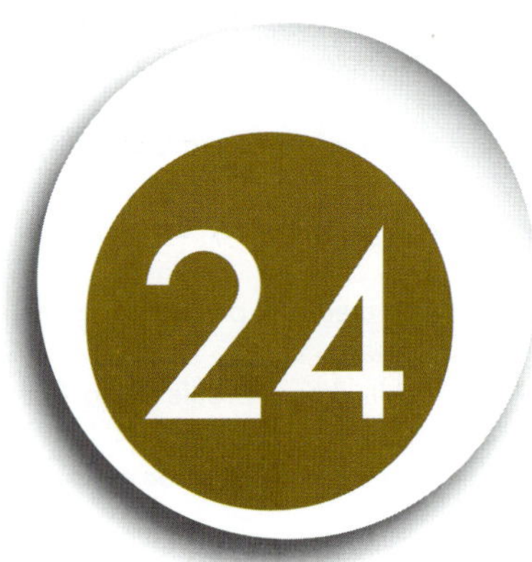

LASIK—Epithelial Ingrowth

Sharon D'Souza and Rohit Shetty

Epithelial ingrowth is an infrequent complication of laser-assisted in situ keratomileusis (LASIK) and usually clinically insignificant. It is a late postoperative complication of LASIK and can develop within 1 month of surgery and up to 5 months after the surgery. Epithelial cells proliferate in the lamellar interface causing opacification of interface and occasional melting of the LASIK flap. Typically, epithelial ingrowth starts at the edge of the flap and extends inwards (<0.5 mm). The ingrowth is insignificant and self-limiting in 14.7% of cases; and only about 1.7% of cases develop significant epithelial ingrowth requiring flap revision.

RISK FACTORS FOR DEVELOPING EPITHELIAL INGROWTH

Preoperative

- Epithelial defect
- Diabetes
- Epithelial ingrowth in other eye

Postoperative

- Epithelial defects
- Flap slippage within 24 hours/flap instability
- Diffuse lamellar keratitis

Intraoperative

- Epithelial defect/excessive irrigation with hydration of the flap
- Poor-quality blade
- Hyperopic LASIK
- Flap complications
- Foreign bodies in the interface

SURGICAL MANAGEMENT — VARIOUS MODALITIES

- Scraping of stromal bed
- Irrigation of stromal bed
- Flap reposition

ADJUVANT TREATMENTS (RECURRENT CASES/HIGH RISK OF RECURRENCE)

- Stromal bed
  - Mitomycin C
  - Alcohol
  - Phototherapeutic keratectomy
  - Nd:YAG (Neodymium-doped yttrium aluminium garnet) laser neodymium-doped yttrium aluminum garnet
- Flap repositioning
  - Suturing
  - Fibrin glue
  - Amniotic membrane graft

CASE STUDY

A 28-year-old male presented with chief complaints of difficulty in opening his eyes in bright light and watering of both the eyes for 3 months. He also complained of gradual and progressive blurring of vision in both the eyes (left eye > right eye) for 2 months. He had undergone LASIK [oculus uterque (OU)] 1 year back. LASIK recorrection was done in [oculus sinister (OS)] 6 months after initial refractive surgery. He developed symptoms 3 months after the recorrective surgery. On examination, his uncorrected visual acuity OD was 6/6, N6,OS was 6/9, N6. Refraction values were OD −0.25 Dsph and OS −0.5 Dsph/ −0.5Dcyl × 80°. A diagnosis of OS epithelial ingrowth (grade 3) post-enhancement LASIK surgery (**Figs 24.1–24.3**) was made. OS flap revision was done by flap lift and scraping along with application of mitomycin (0.02%) and suturing of flap edges.

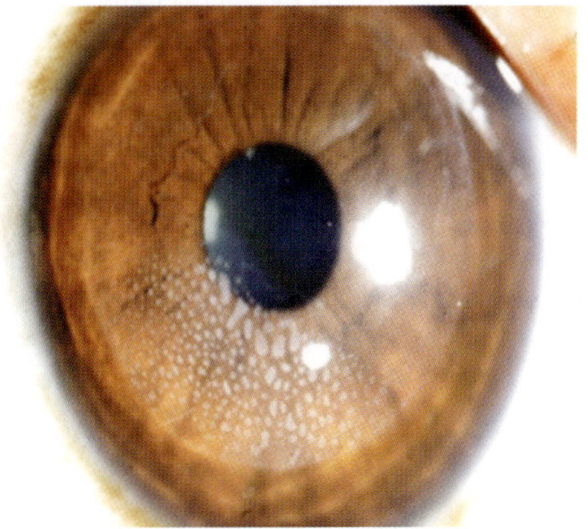

Fig. 24.1 Slit lamp photograph demonstrating epithelial ingrowth below LASIK flap.

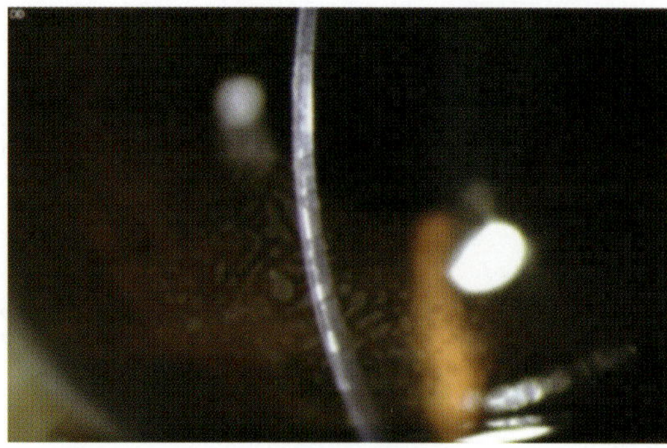

Fig. 24.2 Optical section of epithelial ingrowth.

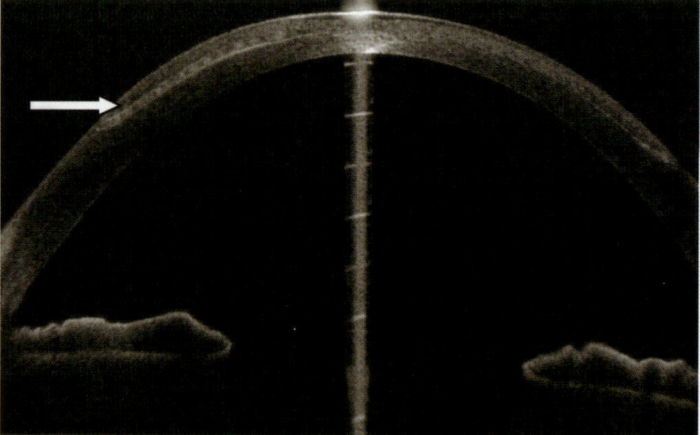

Fig. 24.3 AS-OCT image demonstrating epithelial ingrowth.

FURTHER READING

1. Wang M, Maloney R: Epithelial ingrowth after laser in situ keratomileusis. *Am J Ophthalmol* 129:746–751, 2000.
2. Carr JD: Risk factors for epithelial ingrowth after LASIK. *Invest Ophthalmol Vis Sci* 38(4):S232, 1997.
3. Brightbill FS: Corneal Surgery Theory, Technique, and Tissue, St. Louis: C V Mosby, ed 4, 835, 1986.
4. Tarek A. Post-laser-assisted in situ keratomileusis epithelial ingrowth and its relation to pretreatment refractive error. *Cornea* 30:550–552, 2011.

LASIK Complications—Interface Fluid Syndrome in a Steroid Responder

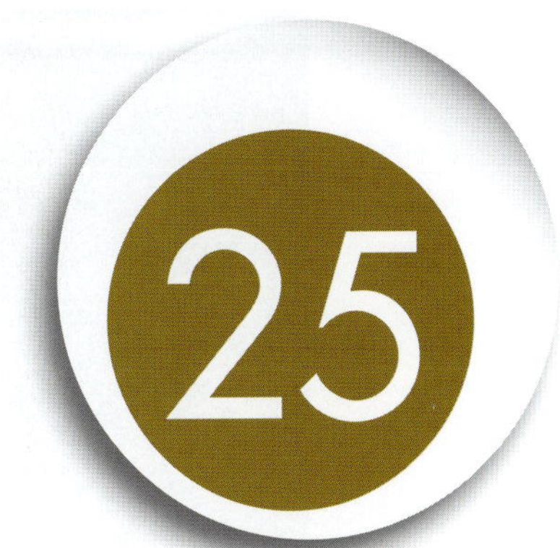

Sharon D'Souza and Rohit Shetty

Laser in situ keratomileusis (LASIK) is one of the most common and popular refractive surgeries performed for various refractive errors including myopia, hyperopia, and astigmatism. In spite of a lot of advancement in technology, flap-related complications can occur even in the hands of the most-experienced surgeon. Interface fluid syndrome (IFS) is one of the flap-related complications that can occur postoperatively in any patient. Patients with IFS usually present to the clinic with blurring of vision, anytime from a week to months after uneventful LASIK surgery. Slit lamp examination reveals a diffuse, nongranular haze in the central and paracentral areas of the flap interface. This haze can be mistaken for diffuse lamellar keratitis (DLK). Corneas with IFS may also have optically clear fluid-filled spaces between the LASIK flap and stromal bed. Steroid-induced ocular hypertension has been suggested to be the most common etiology for IFS, but it may be associated with other etiologies. Treating the primary condition and application of intraocular pressure (IOP)-lowering medication results in resolution of the IFS with no sequelae.

CASE STUDY

A 26-year-old gentleman was referred to our hospital after bilateral uncomplicated LASIK done elsewhere 2 weeks back. The patient had developed acute anterior uveitis postprocedure in the right eye and had been started on topical prednisolone acetate 1% every 2 hours. He presented with a history of pain and redness in the right eye since 1 week and blurred vision oculus dexter (OD) since 3 days. The preoperative intraocular pressure (IOP) was 12 mmHg in both the eyes.

Slit lamp biomicroscopy revealed a diffuse mild haze of the corneal flap in the right eye. Intraocular pressure was found to be 28 mmHg in the right eye and 14 mmHg in the left eye by Goldmann's applanation tonometry. Anterior-segment optical coherence tomography (AS-OCT) scans demonstrated an optically clear space between the LASIK flap and the stromal bed suggestive of fluid (**Fig. 25.1**); spectral-domain optical coherence tomography (SD-OCT) showed diffuse stromal haze suggestive of IFS (**Fig. 25.3**). The patient was administered Timolol (0.5%) eye drops, hypertonic Saline 5% eye drops and the topical steroid was reduced in the right eye. Patient improved symptomatically and repeat scans (**Figs 25.2 and 25.4**) after 1 week revealed no fluid in the interface with decreased corneal edema.

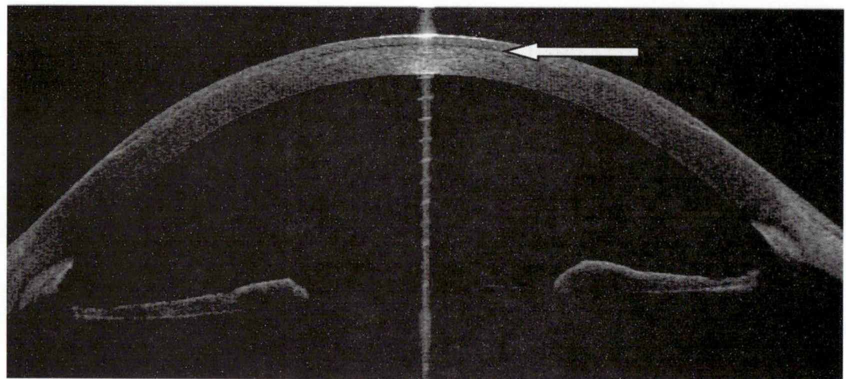

Fig. 25.1 Tomey AS-OCT OD—at presentation.

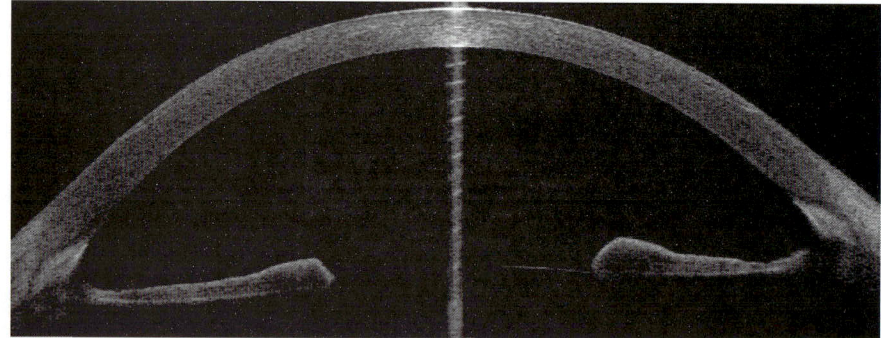

Fig. 25.2 Tomey AS-OCT OD—after 1 week of treatment.

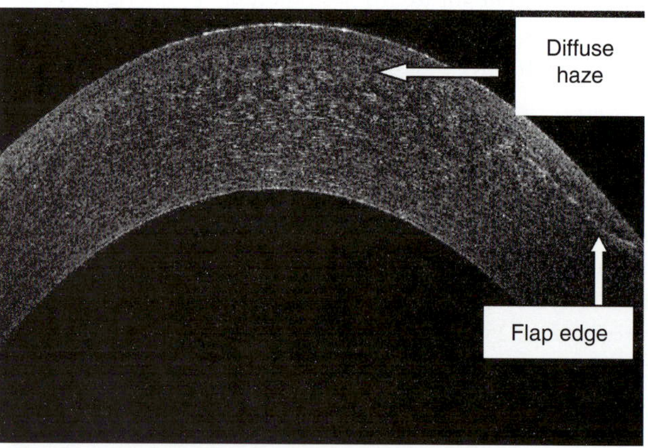

Fig. 25.3 SD-OCT—at presentation.

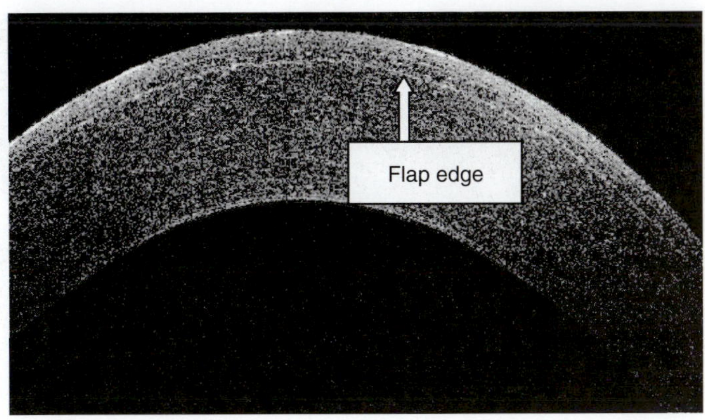

Fig. 25.4 SD-OCT—after 1 week of treatment.

FURTHER READING

1. Sandoval HP, de Castro LE, Vroman DT, et al.: *Refractive Surgery Survey 2004. J Cataract Refract Surg* 31:221–233, 2005.
2. Dawson DG, Schmack I, Holley GP: Interface fluid syndrome in human eye bank corneas after LASIK: causes and pathogenesis. *Ophthalmology* 114:1848–1859, 2007.
3. Lyle WA, Jin GJ: Interface fluid associated with diffuse lamellar keratitis and epithelial ingrowth after laser in situ keratomileusis. *J Cataract Refract Surg* 25:1009–1012, 1999.
4. Fogla R, Rao SK, Padmanabhan P: Interface fluid after laser in situ keratomileusis. *J Cataract Refract Surg* 27:1526–1528, 2001.
5. Buxey K: Delayed onset diffuse lamellar keratitis following enhancement LASIK surgery. *Clin Exp Optom* 87:102–106, 2004.
6. Najman-Vainer J, Smith RJ, Maloney RK: Interface fluid after LASIK: Misleading tonometry can lead to end-stage glaucoma. *J Cataract Refract Surg* 26:471–472, 2000.
7. Portellinha W, Kuchenbuk M, Nakano K, et al.: Interface fluid and diffuse corneal edema after laser in situ keratomileusis. *J Refract Surg* 17(suppl):S192–S195, 2001.
8. Dawson DG, Hardten DR, Albert DM: Pocket of fluid in the lamellar interface after penetrating keratoplasty and laser in situ keratomileusis. *Arch Ophthalmol* 121:894–896, 2003.
9. Lyle WA, Jin GJ, Jin Y: Interface fluid after laser in situ keratomileusis. *J Refract Surg* 19:455–459, 2003.
10. Russell GE, Jafri B, Lichter H, et al.: Late onset decreased vision in a steroid responder after LASIK associated with interface fluid. *J Refract Surg* 20:91–92, 2004.

Limbal Dermoid

Madhusmita Das and Himanshu Matalia

Limbal dermoids are choristomas (dysontogenetic benign tumors) which are tumors that originate from tissues which are uncharacteristic of its anatomical location. Limbal dermoids are seen in 1–3 of 10,000 newborn children and can occur solitarily or in combination with other ocular or extraocular malformation, as in Goldenhar syndrome, oculoauriculovertebral dysplasia, Schimmelpenning–Feuerstein–Mims phakomatosis, or epidermal nevus syndrome. Temporal inferior limbus is the most common location for occurrence of limbal dermoids. Collagenous tissue with hair follicles, sebaceous glands, and nerve tissue is the main composition of the stroma of limbal dermoid. Lipodermoids are commonly localized near the lateral canthus; their stroma consists mainly of fat tissue. Appropriate timing and type of surgical intervention is still a matter of debate in solid corneal dermoids to avoid amblyopia. Anatomically, limbal dermoids have been classified into three grades:

Grade 1: Superficial limbal dermoids

Grade 2: Limbal dermoids involving part of the corneal stroma

Grade 3: Limbal dermoids replacing the cornea and a part of the anterior segment.

CASE STUDY

A 15-year-old girl presented to our cornea clinic with chief complaints of a white mass in [oculus sinister (OS) (left eye)] since birth. She gave a history of undergoing mass excision at a local eye hospital 3 years back, and the mass having come back and gradually increasing in size. Her unaided vision in oculus uterque (OU) was 20/20. Dry retinoscopy readings were OD +0.50 DSph and OS +0.75 DSph/−0.50 D Cyl × 170°. On examination, her anterior segment oculus dexter (OD) was within normal limits and OS showed a whitish mass at the limbus (5.5 mm × 6 mm) with corneal involvement of 2 mm (**Fig. 26.1**). The mass was nontender, soft, with no overlying hair, etc. Dilated fundus examination OU was within normal limits. There was no preauricular skin tag or other significant systemic findings. A provisional diagnosis of OS limbal dermoid (recurrence status post excision elsewhere) was made. Bioptigen imaging of the limbal dermoid (**Fig. 26.2**) was done to make an attempt to evaluate extent and depth of corneal and scleral involvement. A total excision of the dermoid and amniotic membrane graft with fibrin glue and vicryl sutures was done (**Figs 26.3 and 26.4**). Postoperatively, she was advised antibiotic and steroid eye drops and was followed-up at regular intervals in our out patient department (OPD). When seen on her subsequent follow-up, 3 months following surgery, she was doing well and had dry refraction values of +0.25D Cyl × 140° in the operated eye.

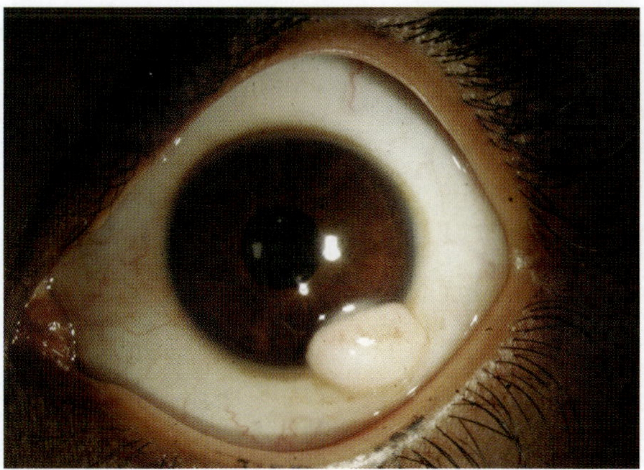

Fig. 26.1 Slit lamp photo—diffuse illumination demonstrating OS limbal dermoid.

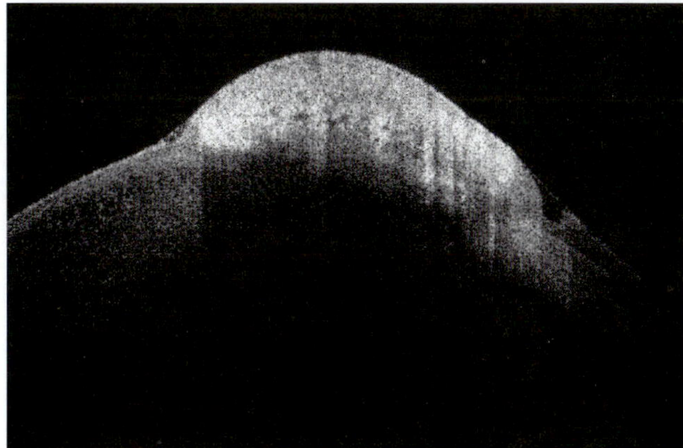

Fig. 26.2 Bioptigen image of OS limbal dermoid showing hyperechoic lesion at limbus and shadowing underneath.

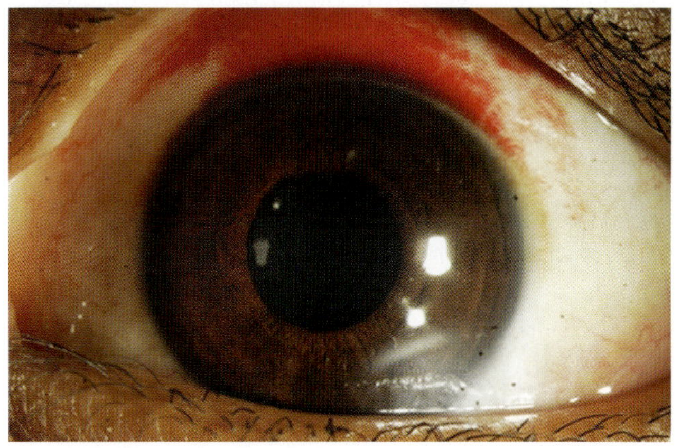

Fig. 26.3 Slit lamp photo OS on the first postoperative day.

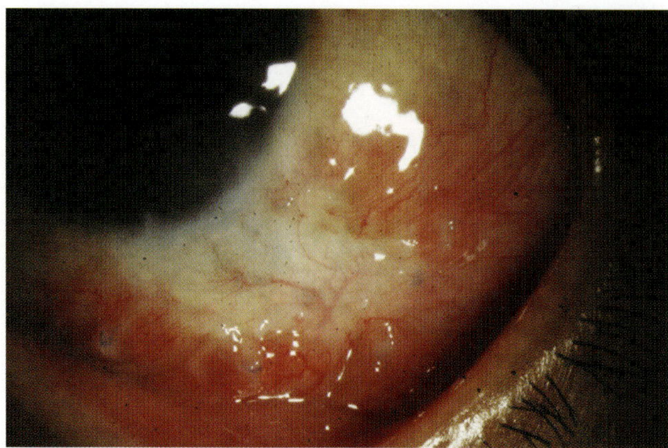

Fig. 26.4 Slit lamp photo OS first postoperative day showing total excision of dermoid from adjacent scleral area and amniotic membrane graft over excised area.

FURTHER READING

1. Pirouzian A, Ly H, Chuck RS, et al.: Fibrin-glue assisted multilayered amniotic membrane transplantation in surgical management of pediatric corneal limbal dermoid: a novel approach. *Graefes Arch Clin Exp Ophthalmol* 249:261–265, 2011.
2. Stergiopoulos P, Link B, Gottfried OH, et al.: Solid corneal dermoids and subconjunctival lipodermoids: impact of differentiated surgical therapy on the functional long-term outcome. *Cornea* 28:644–651, 2009.
3. Shen Y, Chen WI, Wang IJ, et al.: Full-thickness central corneal grafts in lamellar keratoscleroplasty to treat limbal dermoids. *Ophthalmology* 112:1955–1962, 2005.
4. Watts P, Michaeli-Cohen A, Rootman D, et al.: Outcome of lamellar keratoplasty for limbal dermoids in children. *J AAPO* S6:209–215, 2002.
5. Mann I. Developmental abnormalities of the eye, ed 2, Lippincott, 357–364, 1957.

Ocular Surface Squamous Neoplasia

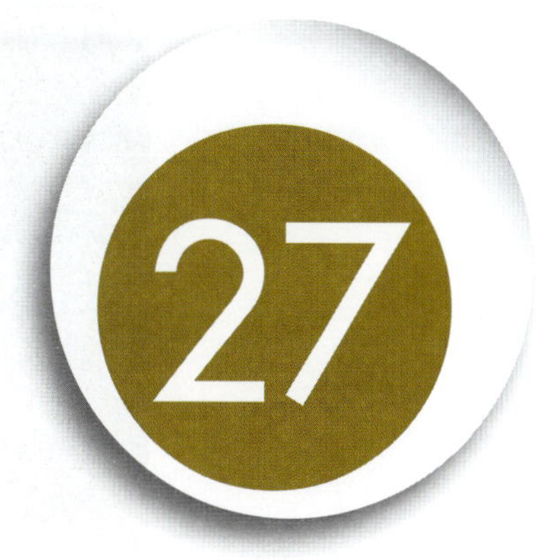

Patrick Oellers, Carol L Karp,
Jared L Matthews, Sander R Dubovy,
and Jianhua Wang

Ocular surface squamous neoplasia (OSSN) is the most common ocular surface tumor with a reported incidence of 0.19–1.9 per 1 million. It represents a spectrum of neoplastic diseases originating from the corneal or conjunctival epithelial cells. When confined to the epithelium, it is referred to as conjunctival or corneal intraepithelial neoplasia (CIN), which can be graded as mild, moderate, severe, or full thickness [carcinoma in situ (CIS)], depending on the degree of epithelial involvement. Squamous cell carcinoma (SCC) refers to epithelial tumors that have breached through the basement membrane of the conjunctiva or Bowman's layer of the cornea, respectively, and invaded into the stroma. Clinically, OSSN presents as a gelatinous, elevated papillary or leukoplakic lesion that is sometimes accompanied by feeder vessels. It arises most commonly near the corneal limbus, but can be found anywhere on the cornea or conjunctiva. On the cornea, it can have a frosted, granular appearance. After diagnosis, treatment is either surgical excision and cryotherapy, topical chemotherapy with Mitomycin-C, 5-fluorouracil, interferon-α-2b drops, interferon-α-2b local injections, or a combination of medical and surgical therapy.

CASE STUDY

A 54-year-old hispanic gentleman presented with a conjunctival lesion on the left eye. He did not have any history of medical problems related to OSSN, including skin cancer or genital warts. He was suffering from a foreign body sensation and redness of the left eye for 2 months, and was referred by his optometrist to our clinic.

Slit lamp examination revealed a normal right eye and a 5.5 mm × 6 mm sessile papilliform lesion on the left eye at the temporal limbus (Fig. 27.1) that was staining with Rose Bengal.

Ultra-high-resolution optical coherence tomography (UHR-OCT) of the lesion and adjacent areas showed a normal corneal epithelium with a sudden transition to a thickened and hyperreflective epithelium at the temporal limbus correlating to the papilliform lesion (Fig. 27.2).

The patient was taken to the operating room the following week. Using Shields' no-touch technique, the lesion was excised with 4-mm-wide conjunctival margins, along with alcohol corneal epitheliectomy, and cryotherapy (double freeze, slow thaw mode) to the conjunctival margins and limbus. The defect was closed using a cryopreserved amniotic membrane.

Pathology of excised conjunctival lesion showed a CIS (Fig. 27.3) with normal conjunctival margins. No invasion into the stroma was identified, and a moderate amount of solar elastosis as well as a moderate chronic lymphatic infiltrate was detected, underlying the neoplastic lesion within the stroma. Corneal cells that were yielded by alcohol epitheliectomy showed no definite cellular atypia.

At follow-up, the patient presented with a nicely healed ocular surface without any signs of recurrence or residual disease.

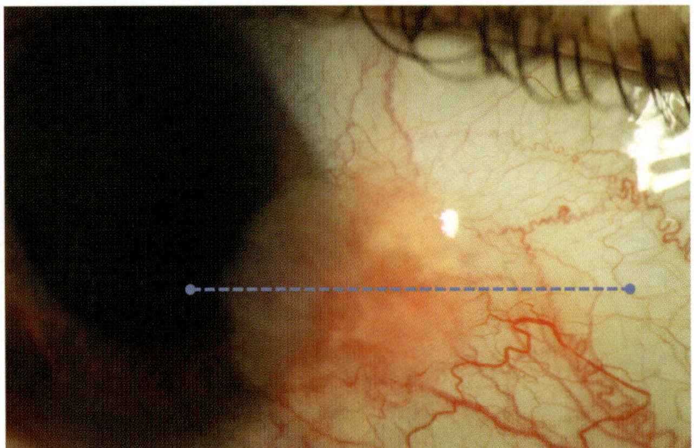

Fig. 27.1 Slit-lamp-photography image showing a 5.5 mm × 6 mm sessile papilliform lesion on temporal limbus of the left eye. The dashed line indicates area scanned by ultra-high-resolution optical coherence tomography (UHR-OCT).

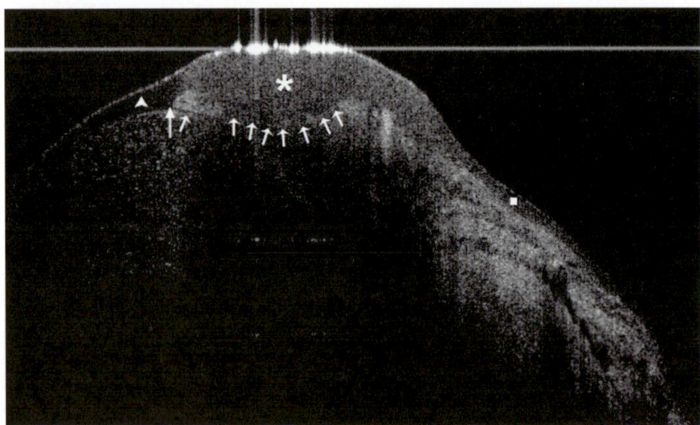

Fig. 27.2 Corresponding ultra-high-resolution optical coherence tomography (UHR-OCT) of the lesion demonstrates a thickened and hyperreflective epithelium of CIN lesion [indicated by an asterix (*)] at limbus compared to dark, hyporeflective, and thin normal epithelium of the cornea (*indicated by arrowhead*) and the thin, hyporeflective conjunctival epithelium (*indicated by square*). There is a characteristic abrupt transition (*indicated by large arrow*) between the normal corneal epithelium and tumor. In several areas, basement membrane can be visualized beneath the lesion suggesting noninvasion (*indicated by small arrows*). The shadow underneath is due to nontranslucency of the lesion.

Ultra-high resolution optical coherence tomography (UHR-OCT) is a valuable tool in detection and management of OSSN. With 2–3-micron resolution, it can be used to initially diagnose conjunctival or CIN, as well as to monitor therapy and possible recurrence. Essentially an "optical biopsy," features of OSSN on optical coherence tomography (OCT) imaging are a sudden transition from normal epithelium towards a more thickened and hyperreflective epithelium. To demonstrate sudden transition between healthy tissue and neoplastic lesion, we suggest showing the lesion next to normal conjunctiva or the cornea in the same image. Subepithelial mass lesions such as pinguecula or pterygia, which are sometimes hard to differentiate from OSSN clinically, demonstrate a circumscribed, subepithelial process with a normal-appearing epithelium on top. In addition to diagnosing CIN at initial presentation, UHR-OCT is capable of detecting subclinical disease during the course of treatment. This is used to follow and guide medical therapy of OSSN lesions until complete resolution. There can be situations when the lesion appears clinically resolved but still shows residual evidence on UHR-OCT. In such cases, the UHR-OCT

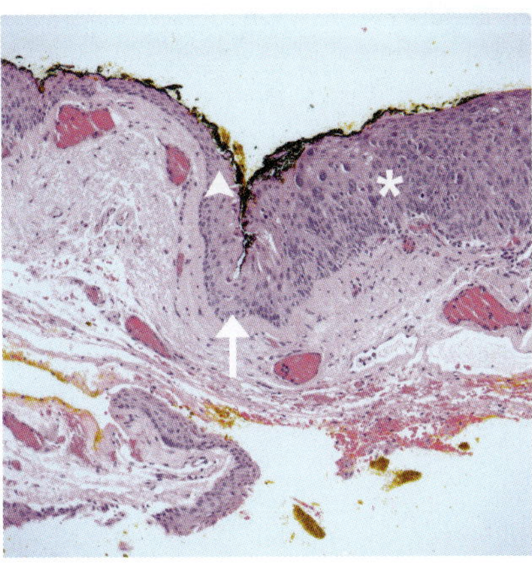

Fig. 27.3 200×-magnified microscopic hematoxylin and eosin (H&E) histologic image of corresponding specimen obtained from surgery shows faulty epithelial maturational sequencing that extends full thickness (CIS indicated by *) adjacent to thinner normal-appearing conjunctival epithelium (*indicated by arrowhead*). The transitional zone between normal conjunctiva and tumor lesion is marked by an arrow. The histopathology correlates nicely with UHR-OCT.

can prevent premature termination of therapy, which would leave cancerous cells behind. After complete treatment response, UHR-OCT can be used in the follow-up period to monitor for recurrences, which may be detected before they become clinically apparent.

In summary, UHR-OCT is an excellent tool to diagnose and follow OSSN, which demonstrates a thickened and hyperreflective epithelium with a sudden transition to normal at the margins.

FURTHER READING

1. Shousha MA, Karp CL, Perez VL, et al.: Diagnosis and management of conjunctival and corneal intraepithelial neoplasia using ultra high-resolution optical coherence tomography. *Ophthalmology* 118(8):1531–1537, 2011.
2. Kieval J, Karp CL, Shousha MA, et al.: Ultra-High resolution coherence tomography for differentiation of ocular surface squamous neoplasia and pterygia. *Ophthalmology* 119(3):481–486, 2012.
3. Giaconi JA, Karp CL: Current treatment options for conjunctival and corneal intraepithelial neoplasia. *Ocul Surf* 1(2):66–73, 2003.
4. Lee GA, Hirst LW: Ocular surface squamous neoplasia. *Surv Ophthalmol* 39(6):429–450, 1995.

Acknowledgments: The authors would like to acknowledge the support of Max Kade Foundation, The Ronald and Alicia Lepke Grant, The Claire and Lee Hager Grant, and the Jimmy and Gaye Bryan Grant.

Pinguecula

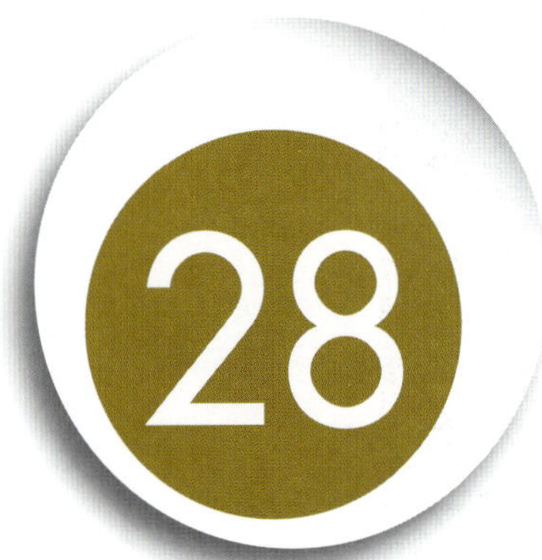

Tarek Ahmed Mohamed and Wael Soliman

Pinguecula is a gray–white nodule of the conjunctiva located in the temporal or the nasal bulbar conjunctiva, not involving the cornea. Histopathology of the pinguecula includes conjunctival epithelial changes, which vary between atrophy, hyperplasia, metaplasia, or dysplasia, in addition to hyalinized subepithelial collagen with elastotic degeneration.

CASE STUDY

A 33-year-old female sought medical advice because she was worried about a small nodule in the white part of her left eye. The nodule was painless and non progressive. Slit lamp examination revealed a small pinguecula (**Fig. 28.1**) and the patient was assured about the benign nature of this nodule.

Spectral-domain optical coherence tomography (SD-OCT) allowed a more detailed visualization of the extent of the lesion. This included localization of the lesion within the conjunctival stroma, which was contained by the corneal limbal boundary.

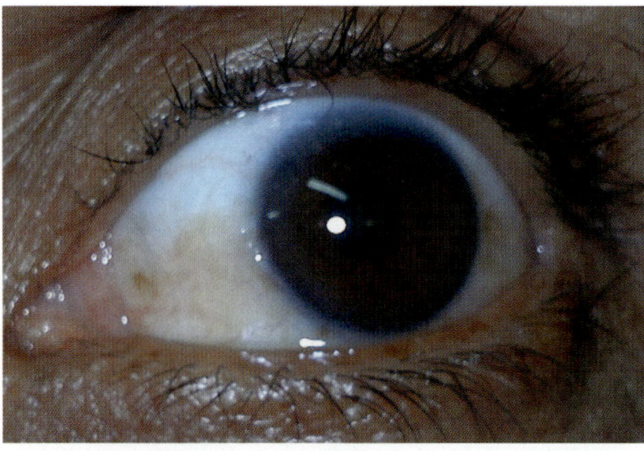

Fig. 28.1 Slit lamp photograph demonstrating nasal pinguecula.

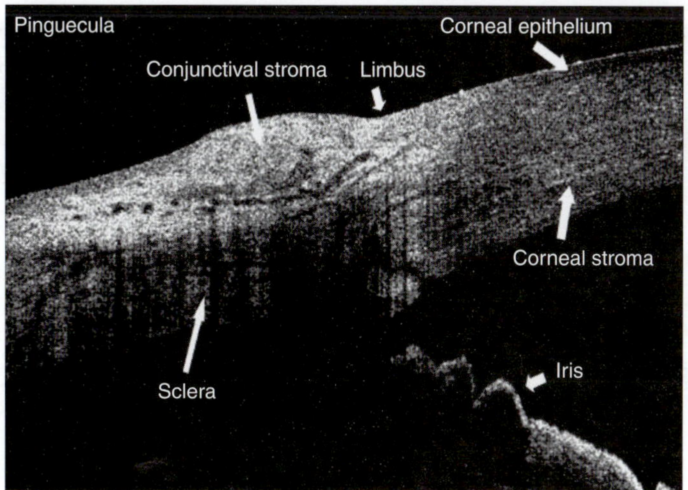

Fig. 28.2 SD-OCT image of pinguecula.

As previously suggested in literature, pingueculae do not invade the corneal limbal barrier. SD-OCT imaging (**Fig. 28.2**) of this lesion further corroborates this finding.

FURTHER READING

1. Archila EA, Arenas MC: Etiopathology of pinguecula and pterygium. *Cornea* 14:543–544, 1995.
2. Sarunic MV, Asrani S, Izatt JA: Imaging the ocular anterior segment with real-time, full-range Fourier-domain optical coherence tomography. *Arch Ophthalmol* 126:537–542, 2008.
3. Soliman W, Mohamed TA: Spectral domain anterior segment optical coherence tomography assessment of pterygium and pinguecula. *Acta Ophthalmol* 90(5):461–465, 2010.

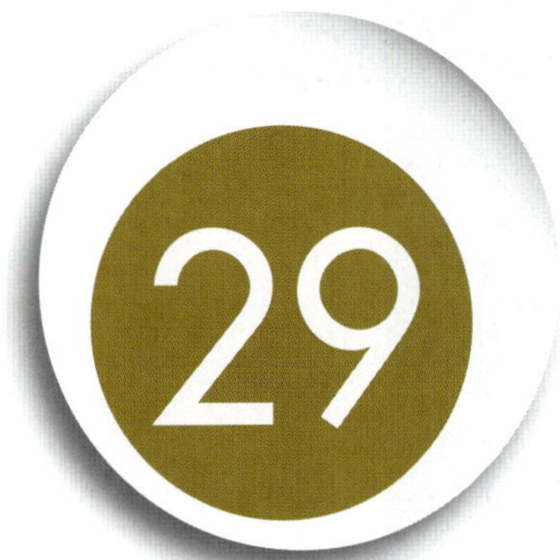

Pterygium

Tarek Ahmed Mohamed and Wael Soliman

Pterygium is a wing-shaped, gray–white thickening located in either the nasal or the temporal limbus, with an apex extending towards the cornea. Superficial blood vessels feature prominently and point towards the apex of the mass. Histologically, pterygium is characterized by elastotic degeneration of conjunctival substantia propria, with associated eosinophilic or basophilic deposits. Epithelial changes are variable and include hyperkeratosis, parakeratosis, or acanthosis.

CASE STUDY

A 45-year-old male farmer presented with a history of an unsightly red growth in the nasal side of his eye of 1-year duration. He claimed that the growth was progressive and had started to affect his vision. He was diagnosed as a case of pterygium (**Fig. 29.1**).

At the extreme superior and inferior periphery of the wing of the pterygium, there were satellites of pterygium masses beyond the apparent peripheral edge of the lesion at the corneal edge of the pterygium (**Figs 29.2 and 29.3**). Therefore, we assumed that excision of the pterygium with a large safety margin at the conjunctival or the corneal sides of the pterygium would reduce recurrence rates, as it would remove the tissue more completely. Anterior-segment spectral-domain optical coherence tomography (SD-OCT) helped us define the full extent of the pterygium not visible clinically.

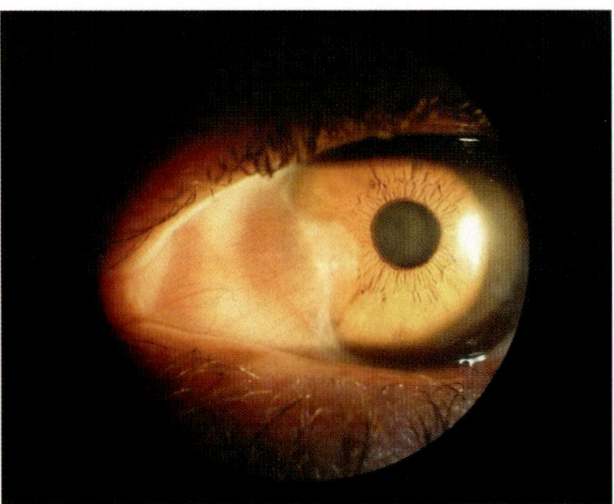

Fig. 29.1 Nasal pterygium.

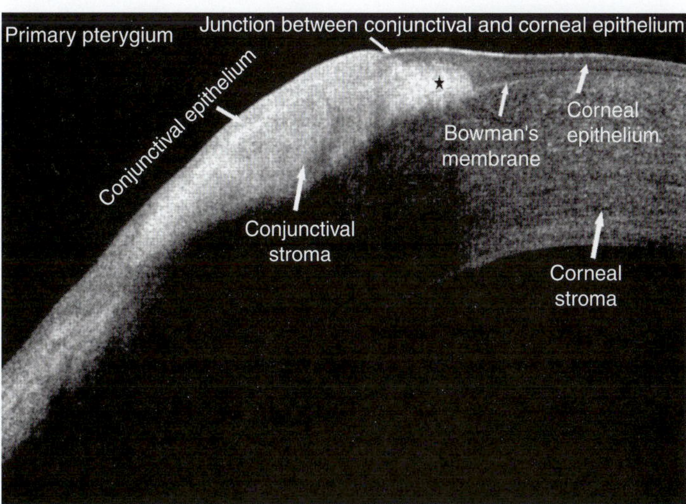

Fig. 29.2 SD-OCT image of the primary pterygium. Spectral-domain optical coherence tomography (SD-OCT) helped us define the true anatomical extent of the mass in relationship to the cornea.

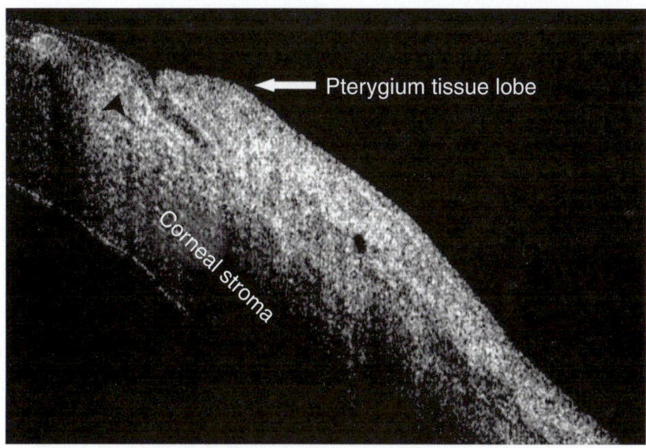

Fig. 29.3 SD-OCT image (high magnification) demonstrating the pterygium tissue lobe.

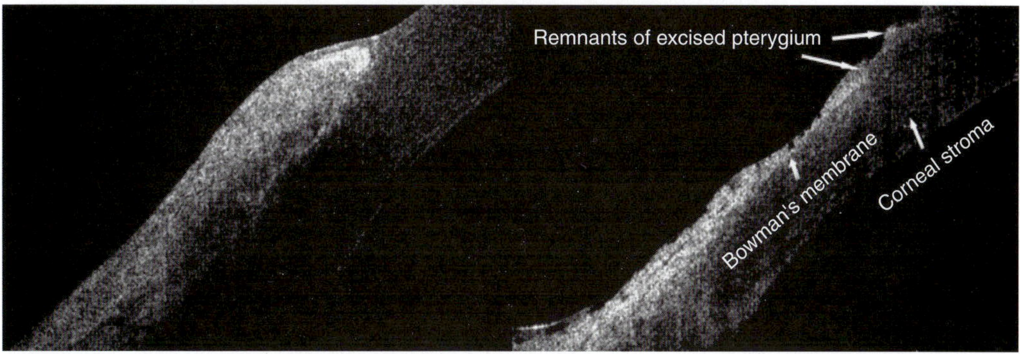

Fig. 29.4 SD-OCT images preoperative (*left panel*) and intraoperative (*right panel*) demonstrating remnants of the excised pterygium seen as hyperlucent areas.

Immediately after simple excision of the primary pterygium with bare sclera, multiple remnants on the corneal and conjunctival surfaces were visible on the anterior segment SD-OCT (**Fig. 29.4**). This elucidates the importance of smoothening the corneal and conjunctival sides after pterygium excision.

The use of a hand-held anterior segment SD-OCT may be of great value in defining the extent of pterygium excision, by providing a real time in vivo image, which ensures complete removal of this lesion. Kheirkhah et al. have demonstrated utility of anterior-segment optical coherence tomography (AS-OCT) in evaluation of the conjunctival graft thickness after pterygium surgery.

FURTHER READING

1. Raizada IN, Bhatnagar NK: Pinguecula and pterygium (a histopathological study). *Indian J Ophthalmol* 24:16–18, 1976.
2. Archila EA, Arenas MC: Etiopathology of pinguecula and pterygium. *Cornea* 14: 543–544, 1996.
3. Soliman W, Mohamed TA: Spectral domain anterior segment optical coherence tomography assessment of pterygium and pinguecula. *Acta Ophthalmol* 90(5):461–465, 2010.
4. Kheirkhah A, Adelpour M, Nikdel M, et al.: Evaluation of conjunctival graft thickness after pterygium surgery by anterior segment optical coherence tomography. *Curr Eye Res* 36(9):782–786, 2011.
5. Kieval JZ, Carp LK, Shosha MA, et al.: UltraHigh resolution optical coherence tomography for differentiation of ocular surface squamous neoplasia and pterygia. *Ophthalmololgy* 119(3):481–486, 2012.

Radial Keratotomy: Acute Hydrops

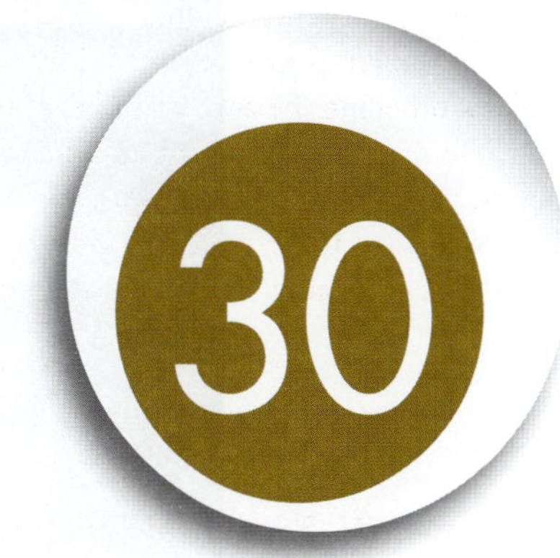

Tushar Agarwal and Amit Sobti

Radial keratotomy (RK) was one of the first refractive surgical procedures. After being in vogue till the 1990s, it went out of repute. This happened due to a progressive hyperopic shift caused by RK, unpredictable visual results due to irregular wound healing, corneal scars, corneal ectasia, risk of endophthalmitis, and corneal infections.

CASE STUDY

A 38-year-old man presented with complaint of sudden onset of whiteness in the right eye. The patient was being treated elsewhere as a case of corneal ulcer with no improvement in symptoms. The patient had undergone RK in both eyes 15 years back. Slit lamp examination showed a white edematous appearance of the cornea with minimal congestion (Fig. 30.1).

Anterior-segment optical coherence tomography (AS-OCT) (Visante) demonstrated an edematous cornea in the center with a localized Descemet's membrane rupture allowing a portal for fluid conduit into the corneal stroma (Fig. 30.2).

Based on clinical examination and AS-OCT findings, a diagnosis of acute hydrops in the right eye was made. The patient was started on a course of prednisolone 1%, homatropine 2%, and oral acetazolamide for a period of 3 weeks. On follow-up, corneal edema disappeared with a visual improvement to 6/36 on Snellen chart.

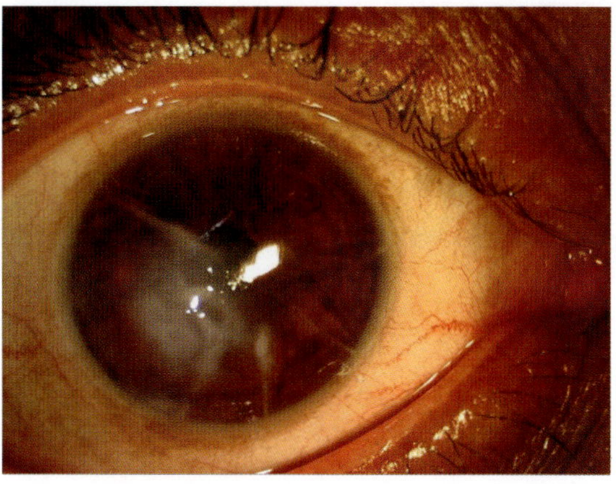

Fig. 30.1 Slit lamp photograph demonstrating corneal hydrops post-RK.

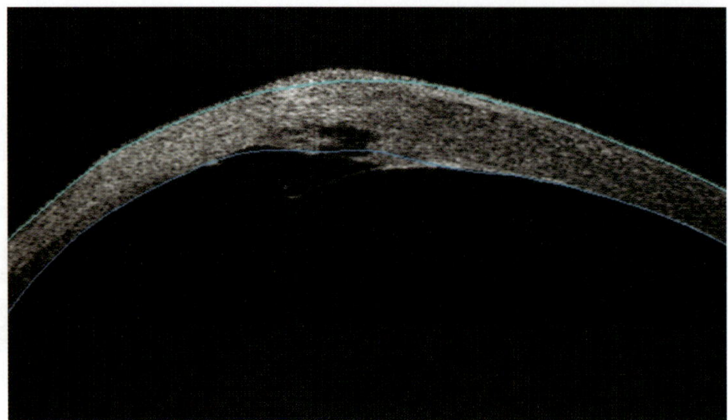

Fig. 30.2 Visante AS-OCT image demonstrating Descemet's membrane rupture and fluid conduit into the corneal stroma.

Though RK is no longer practiced, older patients who have undergone RK can still present with complications. Hydrops, though a rare complication, can be seen in such cases. AS-OCT can be a helpful modality to clearly delineate Descemet's membrane rupture in such cases.

FURTHER READING

1. Binder P, Nayak S, Deg J, et al.: An ultrastructural and histochemical study of long-term wound healing after radial keratotomy. *Am J Ophthalmol* 15:103:432–440,1987.
2. Waring G, Lynn M, McDonnell P: Results of the prospective evaluation of radial keratotomy (PERK) study 10 years after surgery. *Arch Ophthalmol* 112:1298–1308, 1994.
3. Sharma N, Sachdev R, Jindal A, et al.: Acute hydrops in keratectasia after radial keratotomy. *Eye Contact Lens* 36(3): 185–187, 2010.

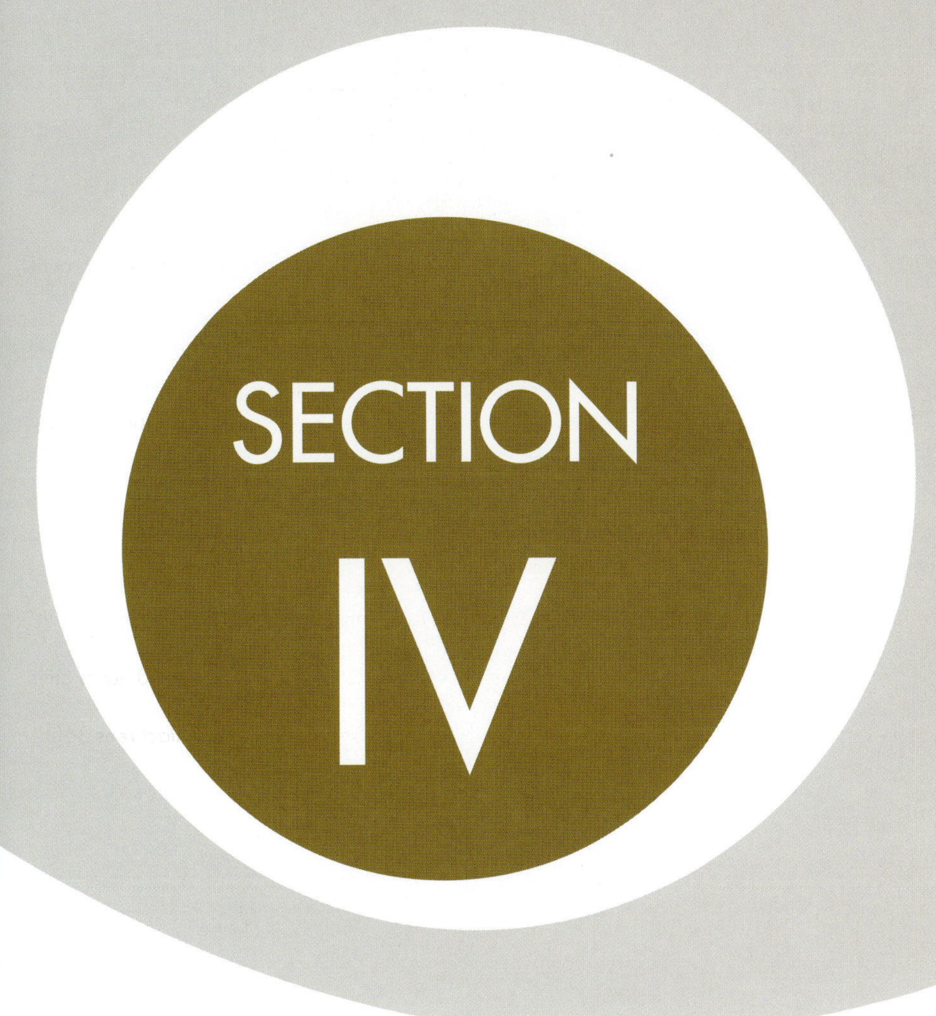

Lens

Aniridia

Mathew Kurien, Sudeep Das, and Rashmi Shetty

Congenital aniridia is a rare ocular malformation that affects development of multiple ocular structures. This abnormality is caused by a mutation in the *PAX6* gene located on chromosome 11p13. Iris hypoplasia is the most obvious sign, but a broad spectrum of disorders can manifest from various mutations in the *PAX6* gene. Many patients develop corneal opacities, cataracts, nystagmus, and foveal and optic nerve hypoplasia. Aniridia typically causes severe visual impairment; foveal hypoplasia is a major factor that can decrease visual function in these patients. Two-third of aniridia cases have autosomal dominant inheritance, while one-third are sporadic.

CASE STUDY

A 25-year-old woman presented to us with decreased vision in both the eyes from birth and increased blurring for past 6 months. On evaluating her, she had nystagmus, almost total aniridia in both eyes (**Figs 31.1 and 31.2**), cataractous lens with absent zonules and foveal hypoplasia in both the eyes. She underwent phacoemulsification with capsular tension rings (CTR) and foldable posterior chamber intraocular lens (PCIOL) implantation in the bag (**Fig. 31.3**). Anterior-segment optical coherence tomography (AS-OCT) postoperatively showed the PCIOL well placed in the capsular bag (**Fig. 31.4**).

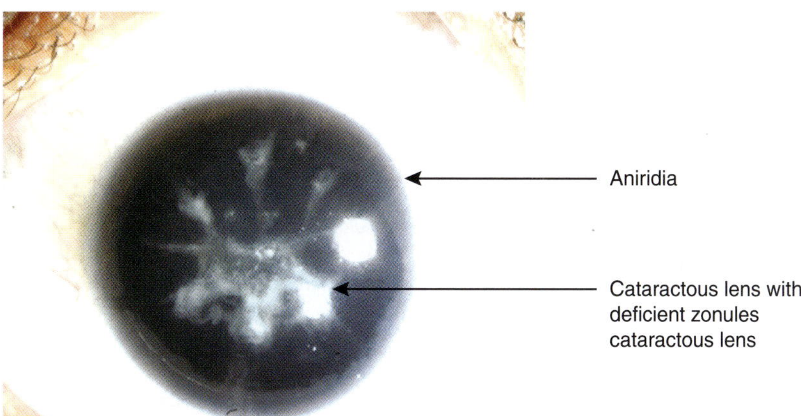

Fig. 31.1 Preoperative slit lamp photograph.

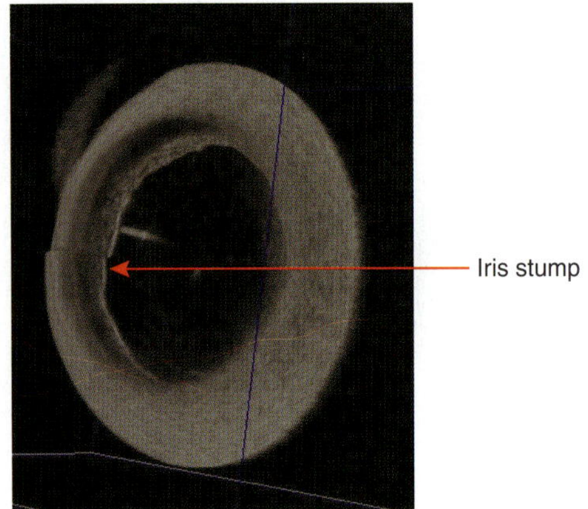

Fig. 31.2 Anterior-segment optical coherence tomography (gonioscopic view) showing an absent iris with only an iris stump seen all around.

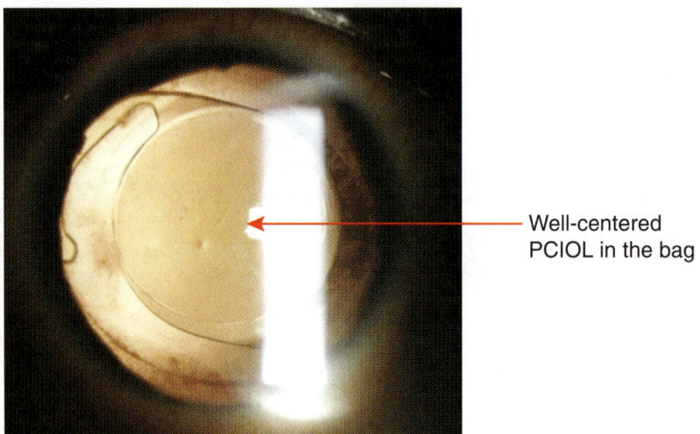

Fig. 31.3 Slit lamp image showing well-centered PCIOL in the bag.

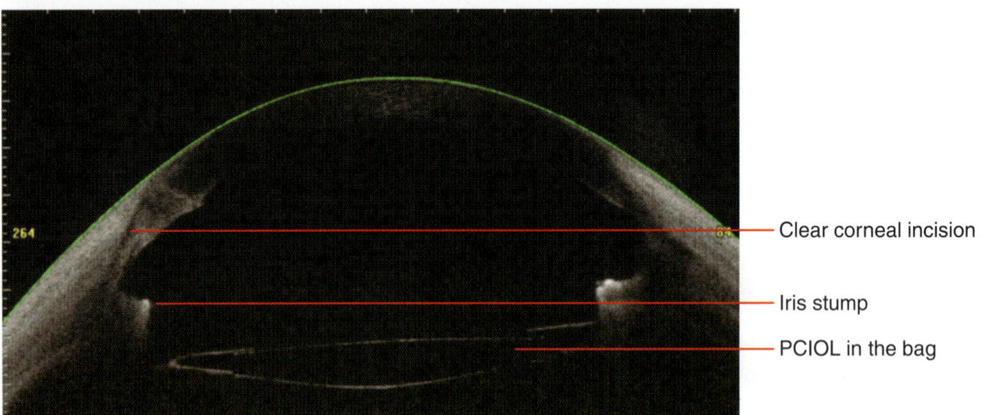

Fig. 31.4 Postoperative AS-OCT image.

DISCUSSION

Until recently, gonioscopy was the only method to study angle in aniridia. AS-OCT provides an easy, noncontact, and examiner-independent method to study the angle structures especially the iris stump remnants in aniridia.

FURTHER READING

1. Prosser J, van Heyninen V: PAX6 mutations reviewed. *Hum Mutat* 11:93–108, 1998.
2. Nelson LB, Spaeth GL, Nowiński TS, et al.: Aniridia. A review. *Surv Ophthalmol* 28:621–642, 1984.
3. Kim JH, Hwang BS, Lee JH, et al.: PAX6 mutations and clinical features of congenital aniridia. *J Korean Ophthalmol Soc* 49:1794–1800, 2008.
4. Muir KW, Duncan L, Enyedi LB, et al.: Central corneal thickness: congenital cataracts and aphakia. *Am J Ophthalmol* 144:502–506, 2007.
5. Reinhard T, Engelhardt S, Sundmacher R.: Black diaphragm aniridia intraocular lens for congenital aniridia: long-term follow-up. *J Cataract Refract Surg* 26:375–381, 2000.

Cataract

Sudeep Das, Mathew Kurien, and Rashmi Shetty

Opacification of any part of the crystalline lens or its capsule is termed cataract. Density of the cataract and pathologies of structures associated with the lens determine the difficulty of the surgery or complications which can occur.

CASE STUDIES

A 45-year-old woman had blurring of vision in both eyes that she noticed 4 months back. Ocular examination showed posterior polar cataract in both the eyes (**Fig. 32.1**). Anterior-segment optical coherence tomography (AS-OCT) showed the cataract as a hyperreflective opacity in the posterior capsule with the capsule itself seen continuously on either side of the cataract as a hyperreflective line (**Fig. 32.2**).

In another illustrative case of posterior polar cataract in a 46-year-old male, AS-OCT image (**Fig. 32.3**) shows that the hyperreflective line representing posterior capsule as being discontinuous with the cataractous opacification. This denotes capsular dehiscence in the center of the pole of the lens.

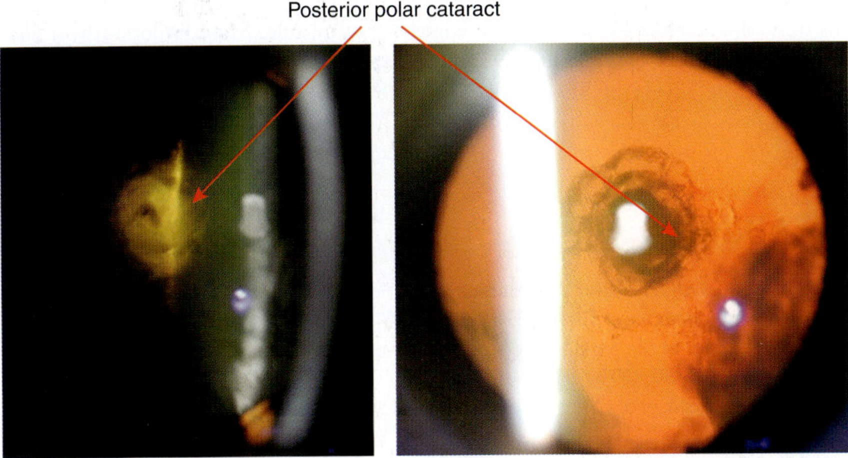

Fig. 32.1 Slit lamp images showing posterior polar cataract.

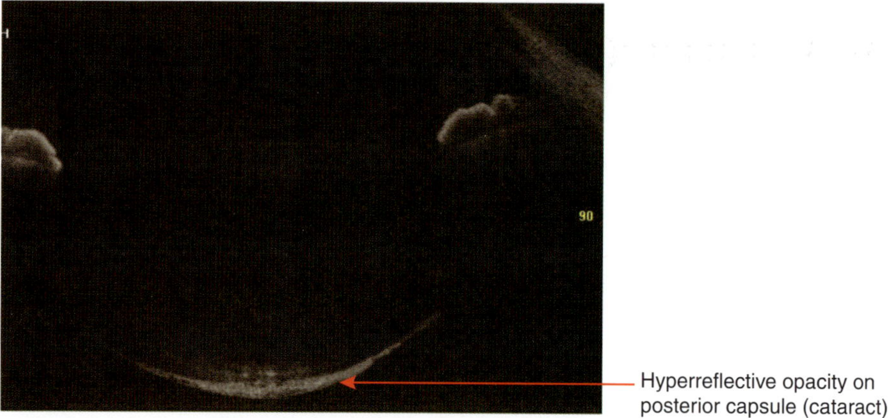

Hyperreflective opacity on
posterior capsule (cataract)

Fig. 32.2 AS-OCT shows a hyperreflective line, denoting an intact posterior capsule. The continuity of this capsule in the center, over the cataractous opacification confirms that there is no dehiscence.

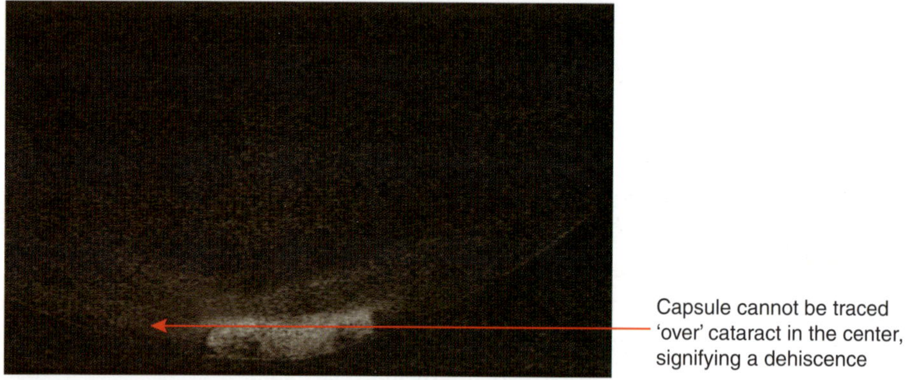

Capsule cannot be traced
'over' cataract in the center,
signifying a dehiscence

Fig. 32.3 AS-OCT showing discontinuity of the capsule (arrow) in the center just adjacent to the cataract suggestive of a pre-existing dehiscence.

DISCUSSION

AS-OCT helps us to localize cataractous change in the lens or the capsule. More importantly, it also helps us to predict posterior capsular integrity (**Figs 32.2 and 32.3**) in posterior polar cataracts and plan for safer surgery taking adequate precautions. Before advent of SD-OCT imaging of the lens, we could not image the posterior capsule categorically in vivo.

FURTHER READING

1. Kumar S, Ram J, Sukhija J, et al.: Phacoemulsification in posterior polar cataract: does size of lens opacity affect surgical outcome? *Clin Experiment Ophthalmol* 38(9):857–861, 2010.
2. Nagappa S, Das S, Kurian M, et al.: Modified technique for epinucleus removal in posterior polar cataract. *Ophthalmic Surg Lasers Imaging* 42(1):78–80, 2011.
3. Das S, Khanna R, Mohiuddin SM, et al.: Surgical and visual outcomes for posterior polar cataract. *Br J Ophthalmol* 92(11):1476–1478, 2008.
4. Wong AL, Leung CK, Weinreb RN, et al.: Quantitative assessment of lens opacities with anterior segment optical coherence tomography. *Br J Ophthalmol* 93(1):61–65, 2009.

Clear Corneal Incision

Sudeep Das, Mathew Kurien, and Ridhima Bhagali

Clear corneal incision is an advantage in phacoemulsification surgery where a foldable lens can be implanted through a small incision, which is bloodless and self-sealing. Nevertheless, if not constructed carefully, it could be disastrous.

CASE STUDY 1

A 70-year-old man underwent clear corneal incision phacoemulsification surgery (**Fig. 33.1**).

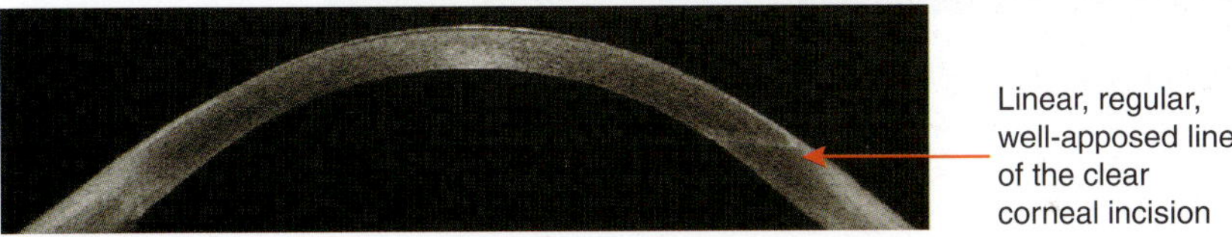

Fig. 33.1 AS-OCT image shows a well-apposed clear corneal wound.

CASE STUDY 2

A 65-year-old diabetic woman underwent phacoemulsification with clear corneal incision. On first postoperative day she had a vision of counting fingers from a distance of 2 meters. A Descemet's membrane (DM) detachment was noted during examination, for which C3F8 gas was injected into the anterior chamber [(AC) (**Figs 33.2–33.4**)].

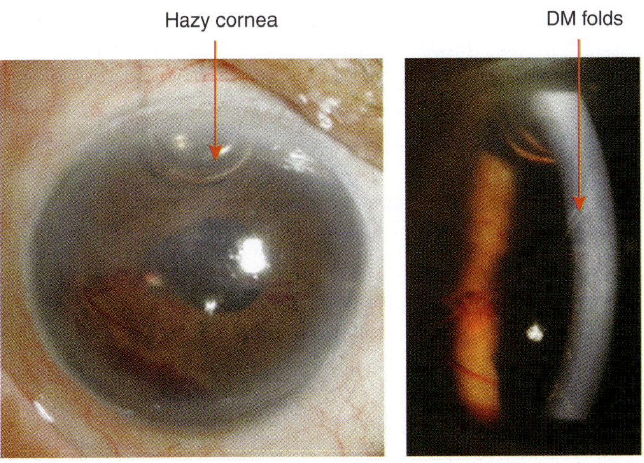

Fig. 33.2 Slit lamp image shows hazy cornea and DM folds and the injected gas bubble.

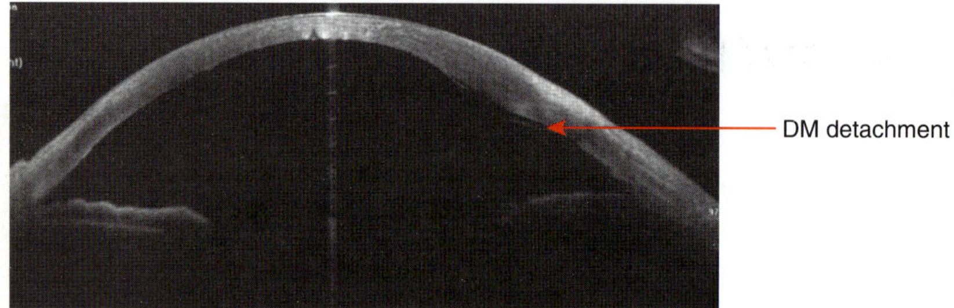

Fig. 33.3 The separation of the Descemet's membrane is seen prior to gas injection on AS-OCT.

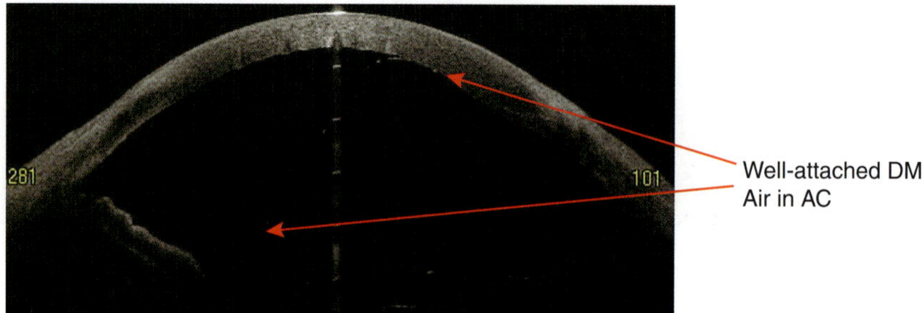

Fig. 33.4 AS-OCT image after C3F8 injection shows well-attached DM and air in AC.

Hence, AS-OCT imaging helps us study the configuration and position of the incision, diagnose, and delineate the extent of complications such as DM detachments and even helps to monitor the successful outcome of management in these cases.

FURTHER READING

1. Can I, Bayhan HA, Celik H, et al.: Anterior segment optical coherence tomography evaluation and comparison of main clear corneal incisions in microcoaxial and biaxial cataract surgery. *J Cataract Refract Surg* 37(3):490–500, 2011.
2. Lyles GW, Cohen KL, Lam D: OCT-documented incision features and natural history of clear corneal incisions used for bimanual microincision cataract surgery. *Cornea* 30(6):681–686, 2011.
3. Fukuda S, Kawana K, Yasuno Y, et al.: Wound architecture of clear corneal incision with or without stromal hydration observed with 3-dimensional optical coherence tomography. *Am J Ophthalmol* 151(3):413–419, 2011.
4. Wylegała E, Nowinska A: Usefulness of anterior segment optical coherence tomography in Descemet membrane detachment. *Eur J Ophthalmol* 19(5):723–728, 2009.
5. Xia Y, Liu X, Luo L, et al.: Early changes in clear cornea incision after phacoemulsification: an anterior segment optical coherence tomography study. *Acta Ophthalmol* 87(7):764–768, 2009.

Alport's Syndrome

Madhusmita Das,
Mathew Kurien,
Rohit Shetty, and Sudeep Das

Alport's syndrome is a rare basement membrane disorder characterized by progressive hereditary nephritis, sensorineural hearing loss, and ocular abnormalities. The inheritance is predominantly X-linked (85%), although it can be autosomal recessive (10%) or autosomal dominant (5%). Homozygote males are usually severely affected but females tend to have a mild form, often with only microscopic hematuria and normal renal function. The typical ocular associations are a dot-and-fleck retinopathy, which occurs in about 85% of affected adult males, anterior lenticonus which occurs in about 25%, and the rare posterior polymorphous corneal dystrophy. The retinopathy and anterior lenticonus are not usually demonstrated in childhood but worsen with time so that the retinal lesion is often present at the onset of renal failure, and anterior lenticonus presents even later. Additional ocular features described in X-linked Alport's syndrome include other corneal dystrophies, microcornea, arcus, iris atrophy, cataracts, spontaneous lens rupture, spherophakia, posterior lenticonus, a poor macular reflex, fluorescein angiogram hyperfluorescence, electrooculogram and electroretinogram abnormalities, and retinal pigmentation. All mutations demonstrated to date in X-linked Alport's syndrome have affected the *COL4A5* gene, which encodes the α5 chain of type IV collagen. This protein is probably common to basement membranes of glomerulus, cochlea, retina, lens capsule, and cornea. However, the α3(IV) and 4(IV) as well as the α5(IV) collagen chains are usually absent from affected basement membranes because abnormal α5(IV) molecule interferes with stability of all three. Loss of these collagen molecules from the affected basement membranes results in an abnormal ultrastructural appearance.

CASE STUDY

A 21-year-old Nigerian male patient presented to our institute with blurring of vision oculus uterque (OU-both eyes) for the last 7 years. He had been prescribed glasses elsewhere; however he was not comfortable with the same. On examination his vision [ocular dexter (OD-right eye)] was 6/12 improving to 6/9 with pin hole (ph) and oculus sinister (OS-left eye) 6/18 improving to 6/9 with ph. Near vision OU was N8. Dry refraction values OD −5.00 DSph/−6.00D Cy × 10° and OS −7 DSph/−5.00D Cy × 160°. He improved to 6/9^{-2} OD with +1.25 DSph and to 6/12^{-1} with +1 DSph OS. He was a known case of Alport's syndrome, had undergone renal transplantation at a multispecialty hospital 1½ years back, and was on oral steroids for the same. His elder brother too had similar ocular complaints and had undergone phacoemulsification with posterior chamber intraocular lens implantation elsewhere. Slit lamp examination OU revealed clear cornea, anterior lenticonus (Fig. 34.1), and clear lens. AS-OCT by Casia Tomey (Fig. 34.2) too revealed the anterior lenticonus, and clear cornea and clear lens. NIDEK OPD-Scan III (Fig. 34.3) was obtained to assess the exact total corneal and internal aberrations and single-step measurement of corneal topography and refractive error data for reduced alignment errors. Dilated fundus examination revealed a RPE hypertrophic patch in the inferotemporal quadrant of the retina. Contact lens (CL) trial was done; however as he was not improving with CL, options of surgery was given. Patient underwent phacoemulsification OD with Toric

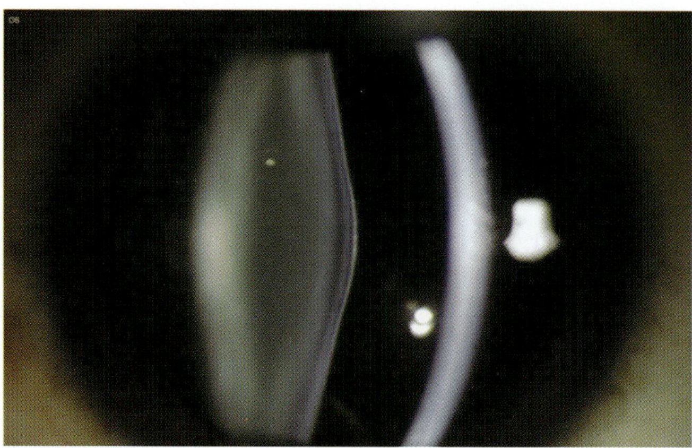

Fig. 34.1 Slit lamp photo demonstrating anterior lenticonus (OS).

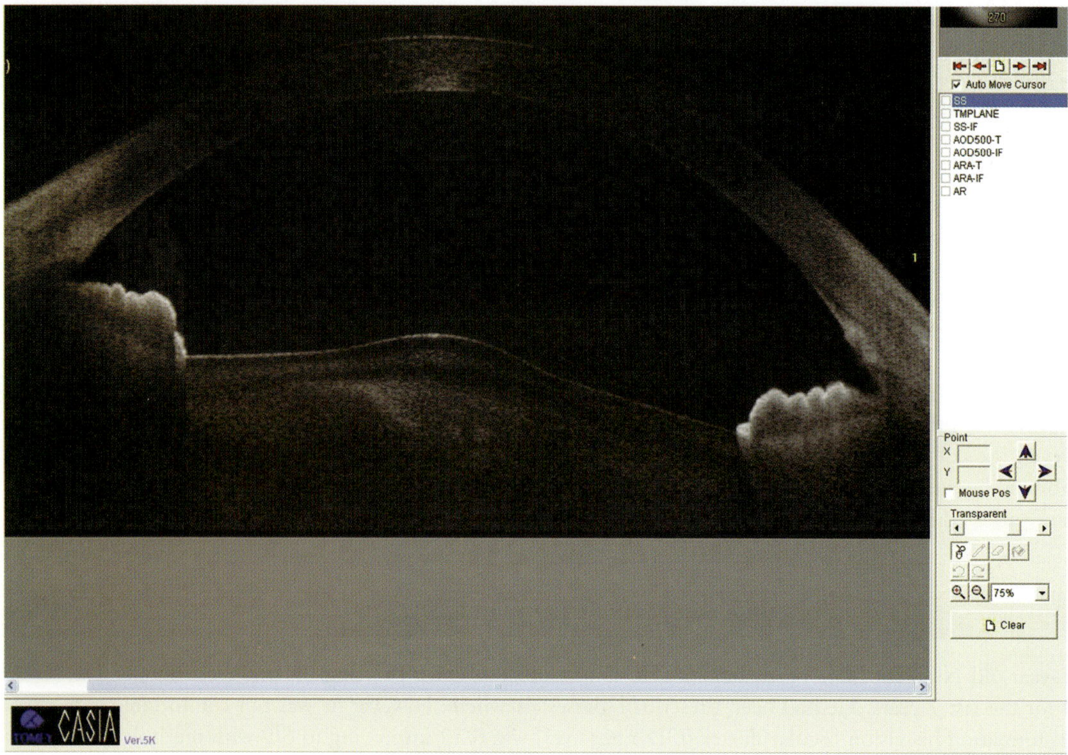

Fig. 34.2 Tomey AS-OCT demonstrating anterior lenticonus and clear cornea (OS).

IOL implantation. His vision OD was $6/6^{-1}$ and N12 at 30 cm, 1 week post surgery. He underwent OS phacoemulsification and Toric IOL implantation after 1 week of the first eye surgery. He had a vision of 6/6 OS and N18 at 30 cm, 1 week postoperatively.

His siblings were called and evaluated at our institute. His sister was found to have OU anterior lenticonus and OU early posterior polymorphous corneal dystrophy. She had hearing problems and is on medical treatment with a nephrologist for her renal pathology. She underwent OU phacoemulsification at our institute and anterior capsule was sent for histopathological analysis at our pathology laboratory. The histopathology of the anterior capsule revealed a stretched lens capsule with mild hyperplasia of lining cuboidal cells (**Fig. 34.4**).

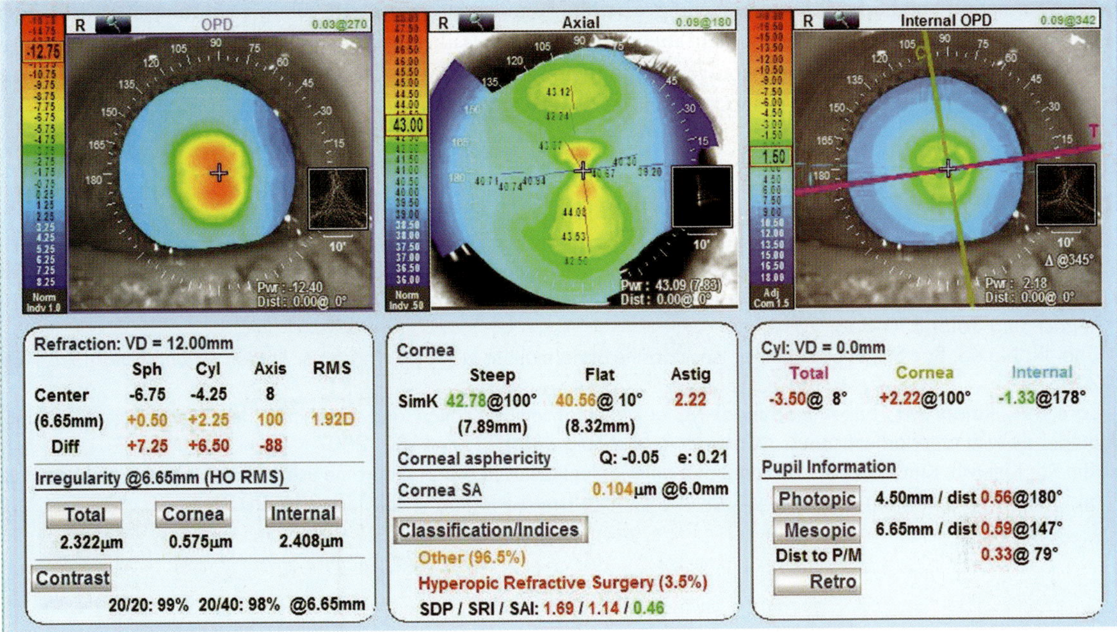

Fig. 34.3 NIDEK OPD-Scan III of OD.

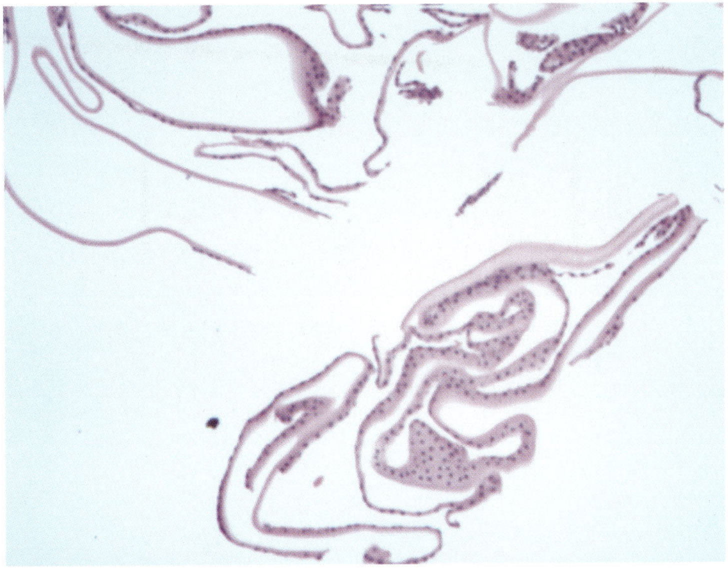

Fig. 34.4 Histopathology of the anterior capsule obtained during phacoemulsification seen by hematoxylin–eosin stain (10×).

DISCUSSION

Wavefront analysis, Scheimpflug imaging technology, and anterior-segment optical coherence tomography (AS-OCT) are effective tools in detection of lens disorders, especially those that are too subtle to be observed by other examination methods. Role of screening of siblings and appropriate referral to nephrologist and/or ENT specialist is of immense importance, when an ophthalmologist is the first doctor whom a patient visits due to visual disturbances. Appropriate preoperative work-up with topography and knowing the total, corneal and internal aberrations helps in selection of an intraocular lens (IOL) that would give best visual results.

FURTHER READING

1. Colville DJ, Savige J: Alport syndrome. A review of the ocular manifestations. *Ophthalmic Genet* 18(4):161–173, 1997.
2. Xu Y, Hersh PS, Chu DS: Wavefront analysis and Scheimpflug imagery in diagnosis of anterior lenticonus. *J Cataract Refract Surg* 36(5):850–853, 2010.
3. Choi JK, Na KS, Bae SH, et al.: Anterior lens capsule abnormalities in Alport syndrome. *Korean J Ophthalmol* 19:84–89, 2005.
4. Zare MA, Rajabi MT, Nili-Ahmadabadi M, et al.: Phacoemulsification and intraocular lens implantation in Alport syndrome with anterior lenticonus. *J Cataract Refract Surg* 33(6):1127–1130, 2007.
5. Kim KS, Kim MS, Kim JM, et al.: Evaluation of anterior lenticonus in Alport syndrome using tracey wavefront aberrometry and transmission electron microscopy. *Ophthalmic Surg Lasers Imaging* 41(3):330–336, 2010.

Phakic Intraocular Lens (pIOL)

Mathew Kurien, Sudeep Das, and Aditi Ghodke

Due to high refractive conditions, such as high myopic astigmatism, some patients are not appropriate candidates for laser-assisted refractive procedures because of increased risk for corneal ectasia and postoperative corneal haze, low visual quality, and unpredictability. Phakic intraocular lens (pIOL) or implantable collamer lens (ICL) is implanted as an alternative treatment to correct ametropia of various refractive ranges. pIOL implantation has several advantages, including rapid visual recovery, excellent refractive accuracy and stability, improved visual acuity, preservation of accommodation, and reversibility. At present, Visian ICL™ (Staar Surgical Company) is the only posterior chamber pIOL approved by the United States Food and Drug Administration (FDA) for treatment of moderate-to-severe myopia.

CASE STUDY

A 24-year-old female patient was keen on getting refractive surgery for high myopic astigmatism. Her refractive error was −13.50 DS/−1.5 DC × 100° in right eye and −12.0 DS/−1.0 DC × 20° in the left eye. Her topography showed

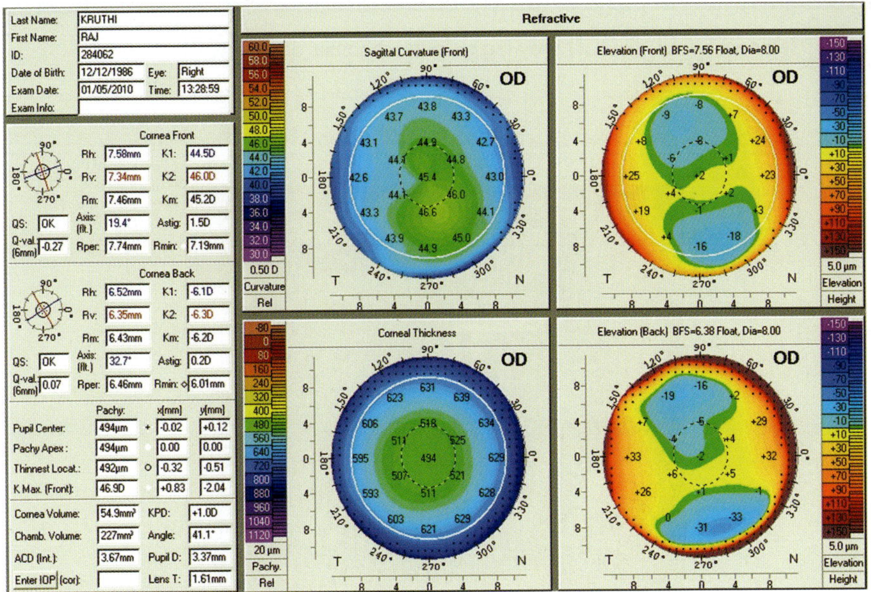

Fig. 35.1 Pentacam showing topography of the right eye.

corneal thickness of 492 μm, as shown (Fig. 35.1). Her anterior chamber depth (ACD) was adequate for pIOL implantation.

On preoperative examination, anterior-segment optical coherence tomography (AS-OCT) was done to measure the ACD, angle-to-angle distance for pIOL sizing. ACD was 3 mm and angle-to-angle diameter was 11.71 mm on AS-OCT (Fig. 35.2).

The patient underwent toric pIOL implantation in both eyes. pIOL is of a foldable collagen copolymer material and is designed to be placed in the posterior chamber, behind the iris, with a haptic zone resting on the ciliary sulcus (Fig. 35.3).

On postoperative follow-up, the ACD and vault were measured using AS-OCT and slit lamp, as shown in Figure 35.4.

On AS-OCT, ACD is 2.164 mm (*red circle*) and ICL vault is 0.529 mm (*yellow arrow*). The white arrow is showing posterior chamber pIOL above crystalline lens (Fig. 35.5).

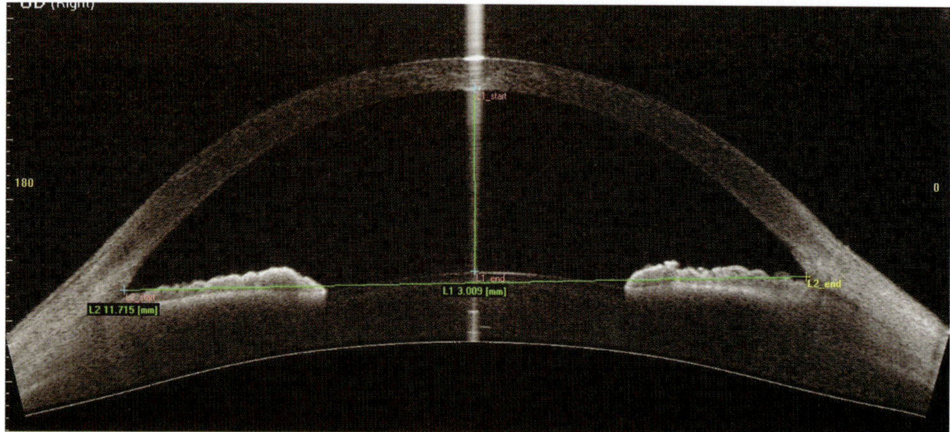

Fig. 35.2 Anterior-segment OCT (AS-OCT) showing anterior chamber depth (ACD).

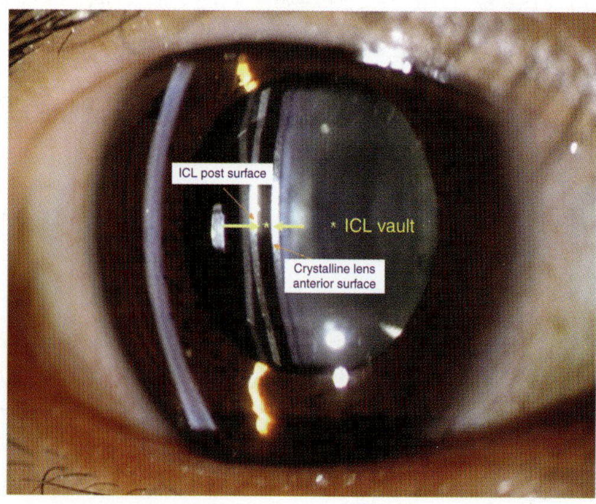

Fig. 35.3 Slit lamp showing phakic IOL vault and crystalline lens.

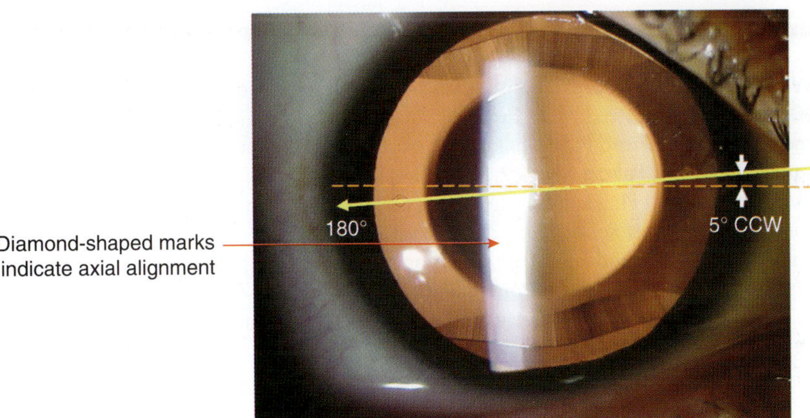

Fig. 35.4 Slit lamp showing toric ICL axis alignment (*yellow arrow*).

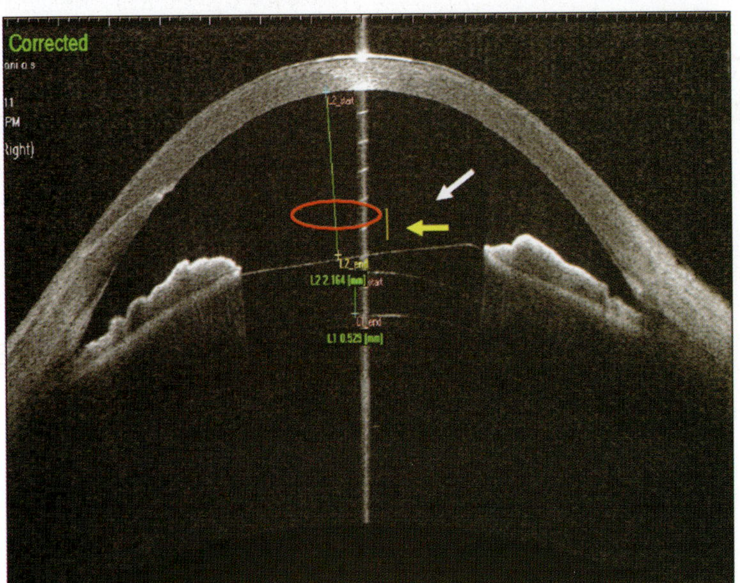

Fig. 35.5 AS-OCT showing phakic intraocular lens (pIOL) placement (*white arrow*) and vault (*yellow arrow*).

DISCUSSION

The "vault" is defined as the distance between the pIOL optic and the crystalline lens. Normally, this vault ranges from 0.25 to 0.75 mm. An oversized pIOL can potentially push the iris, thereby decreasing the size of the angle. An undersized pIOL (<0.125-mm vault), on the other hand, can result in an absent vault, resulting in a pIOL-crystalline lens touch, increasing the risk of early anterior subcapsular cataract.

AS-OCT helps the surgeon determine the correct pIOL sizing preoperatively. Postoperatively, AS-OCT can also be used to follow-up these patients by assessing the vault, ACD, and angles.

FURTHER READING

1. Randleman JB, Woodward M, Lynn MJ, et al.: Risk assessment for ectasia after corneal refractive surgery. *Ophthalmology* 115:37–50, 2008.
2. Gonvers M, Bornet C, Othenin-Girard P: Implantable contact lens for moderate to high myopia; relationship of vaulting to cataract formation. *J Cataract Refract Surg* 29:918–924, 2003.
3. Güell JL, Morral M, Kook D, et al.: Phakic intraocular lenses. Part 1: Historical overview, current models, selection criteria, and surgical techniques. *J Cataract Refract Surg* 36:1976–1993, 2010.
4. Alfonso JF, Fernandez-Vega L, Fernandes P, et al.: Collagen copolymer toric posterior chamber phakic intraocular lens for myopic astigmatism: one year follow-up. *J Cataract Refract Surg* 36:568–576, 2010.
5. Alfonso JF, Lisa C, Palacios A, et al.: Objective vs subjective vault measurement after myopic implantable collamer lens implantation. *Am J Ophthalmol* 147:978–983, 2009.

Subluxated Lens

Sudeep Das, Mathew Kurien, and Ridhima Bhagali

Subluxation of crystalline lens usually occurs because of a large dehiscence or weakness of zonular fibers. *Ectopia lentis* is a term used to describe congenital dislocations. Etiologies include congenital diseases such as Marfan's syndrome, homocystinuria, pseudoexfoliation, and high myopia. Ocular trauma is one of the commonest causes of subluxation. Optical aberrations such as partial aphakia, high myopia, astigmatism, and monocular diplopia are associated with significant impairment of vision. Surgical correction of lens subluxation usually involves the use of capsular tension rings (CTR) with posterior chamber intraocular lenses (IOLs), complete lens removal (ICCE), or implantation of anterior chamber or scleral-fixated IOLs.

CASE STUDY

A 45-year-old male patient presented with a history of progressive diminution of vision in the left eye for the past 6 months. Superior subluxation of crystalline lens with cataractous change was noted on slit lamp examination. The patient had no previous history of trauma. Right eye was normal without lens subluxation. There was more than 180° absence of zonules inferiorly, as shown below (**Fig. 36.1**).

Anterior-segment optical coherence tomography (AS-OCT) was performed for zonular and angle assessment. Red arrow in the picture is showing absence of zonules inferiorly (**Fig. 36.2**). The angles were open. There was no shallowing of anterior chamber.

The lens subluxation may cause many complications; some of which are vision threatening. Lens movement may induce astigmatism and frequent change in refraction. Changes between intermittently phakic and aphakic visual

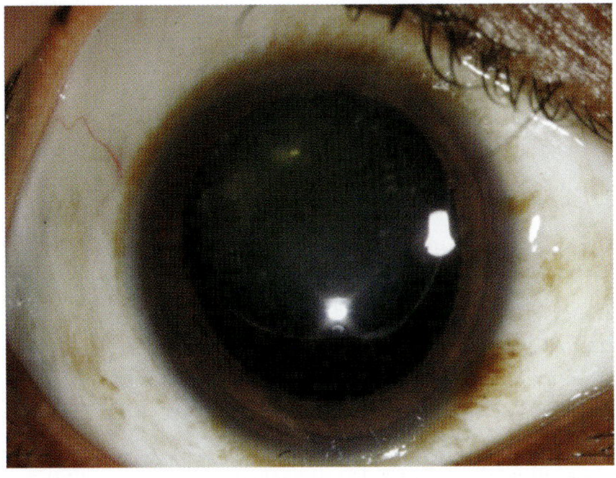

Fig. 36.1 Slit lamp photograph showing superior subluxation of cataractous lens.

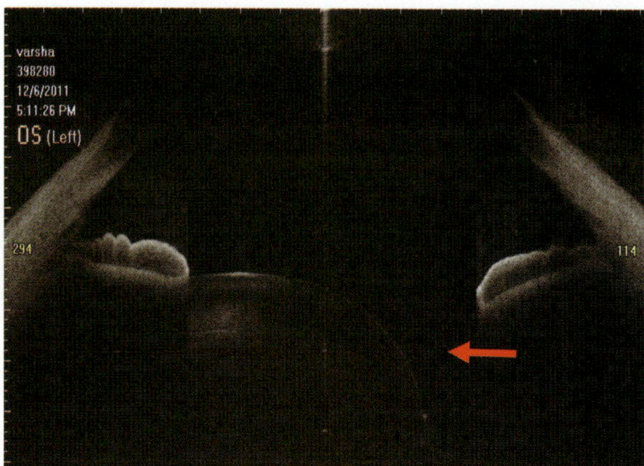

Fig. 36.2 AS-OCT showing absence of zonules with lens subluxation (*red arrow*).

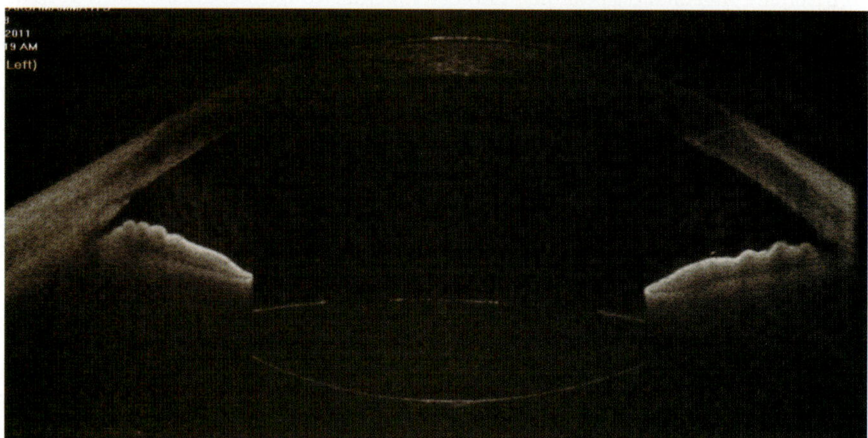

Fig. 36.3 AS-OCT showing scleral-fixated posterior-chamber IOL (SFIOL).

axes may cause marked visual disturbances. Forward dislocation of the lens may precipitate an attack of pupillary block glaucoma or may lead to corneal decompensation. Posterior dislocation of the lens into vitreous may result in uveitis or may even induce a retinal detachment.

This patient underwent ICCE, anterior vitrectomy, and scleral-fixated IOL implantation. The AS-OCT image (Fig. 36.3) shows the scleral-fixated IOL in this case.

FURTHER READING

1. Dureau P: Pathophysiology of zonular diseases. *Curr Opin Ophthalmol* 19:27–30, 2008.
2. Wong AL, Leung CKS, Weinreb RN, et al.: Quantitative assessment of lens opacities with anterior segment optical coherence tomography. *Br J Ophthalmol* 93:61–65, 2009.
3. Wylegala E, Teper S, Nowińska AK, et al.: Anterior segment imaging: Fourier-domain optical coherence tomography versus time-domain optical coherence tomography. *J Cataract Refract Surg* 35:1410–1414, 2009.
4. Praveen MR, Vasavada AR, Singh R: Phacoemulsification in subluxated cataract. *Indian J Ophthalmol* 51(2):147–154, 2003.
5. Cionni RJ, Osher RH: Management of profound zonular dialysis or weakness with a new endocapsular ring designed for scleral fixation. *J Cataract Refract Surg* 24(10):1299–1306, 1998.

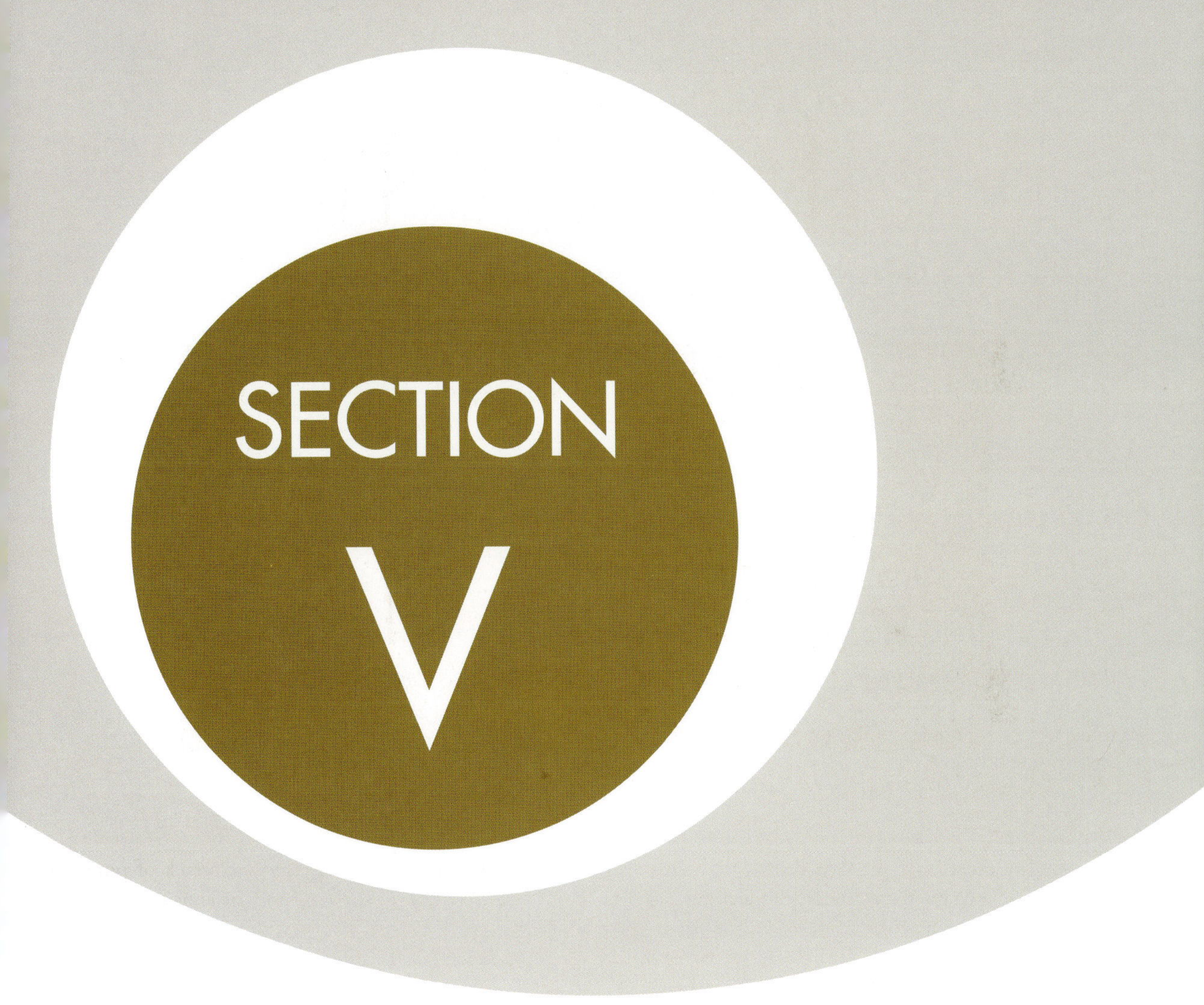

Glaucoma

Angle Imaging

Poemen PM Chan and
Christopher KS Leung

Angle-closure glaucoma represents approximately 25% of glaucoma worldwide and accounts for nearly half of glaucoma blindness. Evaluation of the anterior chamber angle is vital to the detection and diagnosis of angle closure. While gonioscopy is indispensable to visualize the structure and the configuration of the anterior chamber angle, it is limited by being a contact technique, permitting largely qualitative assessment of the angle width. Objective, reproducible, and quantitative measurement of the anterior chamber angle dimensions can only be attained with cross-sectional imaging instruments like the ultrasound biomicroscopy (UBM) and optical coherence tomography (OCT). Compared with UBM, OCT is noncontact, being more efficient in examining the angle configuration at specific meridians in high resolution. The angle opening distance (AOD), the trabecular–iris angle (TIA), the angle recess area (ARA), and the trabecular–iris space area (TISA) are the four standard parameters to document the angle width (**Fig. 37.1**). Most commercially available UBM and OCT instruments allow automatic analysis of these angle parameters once the scleral spur (SS) is located manually (**Fig. 37.2**). Measurement of the angle width is relevant to the evaluation of angle closure as well as assessing the degree of angle opening after laser peripheral iridotomy and cataract extraction.

MEASUREMENTS OF THE ANTERIOR CHAMBER ANGLES

Angle opening distance (AOD) is the perpendicular distance measured from the trabecular meshwork, commonly defined at a distance of 500 μm (AOD 500) anterior to the scleral spur to the anterior iris surface.

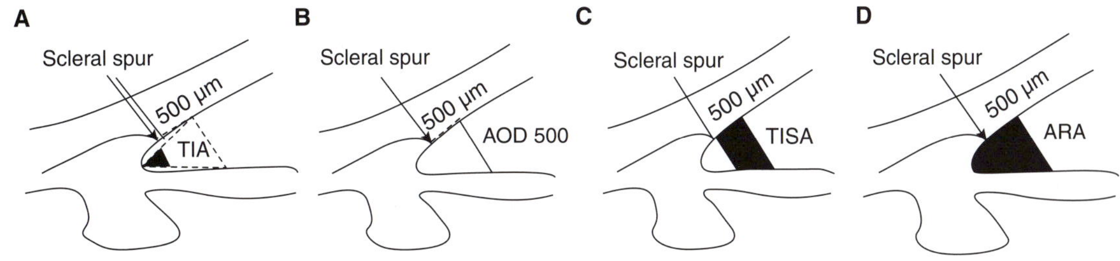

Fig. 37.1 Schematics showing measurement of trabecular–iris angle (TIA) **(A)**, angle opening distance (AOD) **(B)**, trabecular–iris space area (TISA) **(C)**, and angle recess area (ARA) **(D)** at a distance of 500 μm away from the scleral spur (SS). (*Adapted from* Figure 2 in Leung CK, Weinreb RN. Anterior chamber angle imaging with optical coherence tomography. *Eye* 25:261–267, 2010.)

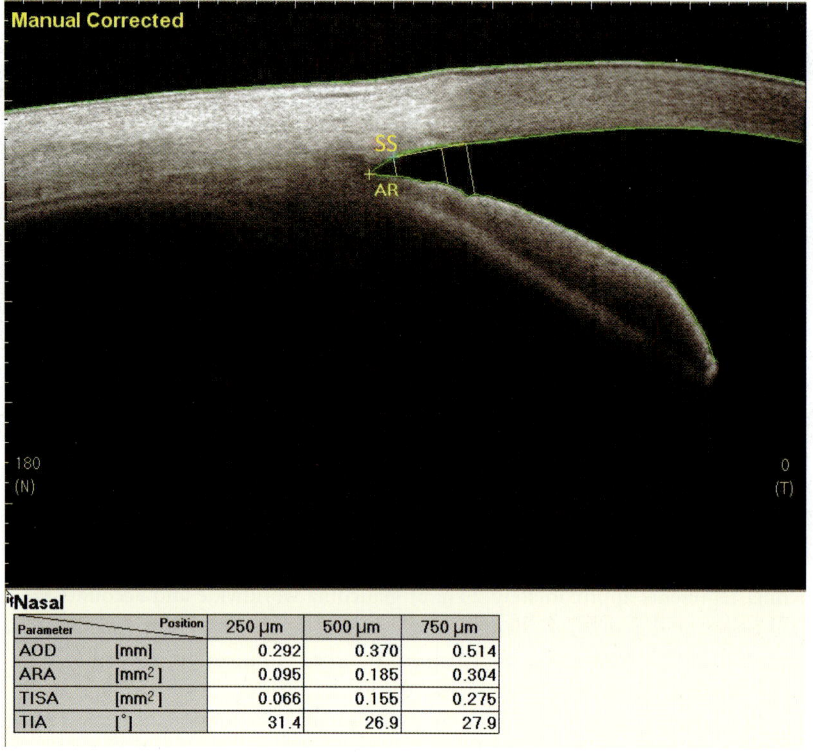

Parameter	Position	250 μm	500 μm	750 μm
AOD	[mm]	0.292	0.370	0.514
ARA	[mm²]	0.095	0.185	0.304
TISA	[mm²]	0.066	0.155	0.275
TIA	[°]	31.4	26.9	27.9

Fig. 37.2 A print screen capture from an anterior-segment optical coherence tomography (The Casia OCT, Tomey, Nogaya, Japan). After the scleral spur (SS) was manually identified, measurements of the angle opening distance (AOD), the trabecular–iris angle (TIA), the angle recess area (ARA), and the trabecular–iris space area (TISA) at 250 μm, 500 μm, and 750 μm away from the SS were automatically generated.

Trabecular–iris angle (TIA) is defined as an angle measured with apex in the iris recess and the arms of the angle passing through a point at 500-μm anterior to the SS (TIA 500) and the point on the iris perpendicularly.

Angle recess area (ARA) represents the area of the angle bounded anteriorly by the AOD.

Trabecular–iris space area (TISA) represents the area bounded anteriorly by the AOD, posteriorly by a line drawn from the SS perpendicular to the plane of the inner scleral wall to the opposing iris, superiorly by the inner corneo-scleral wall, and inferiorly by the anterior iris surface.

During imaging of the anterior chamber angle, it is important to standardize the lighting condition, preferably in complete darkness. This is because the angle width decreases with the pupil size, which is influenced by the amount of light getting into the eye. Angle closure could be missed if imaging is not performed in the dark (Fig. 37.3).

NEW OCT TECHNOLOGIES FOR ANGLE IMAGING

The advent of spectral-domain optical coherence tomography (SD-OCT) has allowed an improved scan speed (27,000–40,000 A-scans/second) and scan resolution (5-μm axial resolution) compared with the time-domain optical coherence tomography (TD-OCT) (200–2000 A-scans/second; axial resolution 18–25 μm). A number of SD-OCT instruments designed for posterior segment imaging, including the Cirrus HD-OCT (Carl Zeiss Meditec, Dublin, CA, USA), the RTVue-100 (Optovue Inc., Fremont, California, USA), and the SPECTRALIS™ OCT

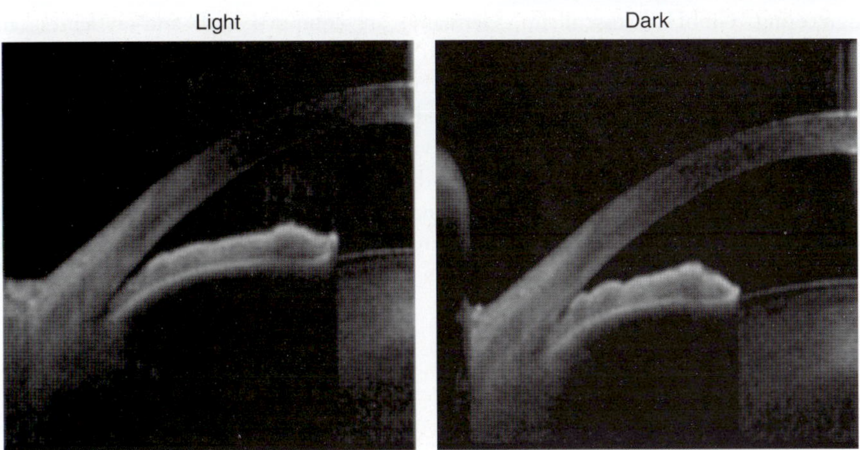

Fig. 37.3 An eye with primary angle closure was imaged in the light (*left*) and in the dark (*right*). While the angle was narrow in the light, appositional angle closure was only detected in the dark.

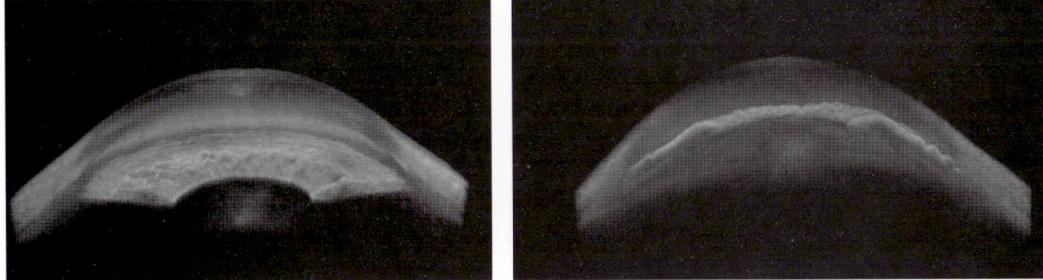

Fig. 37.4 Three-dimensional reconstruction of optical coherence tomography (OCT) images obtained from a swept-source OCT (The Casia OCT, Tomey, Nogaya, Japan) of a normal eye with open angle and an eye with primary angle closure.

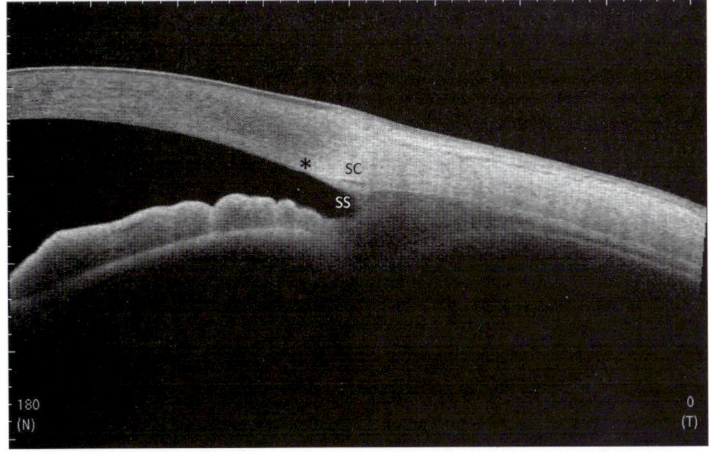

Fig. 37.5 A high-density scan image obtained with a swept-source optical coherence tomography (The Casia OCT, Tomey, Nogaya, Japan) showing the scleral spur (SS), Schwalbe's line (*), and Schlemm's canal (SC).

(Heidelberg Engineering, GmbH, Dossenheim, Germany) are equipped with add-on lenses (anterior-segment module) for anterior segment imaging. The Casia OCT (Tomey, Nagoya, Japan) is a swept-source OCT recently introduced for three-dimensional assessment of the anterior segment structures. With a scan speed of 30,000 A-scans/second, the whole anterior chamber can be imaged in 64 radial scans in 2.5 seconds. The reconstruction of the cross-sectional images can provide three-dimensional visualization of the anterior segment (**Fig. 37.4**). In addition to the sclera spur, the improved scan resolution of the new OCT devices also permits visualization of other angle structures including Schwalbe's line, Schlemm's canal, and collector channels (**Fig. 37.5**). Nevertheless, the clinical significance of detecting these structures remains to be established. All the commercially available anterior-segment OCT instruments provide only partial visualization of the ciliary body. UBM is indispensable for examination of the morphology of the ciliary body.

FURTHER READING

1. Quigley HA, Broman AT: The number of people with glaucoma worldwide in 2010 and 2020. *Br J Ophthalmol* 90: 262–267, 2006.
2. Pavlin CJ, Harasiewicz K, Foster FS: Ultrasound biomicroscopy of anterior segment structures in normal and glaucomatous eyes. *Am J Ophthalmol* 113:381–389, 1992.
3. Radhakrishnan S, Goldsmith J, Huang D, et al.: Comparison of optical coherence tomography and ultrasound biomicroscopy for detection of narrow anterior chamber angles. *Arch Ophthalmol* 123:1053–1059, 2005.
4. Leung CK, Weinreb RN: Anterior chamber angle imaging with optical coherence tomography. *Eye* 25:261–267, 2010.

Anterior Chamber Angle and Iris Configuration Changes After Peripheral Laser Iridotomy

Poemen PM Chan, Cong Ye, and Christopher KS Leung

Laser peripheral iridotomy (LPI) creates an aperture in the peripheral iris with the objective of relieving pupillary block in the management of primary angle closure. While LPI is indicated in eyes with acute angle closure, prophylactic LPI is usually performed in the fellow eyes to reduce risk of acute angle closure. However, in eyes with occludable angles, commonly defined as an eye in which ≥270° of posterior trabecular meshwork cannot be seen, it is not entirely clear whether prophylactic LPI is beneficial or not. Visual disturbances (shadows, halo, ghost images), cataract formation, damage to corneal endothelium, and malignant glaucoma are potential complications following LPI.

In relative pupillary block, there is an increase in resistance to the flow of aqueous humor at the pupillary margin, resulting in a pressure gradient between posterior and anterior chambers. The iris assumes a characteristic anterior bowing appearance and the angles become narrow or closed with a greater pressure posterior to the iris. LPI provides a communication between the posterior and anterior chambers, thereby eliminating the pressure gradient, flattening the iris, and opening up the anterior chamber angle. Anterior-segment optical coherence tomography (AS-OCT) imaging can provide an objective evaluation of morphological changes of the angle configuration and the iris before and after LPI.

CASE STUDY

An 83-year-old Chinese man, who had an episode of acute angle closure of the right eye, had primary angle closure detected in the left eye. Slit lamp examination revealed a shallow anterior chamber (**Fig. 38.1A**) and the trabecular meshwork was not visible with gonioscopy in all quadrants (**Fig. 38.1B**). **Figures 38.2A and B** show the AS-OCT images captured in the dark. The anterior chamber angles (trabecular–iris angle, TIA500) were narrow (temporal, superior, nasal, and inferior angles measured at 180°, 90°, 0°, and 270° were 13.5°, 15.5°, 11.7°, and 6.1°, respectively) and the iris showed an anterior bowing configuration. After LPI, the angles were widened (temporal, superior, nasal, and inferior angles were 24.7°, 21.3°, 24.5°, and 19.9°, respectively) and the iris was flattened. LPI creates a free passage between posterior and anterior chambers, bypassing the iris–lens channel and equalizing the pressure between the two chambers. This reduces the anterior bowing of the peripheral iris and widens angle width.

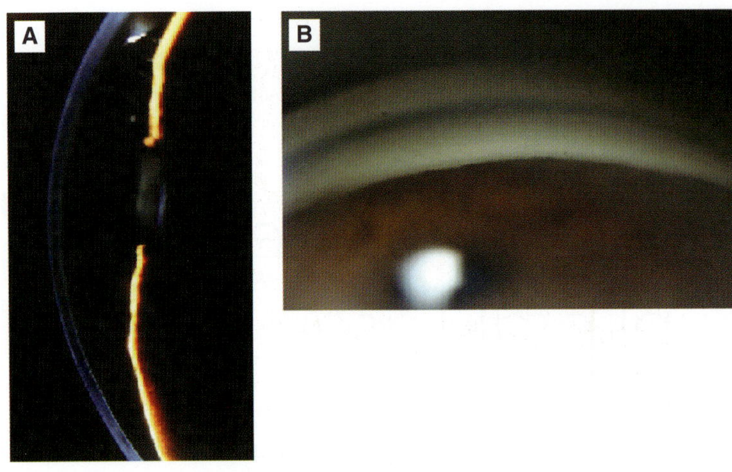

Fig. 38.1 **(A)** An eye with primary angle closure showing a shallow anterior chamber in slit lamp photography. **(B)** The posterior trabecular meshwork cannot be visualized with gonioscopy.

Before laser peripheral iridotomy

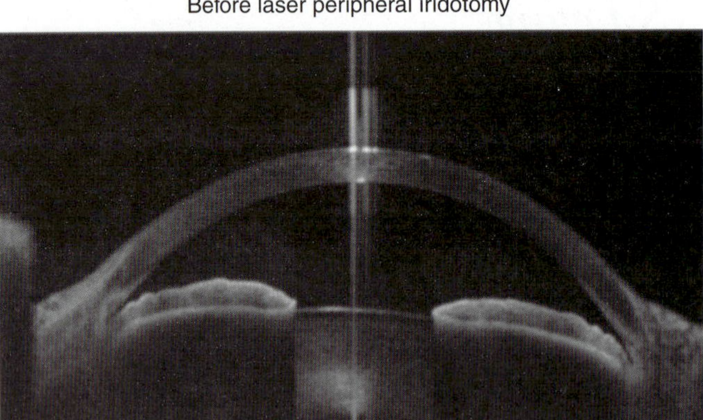

After laser peripheral iridotomy

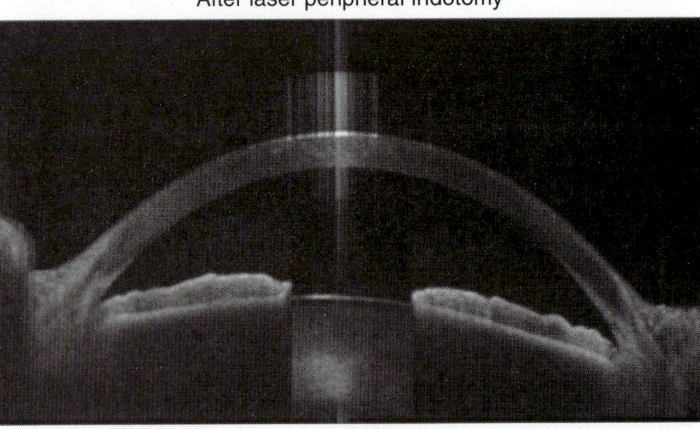

Fig. 38.2 **(A)** The anterior chamber of the same eye in Figure 38.1 imaged by an anterior-segment optical coherence tomography (AS-OCT) at the horizontal meridian. The angles were narrowed (temporal trabecular–iris angle = 13.5°; nasal trabecular–iris angle = 11.7°) and the iris had an anterior bowing appearance because of the pressure gradient between the anterior and posterior chambers. The pressure gradient was eliminated after laser peripheral iridotomy. The angle was opened up (temporal trabecular iris angle = 24.7°; nasal trabecular–iris angle = 24.5°) and the iris was flattened.

Before laser peripheral iridotomy

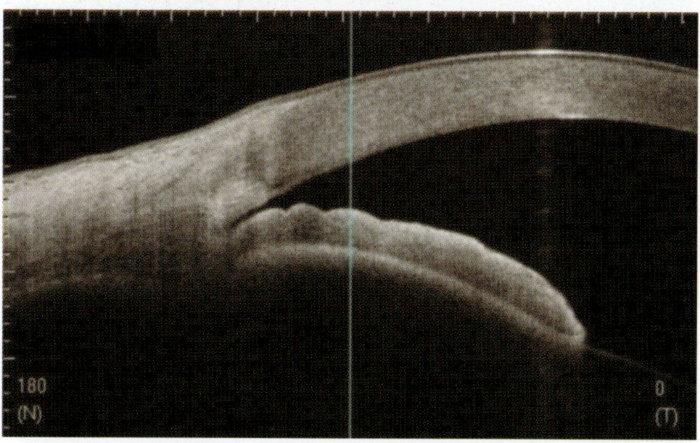

After laser peripheral iridotomy

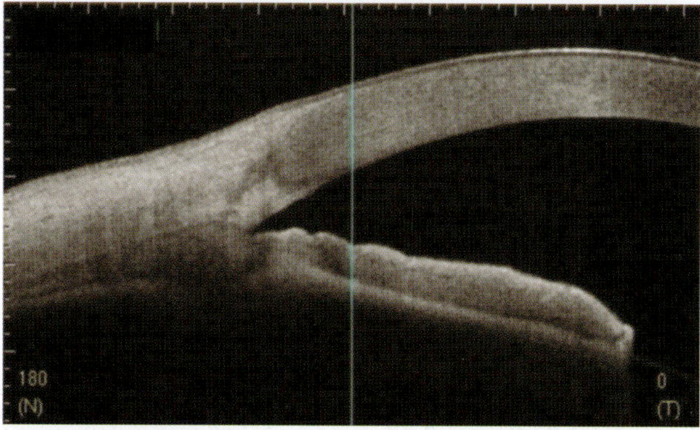

Fig. 38.2 **(B)** The nasal angle of the same eye imaged in a higher resolution.

FURTHER READING

1. How AC, Baskaran M, Kumar RS, et al.: Changes in anterior segment morphology after laser peripheral iridotomy: an anterior segment optical coherence tomography study. *Ophthalmology* 119(7):1383–1387, 2012.
2. Lee KS, Sung KR, Kang SY, et al.: Residual anterior chamber angle closure in narrow-angle eyes following laser peripheral iridotomy: anterior segment optical coherence tomography quantitative study. *Jpn J Ophthalmol* 55(3): 213–219, 2011.

Angle Recession

Rajesh S Kumar and Sathi Devi AV

Angle recession most commonly occurs in case of blunt trauma to the eye. About 6%–7% of eyes with recession have the risk of developing secondary glaucoma; this risk increases if the recession extends 180° or more. The presentation may vary depending on the degree and extent of the recession. It is characterized on gonioscopy by deepening of the anterior chamber, widening of the ciliary body band (thereby leaving it bare in comparison to the rest of the quadrants), and posterior displacement of the iris root.

It is characterized on ultrasound biomicroscopy (UBM) by a posterior displacement, where the iris attaches to the sclera and a wider ciliary body face. In the acute post-traumatic stage, blood could obscure the recessed angle, and performing indentation gonioscopy or even UBM could dislodge blood clots, causing rebleeding. A noncontact imaging device like anterior-segment optical coherence tomography (AS-OCT) could allow visualization of the recession; the newer source—swept OCT would also give information about extent of pathology.

CASE STUDY

A 56-year-old male patient presented with a history of blunt trauma with a shuttlecock; he had pain and redness associated with decrease in vision in his right eye. Visual acuity in his right eye was 6/18 (best corrected); slit lamp examination revealed clear cornea with anterior chamber flare and cells; the iris showed sphincter tears and a subluxed traumatic cataract. Gonioscopy showed angle recession in the superior and inferior quadrants (Fig. 39.1). The media was clear with no treatable retinal lesions; and a healthy optic nerve was seen on dilated fundus evaluation. Left eye was within normal limits.

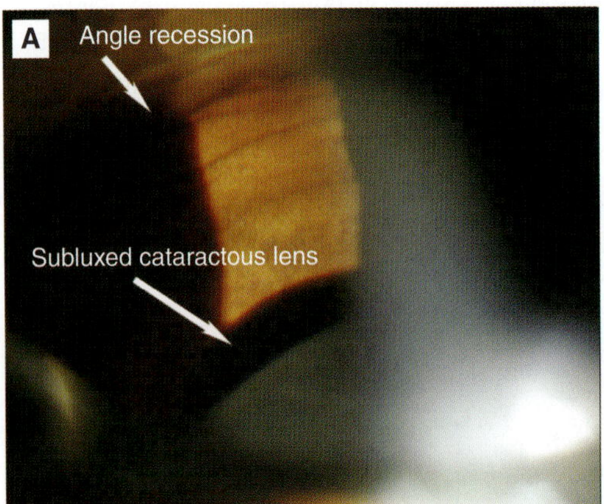

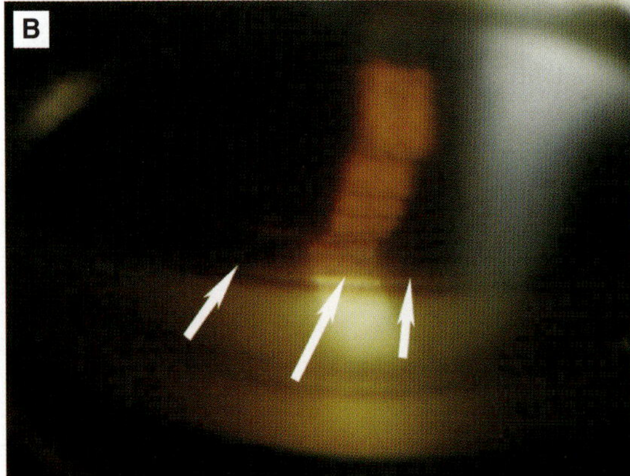

Fig. 39.1 (A) and **(B)** Slit lamp images of the right eye showing angle recession in the superior **(B)** and inferior **(A)** quadrants, and subluxed lens with cataractous changes.

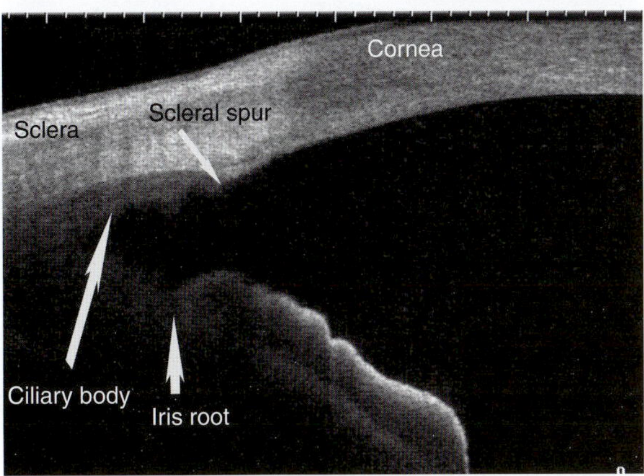

Fig. 39.2 AS-OCT image of a quadrant of the right eye with angle recession showing widening of angle recess and exposure of ciliary body band.

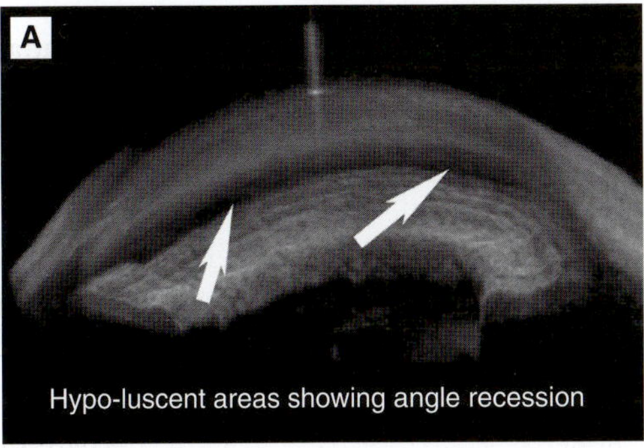

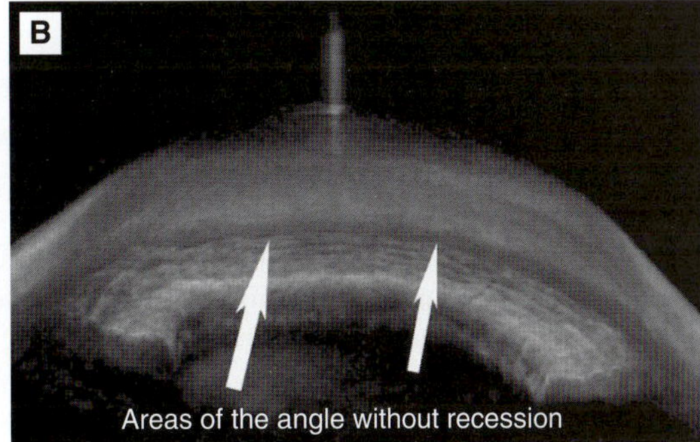

Fig. 39.3 AS-OCT 3-D reconstructed "gonioscopic view" images showing areas of angle with (A) and without (B) recession.

AS-OCT of the right eye demonstrated widening of angle recess with exposure of the ciliary body and iris root positioned further away from the sclera (Fig. 39.2). Three-dimensional gonioscopic reconstructed views of the angle showed a hypolucent area, where the recession was present, compared to areas where there was no recession (Fig. 39.3).

The intraocular pressure (IOP) in the right eye of the patient was recorded to be 32 mmHg; the patient was started on topical IOP-lowering medications. At 2-weeks follow-up, his IOP was 12 mmHg. The patient was advised to undergo cataract extraction with insertion of a capsular tension ring and posterior chamber intraocular lens.

FURTHER READING

1. Tumbocon JAJ, Latina MA: Angle recession glaucoma. *International Ophthalmology Clinics* 3:69–78, 2002.
2. Mooney D: Angle recession and secondary glaucoma. *Br J Ophthalmol* 57:608–612, 1973.

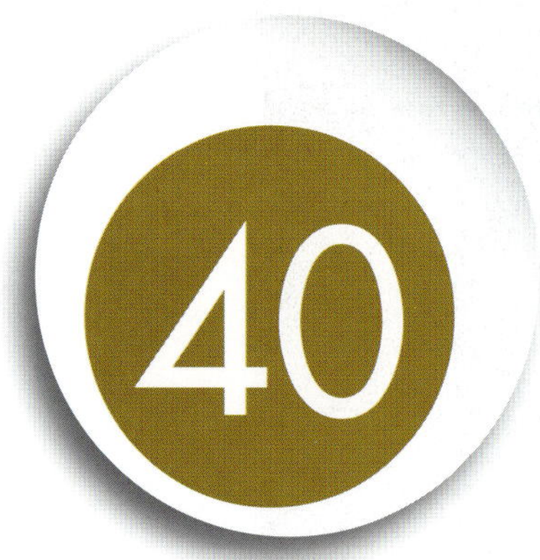

Anterior Chamber Angle—Open and Closed

Lisandro M Sakata

Angle closure process occurs in anatomically predisposed eyes in which contact between peripheral iris and trabecular meshwork represents a mechanical blockage impairing aqueous outflow. This process may eventually lead to intraocular pressure (IOP) increase and glaucomatous optic neuropathy. Thus, the presence of iridotrabecular contact may represent an important risk factor for development of this disease.

Anterior-segment optical coherence tomography (AS-OCT) represents a rapid noncontact method to obtain real-time images of the anterior chamber angles (ACA). These images can be used to qualitatively assess presence of iridotrabecular contact. However, the time-domain–AS-OCT resolution does not permit identification of trabecular meshwork. Thus, the location of scleral spur represents an anatomical landmark, which reveals relative location of the trabecular meshwork that is located approximately between 250- and 500 μm above the scleral spur along the angle wall. A closed ACA on AS-OCT imaging is usually defined by the presence of any contact between the iris and angle wall anterior to the sclera spur (**Figs 40.1–40.3**).

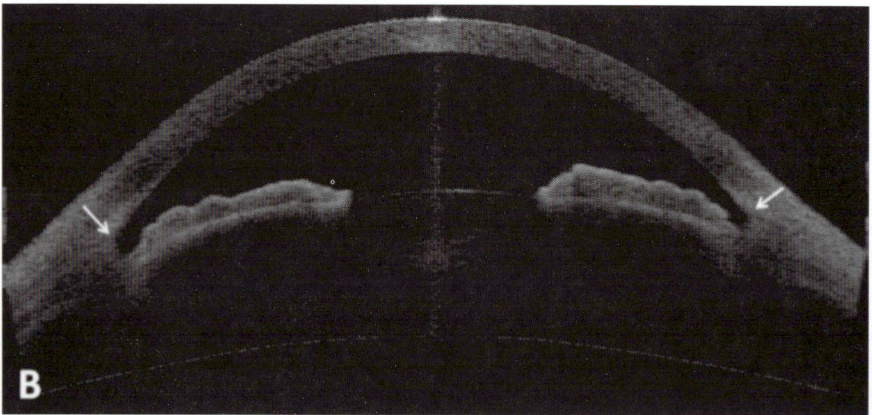

Fig. 40.1 Time-domain AS-OCT image of a 64-year-old Chinese woman with no symptoms, IOP of 16 mmHg, and normal-optic-disc appearance. On gonioscopy, it is possible to see scleral spur in all four quadrants, with no peripheral anterior synechiae. AS-OCT image of the ACA is showing an open angle in both nasal and temporal quadrants. The white arrows show the location of the scleral spur. (Photo courtesy: Dr Tin Aung, Singapore Eye Research Institute.)

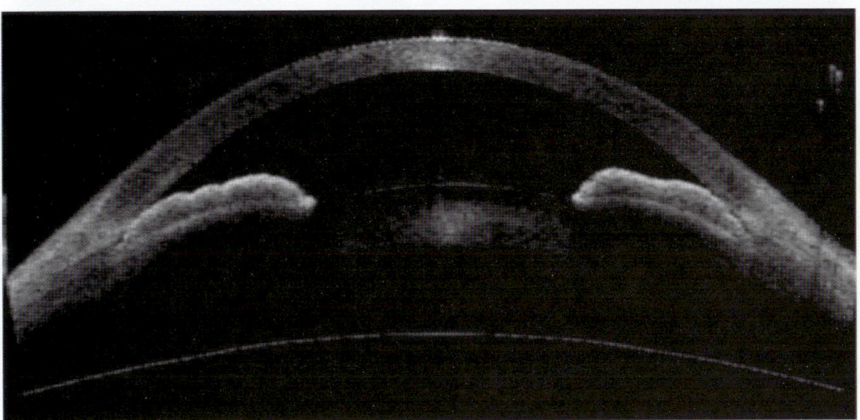

Fig. 40.2 Time-domain AS-OCT image of a 60-year-old Chinese woman with no symptoms, IOP of 12 mmHg, and normal-optic-disc appearance. On gonioscopy, it is not possible to see the posterior trabecular meshwork in three quadrants with no peripheral anterior synechiae. AS-OCT image of ACA is showing a closed angle in both nasal and temporal quadrants. (Photo courtesy: Dr Tin Aung, Singapore Eye Research Institute.)

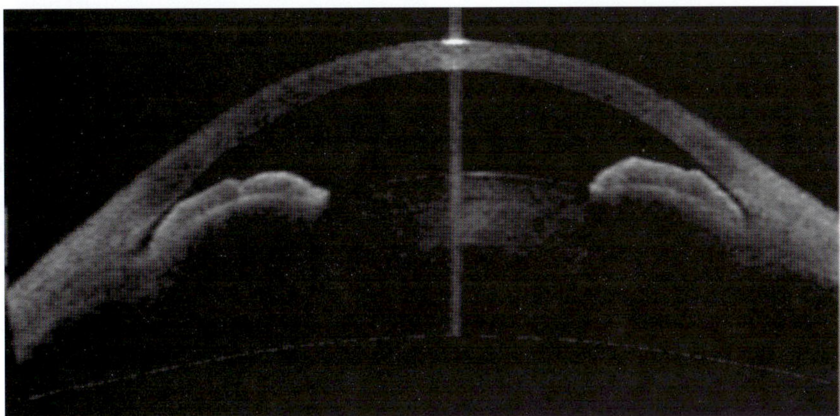

Fig. 40.3 Time-domain AS-OCT image of a 57-year-old Malay man with no symptoms, IOP of 14 mmHg, and normal-optic-disc appearance. Gonioscopy shows a closed angle with nonvisible posterior trabecular meshwork in all four quadrants with no peripheral anterior synechiae. AS-OCT image of the ACA is showing a pronounced convexity of the iris with very narrow but open angle—over-the-hill configuration. (Photo courtesy: Dr Tin Aung, Singapore Eye Research Institute.)

It is interesting to note that even in eyes in which the exact location of scleral spur cannot be determined many AS-OCT images could still be qualitatively graded as having either an open or closed ACA by relying on other morphological landmarks, such as insertion of the iris and peripheral iris profile.

Previous studies observed that AS-OCT imaging seems to be detecting more closed ACA than gonioscopy (Fig. 40.4). It is hypothesized that disagreement between these two techniques may be partially explained by the fact that while AS-OCT uses infrared light and does not require contact with the eye, inadvertent indentation by goniolenses and use of light during gonioscopy may artificially open the ACA. In addition, it is possible that anatomical landmarks for determining the presence of a closed angle may not be the same. A closed ACA in gonioscopy was determined by observation of contact between the iris and the posterior trabecular meshwork; however, in imaging, any contact between the iris and the angle wall anteriorly to the scleral spur would suffice to consider an ACA as closed.

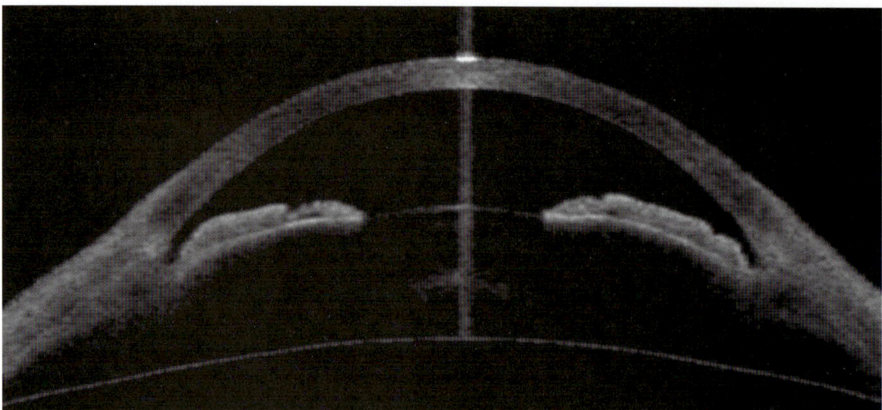

Fig. 40.4 Time-domain AS-OCT image of an 80-year-old Chinese man with no symptoms, IOP of 20 mmHg, and early glaucomatous optic neuropathy. Gonioscopy shows an open angle with visible scleral spur in three quadrants with no peripheral anterior synechiae. AS-OCT image of the ACA is showing an open angle in both the nasal and the temporal quadrants. Despite that, it is not possible to detect the exact location of the scleral spur, particularly on the right angle (artifact on angle wall). (Photo courtesy: Dr Tin Aung, Singapore Eye Research Institute.)

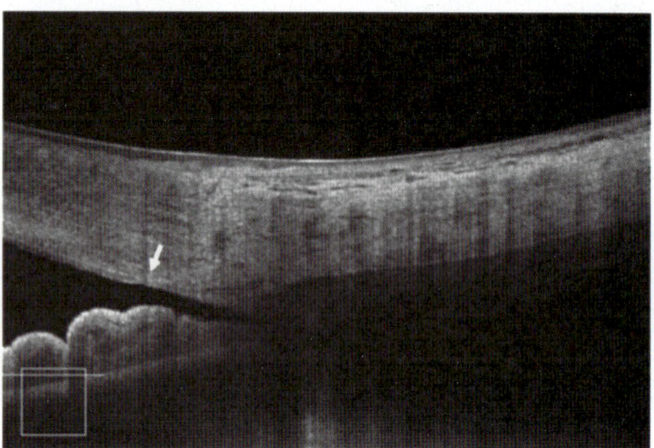

Fig. 40.5 Cross-sectional (not dewarped) high-definition optical coherence tomography images from a Chinese subject with an open ACA, in which it is possible to observe termination of Descemet's membrane (Schwalbe's line – *white arrow*) and also Schlemm's canal. (Photo courtesy: Dr Tin Aung, Singapore Eye Research Institute.)

Recently, the Fourier-domain–OCT-enabled–high-resolution imaging of the ACA became available. This new technology appears to provide enough resolution to identify structures such as Schwalbe's line; and in some cases, the trabecular meshwork and Schlemm's canal (**Fig. 40.5**).

New studies should assess the impact of this new technology in the detection of anterior segment abnormalities; however, until current time, none of the commercially available Fourier-domain OCTs are able to correct the images for the optic distortion of the scanning beam as it passes through the air, cornea, and aqueous humor (images are not "dewarped"; **Figs 40.6 and 40.7**). This represents an important limitation, as this optical distortion may make the ACA appear wider than real. The repositioning of the eye from primary position during image acquisition is recommended by the manufacturers in an attempt to obtain images in which the scanning beam is perpendicular to the ACA region, and thus minimizes distortions at the level of the angle.

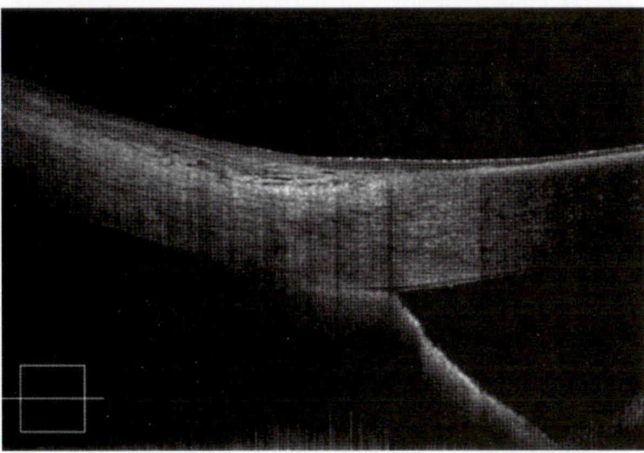

Fig. 40.6 Cross-sectional (not dewarped) high-definition optical coherence tomography image from a Chinese subject with closed angle. On gonioscopy, it was possible to detect the presence of peripheral anterior synechiae at the same quadrant where the image was acquired. (Photo courtesy: Dr Tin Aung, Singapore Eye Research Institute.)

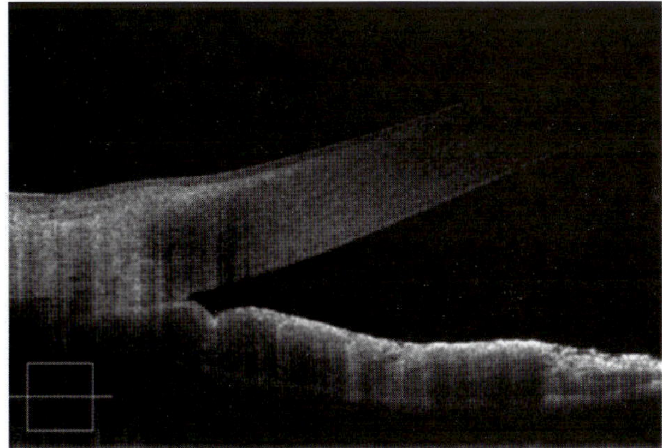

Fig. 40.7 Cross-sectional (not dewarped) high-definition optical coherence tomography images from a Chinese subject with closed ACA. On gonioscopy, it was possible to detect the presence of iridotrabecular contact at the same quadrant where the image was acquired. (Photo courtesy: Dr Tin Aung, Singapore Eye Research Institute.)

CONCLUSION

At the current time, it is not known whether anterior segment imaging is actually detecting eyes at risk of angle closure that are being missed by gonioscopy, or if imaging, for some reason, is overdetecting closed ACA (false-positives cases). It seems that particularities on the methods of assessing and interpreting the ACA configuration of each technique may be accounting for at least some of discrepancies between gonioscopy and imaging exams. Thus, until now, imaging results alone should not guide clinical decisions. Longitudinal studies are required to clarify how the anterior segment imaging findings should be incorporated into clinical decision-making process. Until then, it is important to emphasize that gonioscopy is a required feature of an eye examination and a properly performed dark-room gonioscopy is the reference standard exam to assess the ACA.

FURTHER READING

1. Nolan WP, See JL, Chew PT, et al.: Detection of primary angle closure using anterior segment optical coherence tomography in Asian eyes. *Ophthalmology* 114:33–39, 2007.

2. Sakata LM, Lavanya R, Friedman DS, et al.: Comparison of gonioscopy and anterior segment ocular coherence tomography in detecting angle closure in different quadrants of the anterior chamber angle. *Ophthalmology* 115:769–774, 2008.

3. Leung CK, Li H, Weinreb RN, et al.: Anterior chamber angle measurement with anterior segment optical coherence tomography: a comparison between slit lamp OCT and Visante OCT. *Invest Ophthalmol Vis Sci* 49:3469–3474, 2008.

4. Wong HT, Lim MC, Sakata LM, et al.: High-definition optical coherence tomography imaging of the iridocorneal angle of the eye. *Arch Ophthalmol* 127:256–260, 2009.

Aqueous Drainage Channels

Syril Dorairaj and Vishal Jhanji

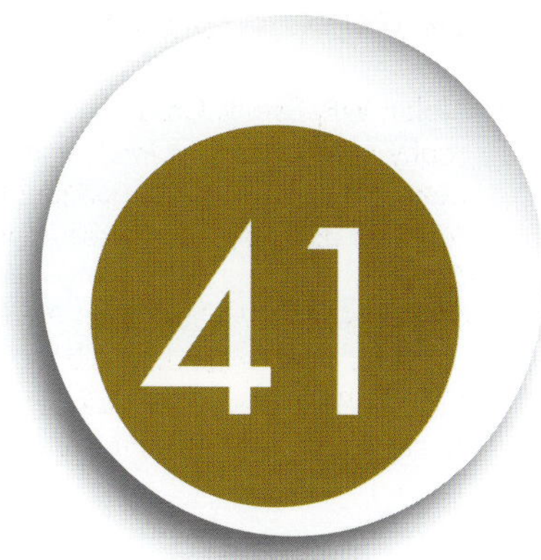

Anterior-segment–Fourier-domain optical coherence tomography (AS–FD-OCT), with its microscopic resolution, can be used to study the structures comprising the main outflow route of the human eye, namely, the trabecular pathway. We reported a technique to improve the quality in the visualization of these microstructures, which can be further enhanced by using serial, radial and tangential scans, and 2-D or 3-D reconstructions (**Fig. 41.1**). This *in vivo* imaging technique of the trabecular pathway led to the following conclusions:

- There is an age-related reduction of Schlemm's canal (SC) dimensions in normal eyes starting in the fourth decade of life; this reduction may appear earlier or progress faster in eyes with primary open-angle glaucoma.

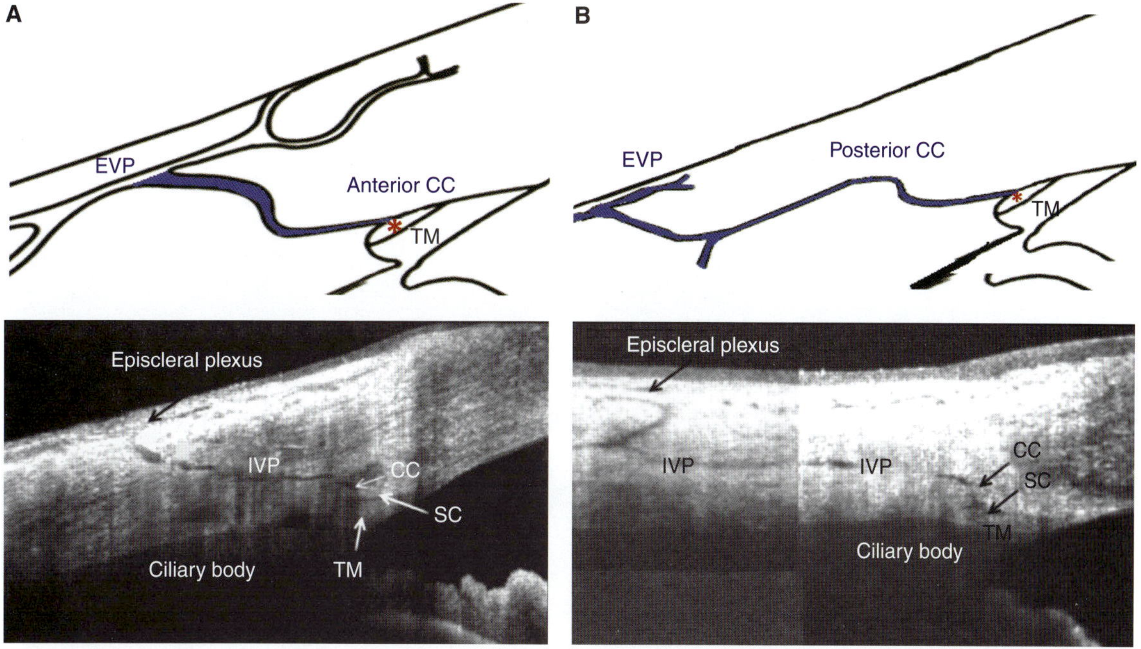

Fig. 41.1 Composite radial images. The CC can be visualized using AS–FD-OCT. According to their course, CC can be classified into anterior (those immediately reaching the episcleral plexus), **(A)** and posterior (those following a loner intrascleral course), **(B)** junctions.

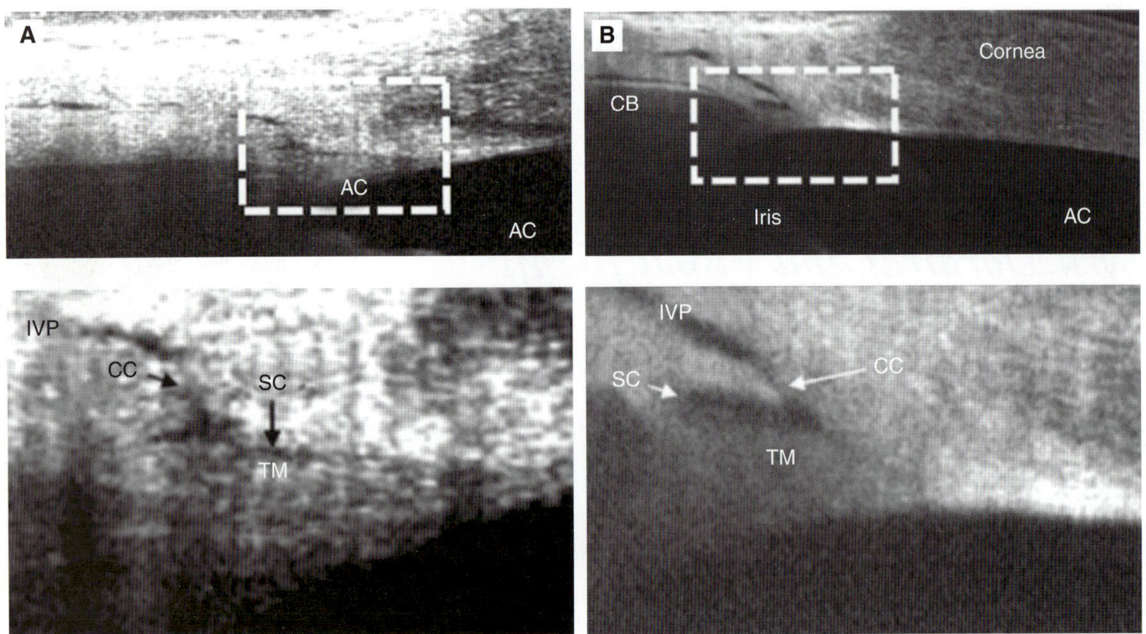

Fig. 41.2 Radial AS–FD-OCT scans capturing the SC–CC junction. A CC exits SC outer wall in the posterior third; the ostium is followed by a narrower section (CC), which then connects to a vessel of the intrascleral venous plexus, which has a wider lumen as compared with the "real" CC. In Figure B, a CC exits SC in the anterior third (towards Schwalbe's line).

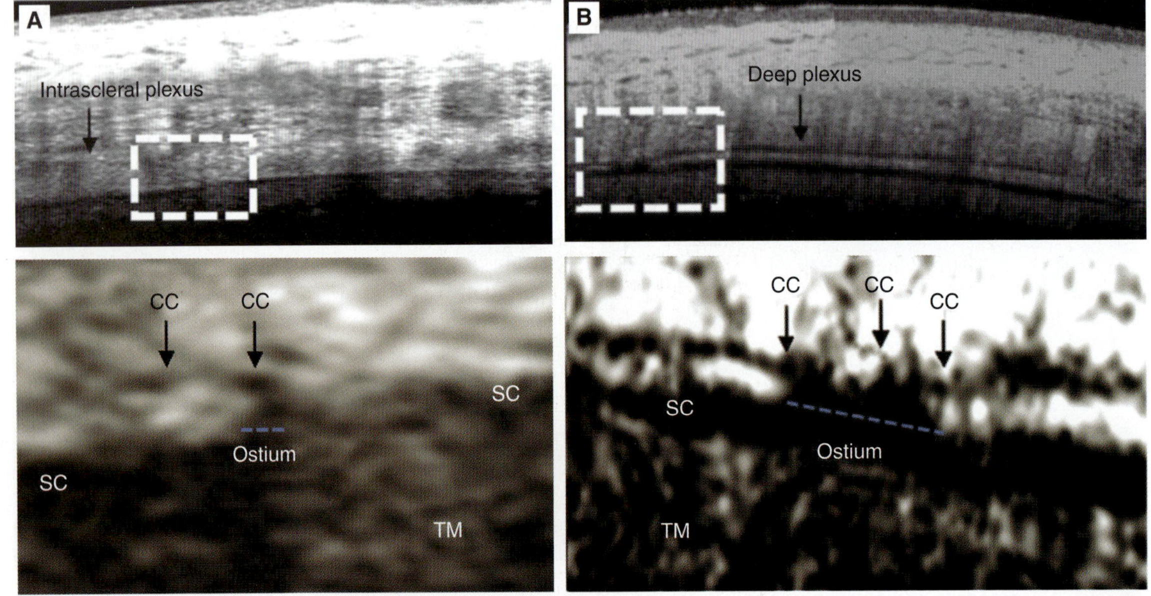

Fig. 41.3 Tangential AS–FD-OCT scans capturing the SC–CC junction. The SC–CC areas of junction can be divided according to their morphometry into small **(A)** and large **(B)**.

- The intertrabecular spaces are lost with age, making the trabecular meshwork appear homogenous and of higher OCT signal intensity in older subjects.
- The collector channels (CC) can be visualized using this technique. They exit Schlemm's canal outer wall and follow an oblique intrascleral course (**Fig. 41.1**). The ostia (SC–CC junction area) appear as dilated areas connecting the CC to SC outer wall (**Figs 41.2 and 41.3**). The SC–CC junctions can also be divided into small and large types (**Fig. 41.3**). Also, they may show a single, double, or multiple CC exiting from these areas. Immediately after connecting with SC, the CC shows a narrower section, which may correspond to what the "real CC" are; this portion connects to the wider intrascleral vessels. Occasionally, the CC can drain directly into the overlying episcleral plexus (**Fig. 41.1B**). Most of them follow an oblique intrascleral course giving secondary and tertiary branches reaching the episcleral several microns after Tenon's insertion (**Fig. 41.1A**). Occasionally, these branches direct towards the suprachoroidal space. Some individuals possess a complete or incomplete deep sclera parallel to circular plexus. In such cases, SC and the CC join through larger ostia and interlinking channels (**Fig. 41.3B**).

The anatomy and physiology of the aqueous outflow pathways of the human eye remain poorly understood. The new technologies or the combination of existent ones will help to better understand these pathways in healthy and glaucomatous eyes.

FURTHER READING

1. Sarunic MV, Asrani S, Izatt JA: Imaging the ocular anterior segment with real-time, full-range Fourier-domain optical coherence tomography. *Arch Ophthalmol* 126(4):537–542, 2008.
2. Leitgeb R, Hitzenberger CK, Fercher AF: Performance of Fourier domain vs time domain optical coherence tomography. *Optics Express* 11(8):889–894, 2003.
3. Castillejos AR, Dorairaj SK, De Moraes CGV, et al.: *In-vivo* imaging of the trabecular pathway and Schlemm's canal with anterior segment Fourier-domain (AS-FDOCT) optical coherence tomography. *Invest Ophthalmol Vis Sci* 2010;51: E-Abstract 3852.

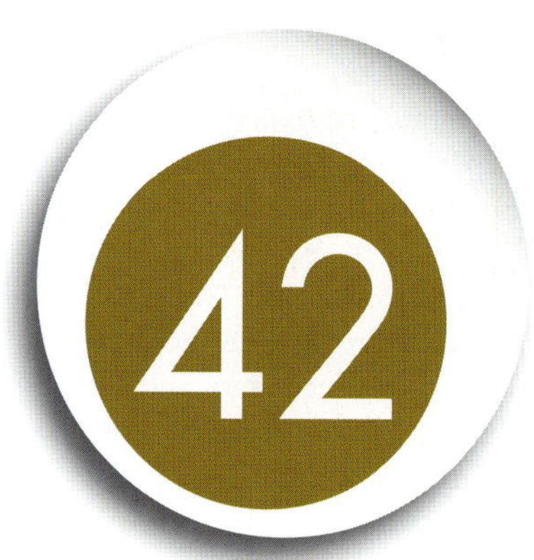

Ciliochoroidal Effusion— Drug Induced

Rajesh S Kumar, Sathi Devi AV, and Dhanraj Rao AS

Acute-onset bilateral angle closure and/or transient myopia has been reported for many drugs, including SSRI (selective serotonin reuptake inhibitors), tricyclic antidepressants, sulfonamides, tetracycline, and some diuretics. The postulated mechanisms by which supraciliary effusions produce angle-closure glaucoma and transient myopia have already been described. The fluid movement in choroidal effusion could be related to drug-induced membrane potential changes or a possible idiosyncratic reaction. The acute myopia seems to be explained by forward displacement of the lens caused by supraciliary effusion, although ciliary body swelling and lens thickening may also play a role.

CASE STUDY

A 25-year-old female presented with a sudden onset of painless progressive decrease of vision in both eyes over 2 days. She was emmetropic previously. There had been no similar episodes. There was no significant ocular history. She had been started on oral topiramate 25 mg once a day for recurrent migraine 15 days back. At presentation, her uncorrected visual acuity was counting fingers close to face in both eyes improving to 6/6 with a refractive correction of –4.25 D. The corneas were clear and pupils were sluggish, but not dilated or fixed. Both anterior chambers were uniformly shallow (**Fig. 42.1A**). Her intraocular pressure (IOP) was recorded as 28 mmHg and 24 mmHg in the right and left eyes, respectively. Gonioscopy revealed bilateral closed angles that opened, with difficulty, to scleral spur on indentation (**Fig. 42.1C**). Dilated fundus examination revealed macular folds in both the eyes, and there was no obvious evidence of retinal elevation. Examination with 78-D lens showed normal optic nerves. Anterior-segment optical coherence tomography (AS-OCT) revealed 360° ciliochoroidal effusion and closed angles (**Figs 42.2A and B**) with scleral thickening (**Fig. 42.2B**). A-scan revealed axial length of 23 mm in both the eyes.

She was advised to discontinue oral topiramate and was started on topical cycloplegics and oral steroids (10 mg per day). Her uncorrected vision had improved to 6/6 in both the eyes without further intervention, 6 days later. IOP was 12 mmHg in both the eyes. The anterior chamber was deep and gonioscopy revealed open angles up to scleral spur in both the eyes (**Figs 42.1B and D**); AS-OCT showed open angles (**Fig. 42.3A**) and only traces of ciliary effusion (**Fig. 42.3B**). Serial AS-OCT showed complete resolution of the supraciliary effusion over a 3-week period. All medications were withdrawn subsequently.

There are multiple published reports of topiramate-induced acute angle closure (mostly bilateral), myopia, and suprachoroidal effusions. All of these pathologies are reversible if recognized early and if the drug is discontinued. The first presenting symptom in most subjects is blurring of vision. Peripheral iridotomy is ineffective for this form of angle closure, as it is not due to pupil block.

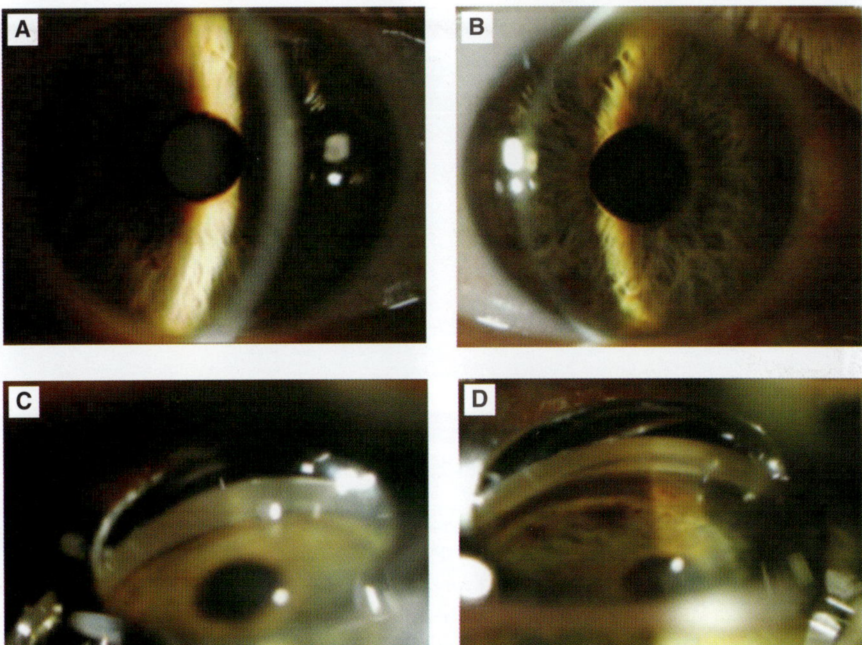

Fig. 42.1 Slit lamp images **(A and B)** day 1 and day 5 gonioscopy images **(C and D)** showing closed angles (day 1) and open angles (day 5).

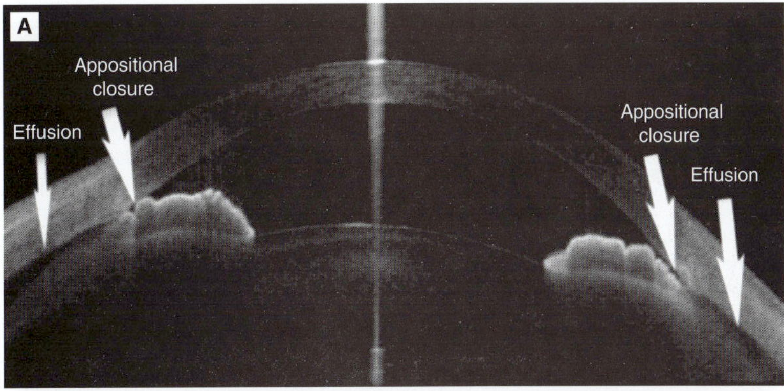

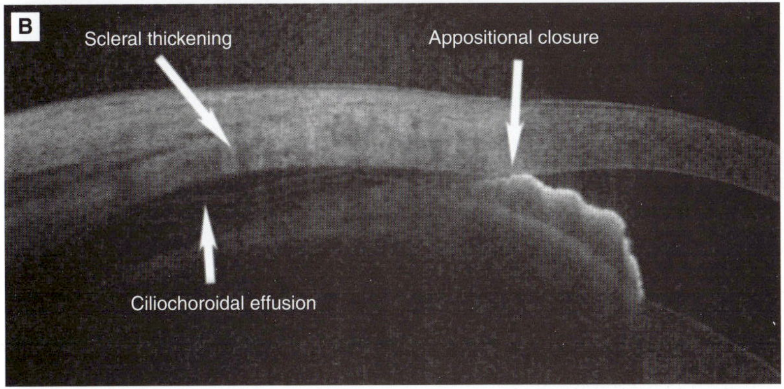

Fig. 42.2 AS-OCT images at presentation: **(A)** overall view (0°–180°) and **(B)** quadrant-specific view.

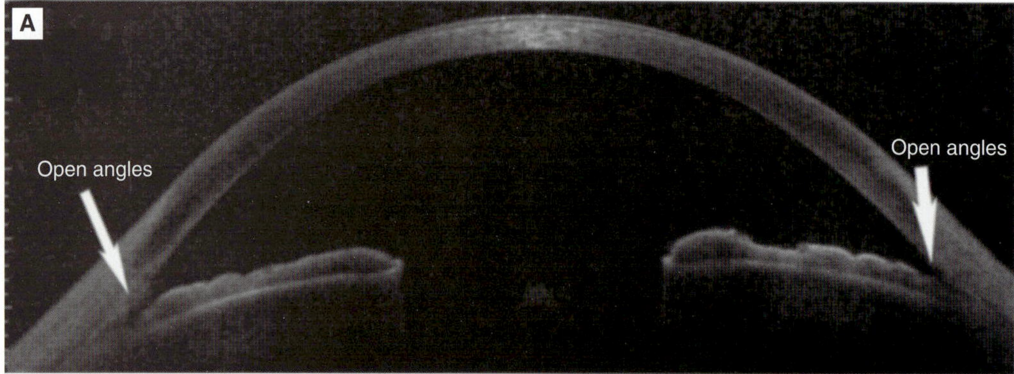

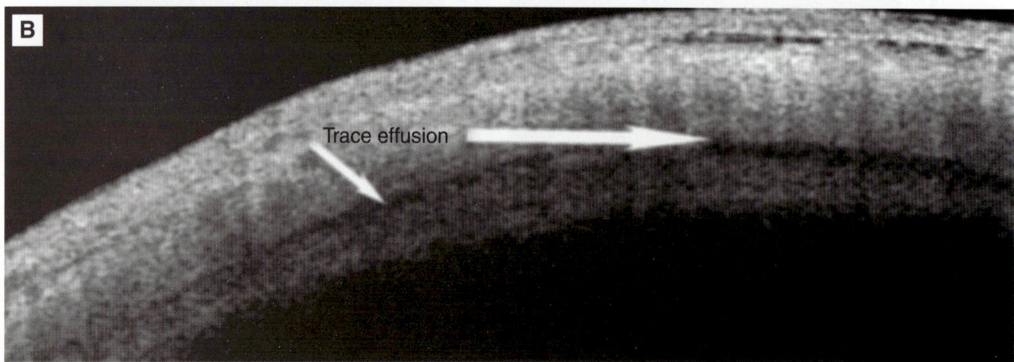

Fig. 42.3 AS-OCT images after 5 days of withdrawing topiramate showing open angles **(A)** and significant decrease in ciliochoroidal effusion **(B)**.

FURTHER READING

1. van Issum C, Mavrakanas N, Schutz JS, et al.: Topiramate-induced acute bilateral angle closure and myopia: pathophysiology and treatment controversies. *Eur J Ophthalmol* 21(4):404–409, Jul 2011.
2. Cole KL, Wang EE, Aronwald RM: Bilateral acute angle-closure glaucoma in a migraine patient receiving topiramate: a case report. *J Emerg Med* 43(2):e89–91, 2012.
3. Levy J, Yagev R, Petrova A, et al.: Topiramate-induced bilateral angle-closure glaucoma. *Can J Ophthalmol* 41(2): 221–225, 2006.

Cyclodialysis Cleft

Rajesh S Kumar, Sathi Devi AV, and Ramgopal Balu

Cyclodialysis clefts are rare entities. A cleft usually develops due to a tear of the circumferential insertion of meridional ciliary muscles that attach to scleral spur. An alternate pathway is created for aqueous humor to drain into the suprachoroidal space that could lead to chronic ocular hypotony. Depending on the extent, intraocular pressure (IOP) could be low (<5 mmHg), causing a shallow anterior chamber, cataract, ciliochoroidal effusion, choroidal folds, and optic nerve head edema. Clefts are most commonly due to blunt trauma; other reported causes are usually postsurgical.

A clinical diagnosis of a cyclodialysis cleft is based on slit lamp findings like iris sphincter tears, hyphema, and hypotony in an eye with a history of trauma/surgery. In the acute phase, presence of anterior chamber inflammation, hyphema, and corneal edema might prevent visualization of anterior chamber angle (ACA) morphology. Since the eye is soft, even if there is no hyphema or other pathology impeding ACA evaluation, gonioscopy would be very difficult to perform due to corneal folds. There are reports of using intracameral viscoelastics along with topical pilocarpine to facilitate gonioscopy and to allow the angle to open completely so as to determine the complete extent of the cleft. Ultrasound biomicroscopy (UBM) is useful in visualizing the ciliary body, but requires contact with the injured eye. Newer imaging methods like the modified Retcam™ provides high-quality photographs of the ACA, but again requires a coupling medium to be used between the probe and the eye. A noncontact imaging technique like AS-OCT could serve as a rapid imaging tool in these cases without causing any discomfort to the patient; it has better resolution than the UBM, but might not allow adequate visualization of the ciliary body.

CASE STUDY

A 35-year-old woman presented with a 12-hour history of sudden, painful loss of vision in her right eye following blunt trauma with a wooden stick. On examination, visual acuity in the right eye was hand movements close to face and projection of light was accurate. Slit lamp examination showed multiple small corneal abrasions, with a 2-mm hyphema and an iridodialysis extending from 4–6 o'clock hour; there was a traumatic cataract with phacodonesis (**Fig. 43.1**). B-scan revealed an intact retina with clear media and no evidence of any intraocular foreign body. IOP at presentation was recorded to be 12 mmHg; gonioscopy was deferred. The patient was treated with topical steroids, antibiotics, and cylcoplegics. IOP was noted to be 6 mmHg at first week visit and dilated fundus evaluation revealed a resolving vitreous hemorrhage, choroidal folds, and macular edema, most probably due to the low IOP. Optic nerve head showed a cup:disc ratio of 0.2, with healthy rims. Gonioscopy revealed a large cyclodialysis cleft, extending for almost 7 clock hours (7 o'–2 o'clock hour); this was confirmed on Retcam™ (**Fig. 43.2**).

AS-OCT images demonstrated disinsertion of the iris root from the scleral wall with a possible communication with the ciliochoroidal space and evidence of ciliochoroidal effusion (**Fig. 43.3**). She was advised cryopexy; when she presented a week later, her IOP was 14 mmHg and best-corrected visual acuity had improved to 6/24; gonioscopy

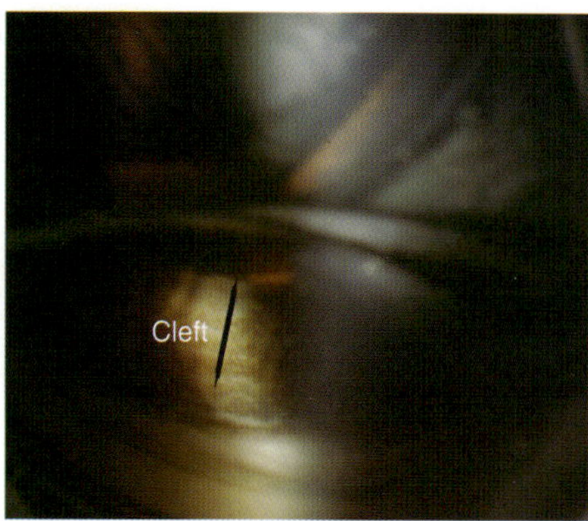
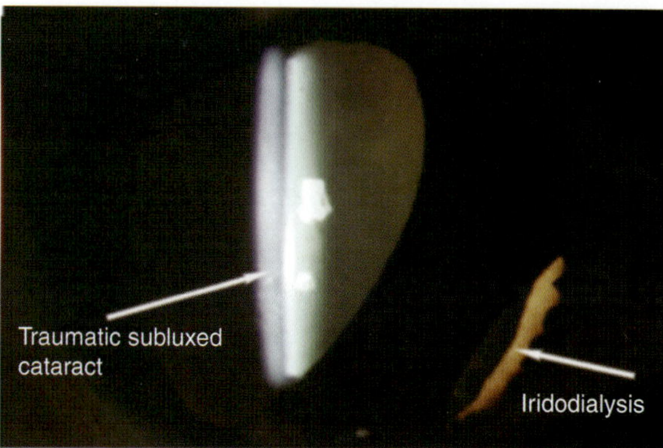

Fig. 43.1 Slit lamp images showing a large cyclodialysis cleft on gonioscopy along with traumatic cataract and iridodialysis.

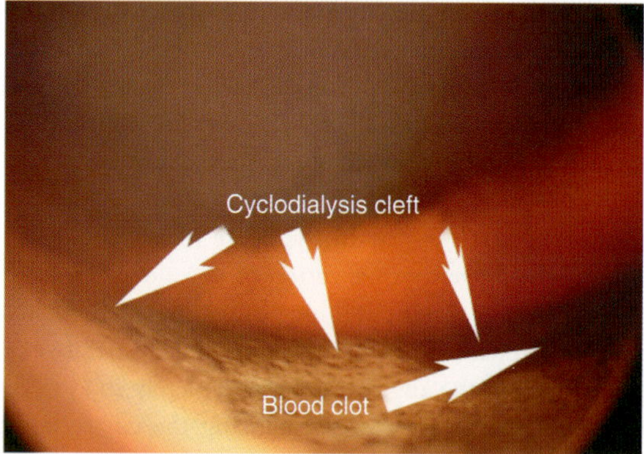

Fig. 43.2 Retcam™ image showing the cleft with a large blood clot.

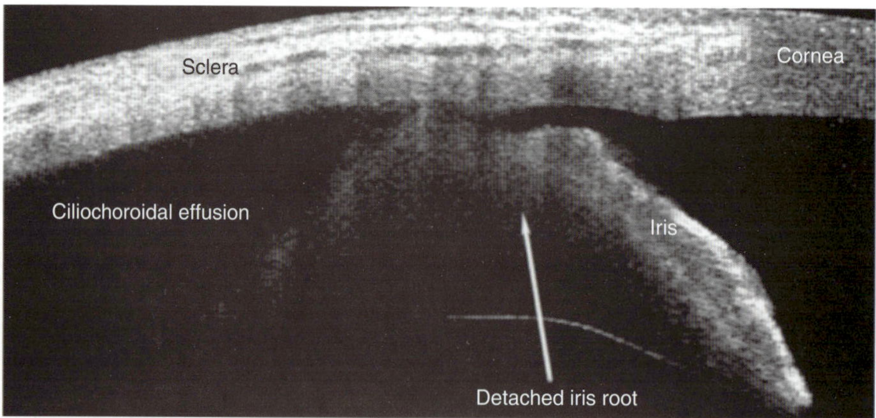

Fig. 43.3 Cyclodialysis cleft can be identified on this AS-OCT image by the presence of detachment of ciliary body from its normal location at scleral spur and ciliochoroidal effusion.

revealed persistent cleft. At 6-months follow-up vision was stable and IOP was 12 mmHg with some retinal pigment epithelial changes noted at the macula; no further intervention was performed.

FURTHER READING

1. Loannidis AS, Barton K: Cyclodialysis cleft: causes and repair. *Curr Opin Ophthalmol* 21:150–154, 2010.
2. Dada T, et al.: Ultrasound biomicroscopy in glaucoma. *Surv Ophthalmol* 56:433–450, 2011.

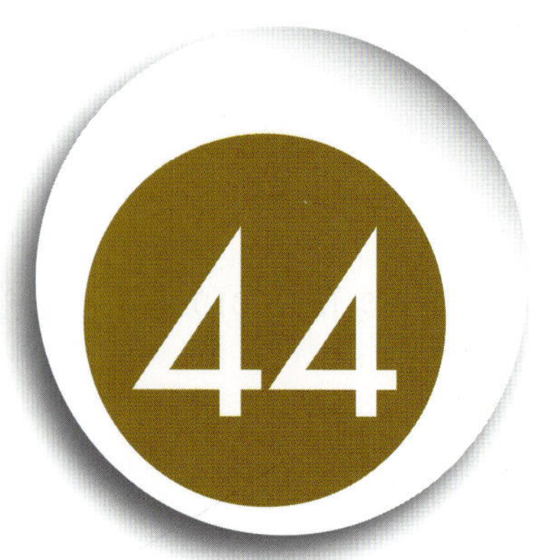

Iridocorneal Endothelial Syndrome

Rajesh S Kumar, Sathi Devi AV, and Narendra KP

The iridocorneal endothelial (ICE) syndrome is characterized by progressive secondary angle-closure glaucoma without pupillary block in association with corneal edema due to abnormal corneal endothelium, varying degrees of iris atrophy, and peripheral anterior synechiae (PAS). There are three established clinical variations described:

- Iris nevus (Cogan–Reese) syndrome
- Chandler's syndrome (CS)
- Essential (progressive) iris atrophy.

The condition is unilateral; it is more commonly seen in women in the third to fifth decade. The posterior corneal surface has a characteristic beaten-metal appearance, and the ICE cells are noted usually on specular microscopy. The fellow eye may also present with subclinical endothelial abnormalities of the cornea.

Glaucoma reportedly occurs in about 50% of eyes and is usually more severe in the eyes that have essential iris atrophy and the Cogan–Reese variants compared to those with CS. The extent of angle closure does not always correlate with increase in intraocular pressure (IOP), as endothelial membrane without the presence of synechial closure may functionally close some angles. Patients often notice some blurring of vision during waking hours due to lid closure and mild corneal edema; the vision usually improves due to corneal "dehydration" after exposure to air. Other signs include irregular shape or position of the pupil (corectopia), multiple iris holes (pseudopolycoria), and stromal atrophy. Although medical management may be effective initially, surgery is usually required. The high failure rate of surgery is attributable to endothelialization occurring over fistula or bleb itself; glaucoma drainage devices might be required in refractory cases.

CASE STUDY

A 38-year-old woman presented with a 6-months history of blurring of vision in her right eye when she woke up every morning; the vision would slowly improve during the day. She had been diagnosed to have "open-angle glaucoma" elsewhere and was on IOP-lowering topical medications. She was a hypertensive and asthmatic on treatment. Her best-corrected distance visual acuity was 6/9 in the right eye; the IOP was recorded to be 26 mmHg on topical latanoprost 0.005% and oral acetazolamide 250 mg thrice a day. On slit lamp exam, the right eye showed the corneal edema, ectropion uvea, multiple iris holes, and atrophic patches with a vertically oval pupil (**Fig. 44.1**) and PAS; gonioscopy revealed almost 270° PAS (**Fig. 44.2**). Her left eye was essentially normal. Her right optic nerve had a cup:disc ratio of 0.7 with superior rim erosion, early inferotemporal rim thinning, and corresponding visual field defects (**Fig. 44.3**). Specular microscopy showed endothelial cell counts of 2555 cells/mm^2 in the left eye and 1464 cells/mm^2 in the right eye. She was diagnosed to have ICE syndrome and underwent YAG laser peripheral iridotomy on the same day.

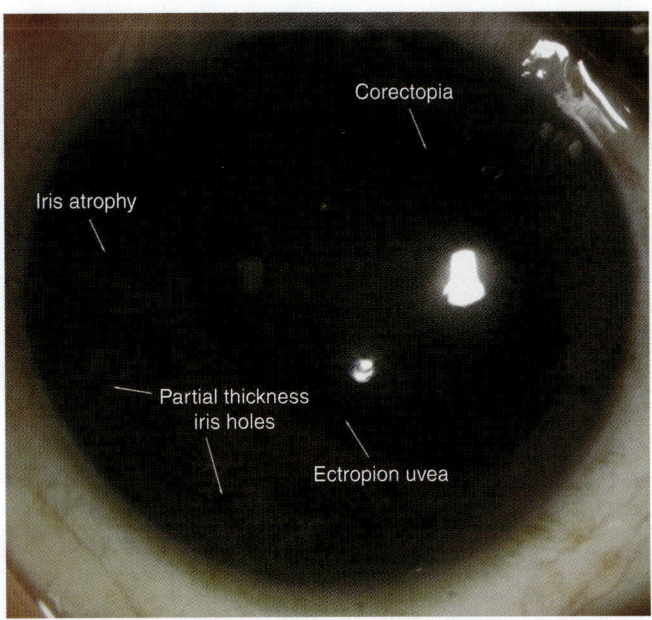

Fig. 44.1 Slit lamp photo of the right eye showing corectopia with areas of iris holes, atrophy, and ectropion uvea.

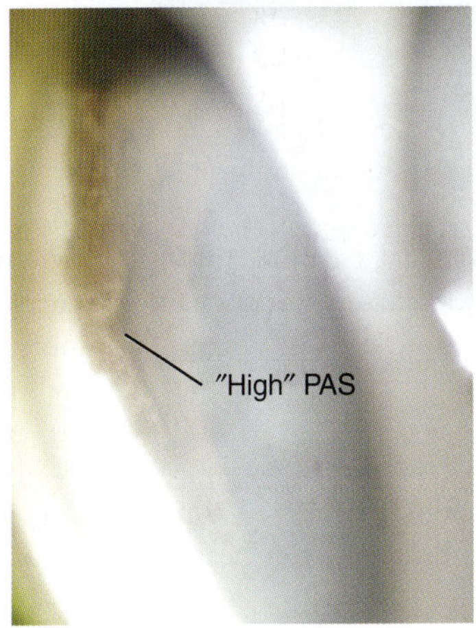

Fig. 44.2 Gonioscopy showing characteristic "high" PAS extending beyond the Schwalbe's line.

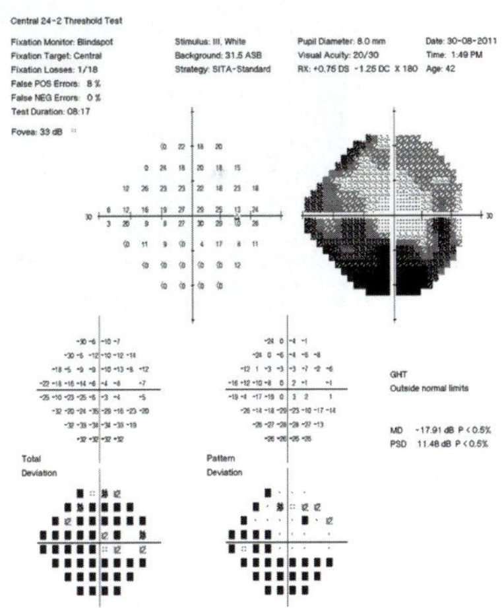

Fig. 44.3 Humphrey visual field (24-2 SITA-standard) demonstrating superior arcuate scotoma.

The anterior-segment optical coherence tomography (AS-OCT) features of the ICE syndrome are shown in the images given below:

- Partial thickness iris holes (**Fig. 44.4**)
- Characteristic "high" PAS (**Fig. 44.4**)
- Ectropion uvea (**Fig. 44.5**)
- Iris atrophy is seen as thinned-out iris when undilated (**Fig. 44.5**).

The right-eye IOP was recorded to be 25 mmHg on maximum medical therapy (without β-blockers given her history of asthma), 3 months after presentation; she underwent trabeculectomy with intraoperative Mitomycin-C

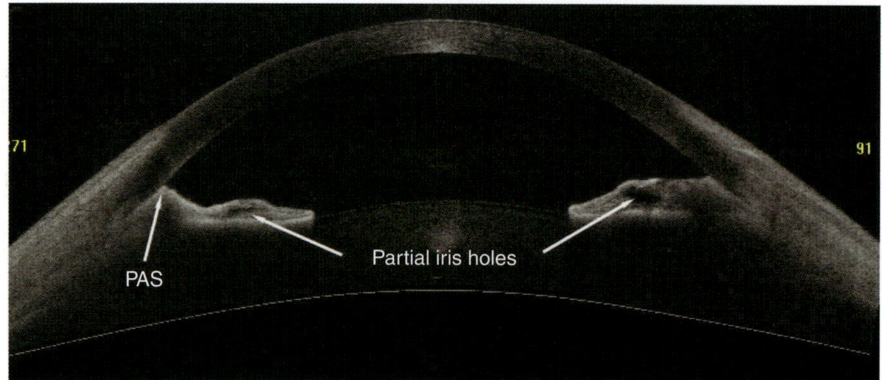

Fig. 44.4 AS-OCT image of the right eye showing PAS and iris holes.

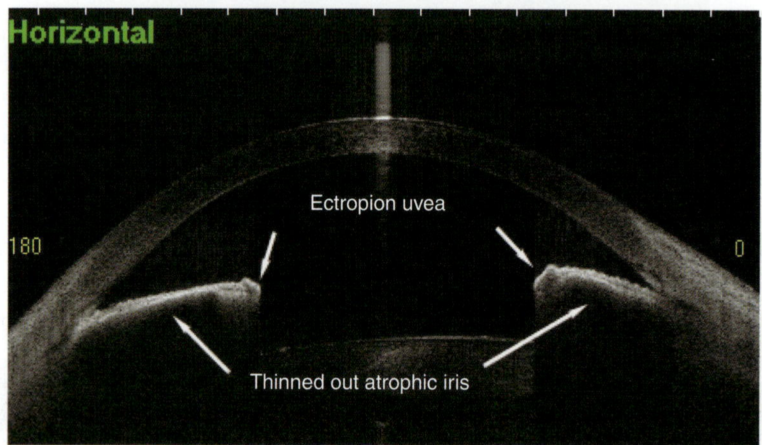

Fig. 44.5 AS-OCT image of the right eye showing thinned-out iris and ectropion uvea.

within 3 days. Her IOP was controlled at 10 mmHg with a diffuse avascular bleb at 6-months follow-up. The AS-OCT demonstrates the entire characteristic signs of the ICE syndrome and can be a useful adjunct tool in documentation of the disease.

FURTHER READING

1. Shields MB, Campbell DG, Simmons RJ: The essential iris atrophies. *Am J Ophthalmol* 85(6):749–759, 1978.
2. Shields MB: Progressive essential iris atrophy, Chandler's syndrome, and the iris nevus (Cogan-Reese) syndrome: a spectrum of disease. *Surv Ophthalmol* 24:3–20, 1979.
3. Doe EA, Budenz DL, Gedde SJ, et al.: Long-term surgical outcomes of patients with glaucoma secondary to the iridocorneal endothelial syndrome. *Ophthalmology* 108:1789–1795, 2001.
4. Lucas-Glass TC, Baratz KH, Nelson LR, et al.: The contralateral corneal endothelium in the iridocorneal endothelial syndrome. *Arch Ophthalmol* 115:40–44, 1997.

Plateau Iris

Rajesh S Kumar and Tin Aung

Gonioscopy is the accepted gold standard for evaluating anterior chamber angle (ACA); however, it does not allow the observer to assess structures posterior to the iris, like ciliary body, and spatial relationship between the ACA structures. Ultrasound biomicroscopy (UBM) allows both qualitative and quantitative imaging of the ACA anatomy, but is cumbersome, and requires an experienced observer and a cooperative subject to get reproducible results. The anterior-segment optical coherence tomography (AS-OCT) is a noncontact, rapid, and reproducible method to view the ACA. However, it is not possible to image the ciliary body in detail using a signal source of 1093-nm diode, as depth of penetration is limited at 2 mm.

Laser peripheral iridotomy (LPI) is the accepted first-line therapy in treating angle closure; however, progression to angle closure/angle-closure glaucoma has been reported by various studies. Nonpupil block mechanisms like the plateau iris that have been reported to be prevalent, especially in the Asian population and could account for disease progression in the presence of a patent LPI.

Gonioscopically, plateau iris has been defined as an ACA with appositional closure, with a flat iris plane, and a relatively deeper central anterior chamber; post-LPI, there is a persistent appositional closure. The UBM is a more appropriate tool to detect the plateau iris, given that it helps define relationship between the iris, trabecular meshwork, and the ciliary body. Recent definitions have included the following criteria for a quadrant of an eye to be classified as the plateau iris:

(A) An anteriorly directed ciliary process supporting peripheral iris as a result of which it is positioned parallel to the trabecular meshwork
(B) The iris root has a steep rise from its point of insertion and a downward angulation
(C) The presence of a flat iris plane centrally
(D) The ciliary sulcus is absent
(E) Iridotrabecular contact (above the level of scleral spur).

CASE STUDY

A 60-year-old Asian Indian man who presented with a 2-year history of recurrent unilateral frontal headaches along with retrobulbar pain was referred for an ophthalmology assessment. He had systemic hypertension, for which he was on medication; he was not on any other long-term treatment. Intraocular pressures (IOPs) were measured at 24 mmHg and 28 mmHg in the right and left eyes, respectively, and angles were grade 0 (360°); there were areas of blotchy pigmentation, without any peripheral anterior synechiae. Optic nerves were healthy in both the eyes. A diagnosis of primary angle closure with suspected intermittent angle-closure attacks was diagnosed and the LPI was performed in both the eyes (**Fig. 45.1**); he was started on brimonidine 0.15% twice a day to lower the IOP. Post-LPI, his IOP did not decrease despite being on the medication; and gonioscopy revealed persistent appositional closure

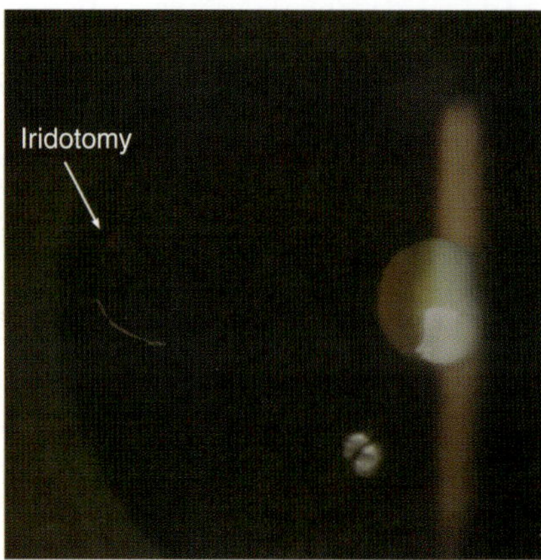

Fig. 45.1 Slit lamp photograph showing an eye with a patent laser peripheral iridotomy.

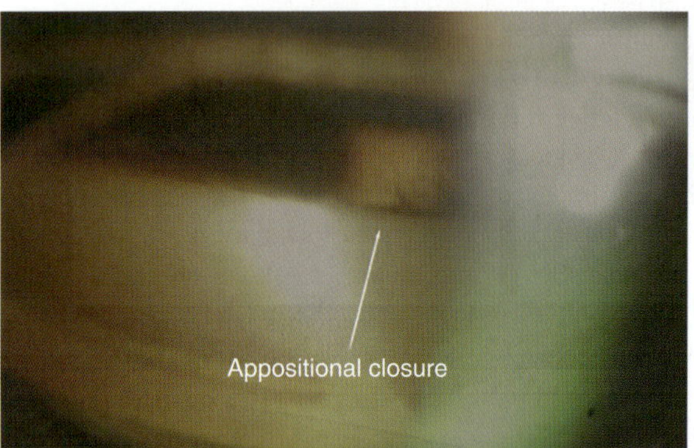

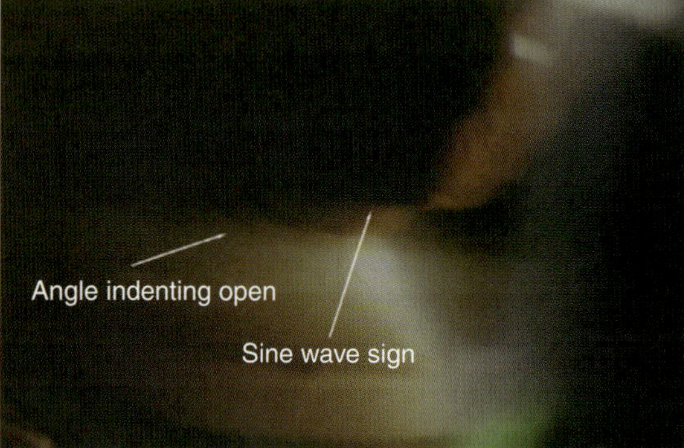

Fig. 45.2 Gonioscopy photographs showing appositional angle closure despite the presence of a patent laser iridotomy and angle opening up with demonstration of sine wave sign on indentation.

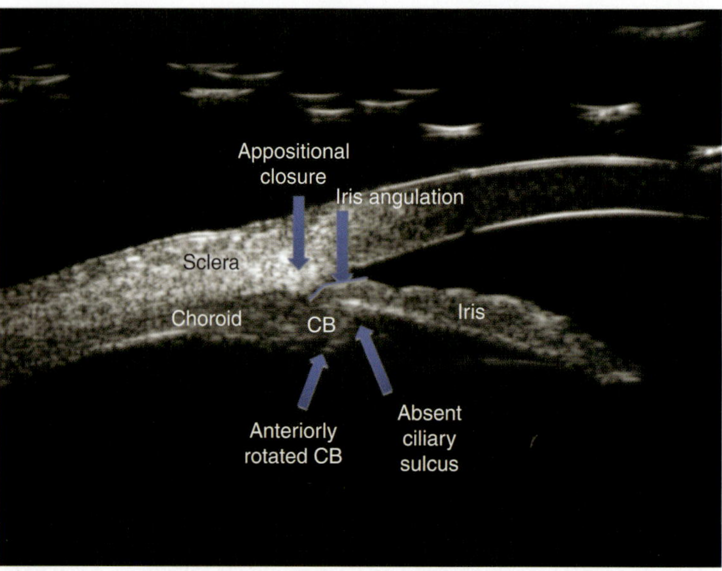

Fig. 45.3 Ultrasound biomicroscopy image demonstrating plateau iris in a quadrant of an eye after laser iridotomy.

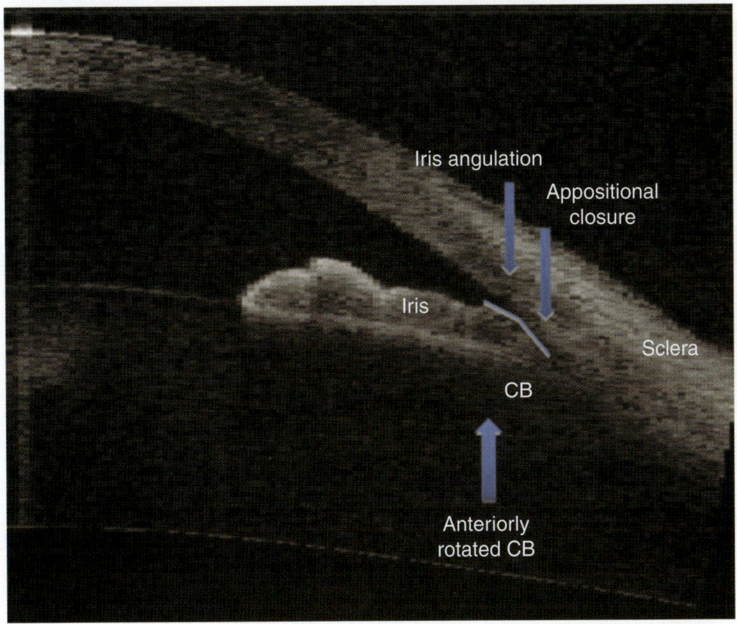

Fig. 45.4 AS-OCT image of the same quadrant showing iris angulation and persistent appositional closure along with anteriorly rotated ciliary body.

over 180° with the iris demonstrating a sinusoidal shape on indentation (sine wave sign) (**Fig. 45.2**). The UBM imaging shows presence of the plateau iris in a quadrant with presence of all described criteria (**Fig. 45.3**).

Figure 45.4 is of the same quadrant highlighting possible landmarks that can be used to identify the plateau iris in the AS-OCT images.

FURTHER READING

1. Snow JT: Value of prophylactic peripheral iridotomy on the second eye in angle closure glaucoma. *Trans Ophthalmol Soc UK* 97(1):189–191, 1977.
2. Wang N, Wu H, Fan Z: Primary angle closure glaucoma in Chinese and Western populations. *Chin Med J (Engl)* 115(11): 1706–1715, 2002.
3. Ritch R: Plateau iris is caused by abnormally positioned ciliary processes. *J Glaucoma* 1(1):23–26, 1992.
4. Kumar RS, Baskaran M, Chew PT, et al.: Prevalence of plateau iris in primary angle closure suspects an ultrasound biomicroscopy study. *Ophthalmology* 115(3):430–434, 2008.

Pseudoexfoliation Syndrome

Rajesh S Kumar and Sathi Devi AV

Pseudoexfoliation syndrome (PXE) is a systemic disorder in which a fibrin-like, proteinaceous substance is present in abnormally high concentrations within ocular tissues. It is one of the common causes of secondary glaucoma.

It is more prevalent in women than men. Age is another major risk factor and it rarely occurs in individuals under the age of 50 years. People living at higher altitudes and those with high exposure to ultraviolet light are also known to be more at risk. About 15%–30% of those with PXE develop glaucoma.

CASE STUDY

An 80-year-old Asian Indian male presented with slowly progressive painless decrease in vision in both the eyes over a 6-month period; there were no other ocular symptoms. Visual acuity at presentation was 6/9 in the right eye and

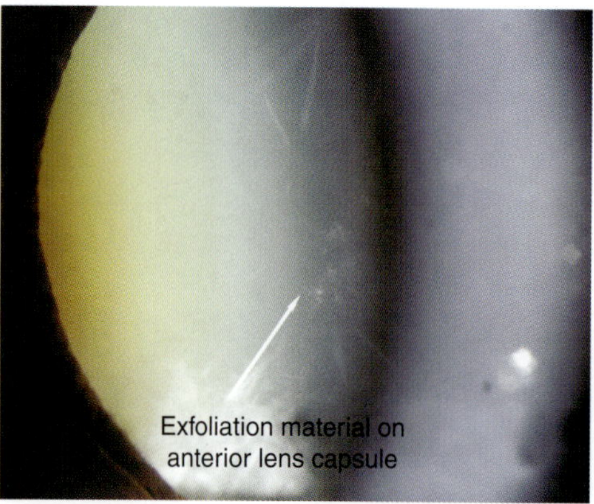

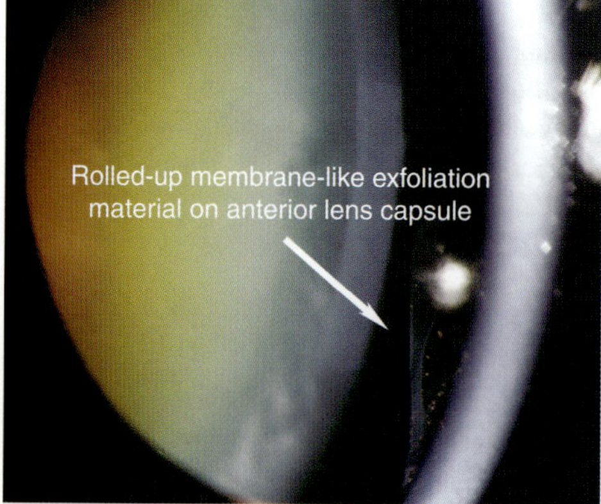

Fig. 46.1 Slit lamp photos showed membrane-like exfoliation material sticking into the anterior chamber.

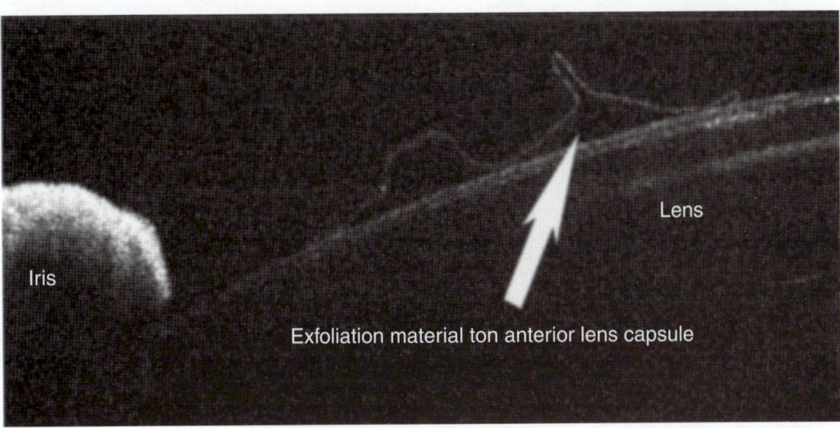

Fig. 46.2 AS-OCT image using hand-held Bioptigen showed rolled-up exfoliation material over anterior lens capsule.

6/12 in the left. He was on treatment for both ischemic heart disease and hypertension for the last 20 years. He had been diagnosed to have the glaucoma in both the eyes and was on treatment with topical brimonidine, dorzolamide, and bimatoprost for the last 2 years.

Ophthalmic examination revealed corneal guttae along with brunescent cataracts in both the eyes. Both the eyes showed pseudoexfoliation material; however, the right eye showed a folded over, transparent, membrane-like structure that appeared to represent true exfoliation of the lens capsule (**Fig. 46.1**); this was seen on AS-OCT as a folded hyperdense structure on the anterior margin of the lens (**Fig. 46.2**).

The right eye also showed subluxation of the lens nasally, with vitreous peaking into the anterior chamber. Intraocular pressures (IOPs) were recorded as 32 mmHg and 20 mmHg on treatment; both eyes had 270° appositional contact without any evidence of peripheral anterior synechiae.

He underwent laser iridotomy in his right eye, following which he underwent phacoemulsification with posterior chamber intraocular lens (with Cionni-capsular tension ring) implantation and trabeculectomy with intraoperative Mitomycin-C application a week later. His postoperative visual acuity was 6/9 at 6 weeks; the IOP was 12–13 mmHg. Although the PXE can be visualized clinically in most instances, the AS-OCT provides a new perspective in identifying and documenting pathology.

FURTHER READING

1. Lee RK: Glaucomas: pseudoexfoliation glaucoma. In: Giacconi JA, Law SK, Coleman AL, Caprioli J, editors, *Pearls of glaucoma management*. Springer-Verlag, Berlin, Heidelberg, 337–343, 2010.
2. Myers J, Katz LJ: Secondary open angle glaucoma. In: Choplin NT, Lundy DC, editors, *Atlas of glaucoma*. Informa Healthcare, UK, 133–149, 2007.
3. Stamper RL, Lieberman MF, Drake MV, editors: Secondary open angle glaucoma. In: *Becker–Shaffer's diagnosis and therapy of the glaucomas*. Mosby Elsevier, UK, 269–270, 2009.

Retinal Nerve Fiber Layer in Glaucoma

Dhanraj Rao AS and
Rajesh S Kumar

Optical coherence tomography (OCT) is one of the objective imaging device technologies available for clinical application in glaucoma. Third-generation Stratus OCT is currently the most widely used device. It relies on time-domain technology, which involves acquiring images by assessing the interference patterns created by echo–time delay of back-scattered light from the subject's retina and those from a moving reflectance mirror. Disadvantages of this technology are lower resolution, slower data acquisition, and motion artifacts. The spectral-domain optical coherence tomography (SD-OCT) is a newer technology that does not depend on the moving reflectance mirror and does not measure reflectivity changes between retinal layers. Instead, the spectrometer detects relative amplitudes of many optical frequencies at the same time within the backscattered light. Thus, multiple points are sampled simultaneously with all the layer depths of each A-scan calculated using Fourier transformation. The SPECTRALIS™ OCT (Heidelberg engineering) scans 100 times faster than the Stratus OCT at 40,000 A-scans/second using an 870-nm light source. A previous study comparing the Stratus and Cirrus SD-OCT demonstrated systematic differences in the retinal nerve fiber layer (RNFL) measurements between the machines. However, there is no published data comparing the Stratus and SPECTRALIS™ in glaucoma till date.

Many studies have reported the diagnostic ability of the OCT parameters. The RNFL thickness in the inferior region of the optic nerve appears to be the best parameter to discriminate between healthy and glaucomatous eyes (sensitivity of 67%–84% and specificity of >90%). This moderate sensitivity and high specificity means that the OCT cannot be used in isolation for the diagnosis of early glaucoma. However, reports have shown a high-positive likelihood ratio of the 6 o'clock parameter; with knowledge of pretest probability, this could be a useful parameter to manage individual patients.

In moderate and severe glaucoma, the OCT might not be of much help as clinical appearance along with visual field is usually sufficient to make a diagnosis. Use of OCT in preperimetric glaucoma is currently limited due to its poor sensitivity in these cases. However, the device could be of help to evaluate progression of disease.

MILD GLAUCOMA IN THE RIGHT EYE

CASE STUDY 1

A 61-year-old female, who came for a routine examination, had intraocular pressures (IOP) of 28 mmHg in the right eye and 25 mmHg in the left eye. Gonioscopy showed open angles. Anterior segment examination was unremarkable. Optic disc in the right eye was medium sized with cup:disc (CD) ratio of 0.5; the neuroretinal rim thickness was equal in the superior and inferior quadrants. There was a splinter hemorrhage crossing the disc margin in the infero-temporal quadrant with an adjacent wedge-shaped nerve fiber layer defect (**Fig. 47.1**). Left disc was essentially normal

(**Fig. 47.2**). The white-on-white perimetry (WWP) in the right eye showed depressed points in the superior arcuate area of the pattern-deviation plot (**Fig. 47.3**) that correlated with the disc findings. This falls under mild category of Hodapp–Parrish–Anderson classification. The WWP in the left eye was essentially normal (**Fig. 47.4**). The Stratus OCT (fast RNFL) scan of the right eye showed mild depression of the inferotemporal TSNIT [(temporal, superior,

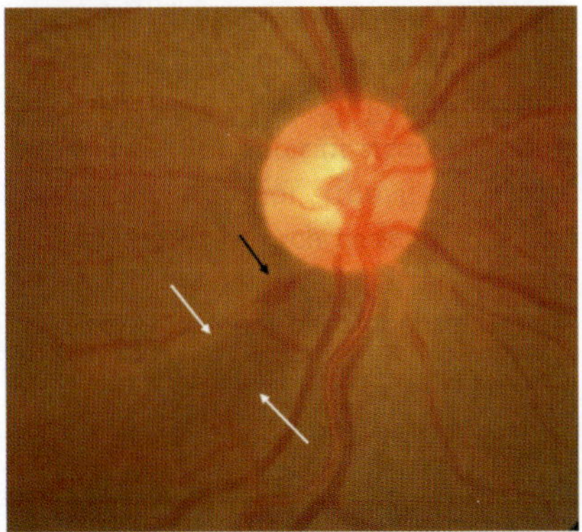

Fig. 47.1 Optic disc of right eye shows a splinter hemorrhage crossing disc margin in the inferotemporal quadrant (*black arrow*) with an adjacent wedge-shaped nerve fiber layer defect (*white arrows*).

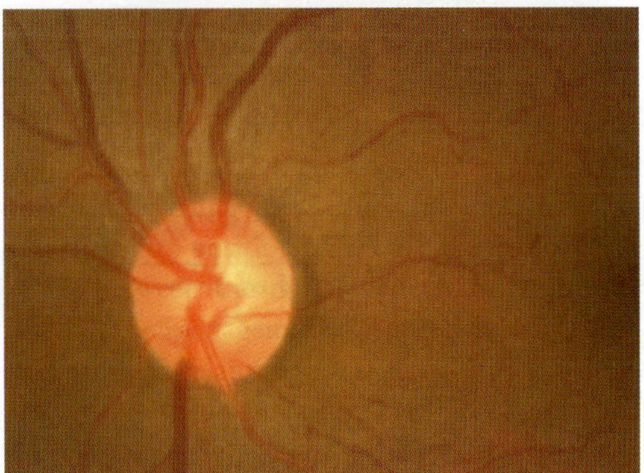

Fig. 47.2 Normal optic disc of the left eye.

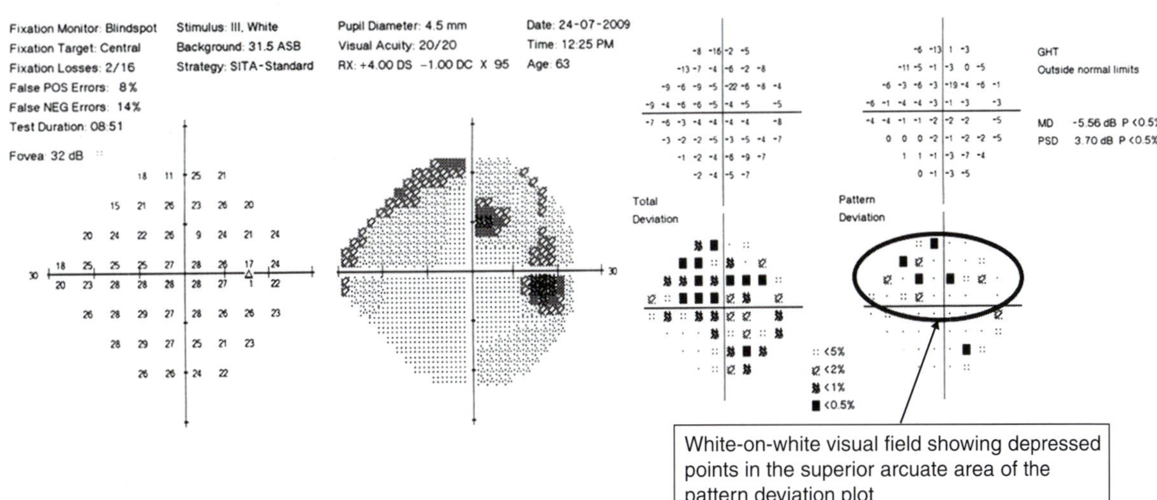

Fig. 47.3 White-on-white visual field showing depressed points in the superior arcuate area of the pattern-deviation plot.

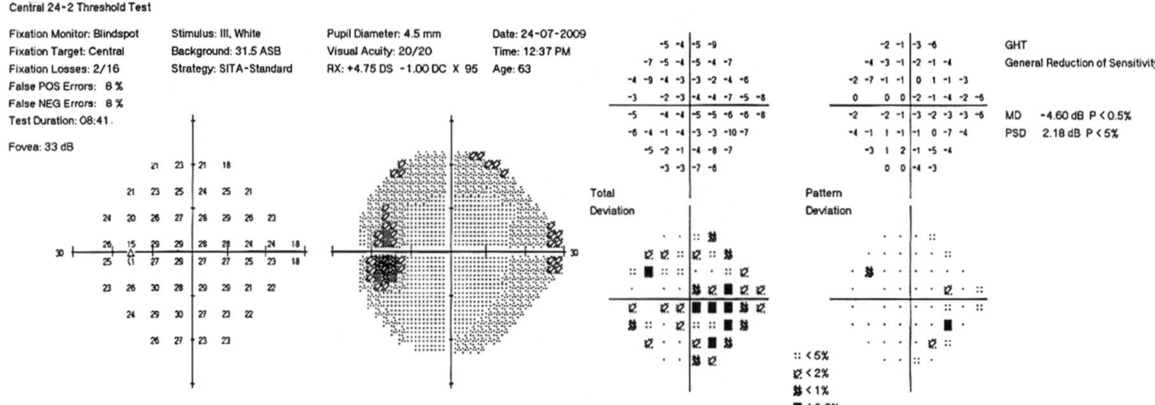

Central 24-2 Threshold Test
Fixation Monitor: Blindspot
Fixation Target: Central
Fixation Losses: 2/16
False POS Errors: 8 %
False NEG Errors: 8 %
Test Duration: 08:41
Fovea: 33 dB
Stimulus: III, White
Background: 31.5 ASB
Strategy: SITA-Standard
Pupil Diameter: 4.5 mm
Visual Acuity: 20/20
RX: +4.75 DS -1.00 DC X 95
Date: 24-07-2009
Time: 12:37 PM
Age: 63
Total Deviation
Pattern Deviation
GHT
General Reduction of Sensitivity
MD -4.60 dB P < 0.5%
PSD 2.18 dB P < 5%
:: < 5%
< 2%
< 1%
< 0.5%

Fig. 47.4 Normal white-on-white visual field of the left eye.

Stratus OCT scan showing mild depression of the inferotemporal TSNIT (not statistically significant but correlates clinically)
Microns
TEMP
SUP
NAS
INF
TEMP
OD
OS
Signal Strength (Max 10) 9
Signal Strength (Max 10) 10
OD Scans used 1, 2, 3
OS Scans used 1, 2, 3
Normal distribution Percentiles
100%
95%
5%
1%
0%

	OD (N=3)	OS (N=3)	OD-OS
Imax/Smax	1.01	0.90	0.11
Smax/Imax	0.99	1.11	-0.12
Smax/Tavg	2.03	2.33	-0.29
Imax/Tavg	2.05	2.09	-0.04
Smax/Navg	2.14	1.76	0.38
Max-Min	108.00	117.00	-9.00
Smax	156.00	162.00	-6.00
Imax	157.00	146.00	11.00
Savg	136.00	147.00	-11.00
Iavg	113.00	128.00	-15.00
Avg.Thick	99.79	109.29	-9.50

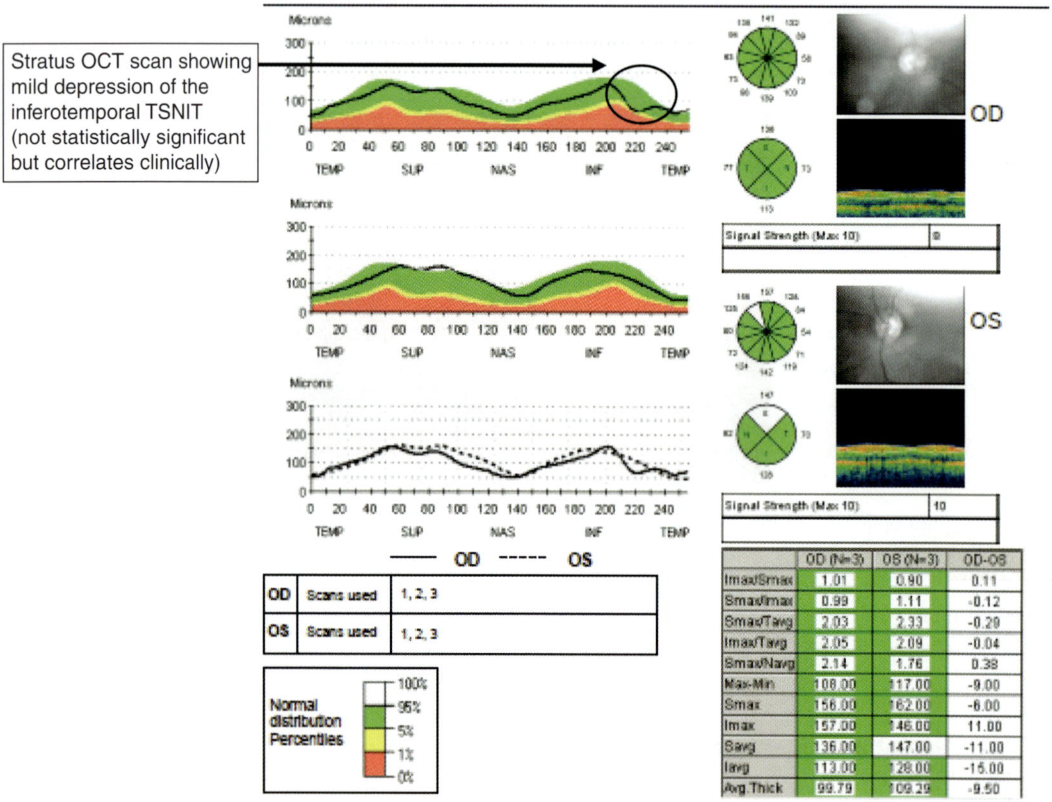

Fig. 47.5 Stratus OCT scan showing mild depression of the inferotemporal TSNIT (not statistically significant but correlates clinically).

nasal, inferior, temporal) not statistically significant but correlates clinically]; though none of the parameters were tagged borderline/abnormal (Fig. 47.5). However, the SPECTRALIS™ OCT did show dipping of the TSNIT graph into red shaded area inferotemporally, and showed borderline RNFL thickness values inferotemporally (Fig. 47.6). This is an example to show that newer imaging modalities like the OCT cannot replace good clinical acumen and that test results will attain clinical significance only when they correlate with the clinical findings.

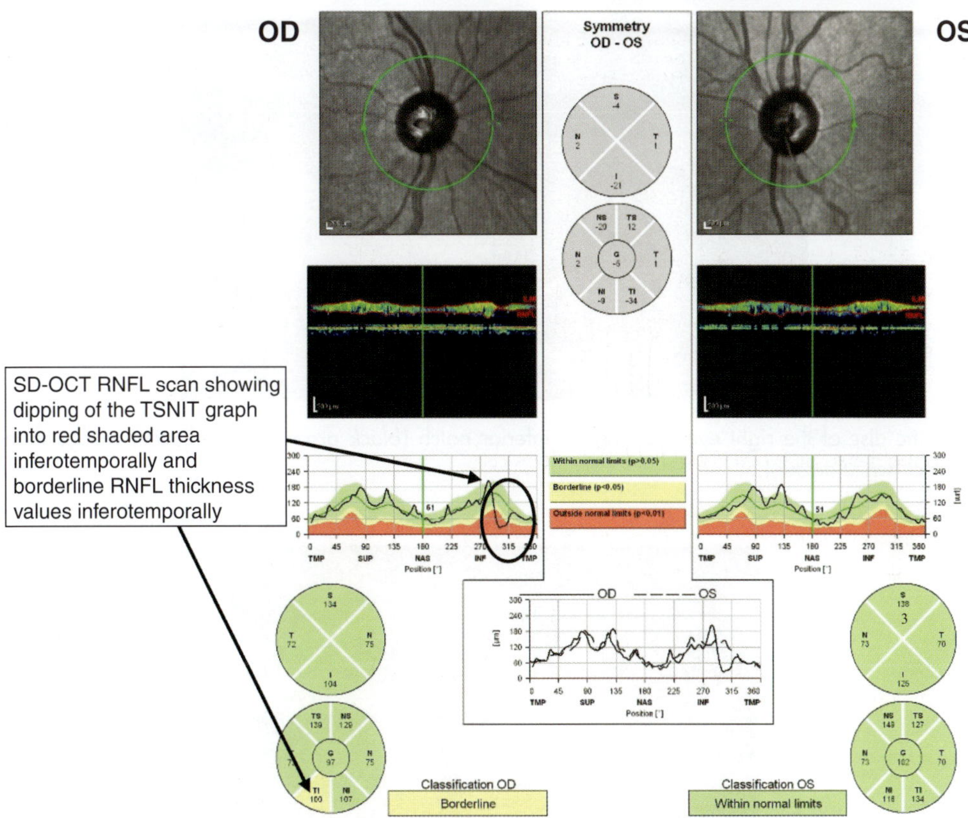

Fig. 47.6 SD-OCT RNFL scan showing dipping of TSNIT graph into the red shaded area inferotemporally and borderline RNFL thickness values inferotemporally.

MODERATE GLAUCOMA IN THE RIGHT EYE AND PREPERIMETRIC GLAUCOMA IN THE LEFT EYE

CASE STUDY 2

A 65-year-old man, who came for a routine eye examination, was detected to have IOPs of 26 mmHg in the right eye and 24 mmHg in the left eye. The gonioscopy showed open angles in both the eyes. The anterior segment was unremarkable in both the eyes. The optic disc in the right eye was medium sized, with a CD ratio of 0.8, inferior notch, and an adjacent area of wedge-shaped nerve fiber layer defect (**Fig. 47.7**). The left optic disc was medium sized, with a CD ratio of 0.7, with the inferior neuroretinal rim being thinner than the superior rim, and a localized wedge-shaped nerve fiber layer defect inferotemporally (**Fig. 47.8**). Primary open-angle glaucoma (POAG) was diagnosed provisionally.

Though the WWP in the right eye had significant false-negatives, the pattern-deviation plot showed significantly depressed points in superior nasal and arcuate areas and inferior nasal area with nasal step. The glaucoma hemifield test (GHT) was classified as outside normal limits (**Fig. 47.9**). The WWP in the left eye was essentially within normal limits (**Fig. 47.10**).

The Stratus OCT (fast RNFL protocol scan) of the right eye showed the following features (**Fig. 47.11**):

1. The loss of double-hump pattern of the RNFL, as seen in the TSNIT graph.
2. Abnormally low inferior RNFL thickness values (coded red), as depicted in the clock hour and quadrant-wise analysis.
3. Abnormally low I_{max} and I_{avg} values.

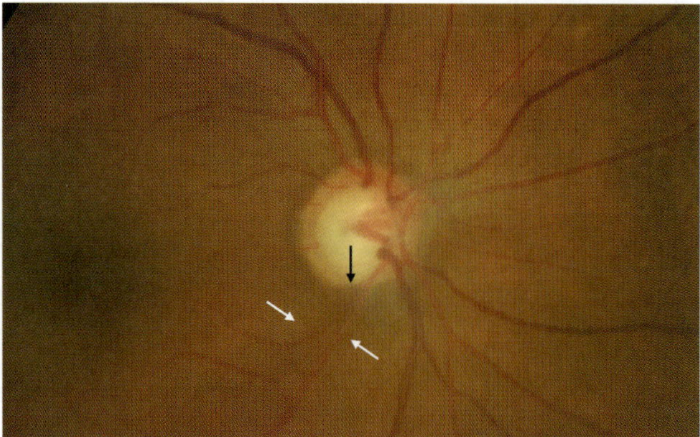

Fig. 47.7 Optic disc of the right eye showing an inferior notch (*black arrow*) with adjacent wedge-shaped nerve fiber layer defect (*white arrows*).

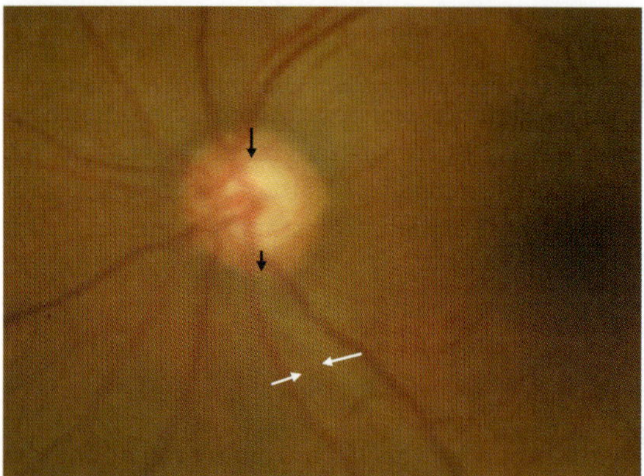

Fig. 47.8 Optic disc of the left eye shows the inferior neuroretinal rim being thinner than the superior neuroretinal rim (*black arrows*), and a localized wedge-shaped nerve fiber layer defect inferotemporally (*white arrows*).

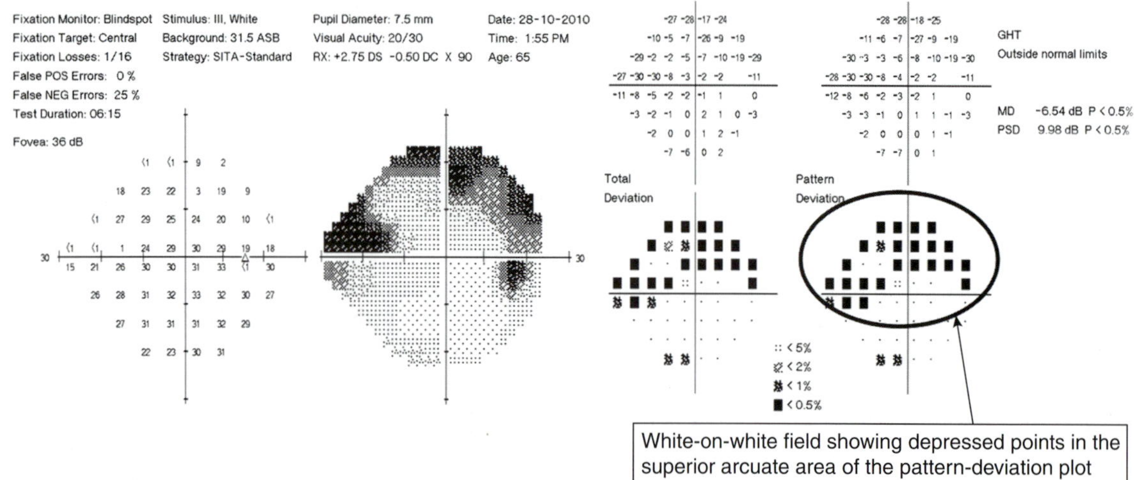

Fig. 47.9 White-on-white field showing depressed points in superior arcuate area of the pattern-deviation plot.

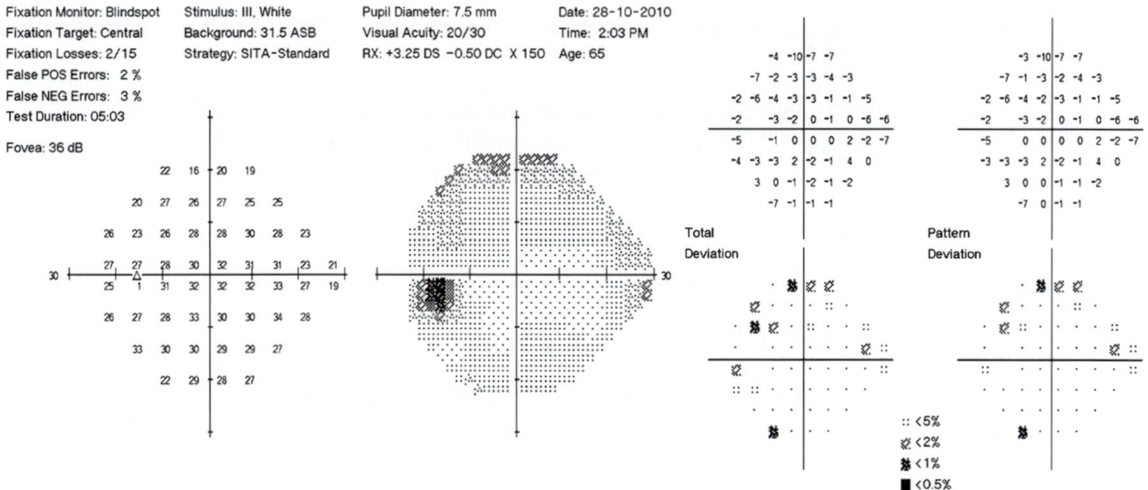

Fig. 47.10 Normal white-on-white visual field of the left eye.

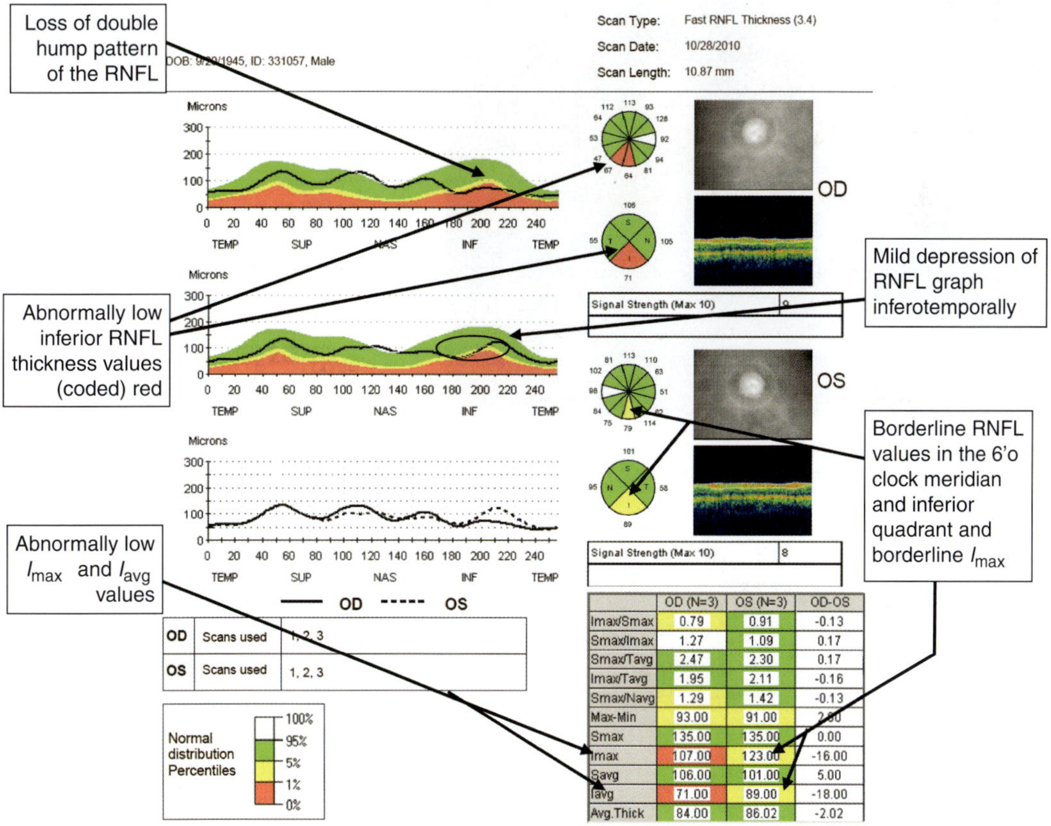

	OD (N=3)	OS (N=3)	OD-OS
Imax/Smax	0.79	0.91	-0.13
Smax/Imax	1.27	1.09	0.17
Smax/Tavg	2.47	2.30	0.17
Imax/Tavg	1.95	2.11	-0.16
Smax/Navg	1.29	1.42	-0.13
Max-Min	93.00	91.00	2.00
Smax	135.00	135.00	0.00
Imax	107.00	123.00	-16.00
Savg	106.00	101.00	5.00
Tavg	71.00	89.00	-18.00
Avg.Thick	84.00	86.02	-2.02

Fig. 47.11 OCT showing clinically explainable features (optic nerve head findings) suggestive of glaucoma in both the eyes.

The clinical appearance of the optic nerve head, OCT features, and visual field correlated well in the right eye.

The OCT of the left eye showed mild depression of the RNFL graph inferotemporally, borderline RNFL values in the 6 o'clock meridian, and inferior quadrant and borderline I_{max} (**Fig. 47.11**). Though the OCT correlated well with the clinical appearance of the optic nerve head, the visual field did not show any corresponding defects.

While severity of the glaucoma fell into moderate category of Hodapp–Parrish classification in the right eye, the left eye had a definite evidence of glaucoma in the form of RNFL defect without any corresponding visual field defect (preperimetric glaucoma).

This patient achieved good IOP control with topical medication (travoprost 0.004% eye drops).

SEVERE GLAUCOMA IN THE RIGHT EYE

CASE STUDY 3

An 80-year-old man, who is a known hypertensive, complained of diminution of vision in the right eye. He had lost vision in the left eye during childhood due to a penetrating injury; the eye was phthisical. On examination, the IOP was 32 mmHg in the right eye. The gonioscopy showed open angles. Anterior segment was unremarkable except for early nuclear sclerosis. The optic disc in the right eye showed advanced glaucomatous damage (**Fig. 47.12A**). Visual

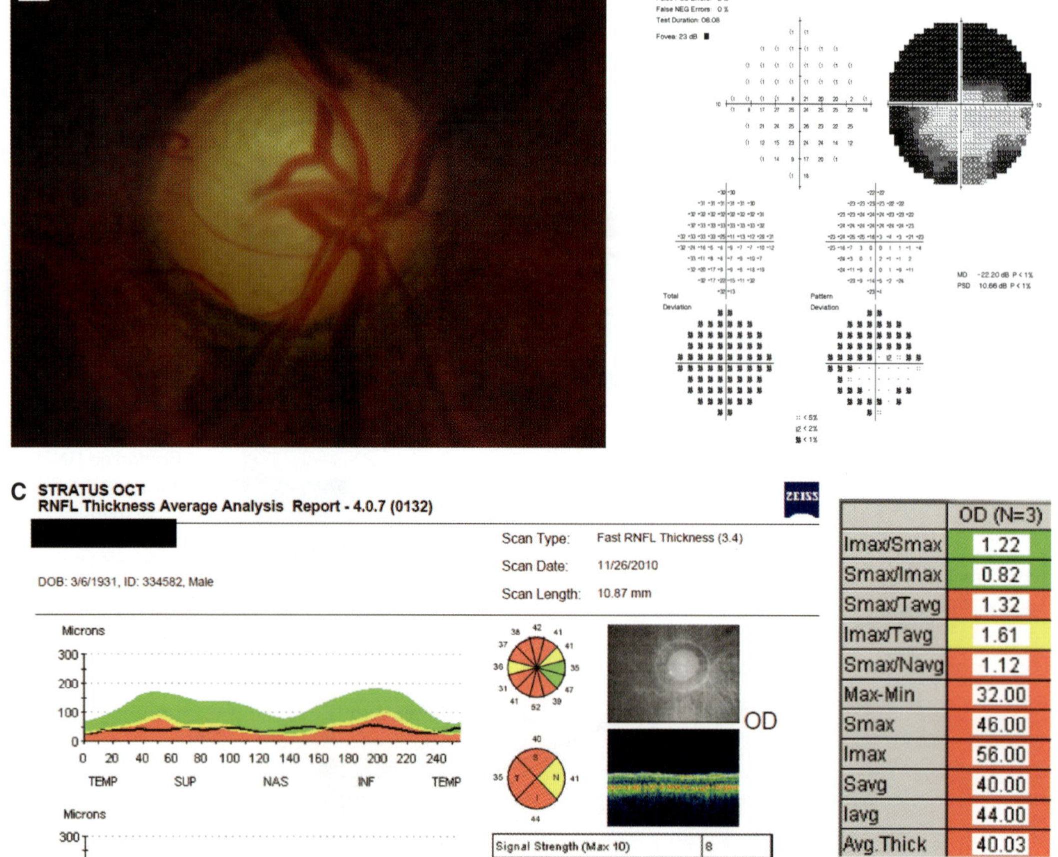

	OD (N=3)
Imax/Smax	1.22
Smax/Imax	0.82
Smax/Tavg	1.32
Imax/Tavg	1.61
Smax/Navg	1.12
Max-Min	32.00
Smax	46.00
Imax	56.00
Savg	40.00
Iavg	44.00
Avg.Thick	40.03

Fig. 47.12 **(A)** Advanced glaucomatous optic atrophy, **(B)** advanced visual field loss with fixation threat, and **(C)** near flattening of the TSNIT graph.

field showed advanced loss with fixation being threatened in the right eye (**Fig. 47.12B**). The OCT showed near flattening of the TSNIT graph, with abnormally thinned RNFL in all quadrants (**Fig. 47.12C**). Although the OCT is very sensitive in detecting severe glaucoma, it is of very little use in these cases as clinical examination itself is sufficient to make the diagnosis.

FURTHER READING

1. Huang D, Swanson EA, Lin CP, et al.: Optical coherence tomography. *Science* 254:1178–1181, 1991.
2. O'Rese J Knight, Chang RT, Feuer WJ, et al.: Comparison of retinal nerve fiber layer measurements using time domain and spectral domain optical coherent tomography. *Ophthalmology* 116:1271–1277, 2009.
3. Schuman JS, Hee MR, Puliafito CA, et al.: Quantification of nerve fiber layer thickness in normal and glaucomatous eyes using optical coherence tomography. *Arch Ophthalmol* 113:586–596, 1995.
4. Nouri–Mahdavi K, Hoffman D, Tannenbaum DP, et al.: Identifying early glaucoma with optical coherence tomography. *Am J Ophthalmol* 137:228–235, 2004.
5. Bowd C, Zangwill LM, Berry CC, et al.: Detecting early glaucoma by assessment of retinal nerve fiber layer thickness and visual function. *Invest Ophthalmol Vis Sci* 42:1993–2003, 2001.
6. Budenz DL, Michael A, Chang RT, et al.: Sensitivity and specificity of the Stratus OCT for perimetric glaucoma. *Ophthalmology* 112:3–9, 2005.
7. Kanamori A, Nakamura M, Escano MF, et al.: Evaluation of the glaucomatous damage on retinal nerve fiber layer thickness measured by optical coherence tomography. *Am J Ophthalmol* 135:513–520, 2003.
8. Parikh RS, Parikh S, Sekhar GC, et al.: Diagnostic capability of optical coherence tomography (Stratus OCT 3) in early glaucoma. *Ophthalmology* 114:2238–2243, 2007.

Bleb Imaging: Effect of Suturolysis

Rajesh S Kumar and Sathi Devi AV

Bleb morphology after trabeculectomy is a useful clinical parameter to determine bleb function, and could be a predictor of long-term success of the procedure.

Ultrasound biomicroscopy (UBM) has been found to be useful in predicting functioning of a bleb. It has also been used to evaluate blebs after interventions such as laser suture lysis. Recent studies have evaluated utility of anterior-segment optical coherence tomography (AS-OCT) for determining bleb structure and found good correlation with clinical findings. The AS-OCT eliminates need for water bath in contact with the globe. This is especially useful while determining bleb morphology that may be altered by contact and also during immediate postoperative period.

CASE STUDY

A 69-year-old woman presented with a history of painless progressive decrease in visual acuity; the only significant history was that her mother had been on treatment for glaucoma for the last 10 years. Her best-corrected visual acuity was 6/6 in both the eyes; there was grade 1 nuclear sclerosis. Intraocular pressures (IOP) in both the eyes were 34–36 mmHg with Goldmann applanation tonometry and gonioscopy revealed open angles. Her optic nerve assessment revealed medium-sized discs with cup:disc ratios of 0.8–0.9 with bipolar erosions in both eyes. She was started

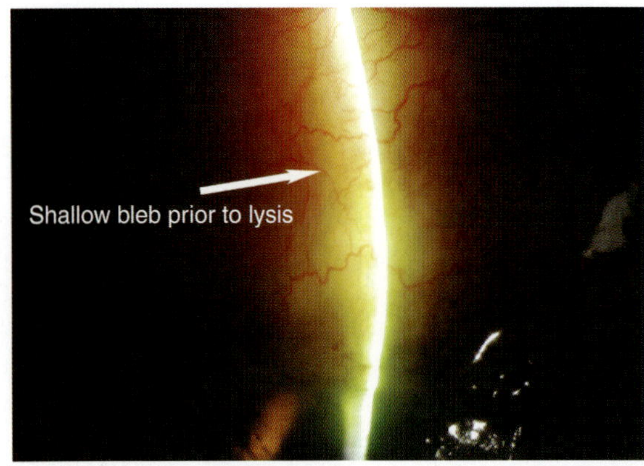

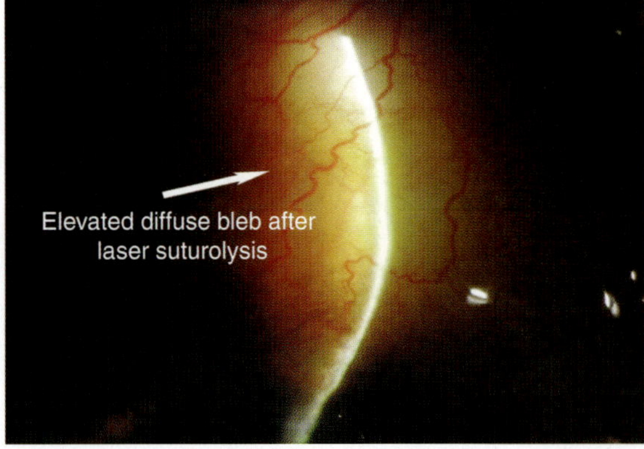

Fig. 48.1 Slit lamp photos showing an increase in bleb height after laser suturolysis.

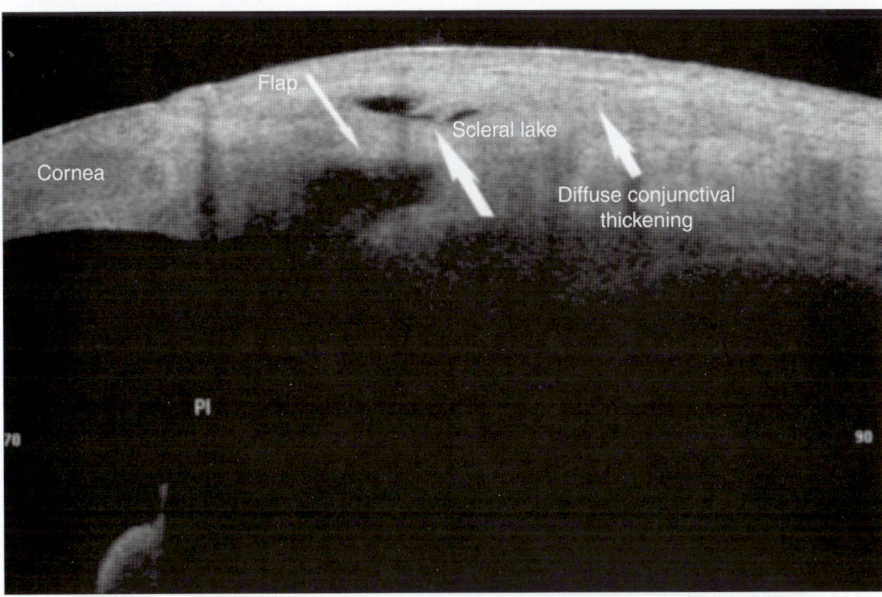

Fig. 48.2 AS-OCT of eye prior to suturolysis showing flap with a small scleral lake and diffuse conjunctival thickening.

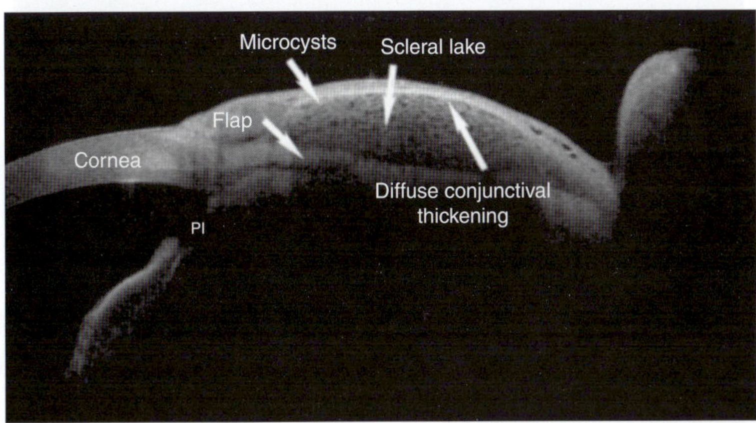

Fig. 48.3 AS-OCT image of eye a week after suturolysis showing a much larger subconjunctival cavity filled, micro-cystic spaces, and diffuse subconjunctival thickening.

on maximum medical therapy topically; her IOP were 24 mmHg and 27 mmHg after 6 weeks. She underwent trabeculectomy with two interrupted non-absorbable sutures along with intra-operative Mitomycin-C (0.4 mg/ml for 2 minutes) in her right eye; at 3-weeks follow-up, her IOP was 19 mmHg with a shallow vascular bleb. Argon suturolysis was performed to cut a single suture; the bleb increased in size on gentle digital massage and IOP was recorded as 12 mmHg (**Fig. 48.1**).

The IOP was stable at 12 mmHg without any medications at 6-months follow-up, with a moderately diffuse vascular bleb. The AS-OCT allows both qualitative and quantitative evaluation of trabeculectomy bleb (**Figs 48.2–48.5**).

Small cystic blebs without microcysts represent a failed procedure, and this could help prognosticate the long-term efficacy of the bleb.

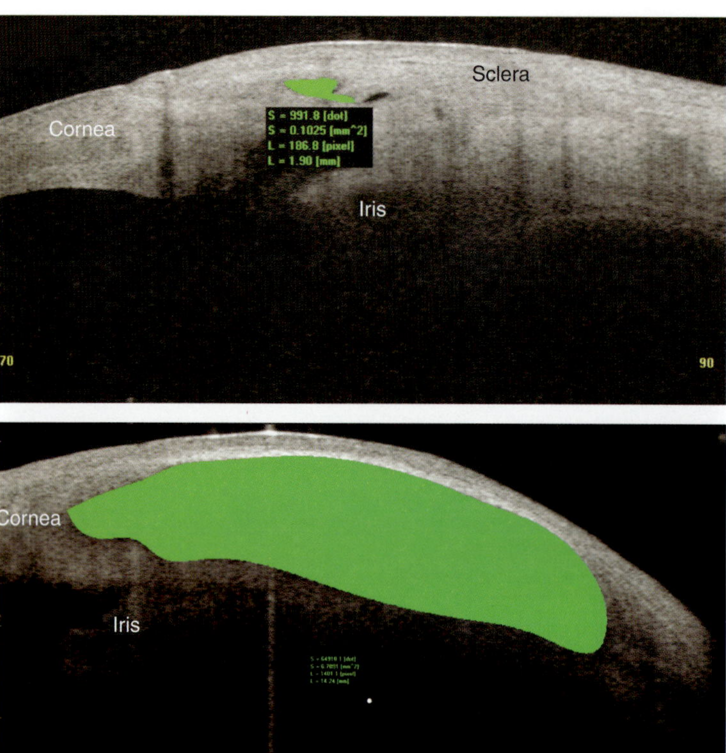

Fig. 48.4 Area analysis performed using built-in software on the machine showed a significant increase in scleral lake after suturolysis.

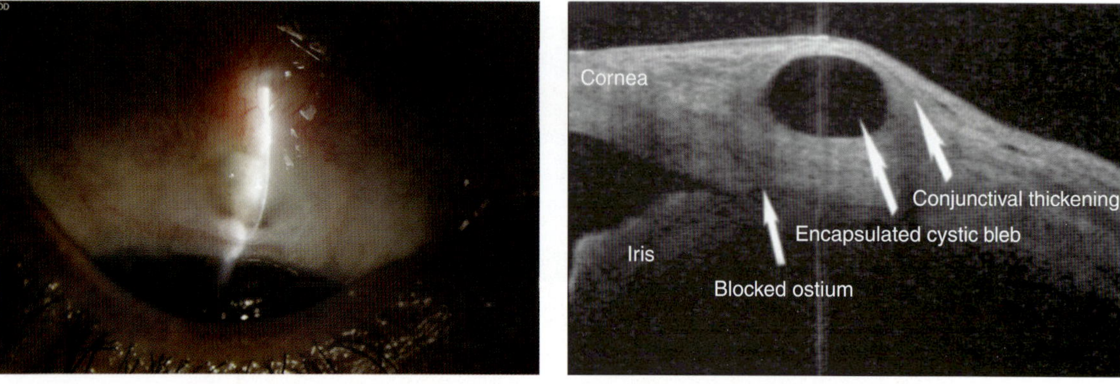

Fig. 48.5 The images above depict an eye 1 year after trabeculectomy that had an encapsulated bleb (slit lamp-left) with a thick wall, high reflectivity, and an enclosed fluid-filled space (AS-OCT image-right).

FURTHER READING

1. Park HY, Ahn MD: Imaging of trabeculectomy blebs with Visante anterior segment optical coherence tomography after digital ocular compression. *Jpn J Ophthalmol* 56(1):38–45, 2012.
2. Sng CC, Singh M, Chew PT, et al.: Quantitative assessment of changes in trabeculectomy blebs after laser suture lysis using anterior segment coherence tomography. *J Glaucoma* 21(5):313–317, 2012.
3. Singh M, Aung T, Friedman DS, et al.: Anterior segment optical coherence tomography imaging of trabeculectomy blebs before and after laser suture lysis. *Am J Ophthalmol* 143(5):873–875, 2007.

Glaucoma Drainage Device—Imaging

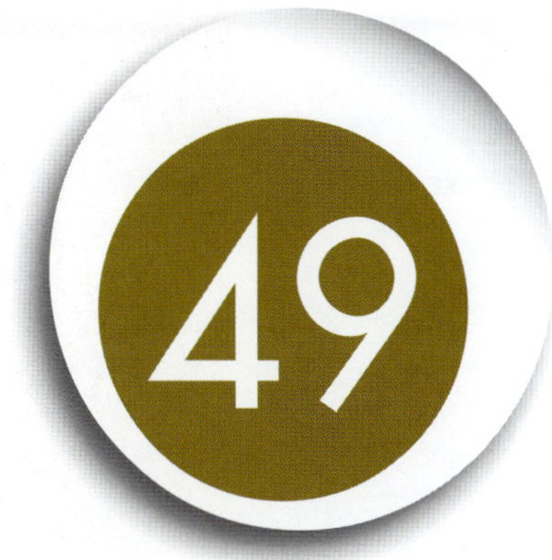

Poemen PM Chan and
Christopher KS Leung

The anterior-segment optical coherence tomography (AS-OCT) is useful to evaluate position and patency of glaucoma drainage devices (GDDs), particularly in the presence of corneal opacity or corneal edema when the slit lamp biomicroscopy only provides limited view of the anterior chamber. Allowing cross-sectional visualization of drainage tube in relation to cornea, iris, and lens, tube malposition can be readily determined. Parameters such as the distance of posterior cornea to tube, tube angle to posterior corneal surface, tube angle to anterior iris, distance from the tube to the anterior iris, and tube length can be measured precisely. However, the clinical impact of these measurements remains to be established. The hypothesis that a shorter distance between the tube and corneal endothelium is associated with a greater extent of corneal endothelial cell loss has not been validated.

TUBE EROSION

CASE STUDY 1

A 65-year-old man with advanced primary open-angle glaucoma had an Ahmed glaucoma valve implant inserted in his left eye. The intraocular pressure was under control with no visual field loss over the past 6 years. **Figure 49.1** shows

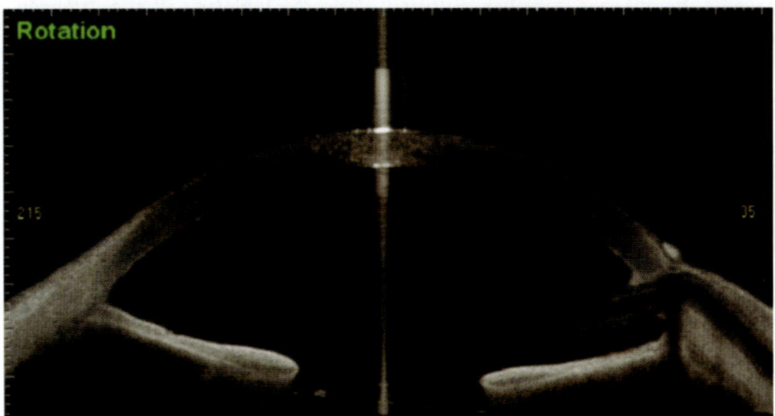

Fig. 49.1 An anterior-segment optical coherence tomography (AS-OCT) image shows the anterior chamber of an eye with a glaucoma drainage device inserted. The drainage tube was patent and well positioned between the cornea and the iris.

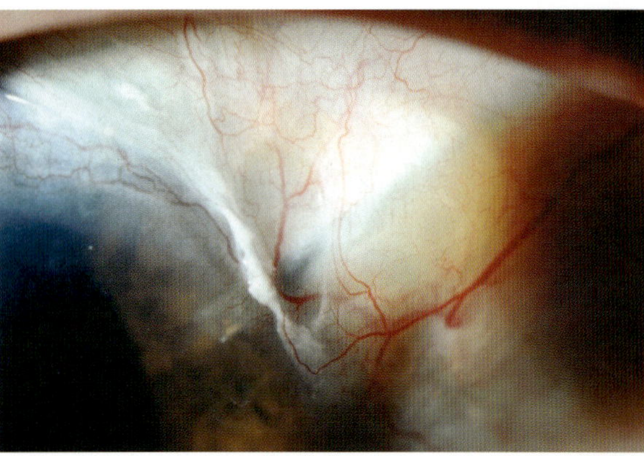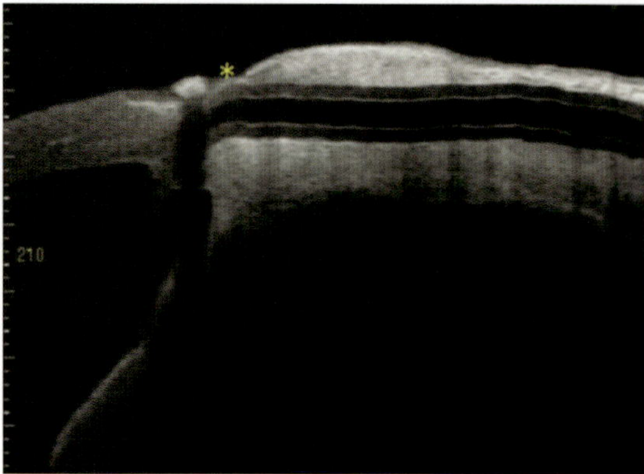

Fig. 49.2 Slit lamp photograph shows early tube erosion at limbus (*left*). Conjunctival thickness (*) measured in optical coherence tomography (OCT) image was 86 μm (*right*).

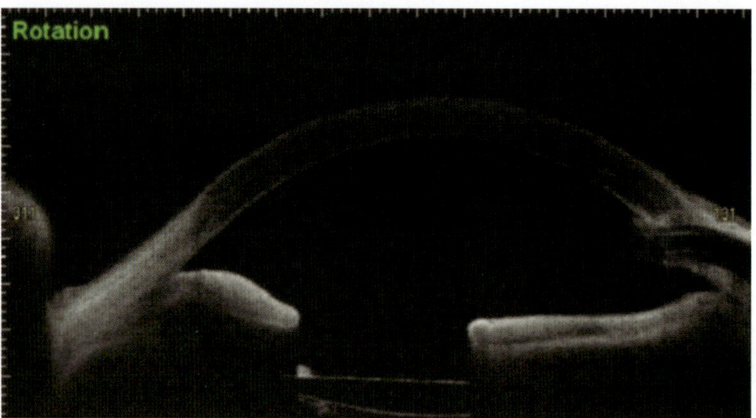

Fig. 49.3 An anterior-segment optical coherence tomography (AS-OCT) image showing tube retraction.

a cross-sectional image of the anterior chamber captured along the long axis of the drainage tube. The tube was well positioned between the cornea and the iris, and there was no abnormal increase in reflectivity in the tube lumen, suggesting tube patency. However, examination of the drainage tube along the scleral bed indicates early erosion at the limbus (**Fig. 49.2**). There was only a thin layer of conjunctiva covering the tube [conjunctival thickness (*) measured in the OCT image = 86 μm]. No leakage was detected.

TUBE RETRACTION

CASE STUDY 2

A 24-year-old woman with juvenile-onset glaucoma had an Ahmed glaucoma valve implanted in her right eye when she was 13 years old. The intraocular pressure (IOP) was then maintained at a level between 14 mmHg and 16 mmHg with two intraocular pressure lowering medications. Notably, the AS-OCT image indicates that although the lumen of the tube was patent, the tube was retracted (**Fig. 49.3**). Serial monitoring of the tube position with AS-OCT would be needed to assist the clinical management.

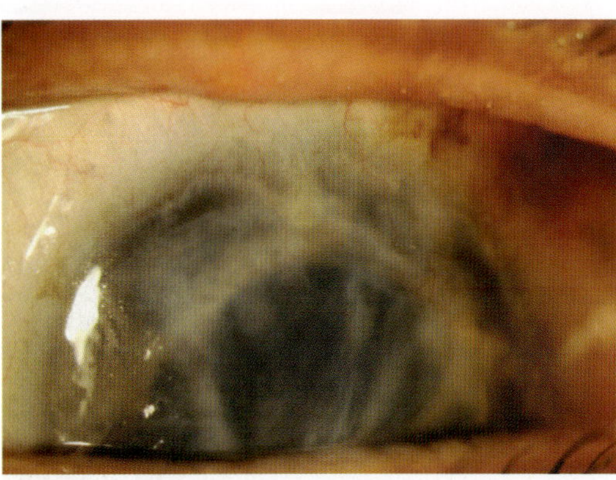 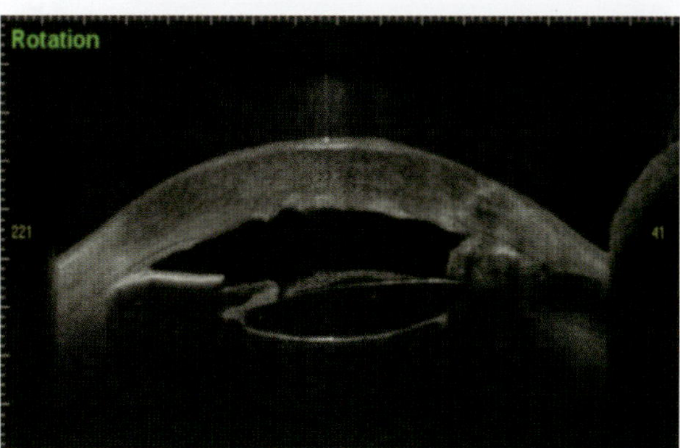

Fig. 49.4 The anterior chamber view is obscured in an eye following cataract extraction and insertion of a Baerveldt glaucoma drainage device, which was complicated by the development of bullous keratopathy (*left*). The anterior-segment optical coherence tomography (AS-OCT) provides visualization of the anterior chamber and drainage tube. The tube was blocked by peripheral anterior synechia. There was no direct communication between the tube and the anterior chamber.

EVALUATING TUBE POSITION IN PRESENCE OF CORNEAL EDEMA/SCAR

CASE STUDY 3

A 56-year-old woman had a longstanding history of chronic angle-closure glaucoma with extensive peripheral anterior synechia. She had cataract extraction with intraocular lens and insertion of a Baerveldt GDD, which was subsequently complicated by the development of bullous keratopathy (**Fig. 49.4**, *left*). With an obscured view of the anterior chamber, it was impossible to visualize the GDD with slit lamp photography. An AS-OCT image (**Fig. 49.4**, *right*) clearly shows that the tube is retracted and no longer in communication with the anterior chamber.

FURTHER READING

1. Hau S, Scott A, Bunce C, et al.: Corneal endothelial morphology in eyes implanted with anterior chamber aqueous shunts. *Cornea* 30:50–55, 2011.
2. Mendrinos E, Dosso A, Sommerhalder J, et al.: Coupling of HRT II and AS-OCT to evaluate corneal endothelial cell loss and in vivo visualization of the Ahmed glaucoma valve implant. *Eye* 23:1836–1844, 2009.
3. Sarodia U, Sharkawi E, Hau S, et al.: Visualization of aqueous shunt position and patency using anterior segment optical coherence tomography. *Am J Ophthalmol* 143:1054–1056, 2007.

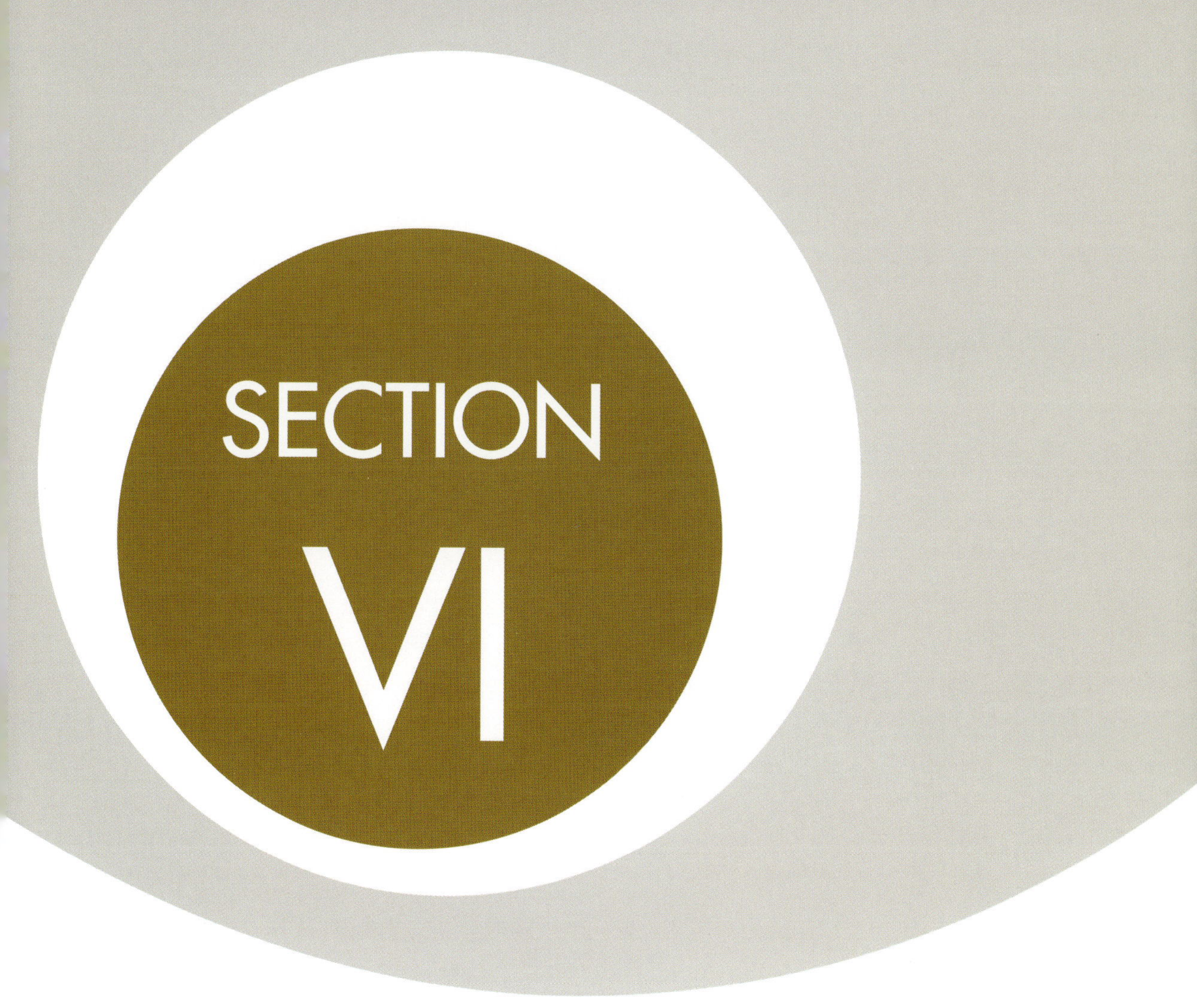

SECTION VI

Retina

Anterior Ischemic Optic Neuropathy

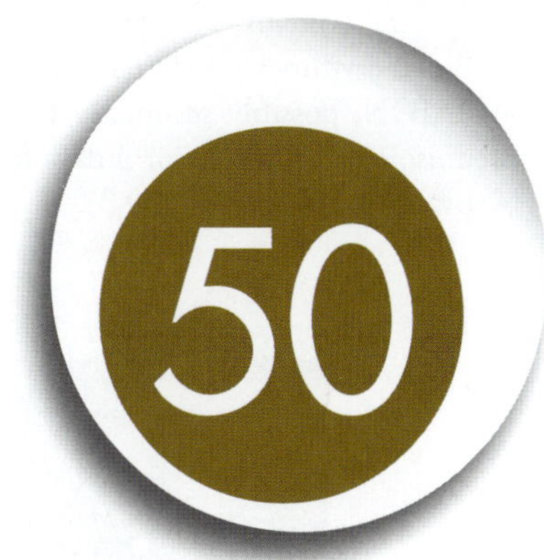

Rajani Battu

Anterior ischemic optic neuropathy (AION) is an acute ischemic infarct of the optic nerve mostly at the lamina cribrosa. Patients present with rapid visual loss; fundus typically shows an acute disc edema, either sectoral or total. AION could be either nonarteritic or arteritic. Nonarteritic AION (NAION) is seen more commonly in patients with an underlying systemic disorder like diabetes or hypertension. Arteritic AION (AAION) seen in elderly is mostly a part of giant cell arteritis and carries a significant risk of blindness in the second eye within days or weeks, if treatment is not instituted urgently. Different patterns of retinal nerve fiber layer (RNFL) changes on OCT have been described in NAION.

CASE STUDY

An 82-year-old man presented with acute, unilateral visual loss of a day's duration. He gave a history of malaise, low-grade fever, and painful jaw movements. Examination in the clinic showed a visual acuity of hand movements close to face in the right eye and 6/6 in the left. There was advanced nuclear sclerosis in both the eyes. There was a relative afferent pupillary defect in the right eye. Fundus of the left eye was normal; fundus of the right eye was as shown in **Figure 50.1**.

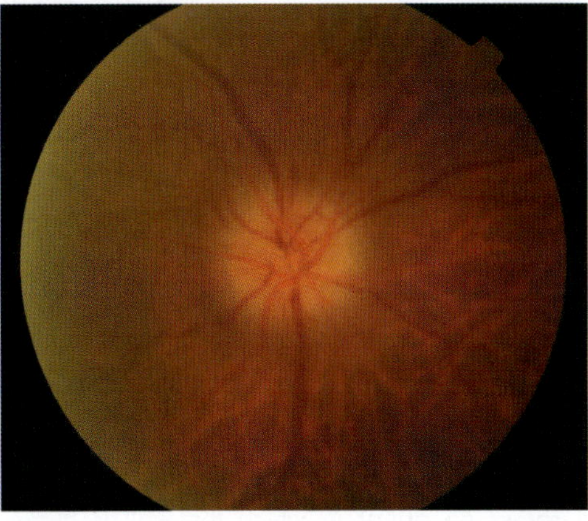

Fig. 50.1 Fundus picture of the right eye showing severe pale disc edema and streak hemorrhages along the disc margin.

Spectral-domain OCT (SD-OCT) showed severe edema of the RNFL (Fig. 50.2).

Blood erythrocyte sedimentation rate (ESR) was 83 mm/hour and the C-reactive protein was positive. A diagnosis of AAION, possibly secondary to giant cell arteritis, was made. The patient was started on intravenous methylprednisolone 1 gm/day for 3 days followed by oral steroids. The patient underwent right superficial temporal artery biopsy the next day (Fig. 50.3).

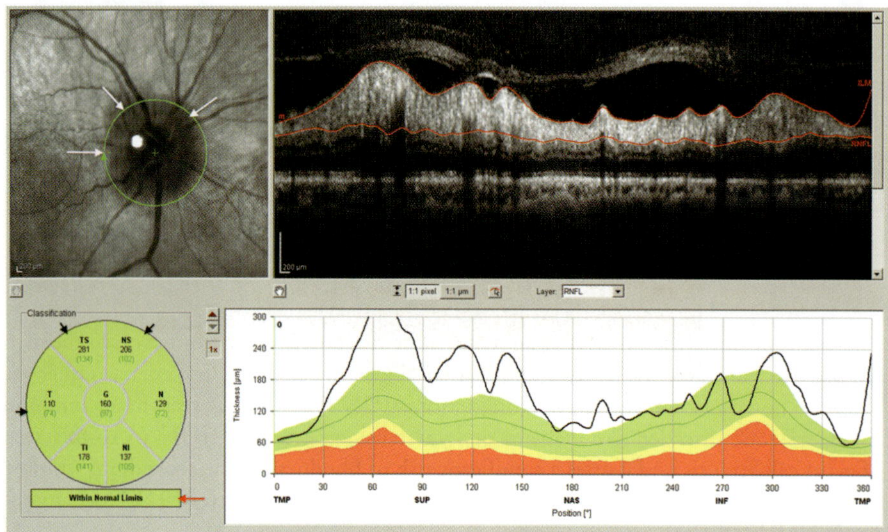

Fig. 50.2 OCT—RNFL analysis of the right eye showing severe peripapillary edema, more in the superior and temporal areas (*white arrows* with the corresponding nerve fiber layer thickness in *black arrows*). The *red arrow* points to the report generated in RNFL scan. It is reported as normal in spite of significant increase in RNFL thickness in this patient. This is because RNFL scans are normally tuned to diagnose glaucomas, a thinning of the retinal nerve fiber is considered abnormal. Any retinal thickness above normal standards continues to be considered normal.

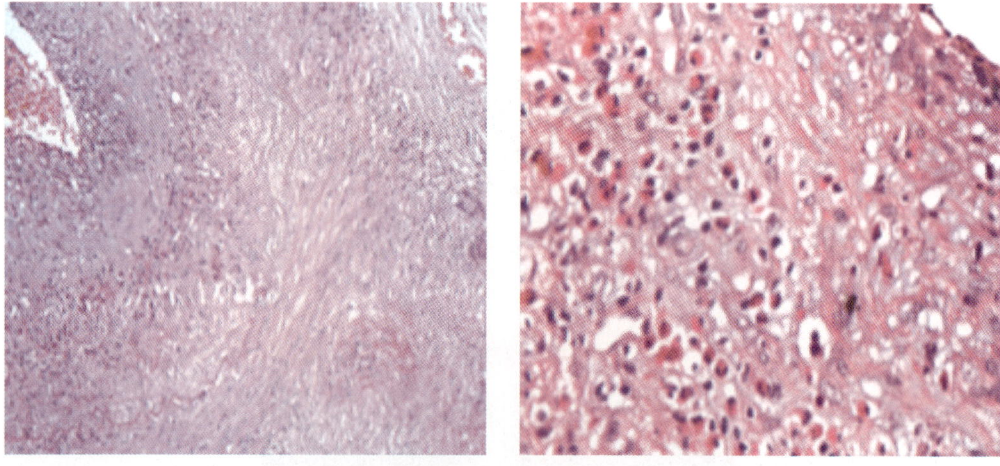

Fig. 50.3 Histopathology section shows an artery in which the wall is thickened and infiltrated by eosinophils, neutrophils, and few lymphocytes. The occasional giant cell is seen. The lumen is narrowed and adventitia shows congestion and dilation of vaso vasorum. Features are suggestive of giant cell arteritis.

The patient was referred to a rheumatologist for the management of giant cell arteritis. Follow-up showed optic atrophy in the right eye (**Fig. 50.4**) and the SD-OCT showed thinning of the RNFL (**Figs 50.5 and 50.6**).

The patient continues to be under the care of his rheumatologist and is being weekly monitored for his ESR and CRP. His vision in the left eye has remained stable at 6/6, with no evidence of AION.

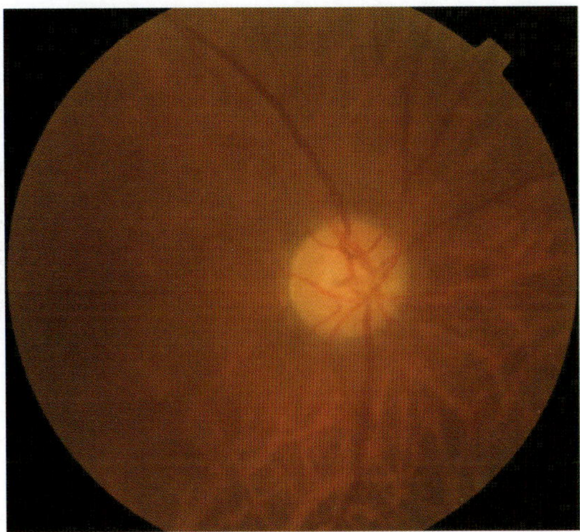

Fig. 50.4 Fundus of the right eye 3 months after treatment was instituted. The disc shows early optic atrophy. The left disc is normal.

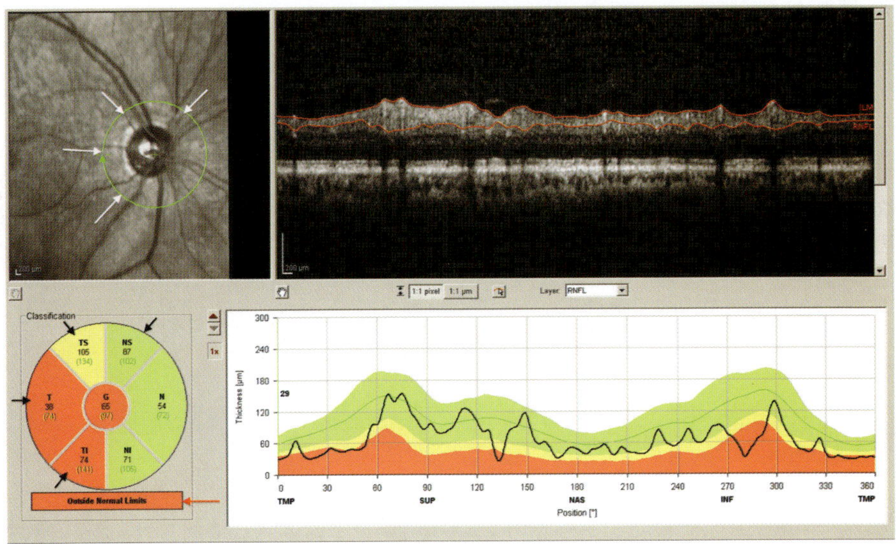

Fig. 50.5 OCT—RNFL analysis of the right eye 1 month after the acute episode. Note that the nerve fiber layer is significantly thinner than normal, the most prominent areas of thinning being in the temporal and inferotemporal areas (*arrows*), possibly signifying the onset of optic atrophy. The red arrow points to the report generated in RNFL scan. This is now reported as "outside normal limits," since the RNFL is thinner than normal.

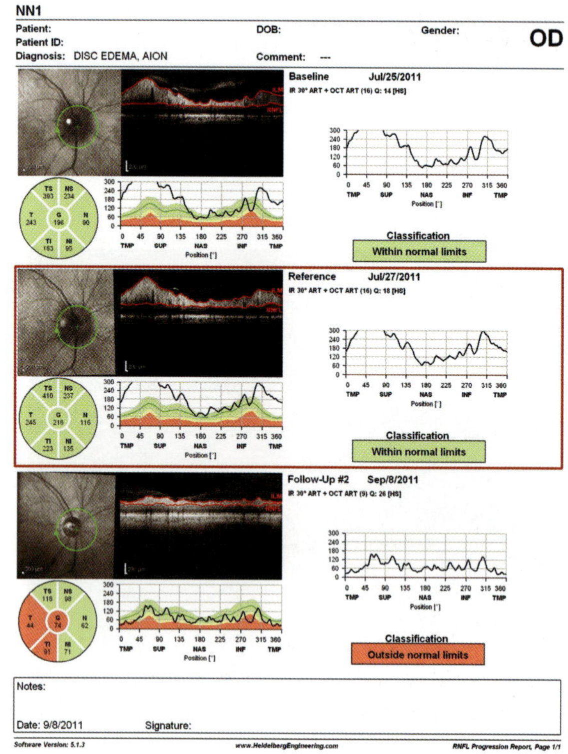

Fig. 50.6 Follow-up scans of the right eye that compares the RNFL thickness in the same eye at two different time frames of examination.

FURTHER READING

1. Hayreh SS: Anterior ischemic optic neuropathy. VIII. Clinical features and pathogenesis of post-hemorrhagic amaurosis. *Ophthalmology* 94(11):1488–1502, 1987.
2. Hayreh SS: Systemic diseases associated with nonarteritic anterior ischemic optic neuropathy. *Am J Ophthalmol* 118(6):766–780, 1994.
3. Fraser JA: The treatment of giant cell arteritis. *Rev Neurol Dis* 5(3):140–152, 2008.
4. Bellusci C: Retinal nerve fiber layer thickness in nonarteritic anterior ischemic optic neuropathy: OCT characterization of the acute and resolving phases. *Graefes Arch Clin Exp Ophthalmol* 246(5):641–647, 2008.

Angioid Streak

Naresh Kumar Yadav and
Santosh Gopi Krishna

Angioid streaks (AS) are irregular, reddish, linear breaks in the Bruch's membrane seen developing radially from the optic disk and may be associated with Pseudoxanthoma elasticum, Ehlers–Danlos syndrome, Paget's disease, and sickle cell anemia. It also appears in patients without any systemic disease. Choroidal neovascular membrane (CNVM) occurs in 42%–86% of patients with angioid streaks. In spite of treatment with conventional laser photocoagulation and photodynamic therapy (PDT) with verteporfin, visual outcomes have been unsatisfactory due to a high rate of recurrence, progression of the CNVM subfoveally, and foveal atrophy. However, with the onset of anti-vascular endothelial growth factor treatments, visual outcome may be favorable, especially in treatment-naive eyes.

CASE STUDY

An 18-year-old boy presented to our clinic with blurred vision in the left eye for 15 days. His best-corrected visual acuity (BCVA) was (6/9) in the right eye and (6/12) in the left eye. Anterior segment was normal. Fundus showed myopia fundii with AS and left-eye CNVM.

As AS are known to have systemic associations, the patient underwent complete systemic evaluation by the physician to rule out any associated conditions; and, there were no systemic associations in this case.

A fundus fluorescein angiogram (FFA) showed classic CNVM. Spectral-domain optical coherence tomography (SD-OCT) showed CNVM complex and intra- and subretinal fluid (**Fig. 51.1**). He underwent three intravitreal bevacizumab injections, following which his vision improved to 6/9.

A repeat FFA showed a scarred CNVM, evident by staining without any active leak; and, SD-OCT showed a scarred and inactive CNVM without any fluid (**Fig. 51.2**).

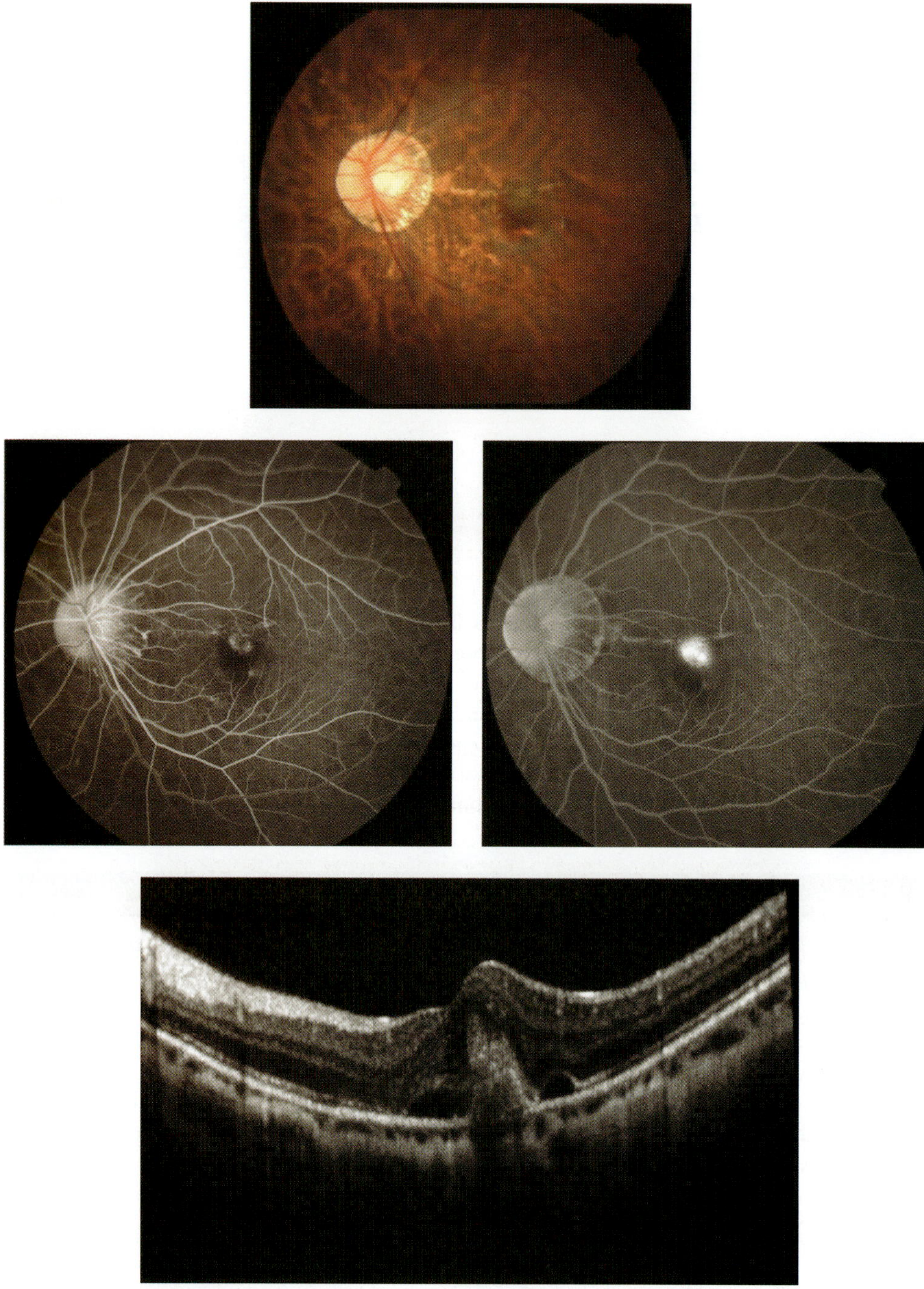

Fig. 51.1 Pretreatment. The above figure shows a myopic fundus with angioid streaks and a CNVM. FFA confirms a classic CNVM and SD-OCT imaging shows a CNVM complex with intra- and subretinal fluid.

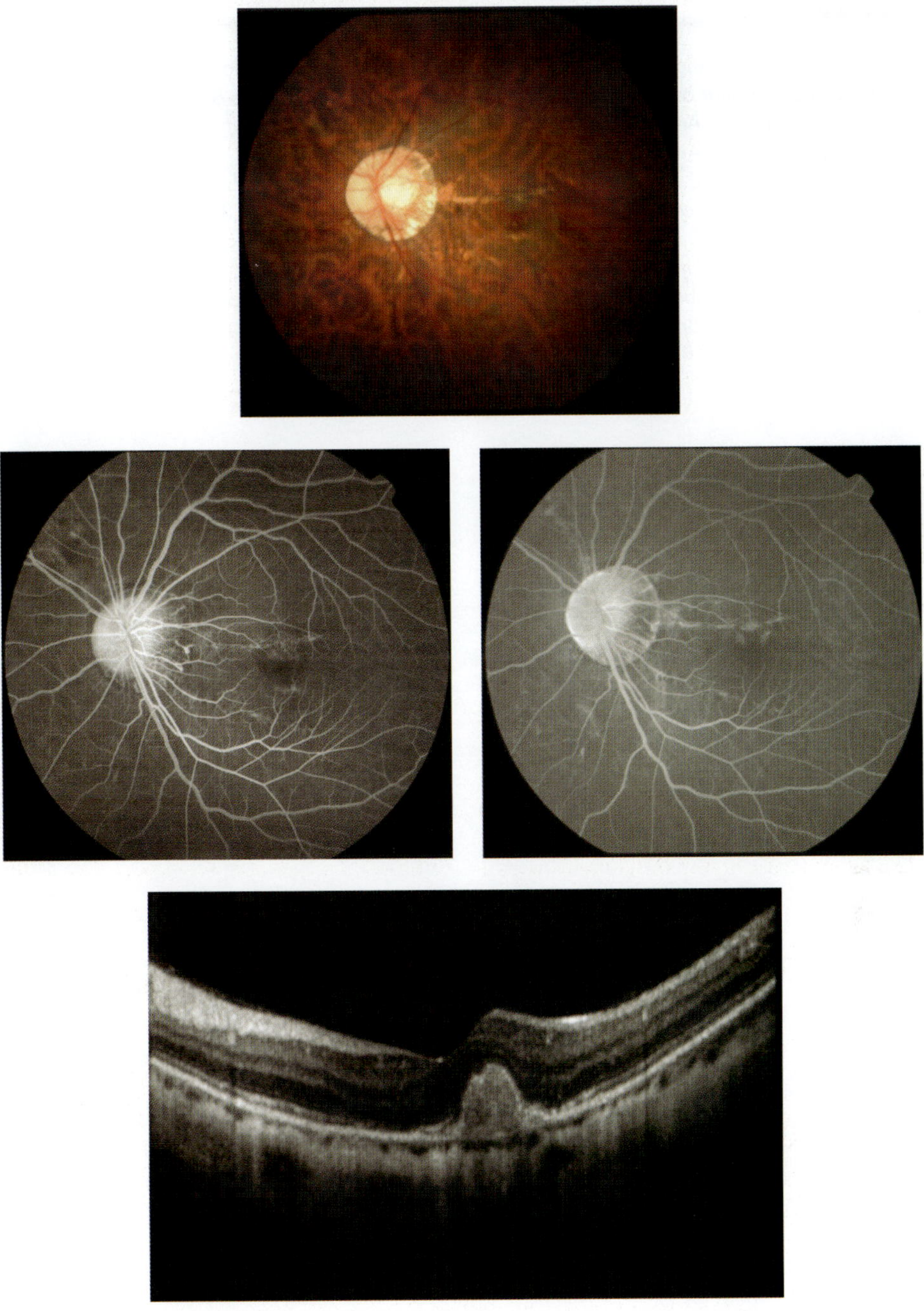

Fig. 51.2 Post-treatment. The above figure shows a scarred CNVM with no active leak but window defects, and late staining on FFA and a scarred CNVM complex with no fluid suggestive of inactive and healed CNVM on SD-OCT post-anti-VEGF (Avastin) therapy.

FURTHER READING

1. Piro PA, Scherga D, Fine SL: Angioid streaks: natural history and visual prognosis. In: Fine SL, Owens SL, editors: *Management of Retinal Vascular and Macular Disorders*. Baltimore, MD: Williams & Wilkins, 1983.
2. Hagedoorn A: Angioid streaks. *Arch Ophthalmol* 21:746–774, 1939.
3. Hagedoorn A: Angioid streaks. *Arch Ophthalmol* 21:935–965, 1939.
4. Clarkson JG, Altman RD: Angioid streaks. *Surv Ophthalmol* 116:235–246, 1982.
5. Klien BA: Angioid streaks: a clinical and histopathologic study. *Am J Ophthalmol* 30:955–968, 1947.
6. Georgalas I, Papaconstantinou D, Koutsandrea C, et al.: Angioid streaks, clinical course, complications, and current therapeutic management. *Ther Clin Risk Manag* 5:81–89, 2009.
7. Wiegand TW, Rogers AH, McCabe F, et al.: Intravitreal bevacizumab (Avastin) treatment of choroidal neovascularisation in patients with angioid streaks. *Br J Ophthalmol* 93:47–51, 2009.

Branch Retinal Artery Occlusion

Priya BV and Kavitha Avadhani

Branch retinal artery occlusion (BRAO) is a common vascular occlusive disorder of the eye. It accounts for 38% of all acute retinal artery obstructions. It presents as an acute painless loss of visual field in the area of distribution of the occluded artery.

These occlusions are caused by embolization, coagulopathies, vasospasm, or vasculitides.

A 35-year-old Asian Indian man presented with complaints of sudden painless blurring of vision in his right eye since 3 days. He gave history of headache since 4 months, and hearing loss in the left ear and slurring of speech since 2 months.

Visual acuity at presentation was 6/6, (near vision–N) N6 in both eyes. Anterior segment examination was normal in both the eyes. On fundus examination of the right eye, whitening of retina was noted along inferior foveal area (Fig. 52.1).

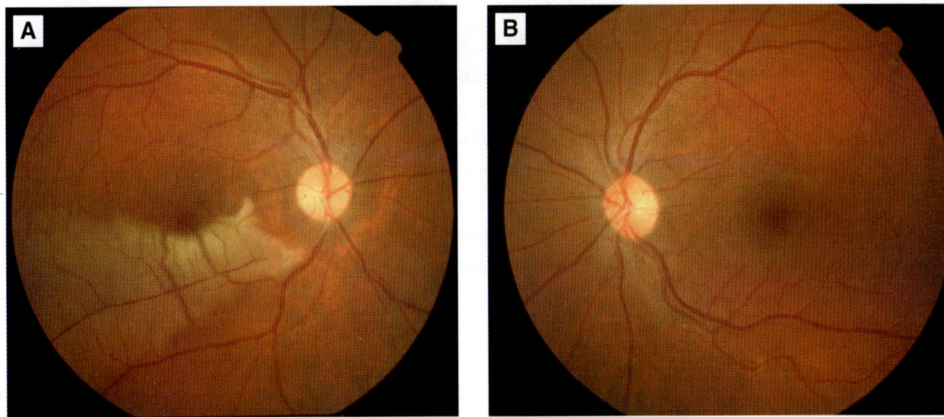

Fig. 52.1 **(A)** Fundus photograph of the right eye showing whitening of retina along the area supplied by the inferotemporal branch retinal artery. **(B)** Fundus photograph of the left eye showing normal posterior pole.

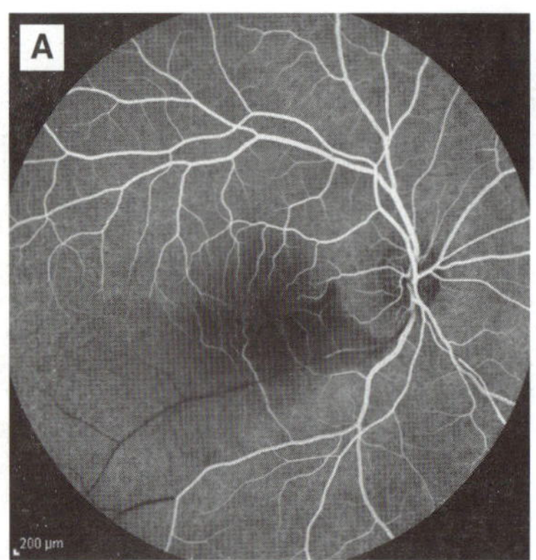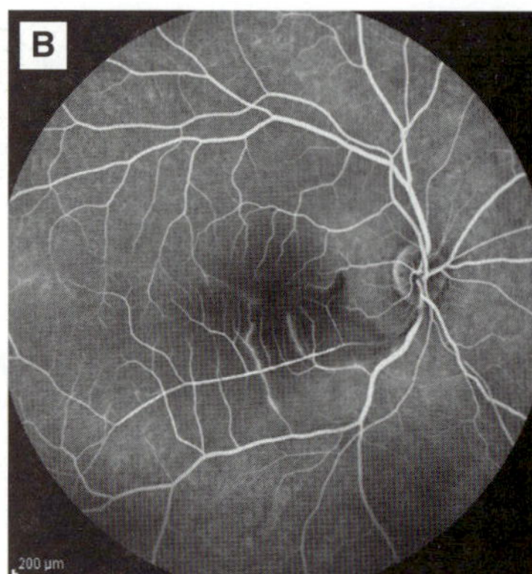

Fig. 52.2 (A) Fundus fluorescein angiogram of the right eye showing hypofluorescence in the inferior perifoveolar retina. **(B)** Fundus fluorescein angiogram of the right eye showing delayed filling of the inferotemporal branch retinal arteriole with perivascular leakage along inferior perifoveolar arterioles.

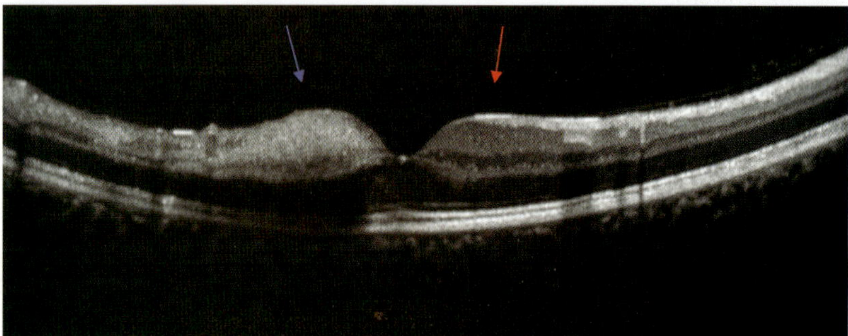

Fig. 52.3 SD-OCT of the right eye of the patient showing increased reflectivity of inner retinal layers with decreased reflectivity of the outer retinal layers due to after shadowing in the inferior perifoveolar retina (*blue arrow*). The superior perifoveal retina shows normal retinal layers (*red arrow*).

Patient underwent fundus fluorescein angiography (FFA) and optical coherence tomography (OCT). FFA showed delayed filling of inferotemporal branch of retinal arteriole with perivascular leakage in inferior perifoveal arterioles (**Fig. 52.2**).

Spectral-domain optical coherence tomography (SD-OCT) (SPECTRALIS™; Heidelberg Engineering, Heidelberg, Germany) of the right eye showed hyperreflectivity, increased thickness of inner retinal layers, and decreased reflectivity of outer retinal layers in the inferior perifoveolar retina as compared to the superior perifoveolar retina (**Fig. 52.3**). Posterior vitreous cells were also noted. SD-OCT scan through the inferotemporal branch retinal artery showed blocked lumen of this vessel, while lumina of adjacent vessels with corresponding after shadowing were clearly seen (**Fig. 52.4**). Foveolar depression was normal. The photoreceptor layer and the retinal pigment epithelium at the fovea were normal. The superior perifoveolar area showed normal retinal layers on OCT.

The patient underwent a thorough medical evaluation, including cardiac and carotid evaluations that were found to be normal. He was also referred to a neurologist in view of other associated symptoms like headache and hearing loss. Susac's syndrome was suspected. MRI brain findings were also suggestive of Susac's syndrome (retinocochleocerebral vasculitis).

He was started on systemic steroids and followed-up regularly. He had improvement in his visual symptoms. Fundus examination on follow-up showed decrease in inferior retinal whitening (**Fig. 52.5**).

OCT at 3-months follow-up showed decrease in inner retinal thickness with development of atrophic inner retina without differentiation between individual layers (**Fig. 52.6**).

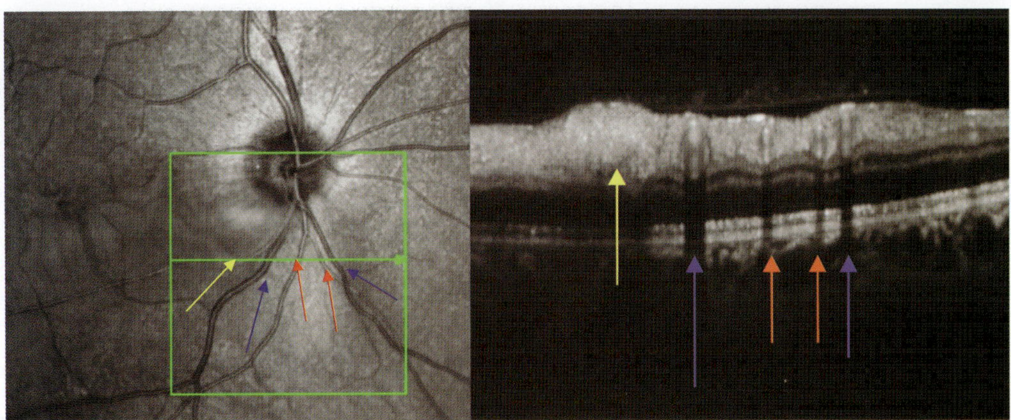

Fig. 52.4 Horizontal SD-OCT scan passing through inferior branches of retinal arteries and veins showing hyper-reflectivity in inner retina corresponding to blocked artery with lumen not visualized (*yellow arrows*), while adjacent retinal arteries and veins were seen as hyporeflective areas in inner retina with after shadowing suggestive of patent lumina (*red and blue arrows, respectively*).

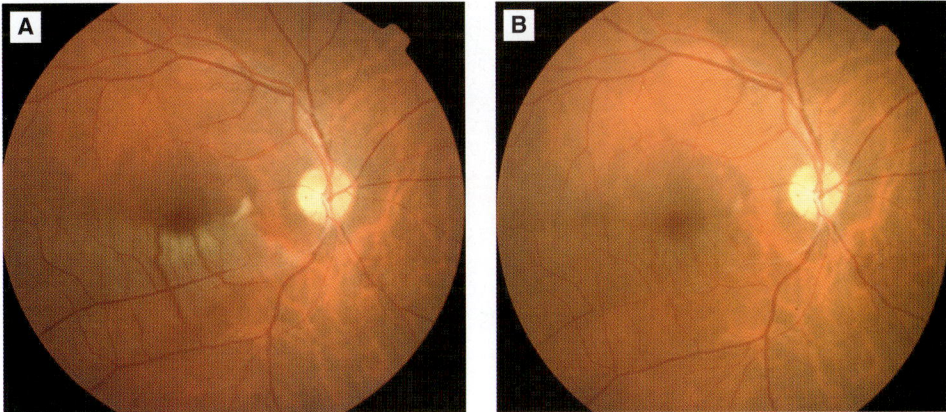

Fig. 52.5 Fundus photograph of the right eye of the patient at 1 month (**A**) and 3 months (**B**) after initial presentation showing reduction in retinal whitening.

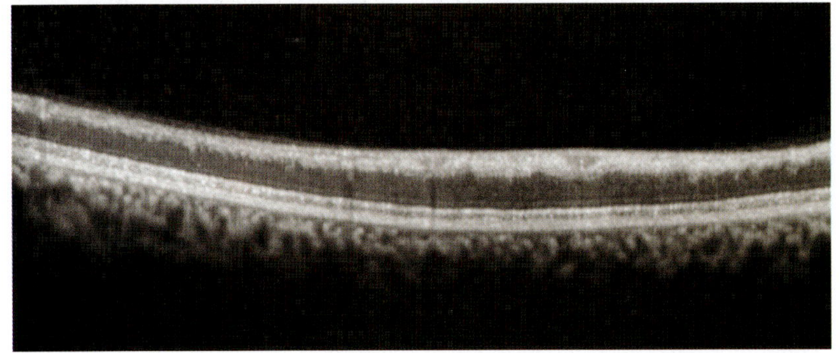

Fig. 52.6 SD-OCT done at 3 months after initial presentation showing atrophic inner retina without distinction between individual layers.

FURTHER READING

1. Murthy RK, Grover S, Chalam KV: Sequential spectral domain OCT documentation of retinal changes after branch retinal artery occlusion. *Clin Ophthalmol* 26;4:327–329, 2010.
2. Mason JO 3rd, Shah AA, Vail RS, et al.: Branch retinal artery occlusion: visual prognosis. *Am J Ophthalmol* 146(3): 455–457, 2008.
3. Shah VA, Wallace B, Sabates NR: Spectral domain optical coherence tomography findings of acute branch retinal artery occlusion from calcific embolus. *Indian J Ophthalmol* 58(6):523–524, 2010.
4. Ritter M, Sacu S, Deák GG, et al.: In vivo identification of alteration of inner neurosensory layers in branch retinal artery occlusion. *Br J Ophthalmol* 96(2):201–207, 2012.

Branch Retinal Vein Occlusion

Mahesh Chandargi

Branch retinal vein occlusion (BRVO) is a common retinal vascular disease, most common in the sixth to seventh decade. Common risk factors are systemic hypertension, diabetes, hyperlipidemia, glaucoma, and smoking. Younger patients must be worked-up for coagulative/inflammatory causes. BRVO can involve major veins—temporal or nasal—and minor veins like macular branches and small tributaries. BRVOs occur at arteriovenous intersections. Features include quadrantic distribution of hemorrhages, soft exudates, dilated/tortuous vessels, hard exudates, macular edema, and late stages are characterized by sclerosed collaterals and sheathed veins. BRVO can cause drop in vision due to macular edema, macular ischemia, vitreous hemorrhage, or foveal traction due to epiretinal membranes and retinal detachments. Treatment options include lasers—grid/sectoral, intravitreal anti-VEGF (anti-vascular endothelial growth factor) injections, intravitreal steroid injections, or vitrectomy.

CASE STUDY 1

A 62-year-old Asian Indian man presented with diminished left eye vision since 3 weeks. BCVA was 20/20 in the right eye and 20/40 in the left eye. Anterior segment examination revealed pseudophakia in both eyes. Fundus showed macular, flame-shaped hemorrhages, cotton-wool spots, and foveal edema suggestive of superior macular branch vein occlusion with foveal edema in the left eye. Fundus fluorescein angiography (FFA) confirmed diagnosis with late leak at the fovea. Spectral-domain optical coherence tomography (SD-OCT) revealed left-eye cystic spaces with loss of foveal contour. He underwent intravitreal injection of Bevacizumab; on follow-up SD-OCT showed resolved cystoid edema and restored foveal contour (**Fig. 53.1**).

CASE STUDY 2

A 66-year-old Indian man, a known hypertensive, complained of defective vision in both eyes (right more than left) since 4 months. BCVA was 20/200 in the right eye and 20/40 in the left eye. Anterior segment showed immature cataract (nuclear sclerosis grade 2) in both the eyes. Fundus revealed right-eye soft exudates, superficial hemorrhages, dilated veins in the superotemporal quadrant with dull foveal reflex suggestive of superotemporal BRVO with macular edema. FFA of the right eye revealed blocked fluorescence, capillary dropout areas, and late leak at the fovea. SD-OCT showed cystoid macular edema. He underwent two injections of intravitreal bevacizumab and one injection of triamcinolone acetonide. Post-treatment SD-OCT showed regained foveal contour and resolved cystic spaces (**Fig. 53.2**).

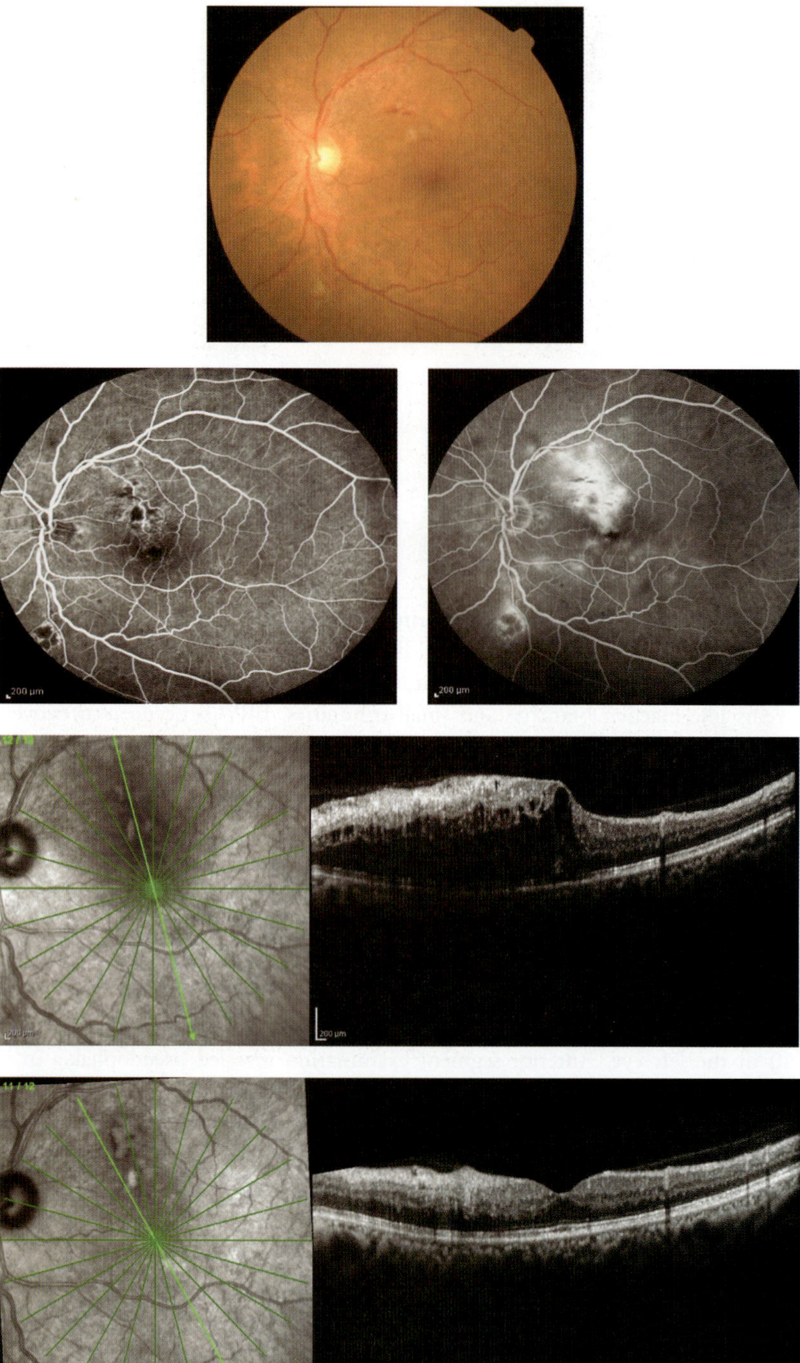

Fig. 53.1 Fundus photo showing soft exudate with flame hemorrhages at the macula with a dull foveal reflex suggestive of macular BRVO and edema. FFA showing capillary dropout areas and late leak. SD-OCT reveals cystoid edema and altered foveal contour at presentation (*above*); post-treatment SD-OCT (*below*) showing resolved edema with regained foveal contour.

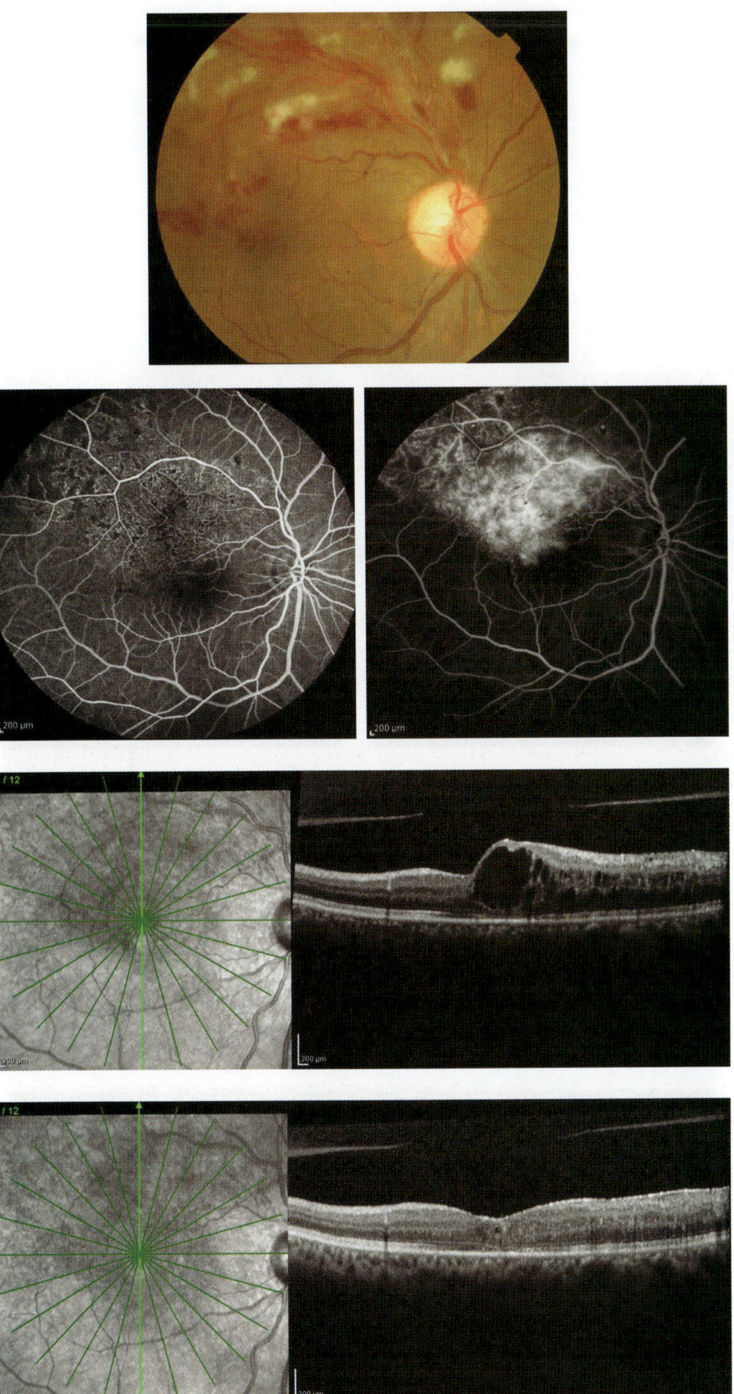

Fig. 53.2 Fundus photo showing dilated vessels, cotton-wool spots, retinal hemorrhages, and macular thickening suggestive of STBRVO with macular edema. FFA showing blocked fluorescence, capillary nonperfusion areas, and late leak. SD-OCT showing cystic spaces and loss of foveal contour at presentation (*above*); post-treatment SD-OCT (*below*) showed resolved edema and foveal contour.

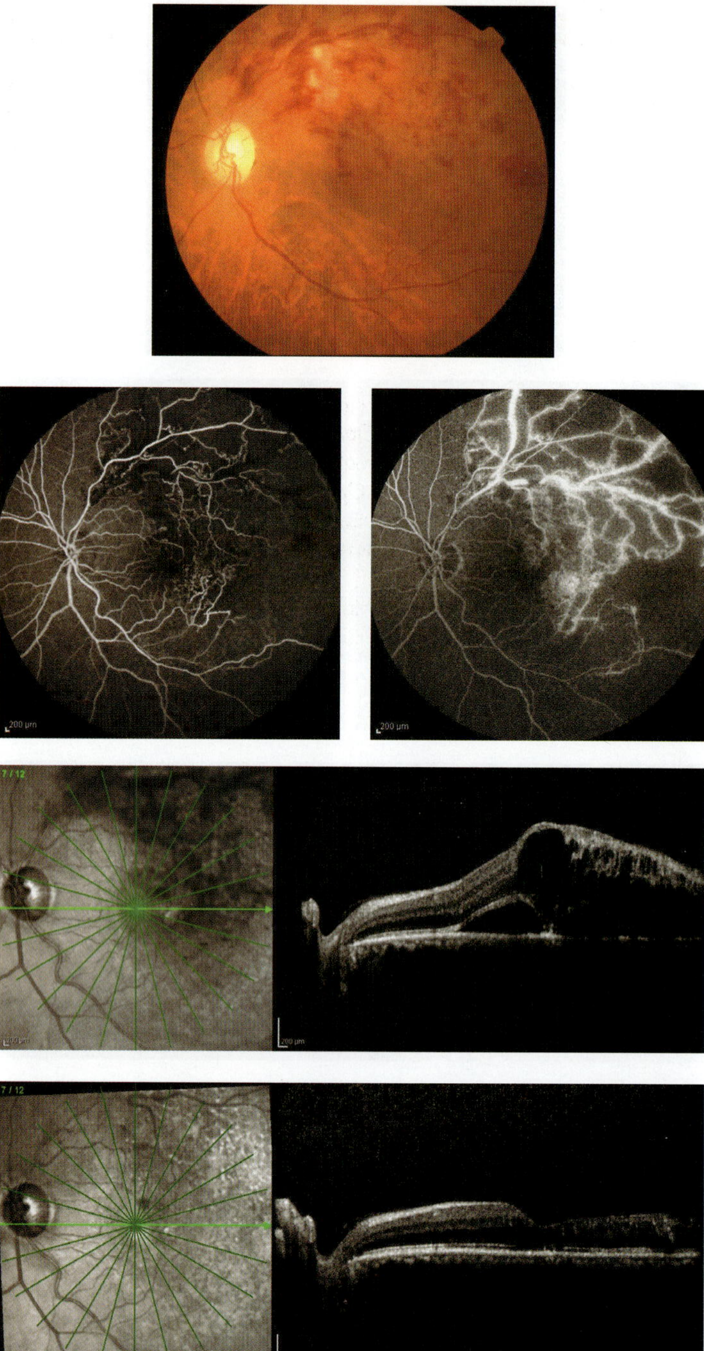

Fig. 53.3 Fundus photo showing left-eye retinal hemorrhages, soft exudates, dilated vessels in superotemporal quadrant, and macular edema. FFA showing blocked fluorescence, capillary dropout areas, vessel staining, and late leak. SD-OCT (*above*) showing cystoid edema, loss of foveal contour, and subfoveal fluid at presentation. Post-treatment SD-OCT (*below*) showing resolved edema and subfoveal fluid.

A 70-year-old Asian south Indian woman walked in with a history of blurred left eye vision since 6 weeks. BCVA was 20/20 in the right eye and 20/200 in the left eye. On examination, the right eye was diagnosed with pseudophakia and the left eye had posterior subcapsular cataract; fundus examination of the left eye revealed retinal hemorrhages in the superotemporal quadrant with macular edema. SD-OCT showed cystoid macular edema, subfoveal fluid, and loss of foveal contour. She received two intravitreal injections of ranibizumab in the left eye. Follow-up SD-OCT revealed resolved cystic spaces and subretinal fluid with normalized foveal contour (**Fig. 53.3**).

FURTHER READING

1. Yunoki T, Miyakoshi A, Nakamura T, et al.: Treatment of macular edema due to branch retinal vein occlusion with single or multiple intravitreal injections of bevacizumab. *Jpn J Ophthalmol* 56(2):159–164, 2012.
2. Donati S, Barosi P, Bianchi M, et al.: Combined intravitreal bevacizumab and grid laser photocoagulation for macular edema secondary to branch retinal vein occlusion. *Eur J Ophthalmol* Nov 2011 18:0. doi: 10.5301/ejo.5000085.
3. Jaissle GB, Szurman Peter, Nicolas Feltgen, et al.: Predictive factors for functional improvement after intravitreal bevacizumab therapy for macular edema due to branch retinal vein occlusion. Retinal Vein Occlusion Study Group. *Graefes Arch Clin Exp Ophthalmol* 249(2):183–192, 2011.
4. Gregori NZ, Rattan GH, Rosenfeld PJ, et al.: Safety and efficacy of intravitreal bevacizumab (Avastin) for the management of branch and hemiretinal vein occlusion. *Retina* 29(7):913–925, 2009.
5. RETINA; Elsevier Mosby, Vol 2, ed 4, 1349–1355.

Hydroxychloroquine Retinopathy

Yoshihiro Yonekawa,
Demetrios G Vavvas, and
RV Paul Chan

Chloroquine (Aralen; Sanofi-Aventis, New Jersey, USA) and hydroxychloroquine (Plaquenil; Sanofi-Aventis, New Jersey, USA) retinal toxicities manifest classically as bull's-eye maculopathies (BEM). Chloroquine retinopathy was first described in the 1950s in patients being treated for malaria. Hydroxychroloquine is a chloroquine metabolite and is considered less toxic. In industrialized countries, hydroxychloroquine is commonly used for its anti-inflammatory properties in the treatment of autoimmune disorders, such as systemic lupus erythematosus and rheumatoid arthritis.

A bull's-eye appearance of fundus is a late finding in hydroxychloroquine toxicity, and visual recovery is unlikely at that stage. The most effective method of management is to discontinue the drug to prevent further visual loss, but the retinopathy can still progress. The best chance for visual preservation is early detection and early cessation or substitution of the offending medication.

Capturing preclinical signs of disease has now become possible with fundus autofluorescence, multifocal ERG (mfERG), and the focus of this book, spectral-domain optical coherence tomography (SD-OCT). Fundus autofluorescence is less invasive and faster than angiography. Increased autofluorescence from outer-segment debris is seen in earlier stages, while retinal pigment epithelium (RPE) depigmentation/atrophy in late stages is present with reduced autofluorescence. mfERG is also a sensitive test that allows early detection of local topographical ERG depressions.

SD-OCT allows high-resolution–cross-sectional imaging of retinal tissue. In 2007, Rodriguez-Padilla, et al. examined 15 patients with hydroxychloroquine retinopathy using a research prototype ultra-high-resolution SD-OCT, and noted a loss of the photoreceptor inner segment–outer segment (IS–OS) junction and thinning of the perifoveal outer nuclear layer. Advanced cases had more severe disruption of the IS–OS junction with irregular scattering bands. Of note, most of these changes spared the foveal center to create the bull's-eye appearance. Similarly, a series of eight patients on chronic chloroquine treatment also demonstrated that the earliest sign of toxicity was loss of the outer nuclear layer thickness; the fovea became affected as well in the most-severe case.

In a case-control study of eight patients with chronic hydroxychloroquine exposure without clinical signs of toxicity and eight controls, Pasadhika et al. recently found that the ganglion cell and inner plexiform layers were thinned even when there were no abnormalities in the photoreceptors or RPE. Pasadhika's team used an image segmentation technique that showed selective thinning of those layers in the perifoveal area. The same group also reported a thinning of the retinal nerve fiber layer and ganglion cell layer in the peripapillary region; although this phenomenon was only seen in patients with clinically evident fundus changes.

CASE STUDY

A 55-year-old woman presented with blurred vision in both eyes. She had a history of rheumatoid arthritis, and had been on hydroxychloroquine 200 mg twice a day for 17 years. Her lean body weight was 45 kg. She also had a history of sinonasal carcinoma, for which she underwent chemoradiation. Visual acuity in the right eye [oculus dexter (OD)] was 20/63 − 1, pinhole (PH) 20/40, and left eye [oculus sinister (OS)] was 20/100 − 1, PH 20/32. Pseudoisochromatic color plates were depressed: OD 3/15 and OS 1/15.

Ophthalmoscopy revealed RPE depigmentation in a bull's-eye configuration in both eyes (**Fig. 54.1**). The left eye also showed signs of radiation damage, including attenuated vessels and disc pallor. Fluorescein angiograms showed window defects in both maculae in a bull's-eye pattern (**Fig. 54.1**). SD-OCT showed a loss of photoreceptor and RPE structures in a concentric pattern in both eyes, with blunting of the foveal pit in the left eye (**Fig. 54.2**). The thinning of the outer retinal layers appeared to cause a "sink-hole" effect on inner retinal layers, particularly in the left eye, as previously described by Stepien et al. Retinal thickness analysis map also demonstrated bilateral perifoveal thinning.

The American Academy of Ophthalmology (AAO) published screening guidelines for chloroquine/hydroxychloroquine retinopathy in 2002 and an update in 2011. The 2002 consensus statement established daily dosing recommendations and defined high-risk characteristics. The contents are summarized in **Table 54.1**.

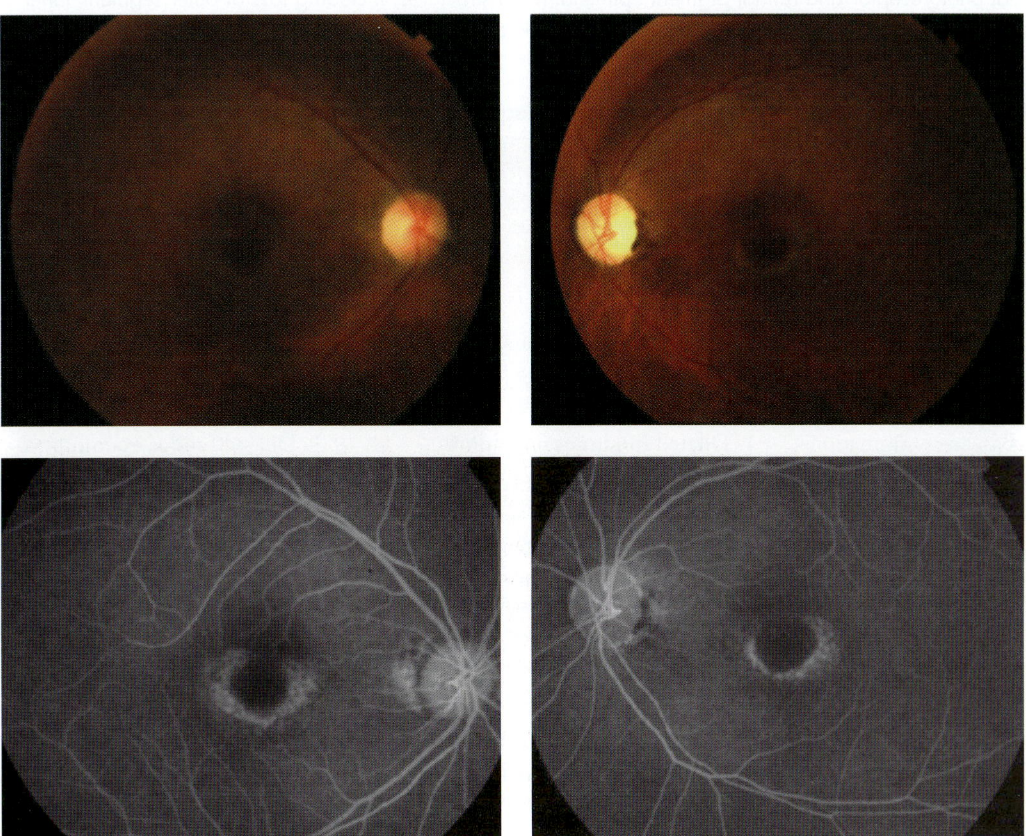

Fig. 54.1 (*Above, left*): Color fundus photograph of the right eye showing an annular macular depigmentation consistent with the bull's-eye maculopathy seen in hydroxychloroquine retinopathy. (*Above, right*): Color fundus photograph of the left eye, also showing a bull's-eye maculopathy. Optic nerve pallor is from radiation papillopathy. (*Below, left*): Arteriovenous phase fluorescein angiograph (FA) of the right eye at 20.5 seconds, showing a concentric retinal pigment epithelial (RPE) window defect. (*Below, right*): Arteriovenous phase FA of the left eye at 1 minute 14.4 seconds, also showing the concentric transmission increase caused by RPE atrophy.

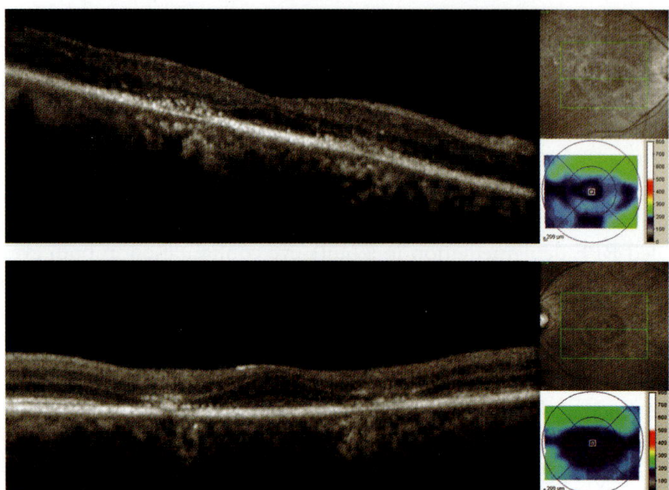

Fig. 54.2 SD-OCT of the right eye (*above*) and left eye (*below*) in hydroxychloroquine retinopathy, showing loss of perifoveal photoreceptor and retinal pigment epithelial (RPE) structures, including loss of outer segment–inner segment (OS–IS) junction. RPE mottling is also evident. Retinal thickness analysis maps shows generalized thinning of maculae.

Table 54.1 American Academy of Ophthalmology Screening Guidelines

	2002	2011

Dosing	Hydroxychloroquine:
	  6.5 mg/kg/day
	Chloroquine:
	  3.0 mg/kg/day
		Hydroxychloroquine:
		  1000 gm cumulative
		Chloroquine:
		  460 gm cumulative

High risk characteristics	>6.5 mg/kg/day, >5 years, obese, hepatic and/or renal disease, age >60 years, concurrent retinal disease	Same
Baseline examination	1. Dilated fundus examination 2. Amsler or HVF 10-2	1. Dilated fundus examination 2. HVF 10-2 3. SD-OCT, mfERG, or FAF

mg, milligrams; kg, kilograms, gm, grams; HVF, humphrey visual field; SD-OCT, spectral domain optical coherence tomography; mfERG, multifocal electroretinography; FAF, fundus autofluorescence.
Adapted from Marmor MF et al.: Recommendations on screening for chloroquine and hydroxychloroquine retinopathy. *Ophthalmol* 109:1377–82, 2002, and Marmor MF et al.: Revised recommendations on screening for chloroquine and hydroxychloroquine retinopathy. *Ophthalmol* 118:415–22, 2011 with permission from Elsevier.

The patient described above was on hydroxychloroquine for 17 years at a dose of approximately 9 mg/kg/day, for a cumulative dose of 2482 gm, both of which are well over recommended guidelines. With her lean weight of 45 kg, the daily dose should have been under 300 mg/day, but cumulative limit of 1000 gm would still be reached at approximately 9 years.

CONCLUSION

SD-OCT is an accurate and efficient modality to aid in the diagnosis and monitoring of hydroxychloroquine retinopathy when utilized in conjunction with the ophthalmoscopic examination. Cardinal findings that most reports have emphasized are disruption of the IS–OS junction and photoreceptor outer segments, and RPE changes.

FURTHER READING

1. Rodriguez-Padilla JA, Hedges TR, 3rd, Monson B, et al.: High-speed ultra-high-resolution optical coherence tomography findings in hydroxychloroquine retinopathy. *Arch Ophthalmol* 125:775–780, 2007.
2. Kellner S, Weinitz S, Kellner U. Spectral domain optical coherence tomography detects early stages of chloroquine retinopathy similar to multifocal electroretinography, fundus autofluorescence and near-infrared autofluorescence. *Br J Ophthalmol* 93:1444–1447, 2009.
3. Pasadhika S, Fishman GA, Choi D, et al.: Selective thinning of the perifoveal inner retina as an early sign of hydroxychloroquine retinal toxicity. *Eye (Lond)* 24:756–762, 2010.
4. Pasadhika S, Fishman GA. Effects of chronic exposure to hydroxychloroquine or chloroquine on inner retinal structures. *Eye (Lond)* 24:340–346, 2010.
5. Stepien KE, Han DP, Schell J, et al.: Spectral-domain optical coherence tomography and adaptive optics may detect hydroxychloroquine retinal toxicity before symptomatic vision loss. *Trans Am Ophthalmol Soc* 107:28–33, 2009.
6. Marmor MF, Carr RE, Easterbrook M, et al.: Recommendations on screening for chloroquine and hydroxychloroquine retinopathy: A report by the American Academy of Ophthalmology. *Ophthalmology* 109:1377–1382, 2002.
7. Marmor MF, Kellner U, Lai TY, Lyons JS, Mieler WF: Revised recommendations on screening for chloroquine and hydroxychloroquine retinopathy. *Ophthalmology* 118:415–422, 2011.

Acknowledgment: We would like to thank Demetrios Vavvas, MD, PhD, for providing the cases for this chapter.

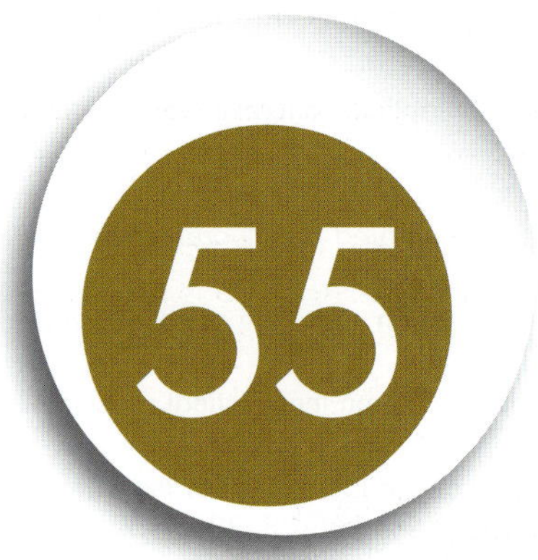

Central Retinal Artery Occlusion

Supriya Dabir and Kanav Gupta

Central retinal artery occlusion (CRAO) leads to sudden, painless loss of vision due to decrease in blood supply to the inner layers of retina.

Central retinal artery is the first intraorbital branch of the ophthalmic artery, which enters the optic nerve and supplies the retina. Short posterior ciliary arteries branch out of the ophthalmic artery and supply the choroid. Cilioretinal branches from the short posterior ciliary artery are the anatomical variations that also supply the macula. Approximately 14% of the population has the cilioretinal artery and it is involved in almost a quarter of the eyes detected with acute CRAO.

CASE STUDY

A 45-year-old man came with sudden onset, painless loss of vision in his right eye since 8 hours. He was a known patient of rheumatic heart disease on treatment.

On examination, his best-corrected vision was 6/6, N6, and counting finger 1 meter in the right and left eye, respectively. Pupillary examination showed a left relative afferent pupillary defect. Anterior segment was normal. Intraocular pressure was 10 and 12 mmHg in the right and left eye, respectively. On fundus examination in the left eye, there were multiple scattered patches of retinal opacification all over the posterior pole with a cherry-red spot at fovea. Box-carring ("cattle-trucking") of blood column in retinal vessels was seen (Fig. 55.1). The right eye was normal.

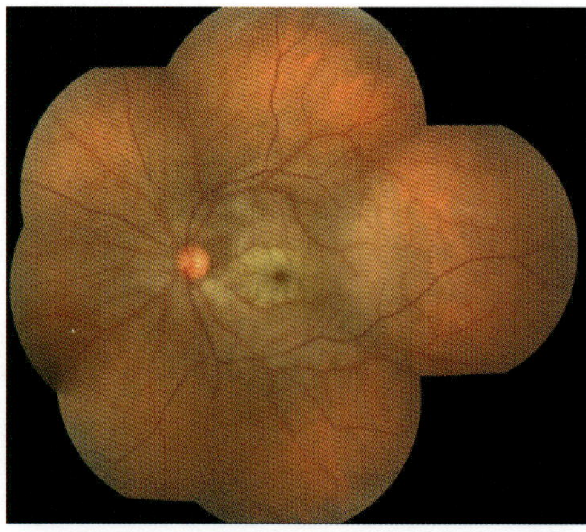

Fig. 55.1 Montage fundus photograph of the left eye shows multiple scattered patches of retinal opacification all over the posterior pole with a cherry-red spot at the fovea.

He was given an ocular massage, and anterior chamber tap was done under aseptic precautions, and he was started on intraocular pressure lowering medication.

He then underwent ocular investigations the next day. On fundus fluorescein angiography, there was delayed, sluggish, and irregular filling of the arterioles (22 msec), and abnormally delayed arteriovenous transit time (>47 msec) with late staining of the disc in the left eye (Fig. 55.2).

A horizontal spectral-domain optical coherence tomography (SD-OCT) scan through the fovea revealed diffuse thickening of the neurosensory retina. Hyperreflectivity of the inner retinal layers corresponded to retinal ischemia and decreased backscattering from retinal photoreceptors was due to fluid accumulation and retinal edema (Fig. 55.3).

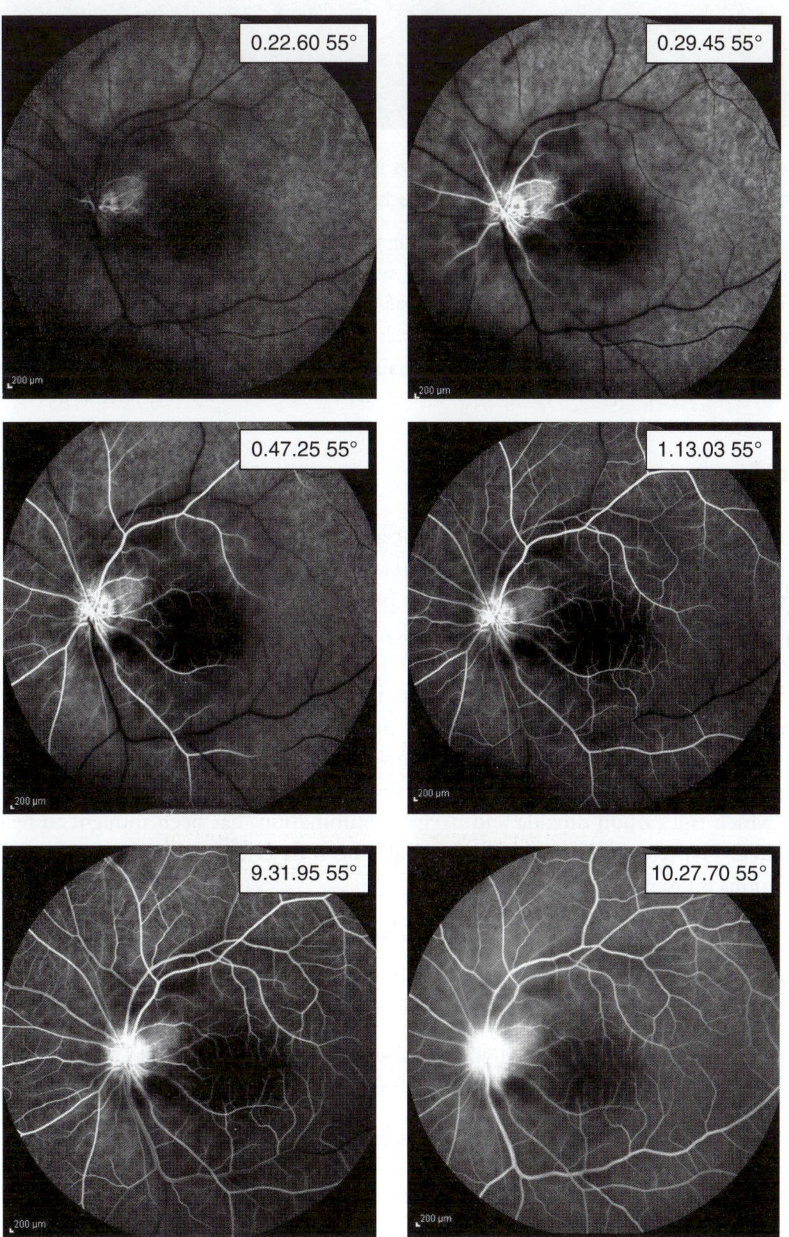

Fig. 55.2 Fundus fluorescein angiography (FFA) shows delayed arm–retina time, slow and sluggish arterial filling, and delayed arteriovenous transit time. There is late staining of the disc.

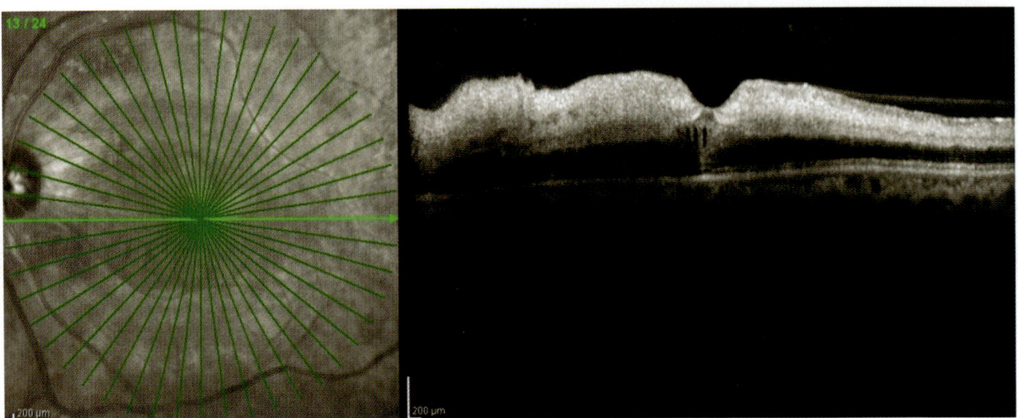

Fig. 55.3 Horizontal SD-OCT scan through macula shows increased reflectivity of the inner neurosensory retina due to ischemia and decreased reflectivity of outer layers due to edema.

The patient was given a thorough cardiac work-up with blood investigations, echocardiography, and carotid doppler. Mild mitral and aortic regurgitation was seen, with no evidence of vegetations or embolus. He was subsequently put on anticoagulation treatment.

On subsequent follow-up till 6 months, his vision remained unchanged.

DISCUSSION

Systemic cardiovascular diseases have a very strong association with CRAO. Associations of arterial hypertension, diabetes mellitus, hyperlipidemia, carotid artery disease, coronary artery disease, cerebrovascular accident, and tobacco smoking are significantly more common in these patients.

Acute presentation of a CRAO is an ocular emergency. Some interventions are recommended in an attempt to restore blood flow to the retina. Absence of an embolus in the retinal artery does not exclude its presence, but it could have migrated beyond the retinal vessels. Maneuvers include ocular-digital massage with or without an anterior chamber paracentesis, with or without oral medications such as acetazolamide to lower the intraocular pressure. It is based on the hypothesis that increase in pressure followed by a sudden return to normal pressure may push the embolus away along the vascular pathway into a distal branch decreasing the compromise to the retinal blood supply. Carbogen therapy, which is a carbon dioxide and oxygen combination, has been thought to help dilate vasculature and may be considered. Hyperbaric oxygen therapy has also been described as a possible intervention. Treatment of the comorbid conditions is essential.

FURTHER READING

1. Hayreh SS, Zimmerman MB: Central retinal artery occlusion: visual outcome. *Am J Ophthalmol* 140:376–391, 2005.
2. Hayreh SS, Patricia A. Podhajsky: Retinal artery occlusion. Associated systemic and ophthalmic abnormalities. *Ophthalmology* 116:1928–1936, 2009.
3. Duker JS, Sivalingam A, Brown GC, et al.: A prospective study of acute central retinal artery obstruction: the incidence of secondary ocular neovascularization. *Arch Ophthalmol* 109:339–342, 1991.
4. Babikian V, Wijman CA, Koleini B, et al.: Retinal ischemia and embolism: etiologies and outcomes based on a prospective study. *Cerebrovasc Dis* 12:108–113, 2001.
5. Cheung N, Lim L, Wang JJ, et al.: Prevalence and risk factors of retinal arteriolar emboli: the Singapore Malay Eye Study. *Am J Ophthalmol* 146:620–624, 2008.
6. Hayreh SS. Pathogenesis of occlusion of the central retinal vessels. *Am J Ophthalmol* 72:998–1011, 1971.

Central Retinal Vein Occlusion

Supriya Dabir and Kanav Gupta

Central retinal vein occlusion (CRVO) is one of the most common vascular diseases of the eye. The pathogenesis is multifactorial with both local and systemic factors involved. The prevalence of CRVO was estimated to be 0.4% according to the Blue Mountains Eye Study.

CASE STUDY

A 55-year-old male, with known type-2 diabetes mellitus, hypertension, and dyslipidemia, presented with best-corrected visual acuity (BCVA) 3/60 and 6/6 in the right eye and left eye, respectively. Anterior segment was normal and gonioscopy showed open angles. On fundus examination of the right eye, media was clear. The retinal veins were dilated and tortuous with multiple intraretinal hemorrhages, cotton-wool spots, and macular edema, as seen in Figure 56.1. The left eye was normal.

Fundus fluorescein angiogram (FFA) of the right eye showed distorted foveal avascular zone more than 15 DD of capillary nonperfusion (CNP) areas in the periphery, areas of blocked fluorescence were seen corresponding to the intraretinal hemorrhages, suggesting the ischemic nature of the occlusion, as seen in Figure 56.2.

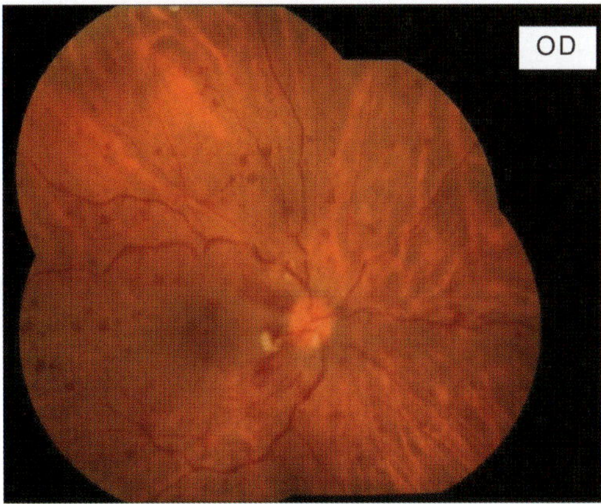

Fig. 56.1 Montage fundus photograph showing dilated and tortuous retinal veins with multiple intraretinal hemorrhages, cotton-wool spots, and macular edema.

The radial spectral-domain optical coherence tomography (SD-OCT) scan of the macula showed large cystoid spaces, involving inner retinal layers. In the early stage, fluid accumulates intracellularly within the muller cells. As it persists, necrosis of the muller cells occurs, leading to the formation of large cystoid cavities or cystoid macular edema. Also seen is the irregularity of the inner segment–outer segment (IS–OS) junctional layer. Edema in the outer retina leading to disruption of photoreceptors might be expected to be more disruptive to visual processing than that of the inner retina due to the ionic imbalance caused by the accumulation of the extracellular fluid.

Central foveal thickness (CFT) was 444 microns with the thickness map showing mean central maximum thickness of 479 microns and mean central minimum thickness of 333 microns. A pseudocolor map reflects the same, as seen in **Figure 56.3**.

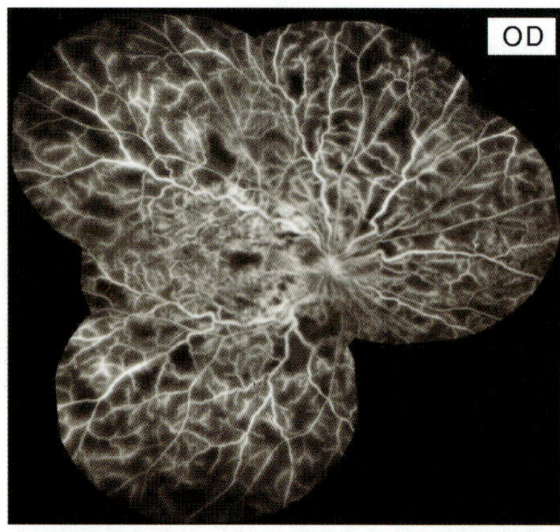

Fig. 56.2 The fundus fluorescein angiogram (FFA) with distorted foveal avascular zone perivascular staining and more than 15 disc diameters of CNP areas in the periphery.

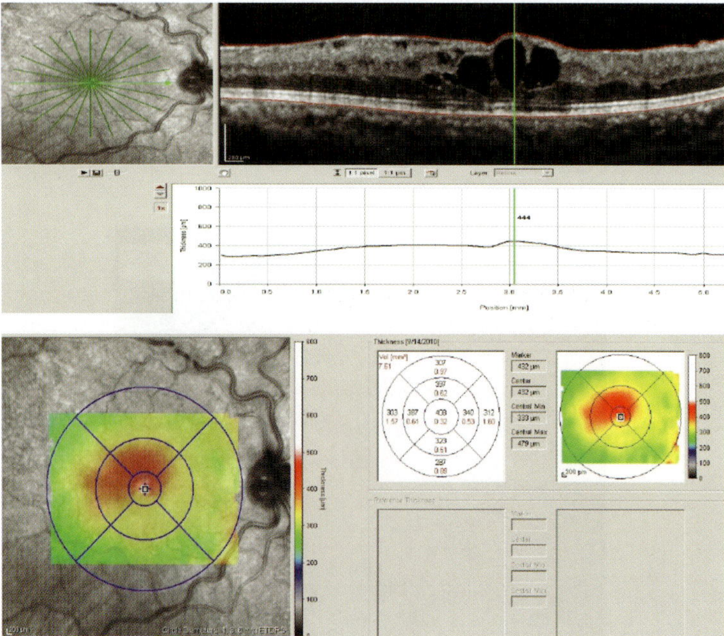

Fig. 56.3 A radial SD-OCT showing intraretinal cysts, epiretinal membrane, and disruption of IS–OS layers. The pseudocolor map shows hot colors in areas of edema.

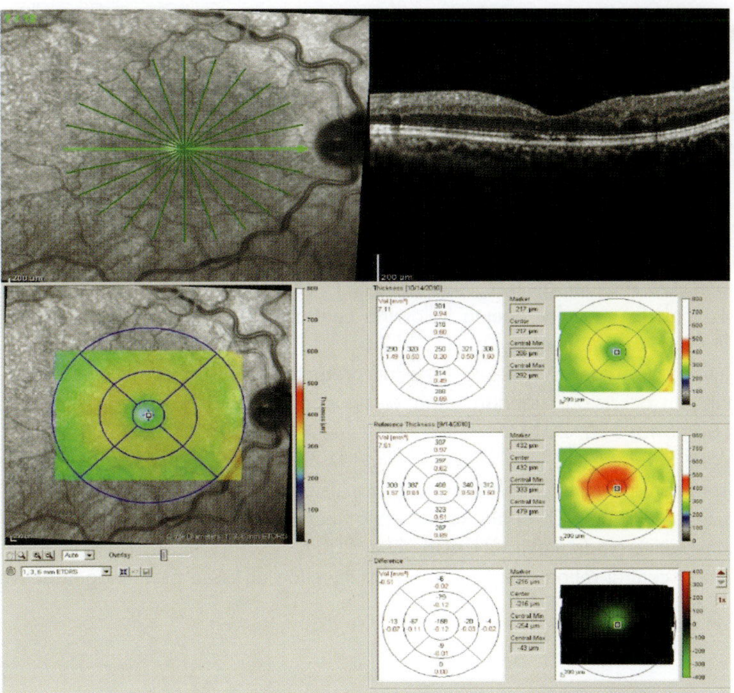

Fig. 56.4 Shows a radial SD-OCT, showing resolution of intraretinal cysts and a normal foveal contour post-treatment. The IS–OS junction, however, remains disrupted. The pseudocolor map reflects the resolution of the hot colors.

After a single dose of intravitreal injection of bevacizumab, the CFT reduced to 201 microns with resolution of cystic spaces. The irregularity of the IS-OS junction remained so. The comparison scan shows the difference map, as seen in **Figure 56.4**.

At 3-months follow-up, the patient however developed neovascularization of the iris in two quadrants, open angles were seen on gonioscopy, and subsequently underwent panretinal photocoagulation.

DISCUSSION

CRVO is the most common cause of visual loss in patients above 50 years of age. It is a multifactorial disorder with local, systemic, and haematological risk factors. It is significantly more common in patients with raised intraocular pressure. It should be differentiated as either ischemic or nonischemic for better management and prognosis. Ischemic CRVO carries a much higher risk of NVG, whereas nonischemic may be an incidental finding.

Peripheral fundus angiograms are of extreme importance, and a criterion of 10 disc diameter or more of retinal capillary obliteration is a sign of ischemic CRVO. The SD-OCT helps to evaluate the macular edema and also highlights any tractional component such as epiretinal membrane. Macular edema is seen in both types of CRVO. This with chronicity can lead to cystoid degeneration, macular scarring, and cellophane maculopathy. SD-OCT also helps to evaluate the effect of treatment and associated visual prognosis.

Many approaches for the treatment of macular edema in CRVO have been tried like macular grid photocoagulation, intravitreal injections of triamcinolone acetonide, and anti-vascular endothelial growth factors. Pan retinal photocoagulation has been used in high-risk eyes and also in the presence of neovascularisation. In refractory cases of NVG, eventually a trabeculectomy may need to be done. In cases of poor visual prognosis cyclocryotherapy may be attempted.

FURTHER READING

1. Hayreh SS: Classification of central retinal vein occlusion. *Ophthalmology* 90:458–474, 1983.
2. Hayreh SS: Management of central retinal vein occlusion. *Ophthalmologica* 217:167–188, 2003.
3. Interventions for Central Retinal Vein Occlusion: An evidence-based systematic review endothelial growth factor agents. *Ophthalmology* 114:507–519, 2007.
4. Central Vein Occlusion Study Group. Central vein occlusion study of photocoagulation therapy: baseline endings. Online *J Curr Clin Trials* [serial online] Doc. No. 95, Oct 14, 1993.
5. Evaluation of grid pattern photocoagulation for macular edema in central vein occlusion: the Central Vein Occlusion Study Group M report. *Ophthalmology* 102:1425–1433, 1995.
6. Brown DM: Ranibizumab for macular edema following central retinal vein occlusion: six-month primary end point results of a phase III study. *Ophthalmology* 117(6):1124–1133, Jun 2010.
7. Scott IU, VanVeldhuisen PC, Oden NL, et al.: Baseline predictors of visual acuity and retinal thickness outcomes in patients with retinal vein occlusion: standard care versus corticosteroid for retinal vein occlusion study report 10. *Ophthalmology* 118(2):345–352, 2011.
8. Leonard BC, Coupland SG, Kertes PJ, et al.: Long-term follow-up of a modied technique for laser-induced chorioretinal venous anastomosis in nonischemic central retinal vein occlusion. *Ophthalmology* 110:948–954, 2003.
9. Opremcak EM, Bruce RA, Lomeo MD, et al.: Radial optic neurotomy for central retinal vein occlusion: a retrospective pilot study of 11 consecutive cases. *Retina* 21:408–415, 2001.
10. Weiss JN. Treatment of central retinal vein occlusion by injection of tissue plasminogen activator into a retinal vein. *Am J Ophthalmol* 126:142–144, 1998.

Central Serous Chorioretinopathy

Manish Nagpal, Navneet Mehrotra, Harsh Yadav, and Jainendra Rahud

Central serous chorioretinopathy (CSCR) is a self-limiting disease with a fairly good prognosis; it commonly occurs during the active part of life from 20–50 years of age. The disease is stress related and type-A personalities are more prone to it. Recurrences are common. The condition is bilateral in 5%–35% of cases. Patients with CSCR complain of decreased or blurred vision, metamorphosia, micropsia, and paracentral scotomas.

Two types of leakages are well documented in literature on fluorescein angiography. Most common is the inkblot leakage (93%) and the second type is the smokestack pattern (7%–20% cases).

Most leakage points are within a 1-mm area around fovea; but they can occur in an area greater than 3 mm from foveal avascular zone (FAZ) in 11.8% cases. In less than 10% cases, the leakage point is found in the fovea. The following is a case of CSCR-manifested leakage of dye arising from under a blood vessel.

CASE STUDY

A 48-year-old female presented with diminished vision since 5 days in the left eye with a best-corrected visual acuity of 6/60 (Figs 57.1 and 57.2).

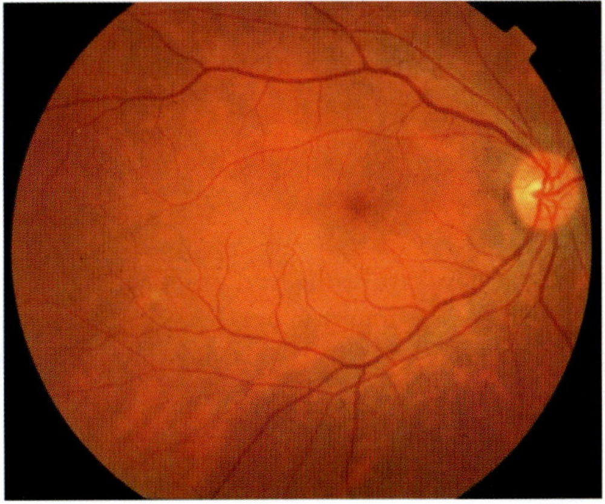
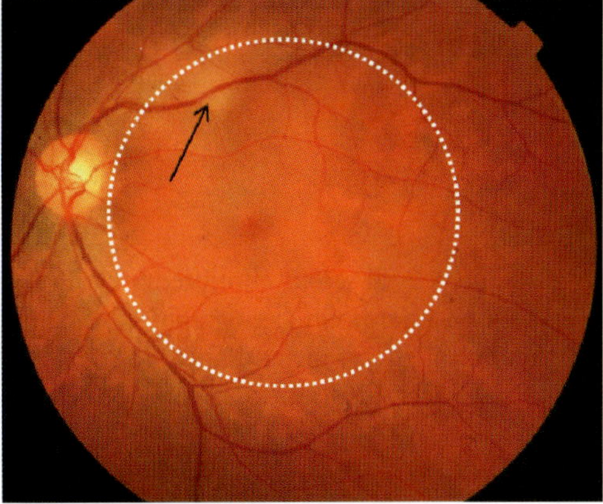

Fig. 57.1 The right-eye fundus was within normal limits. Fundus examination of the left eye showed round, well-delineated area of subsensory fluid in the form of serous retinal detachment in the macular region (*white circle*). Upper limit of serous detachment was crossing the superior arcade and showed a well-defined, elevated, grayish-white lesion just under the superior arcade (*black arrow*).

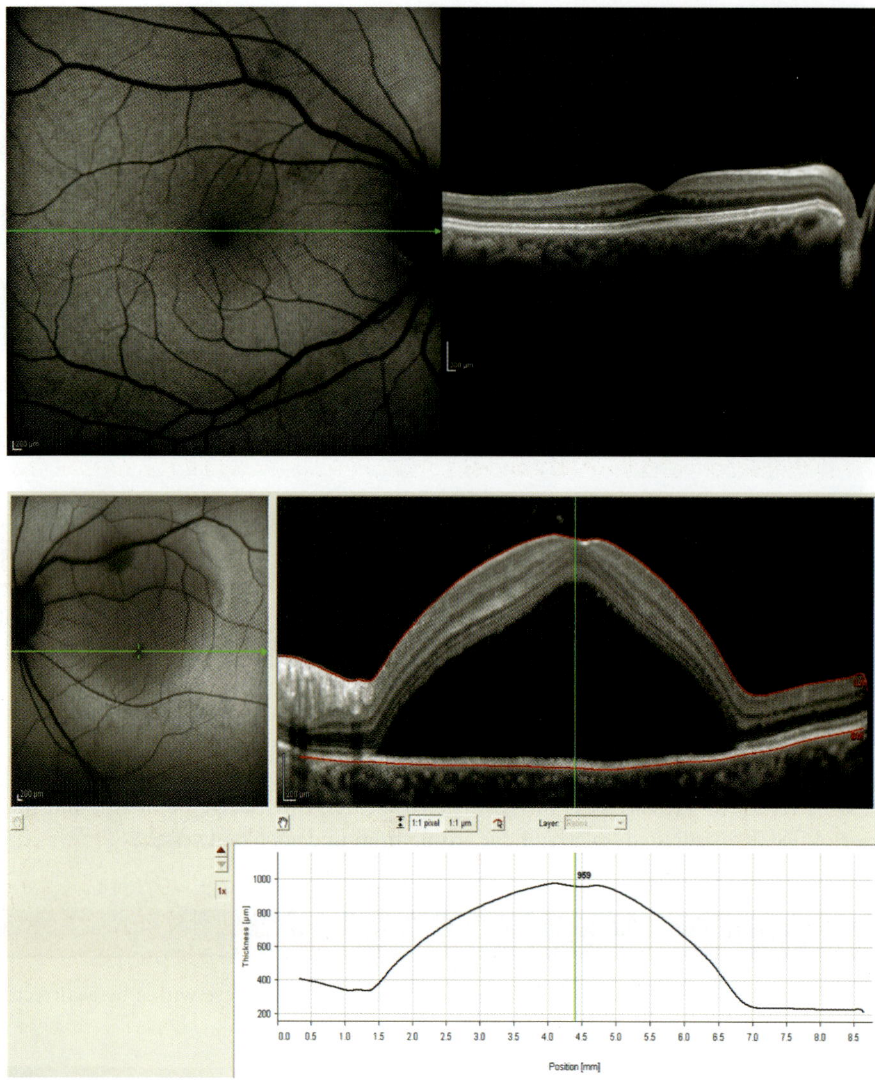

Fig. 57.2 Right-eye OCT showed normal foveal contour, left-eye OCT showed serous retinal detachment with retinal thickness of 959 microns.

Eyes with acute central serous chorioretinopathy (CSC) have focal leakage at the level of retinal pigment epithelium (RPE) seen on fluorescein angiography (FA). Indocyanine green angiography in eyes with CSC shows multiple areas of inner choroidal staining. Detailed optical coherence tomography (OCT) scan passing through the point of leakage in FA gives additional information about morphologic changes at the site of leakage (**Fig. 57.3**). There have

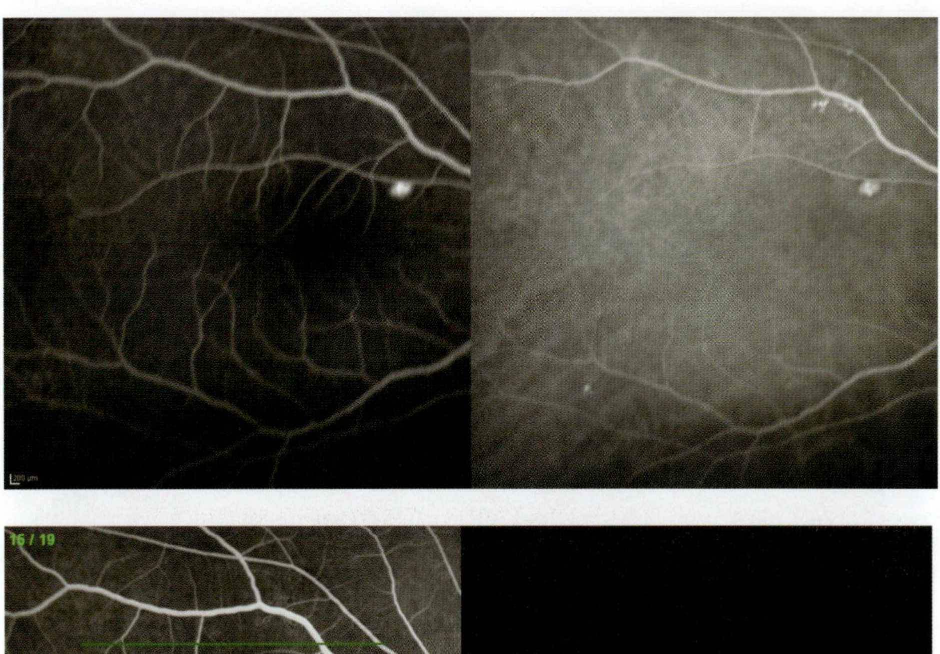

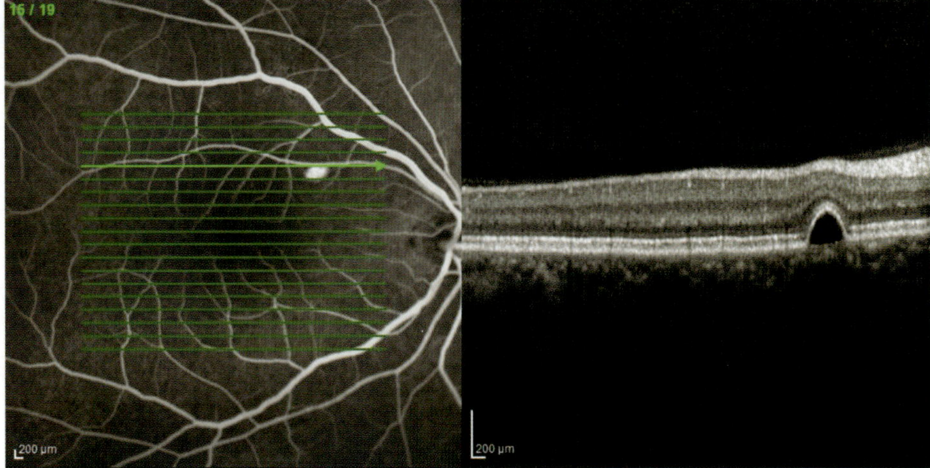

Fig. 57.3 Right eye combined fluorescein/indocyanine green angiogram FA–ICG showed leakage. SD-OCT at the leakage point showed pigment epithelial detachment (PED).

been reports with Fourier-domain OCT examinations showing RPE defect within pigment epithelial detachment (PED) at a leakage site through which fluid might pass from sub-RPE to subretinal area.

Our patient had leakage under a blood vessel (**Fig. 57.4**). The detailed OCT scan passing through the leakage site showed PED with retinal dipping (**Fig. 57.5**). Following laser treatment at the leakage point, CSR resolved with residual PED (**Figs 57.6 and 57.7**).

Although histopathologic studies of CSC are limited, spectral-domain optical coherence tomography (SD-OCT) showed precise morphologic changes in acute CSC. Detailed OCT scan through the leakage site showed presence of a minute RPE defect through which choroidal exudation leaks into the subretinal space. These changes may further help us to enhance our understanding of fluid dynamics in patients with CSC.

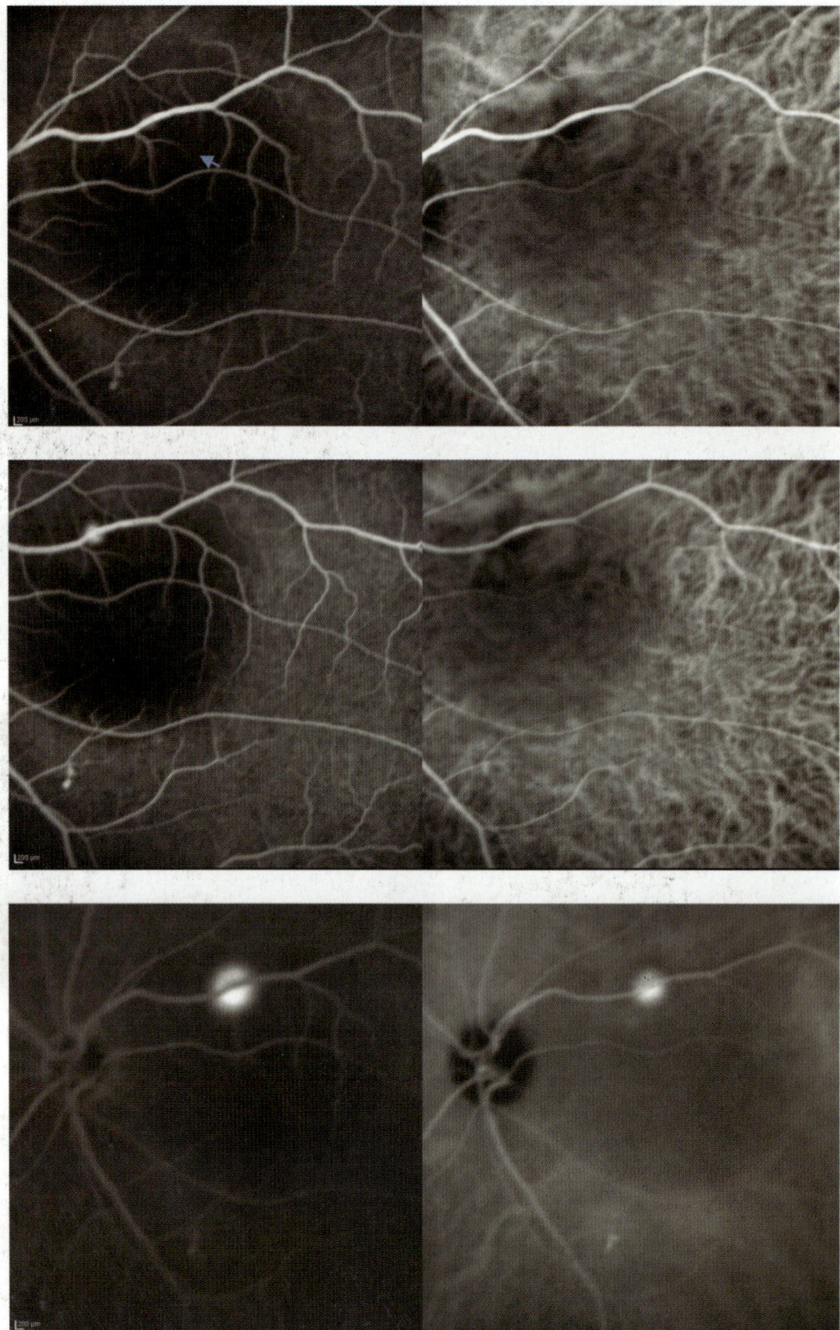

Fig. 57.4 Left-eye FA showed hyperfluorescent spot increasing in size and intensity beneath the superior arcade; corresponding ICGA showed hypofluorescent area with late hyperfluorescence.

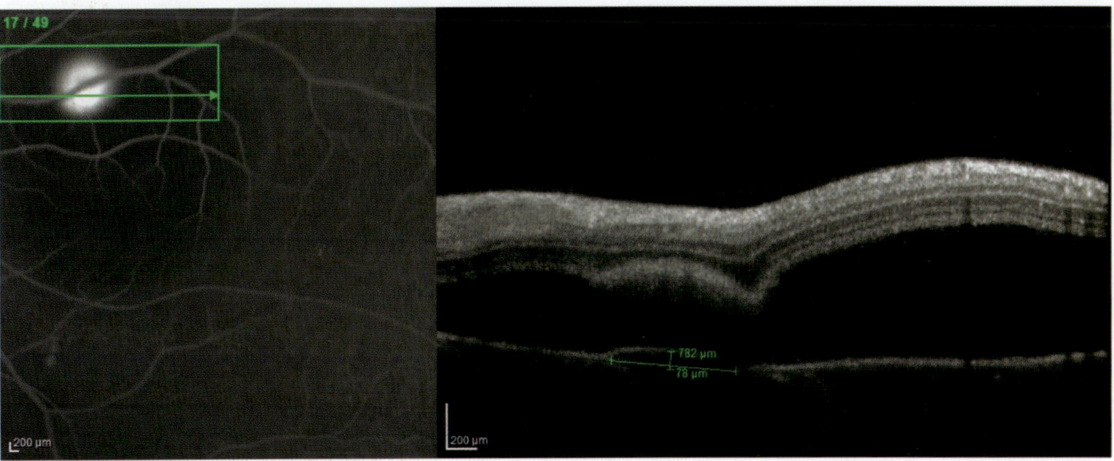

Fig. 57.5 Simultaneous FA and OCT showed PED at leakage point with hyperreflectivity in subsensory space. We treated patient with focal laser in left eye; after 1 month he improved to a visual acuity of 6/9.

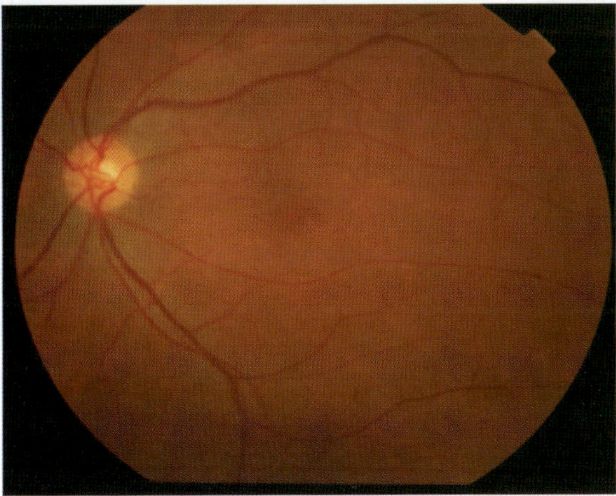

Fig. 57.6 Color photo of left eye after 1 month showing resolved CSR.

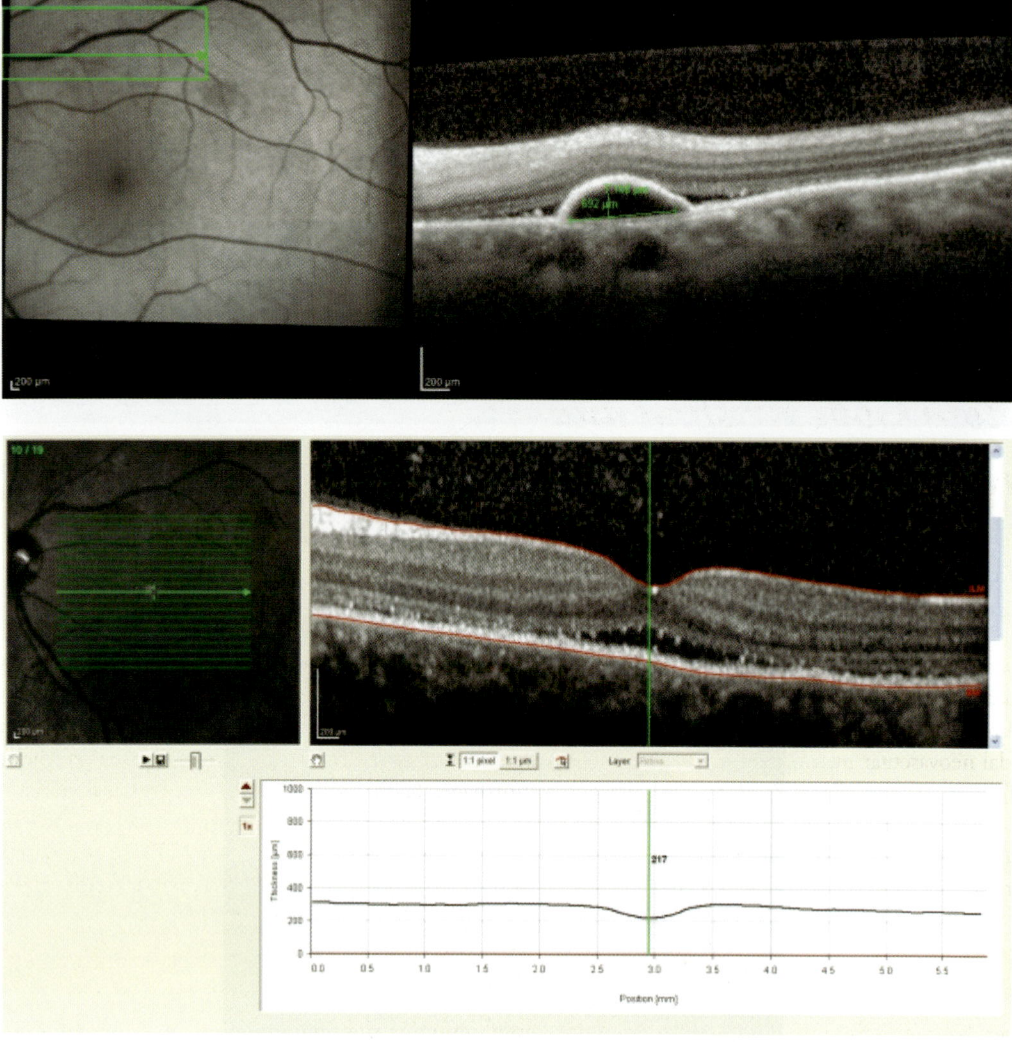

Fig. 57.7 Post-treatment 1-month follow-up OCT at leakage point (*above*) showed PED (pigment epithelial detachment) with resolution of subsensory fluid and reduction of thickness to 217 microns.

FURTHER READING

1. Balacco-gabrieli C, Asciano F, Reibaldi A, et al.: Central serous retinopathy. Etiopathogenetic and clinical considerations. *Ophthalmologica* 181:251–260, 1980.
2. Guyer DR, Yannuzzi LA, Slakter JS, et al.: Digital indocyanine green videoangiography of central serous chorioretinopathy. *Arch ophthalmol* 112:1057–1062, 1994.
3. Piccolino FC, Borgia I: Central serous chorioretinopathy and indocyanine green angiography. *Retina* 14:231–242, 1994.
4. Yannuzzi LA, Shakin JL, Fisher YL, et al.: Peripheral retinal detachments and retinal pigment epithelial atrophic tracts secondary to central serous pigment epitheliopathy. *Ophthalmology* 91:1554–1572, 1984.

Choroidal Neovascularization— Wet Age-related Macular Degeneration

Santosh Gopi Krishna and
Naresh Kumar Yadav

Age-related macular degeneration (AMD) is a major cause of severe visual loss in the elderly. Wet AMD is the severe and exudative form. It results from pathological growth of new blood vessels from pre-existing choroidal vessels into the subretinal space. Ten percent of AMD patients manifest the neovascular form. Neovascular AMD comprises choroidal neovascular membrane (CNVM), pigment epithelial detachment (PED), retinal pigment epithelial (RPE) tears, fibrovascular disciform scarring, and vitreous hemorrhage. The pathogenesis lies in aging and genetic changes in the RPE–Bruchs'–choriocapillaris complex with various angiogenic factors playing a role. Various treatment protocols include focal laser, photodynamic therapy (PDT), transpupillary thermotherapy (TTT), radiotherapy, and the current mainstay of management—intravitreal anti-VEGF (anti-vascular endothelial growth factor) injections.

CASE STUDY 1

A 76-year-old Asian Indian man presented with decreased vision in the right eye. His best-corrected visual acuity (BCVA) was 20/100 in the right eye and 20/20 in the left eye. Anterior segment showed both eyes (BE) pseudophakia. Fundus showed right-eye macular geographic atrophy with fluid suggestive of CNVM and left eye (LE) drusen suggestive of dry AMD. A fundus fluorescein angiogram (FFA) revealed right-eye occult CNVM and left-eye dry AMD (Fig. 58.1). Spectral-domain optical coherence tomography (SD-OCT) showed right-eye PEDs with subretinal fluid and left-eye dry AMD. He received four intravitreal bevacizumab injections leading to scarring of the CNVM and a BCVA of 20/200.

CASE STUDY 2

A 66-year-old Asian Indian woman presented with complaints of blurred vision in the left eye. The BCVA was 20/40 in the right eye and 20/200 in the left eye. Anterior segment showed BE early cataract. Fundus showed dry AMD changes in the right eye and macular RPE atrophy, and scarring with grayish CNVM, and bleed in the left eye. FFA revealed dry AMD in the right eye and multiple areas of leak with late staining suggestive of occult CNVM (Fig. 58.2).

SD-OCT imaging showed right-eye dry AMD changes with left-eye RPE–CNVM complex with intra and subretinal fluid. She underwent three injections of intravitreal bevacizumab in the left eye, following which the CNVM was scarred and BCVA of 20/200 was maintained.

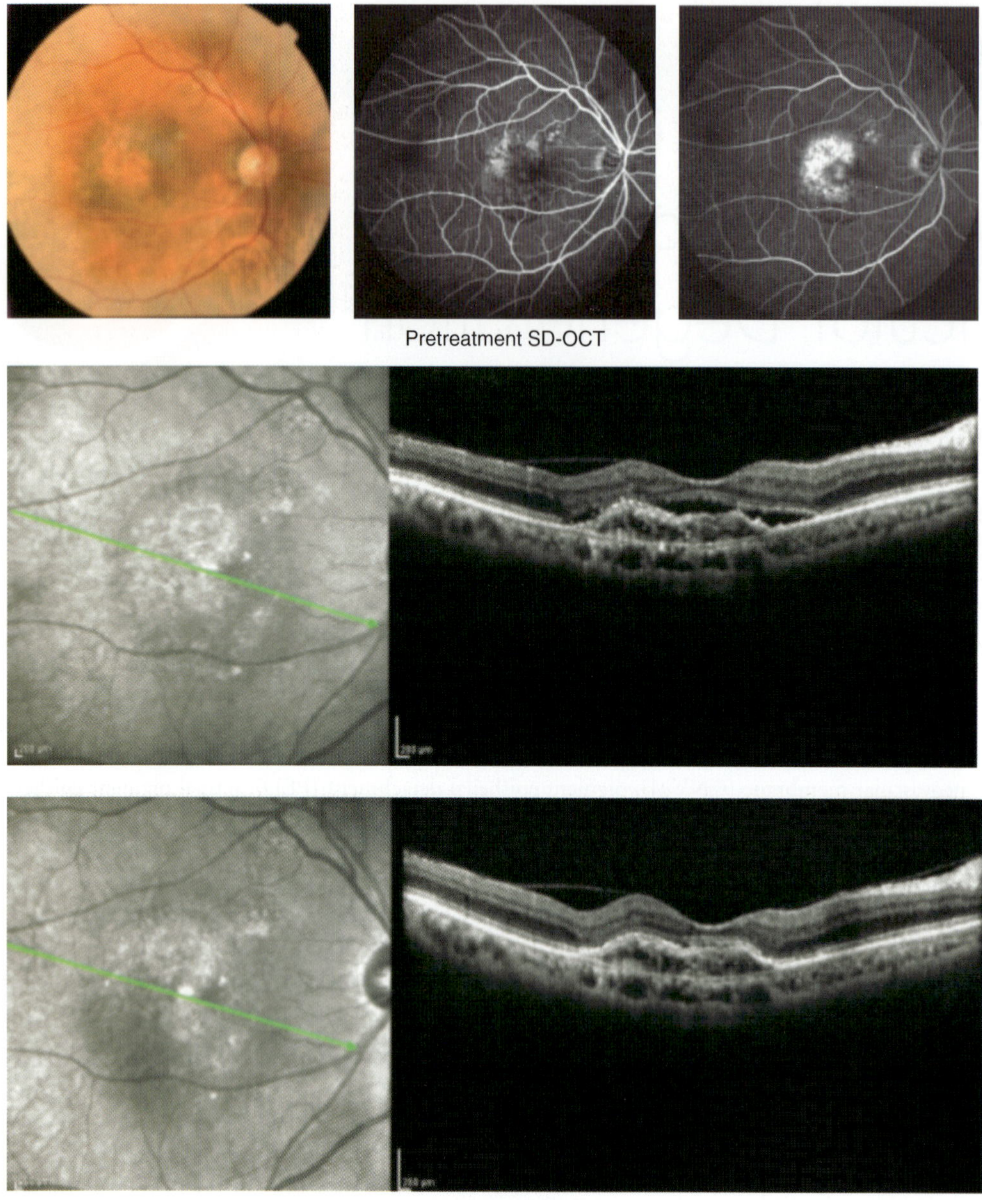

Pretreatment SD-OCT

Post-treatment SD-OCT

Fig. 58.1 Fundus photo showing right-eye macular geographic atrophy with fluid suggestive of CNVM. FFA showing early (*upper middle*) hyperfluorescence with a late (*upper right*) leak suggestive of an occult CNVM. Pretreatment SD-OCT image showing PED–CNVM complex and subretinal fluid. A post-treatment SD-OCT showing significant scarring with decrease in fluid.

CASE STUDY 3

An 80-year-old Asian Indian man presented with blurred vision BE, right eye > left eye. BCVA was 20/200 in the right eye and 20/50 in the left eye. Anterior segment showed posterior subcapsular cataract with grade 2 nuclear sclerosis in BE. Fundus showed a dull foveal reflex with a grayish membrane and fluid in the right eye, and a dull

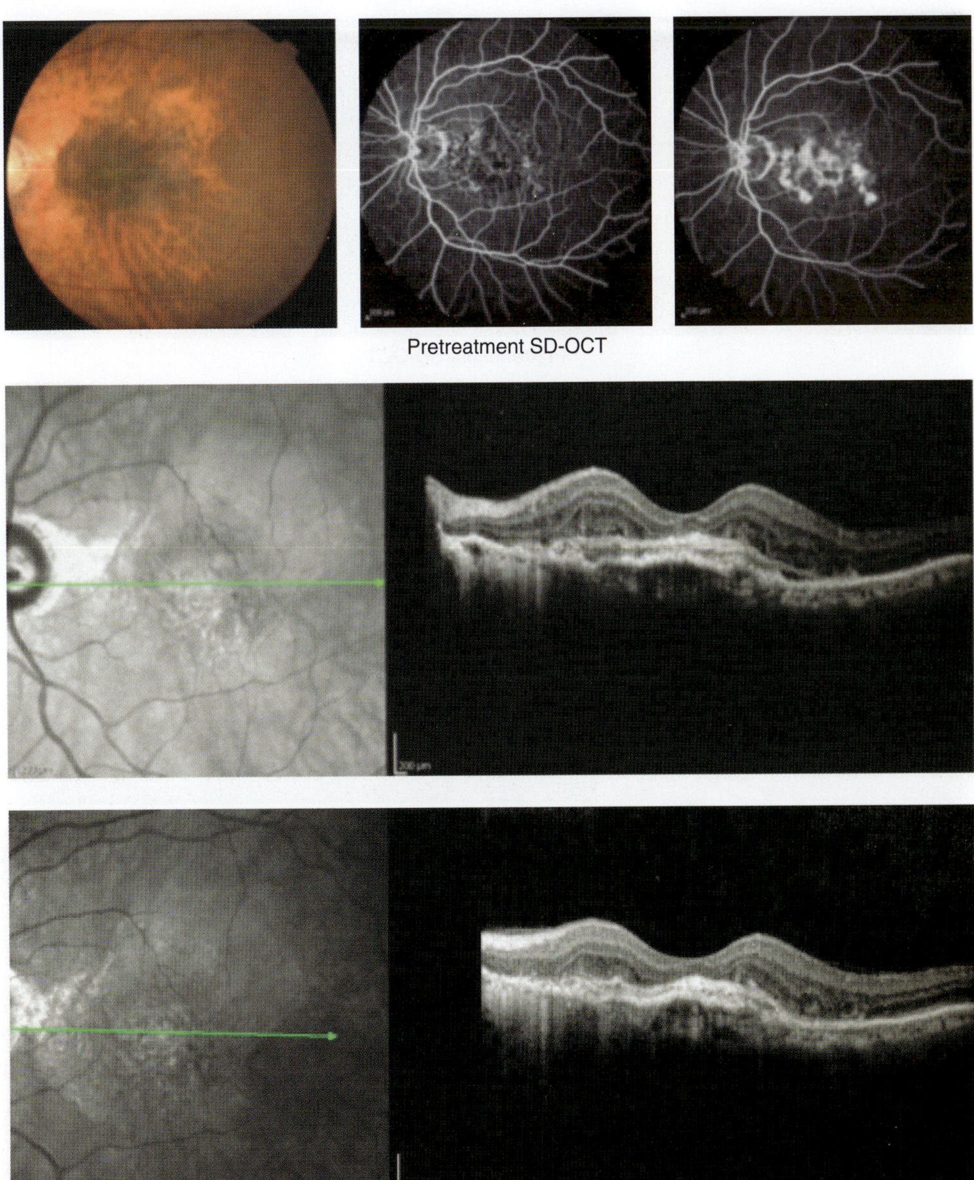

Fig. 58.2 The above fundus photograph shows left-eye macular geographic RPE atrophy and scarring with grayish membrane and bleed suggestive of CNVM. FFA shows multiple leaks confirming an occult CNVM. SD-OCT imaging shows a RPE–CNVM complex with intra- and subretinal fluid. A post-treatment (bevacizumab) SD-OCT shows scarring of the CNVM.

foveal reflex with dry AMD changes in the left eye. FFA showed features suggestive of classic CNVM in the right eye and dry AMD in the left eye (**Fig. 58.3**).

SD-OCT showed clumped RPE–CNVM complex with gross intraretinal fluid spaces in the right eye and dry AMD changes in the left eye. He underwent three injections of intravitreal bevacizumab, following which the CNVM showed decreasing fluid and scarring.

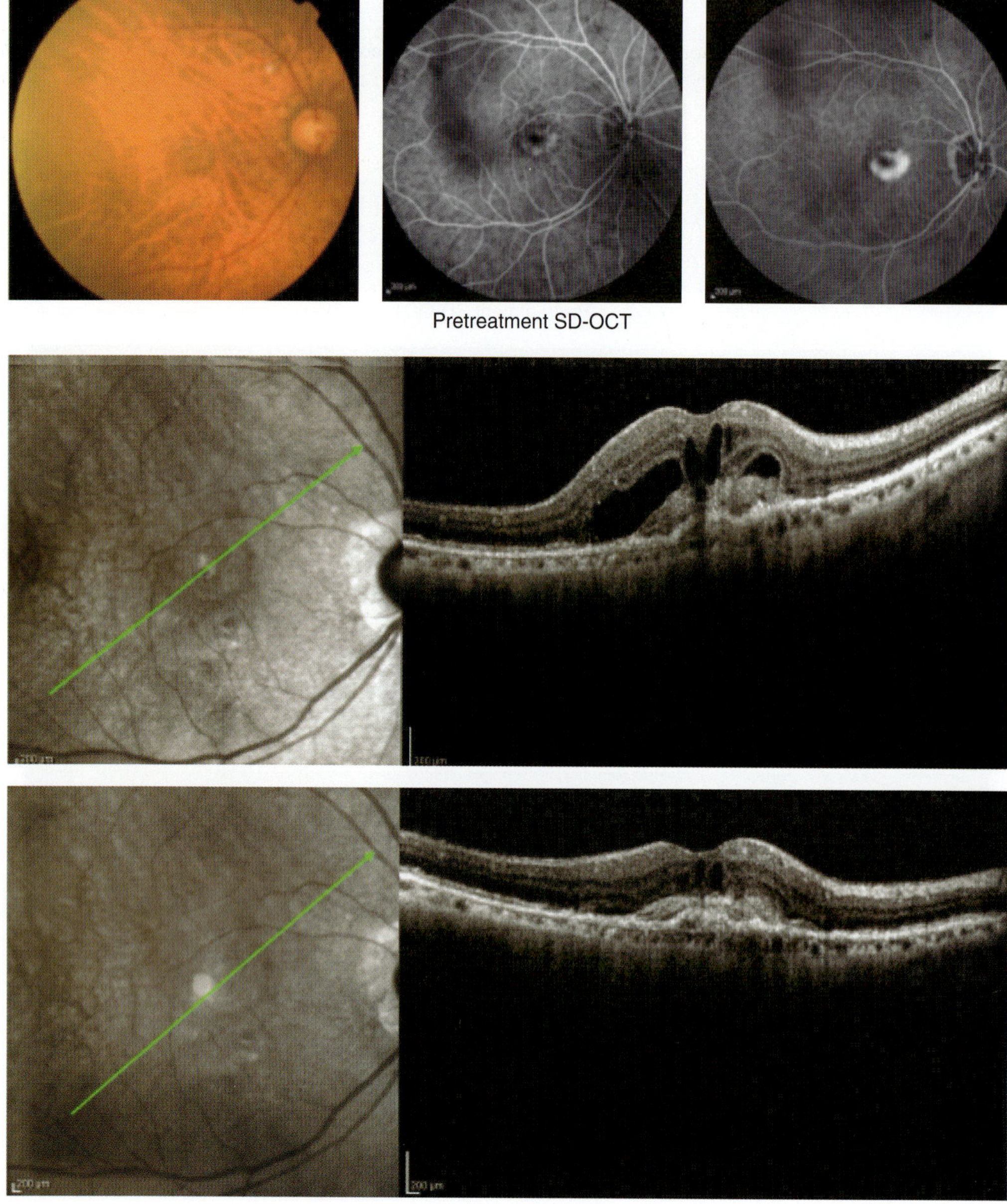

Fig. 58.3 The fundus photo shows a dull foveal reflex with a grayish membrane and fluid. FFA shows features suggestive of classic CNVM. Pretreatment SD-OCT image shows clumped RPE–CNVM complex with gross intraretinal fluid spaces. A post-treatment SD-OCT shows decreasing fluid spaces with scarring of the CNVM.

FURTHER READING

1. Eye disease Prevalence Research Group. Prevalence of age related macular degeneration in US. *Arch Ophthalmol* 122: 564–572, 2004.

2. Ferris FL III, Fine SL, Hyman LA: Age-related macular degeneration and blindness due to neovascular maculopathy. *Arch Ophthalmol* 102:1640–1642, 1984.

3. Age-Related Eye Disease Study Research Group: Risk factors associated with age-related macular degeneration. A case control study in the age-related eye disease study: age-related eye disease study report number 3. *Ophthalmology* 107:2224–2232, 2000.

4. Macular Photocoagulation Study Group, 1994. Laser photocoagulation for juxtafoveal choroidal neovascularization. Five-year results from randomized clinical trials. *Arch Ophthalmol* 112:500–509, 1994.

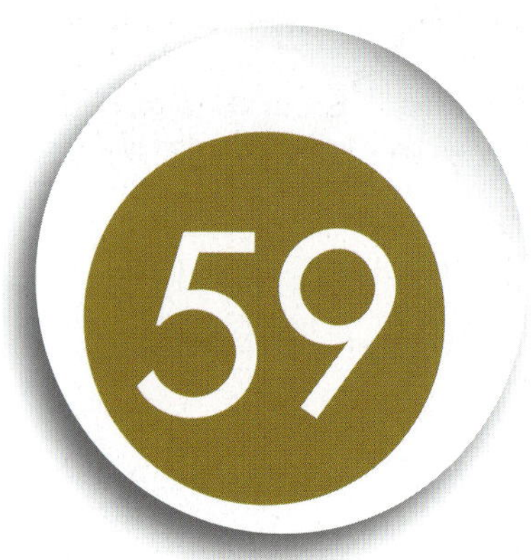

Choroidal Neovascularization—Myopia

Naresh Kumar Yadav

High myopia is especially common in Asia; countries like Singapore have a prevalence of 9%. Choroidal neovascularization (CNV) with chorioretinal atrophy is the most common cause of poor vision in patients with pathologic myopia and CNV will develop in 5%–10% of such eyes. Visual acuity in almost all eyes with myopic CNV will drop to 20/200 or less, if left untreated.

Several treatment options like laser photocoagulation, photodynamic therapy (PDT), and surgical extraction of CNV have been tried for myopic CNV. PDT has been a standard treatment for myopic CNV. However, despite PDT, more than 50% of the eyes have persistent leakage from the CNV, and 13% develop visual loss of three or more lines at 1 year. The recent discovery of vascular endothelial growth factor (VEGF) and its role in the pathogenesis of ocular neovascularization has led to anti-VEGF agents being used to treat myopic CNV.

CASE STUDY

A 34-year-old Indian male presented with complaints of distortion of straight lines in the right eye, since 2 weeks. The best-corrected visual acuity (BCVA) was 6/24, N12 in the right eye and 6/9, N6 in the left eye. The refractive error was −15 D in both the eyes. The patient was diagnosed to have myopic choroidal neovascular membrane and underwent fundus fluorescein angiography (FFA), as well as spectral-domain optical coherence tomography (SD-OCT) (**Fig. 59.1**).

The patient responded well to intravitreal Lucentis® and the BCVA improved to 6/9, N6. The post-treatment images are as below (**Fig. 59.2**).

FFA findings should be relied on more than optical coherence tomography (OCT) in determining retreatment because myopic CNVs are usually not accompanied by frank subretinal fluid. This case demonstrates the efficacy and safety of intravitreal anti-VEGF (Lucentis®) in the management of myopic CNV.

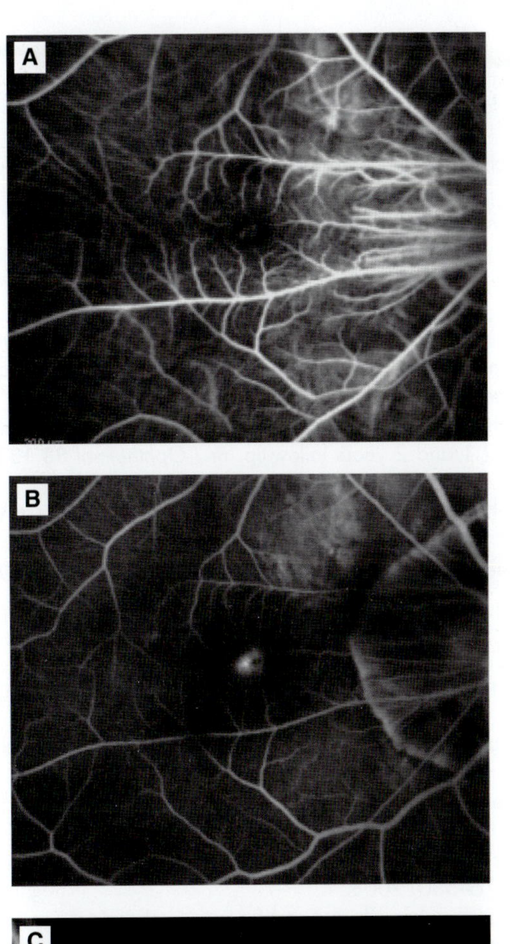

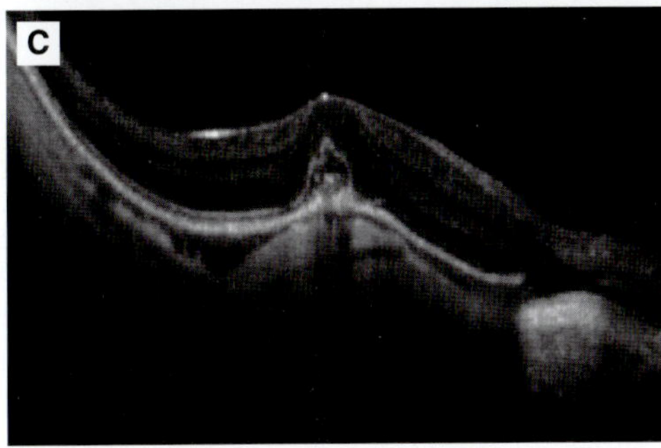

Fig. 59.1 (A) Early-phase FFA showing a classic subfoveal choroidal neovascular membrane with **(B)** leakage in the late phase. **(C)** SD-OCT showing a localized hyperreflective lesion with few pockets of intraretinal edema.

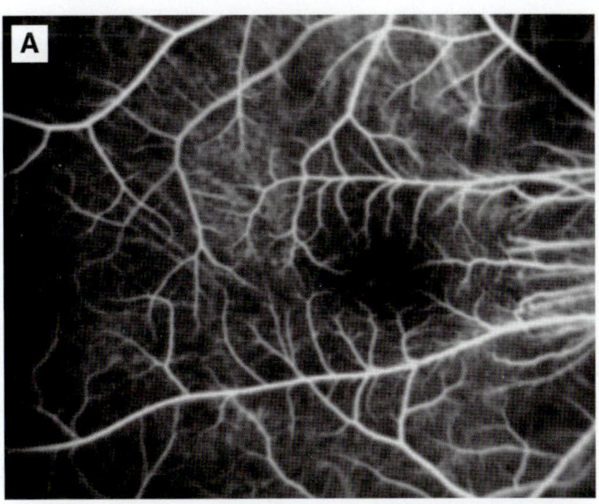

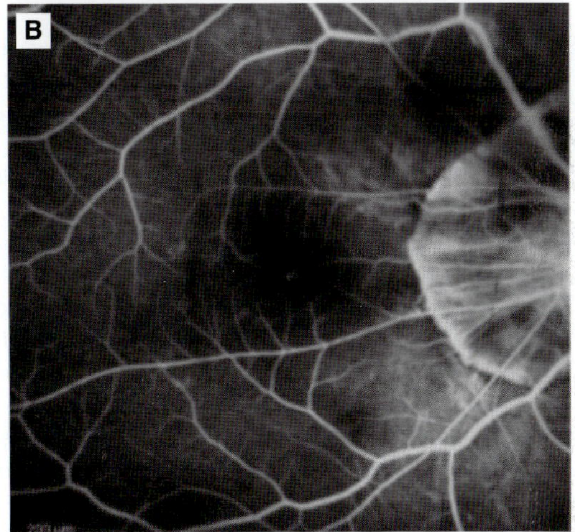

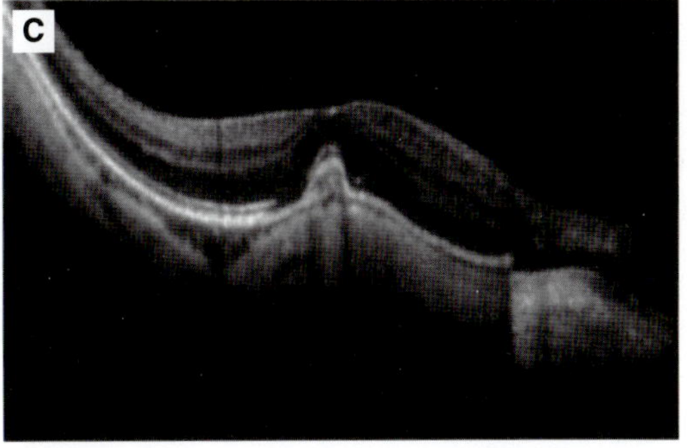

Fig. 59.2 (A) Early- and **(B)** late-phase FFA showing staining of scar tissue with no evidence of leakage. **(C)** Post-treatment SD-OCT showing resolution of intraretinal edema and a hyperreflective lesion corresponding to fibrosed CNV.

FURTHER READING

1. Wong TY, Foster PJ, Hee J, et al.: Prevalence and risk factors for refractive errors in adult Chinese in Singapore. *Invest Ophthal Vis Sci* 41:2486–2494, 2004.

2. Avila MP, Weiter JJ, Jalkh AE, et al.: Natural history of choroidal neo vascularisation in degenerative myopia. *Ophthalmology* 91:1573–1578, 1984.

3. Soubrane G, Coscass GJ: CNV membrane in degenerative Myopia. In: Ryan SJ, editors Retina, ed 4. Philadelphia. Pa; Elsevier Mosby:1115–1133, 2006.

4. Yoshida T, Ohno-Matsui K, Yasuzumi K, et al.: Myopic choroidal neovascularisation. A 10-year follow-up. *Ophthalmology* 110:1297–1305, 2003.

5. Cohen SY, Bulika A, Dubois L, et al.: PDT for juxta foveal CNV in myopic eyes. *Am J Ophthalmol* 136:371–374, 2003.

6. Bandello F, Lanzetta P, Battaglia Parodi M, et al.: Photodynamic therapy of subfoveal recurrences after laser photocoagulation of extrafoveal CNV in pathologic myopic eyes. *Graefes Arch Clin Exp Ophthal* 241:567–570, 2003.

7. Lams DS, Chan WM, Liu DT, et al.: Photodynamic therapy with verteporfin for subfoveal choroidal neo vascularisation of pathologic myopia in Chinese eyes. A prospective series of 1 and 2 years follow-up. *Br J Ophthalmol* 88:1315–1319, 2004.

8. Ruiz-Moreno JM, Montero JA: Long-term visual acuity results after argon laser photocoagulation of juxtafoveal CNV in highly myopic eyes. *Eur J Ophthalmol* 12:117–122, 2002.

9. Ruiz-Moreno JM, de la Vega C: Surgical removal of subfoveal CNV in highly myopic patient. *Br J Ophthalmol* 85:1041–1043, 2001.

10. VIP study group. PDT of sub foveal CNV in pathologic myopia with verteporfin: 1 year of a randomized clinical trial- VIP report No-1. *Ophthalmology* 108:841–852, 2001.

11. VIP study group. PDT of sub foveal CNV in pathologic myopia with verteporfin: 1 year of a randomized clinical trial- VIP report No-3. *Ophthalmology* 110:667–673, 2001.

12. Yamamoto I, Rogers AH, Reichel E, et al.: Intravitreal bevacizumab as treatment for subfoveal choroidal neovascularisation secondary to pathological myopia. *Br J Ophthalmol* 91:157–160, 2007.

13. Sakaguchi H, Ikuno Y, Gomi F, et al.: Intravitreal injection of bevacizumab for choroidal neo vascularisation associated with pathological myopia. *Br J Ophthalmol* 91:161–165, 2007.

14. Marc-Andre' Rheaume and Mikael Sebag: Intravitreal bevacizumab for the treatment of choroidal neovascularization associated with pathological myopia. *Can J Ophthalmol* 43:576–580, 2008.

15. Wai-Man Chan, Timothy YY Lai, David T L Liu, et al.: Intravitreal Bevacizumab (Avastin) for myopic choroidal neovascularization: Six months results of a prospective pilot study. *Ophthalmology* 114:2190–2196, 2007.

Choroidal Osteoma

*Subhashchandra HD and
Kavitha Avadhani*

- The choroidal osteoma is a benign, ossifying tumor of the choroid that is typically found in young, healthy women in the second or third decade of life. Its pathogenesis is unknown. This tumor is clinically unilateral in 75% of cases and tends to be located in the juxtapapillary region.
- Growth, decalcification, subretinal fluid, hemorrhage, and choroidal neovascular membrane (CNVM) are known complications of choroidal osteoma. CNVM is seen in one-third of patients and is a major cause of visual impairment.
- The choroidal osteoma must be differentiated from other intraocular tumors as well as cases of dystrophic and metastatic calcification. Ultrasonography and computed tomography may help in the diagnosis by demonstrating a calcified plaque at the level of the choroid. Fluorescein angiography and indocyanine green (ICG) video angiography may demonstrate choroidal neovascularization, which may be amenable to treatment by laser photocoagulation.
- Spectral-domain-optical coherence tomography (SD-OCT) provides deeper and higher resolution images of the choroidal osteoma when compared with time-domain optical coherence tomography (TD-OCT).

CASE STUDY

- A 23-year-old Asian Indian male presented to us with progressive defective vision in the right eye since 4 months. He gave a history of having received three intravitreal injections of bevacizumab in the same eye.
- Ocular examination revealed best-corrected visual acuity (BCVA) of 20/80 in the right eye (RE) and 20/20 in the left eye (LE). Pupillary reactions and slit lamp biomicroscopic examination of the anterior segment were normal in both eyes. Fundus examination of the LE was normal, while the RE showed a yellowish-orange lesion of 14 disc diameter (DD) having well-defined scalloped margins with pseudopod extensions superiorly and nasally to the disc and in fovea (Fig. 60.1).
- Fundus fluorescein angiography (FFA) of the right eye showed early hyperfluorescence with increase in hyperfluorescence in the late phases suggestive of tumor staining with irregularities in retinal pigment epithelium. The left eye was angiographically normal (Fig. 60.2).

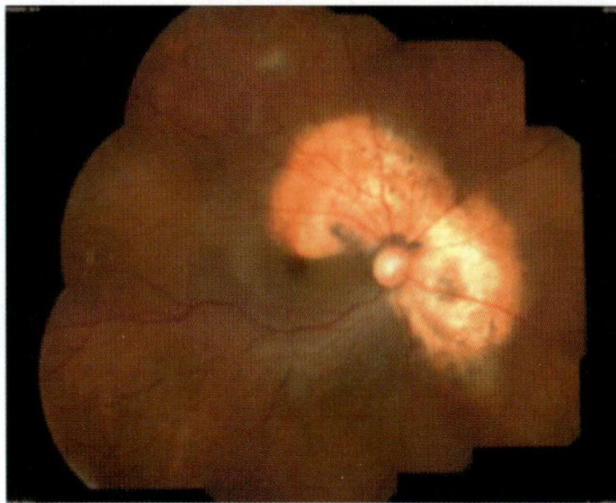

Fig. 60.1 Fundus photo of the right eye showing a well-defined orangish lesion with scalloped margins.

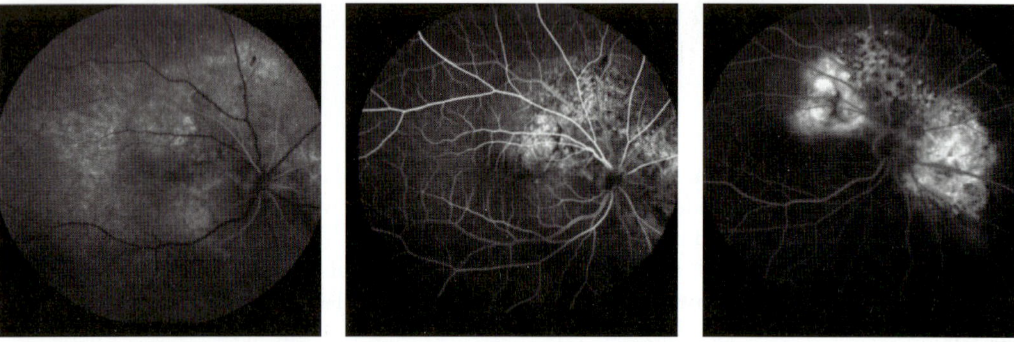

Fig. 60.2 FFA of the right eye in early and late phases showing the lesion.

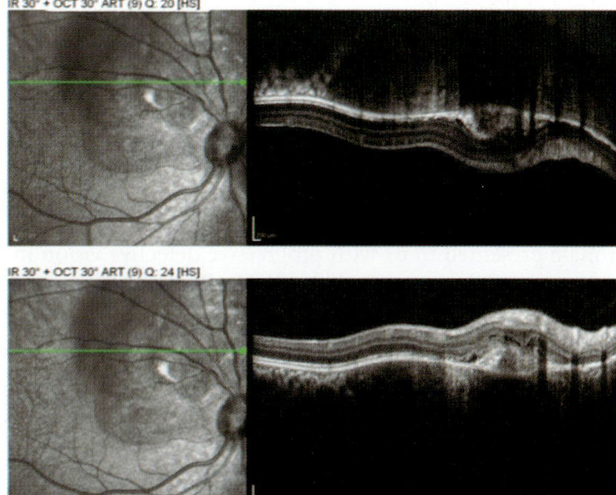

Fig. 60.3 Enhanced depth imaging (*above*) showing a hyporeflective, well-circumscribed lesion in the choroid replacing the normal choroidal architecture. Hyperreflectivity is seen in the Bruch's membrane with backscattering suggestive of calcification. The scan below clearly shows a choriodal neovascular membrane in the adjacent retina.

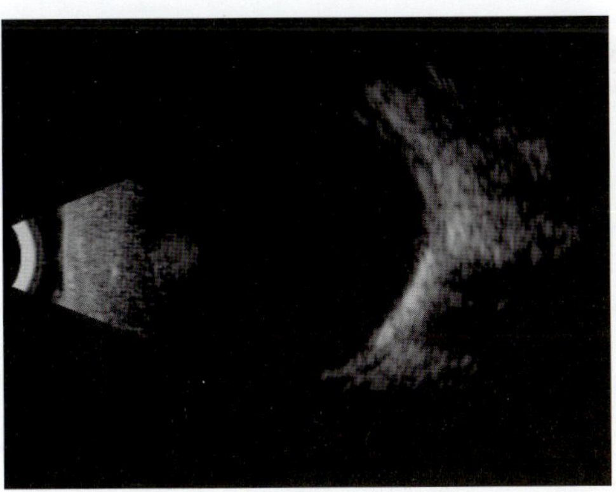
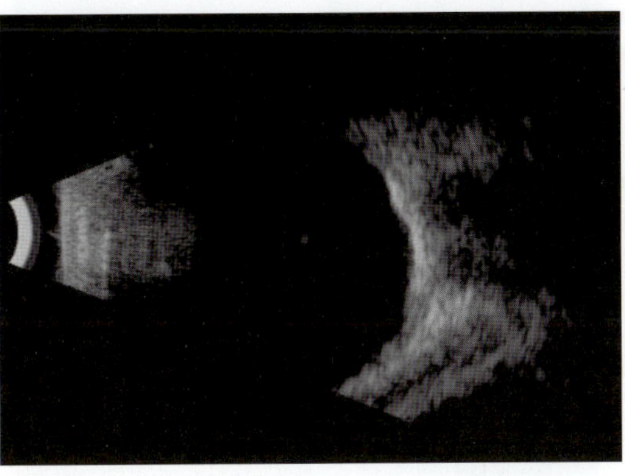

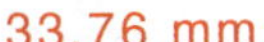

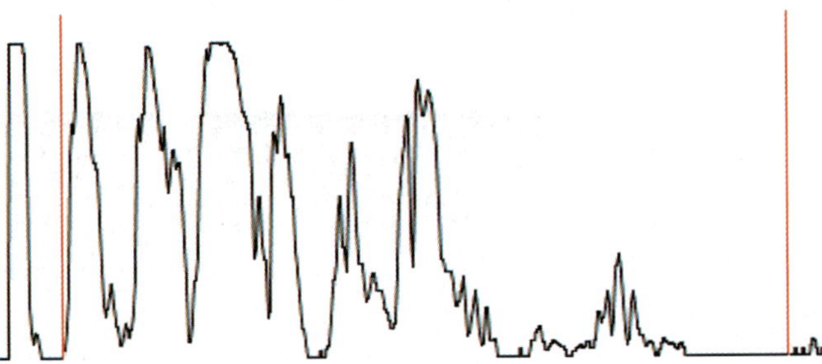

Fig. 60.4 Ultrasound A and B scan showing a highly reflective lesion and orbital shadowing.

- Spectral-domain optical coherence tomography (SD-OCT) showed that the tumor was hyperreflective suggestive of calcification and had hyporeflective areas with the presence of a CNVM and minimal subretinal fluid (Fig. 60.3).
- Enhanced depth imaging technique using SD-OCT demonstrates replacement of normal choriocapillaris with a dense hyporeflective mass with a scalloped posterior border and hyperreflective echoes in the choroid suggestive of calcification.
- B-scan ultrasonography showed a highly reflective mass lesion around 2 mm in basal dimension in the posterior pole and shadowing of orbital soft tissues posterior to the lesion. A-scan ultrasonography showed a high spike corresponding to the anterior surface of the lesion suggestive of choroidal osteoma (Fig. 60.4).

FURTHER READING

Chen J, Lee L, Gass JD: Choroidal osteoma: evidence of progression and decalcification over 20 years. *Clin Exp Optom* 89:90–94, 2006.

Diabetic Retinopathy— Macular Edema Subtypes: Cirrus™ SD-OCT

Vishali Gupta and Amod Gupta

Diabetic macular edema is the most common cause of moderate visual loss in diabetics. The disease is multifactorial in etiology with a number of systemic factors including hypertension, poor metabolic control of diabetes, dyslipidemia, and nephropathy playing a role in its pathogenesis. Additionally, taut posterior hyaloid membrane could cause traction on the macula resulting in tractional variety of macular edema.

On optical coherence tomography (OCT), diabetic macular edema had four distinct patterns:

- Sponge-like retinal thickness
- Cystoid macular edema
- Serous retinal detachment
- Vitreomacular traction

OCT is very useful in monitoring response to any intervention, including the ability to study structural alterations. This indeed gives an ultrastructural detail of changes taking place within the retinal layers. OCT also helps in quantifying retinal thickness. One can measure central foveal thickness in microns and measure retinal volume. In addition, retinal mapping gives quadrant-wise information about retinal thickness. The quantification makes it easier to monitor response to therapy. Fast macular scan protocol can be analyzed, including comparison with normative data and change between different visits. However, the most important role of OCT lies in the identification of vitreomacular traction that becomes an indication for pars plana vitrectomy.

SPONGE-LIKE THICKNESS

CASE STUDY 1

A 54-year-old man was seen with clinically significant macular edema in the left eye (**Fig. 61.1**) that showed a diffuse leak on fluorescein angiogram (**Fig. 61.2**). OCT line scan (**Fig. 61.3**) showed sponge-like thickening of the retina with intraretinal hard exudates (*black arrows*). The *yellow arrows* indicate presence of posterior hyaloid. OCT thickness map showed increased thickness that is maximum inferonasal to the fovea (**Fig. 61.4**), corresponding with the fundus and fluorescein angiogram.

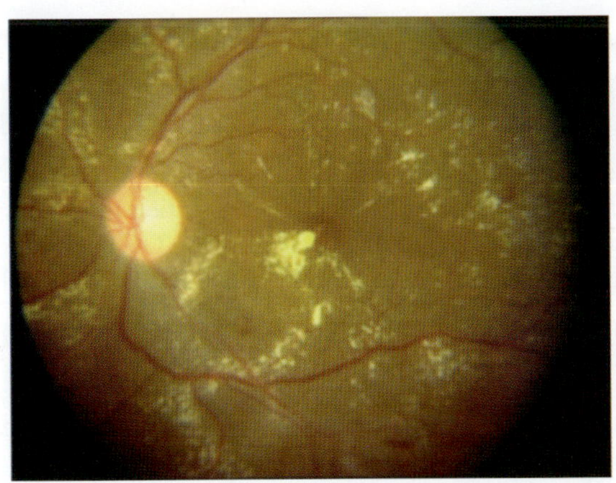

Fig. 61.1 Color fundus photograph of the left eye shows clinically significant macular edema with circinate maculopathy.

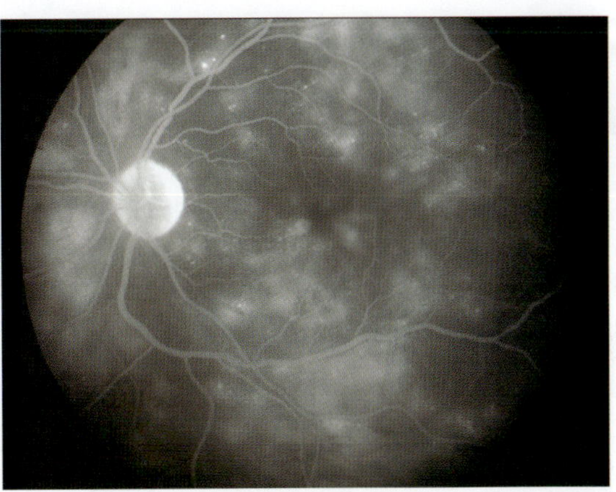

Fig. 61.2 Fundus fluorescein angiogram shows leakage confirming the macular edema.

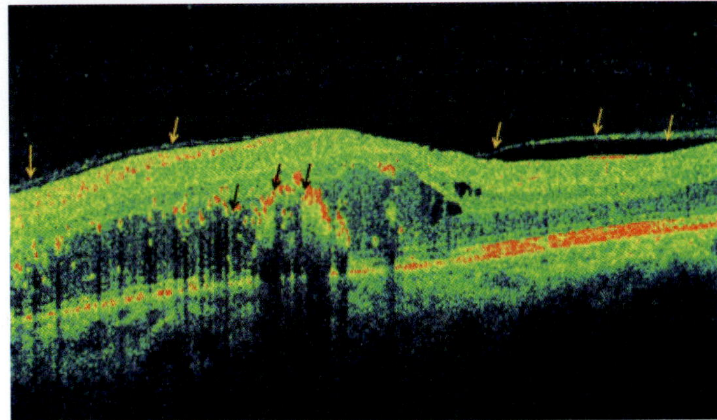

Fig. 61.3 OCT raster line scan shows sponge-like thickening of the retina with intraretinal hard exudates (*black arrows*). The *yellow arrows* indicate presence of posterior hyaloid.

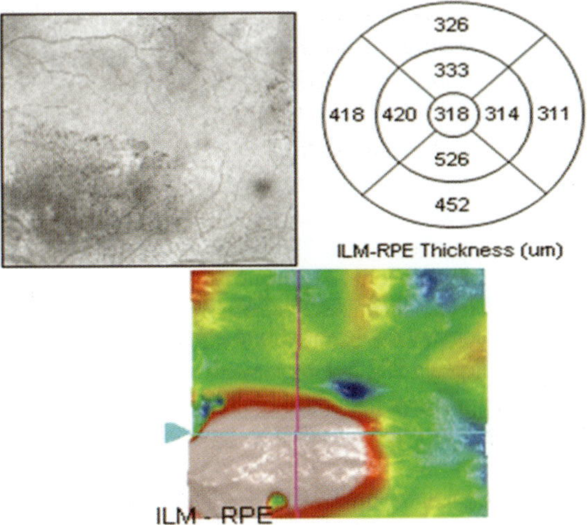

Fig. 61.4 OCT thickness map shows increased thickness that is maximum inferonasal to the fovea.

CYSTOID MACULAR EDEMA

CASE STUDY 2

A 67-year-old woman with type-2 diabetes mellitus was seen with complaints of difficulty in doing near work. Fundoscopy of the right eye showed dull foveal reflex with scars of previous grid laser photocoagulation temporally (**Fig. 61.5**). OCT line scan showed the presence of cystoid spaces within the retinal layers (**Fig. 61.6**). OCT printout (**Fig. 61.7**) showed retinal map indicating retinal thickness in nine quadrants with internal limiting membrane–retinal

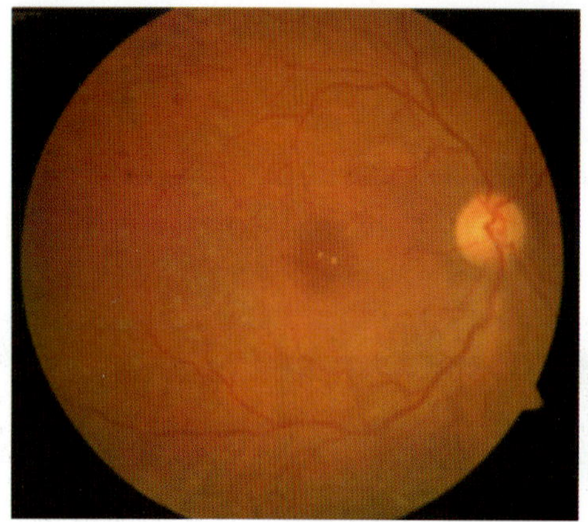

Fig. 61.5 Color fundus photograph of the right eye shows dull foveal reflex with scars of previous grid laser photocoagulation temporally.

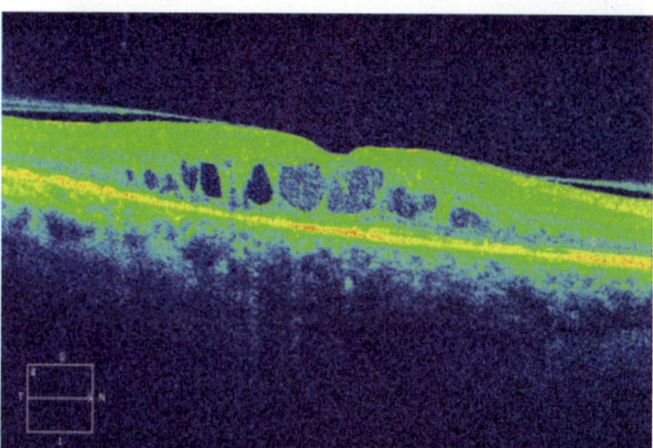

Fig. 61.6 OCT raster line scan shows presence of cystoid spaces within the retinal layers. Posterior hyaloids can be seen attached to the fovea.

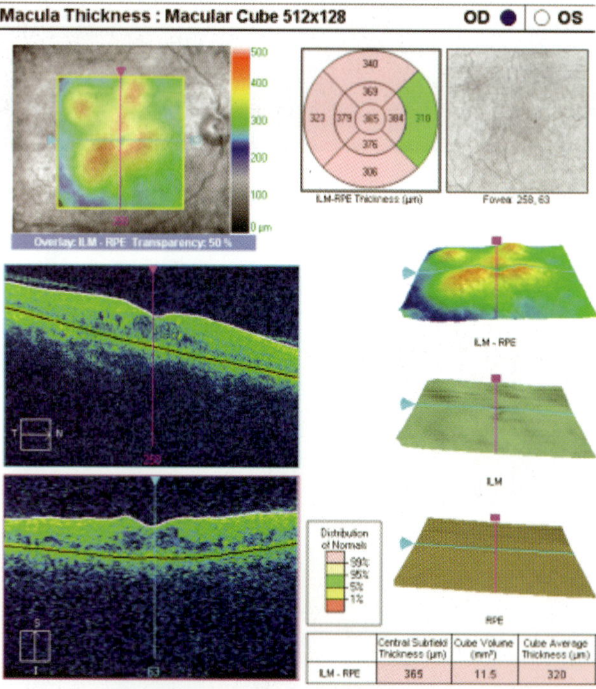

Fig. 61.7 OCT printout shows retinal map indicating retinal thickness in nine quadrants with internal limiting membrane–retinal pigment epithelial (ILM–RPE) map, indicating areas of retinal thickness. The top left picture indicates superimposition of ILM–RPE map on OCT fundus for point-to-point registration.

pigment epithelial (ILM–RPE) map, indicating areas of retinal thickness. The top left picture indicates superimposition of ILM–RPE map on OCT fundus for point-to-point registration.

SUBFOVEAL SEROUS DETACHMENT

CASE STUDY 3

A 45-year-old man with type-2 diabetes mellitus was seen with cataract and diabetic macular edema (Fig. 61.8). Fundus fluorescein angiogram showed diffuse leakage with cystoid macular edema in the late phase (Fig. 61.9). OCT line scan (Fig. 61.10) showed cystoid spaces with a pocket of subretinal fluid under the fovea (*yellow arrow*). The *white arrows* indicate detached posterior hyaloid. OCT printout (Fig. 61.11) shows retinal map indicating retinal thickness in nine quadrants with ILM–RPE map, indicating areas of retinal thickness. The top left picture indicates superimposition of ILM–RPE map on OCT fundus for point-to-point registration. The white color on thickness map indicates retinal thickness of more than 500 microns.

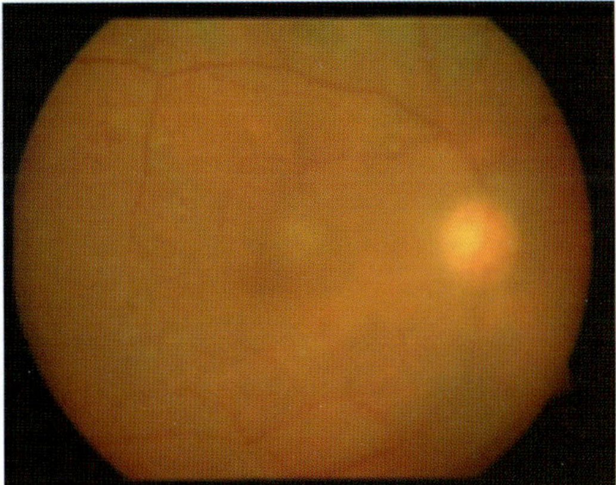

Fig. 61.8 Color fundus photograph of the right eye shows dull foveal reflex with grid laser scars seen temporal to fovea.

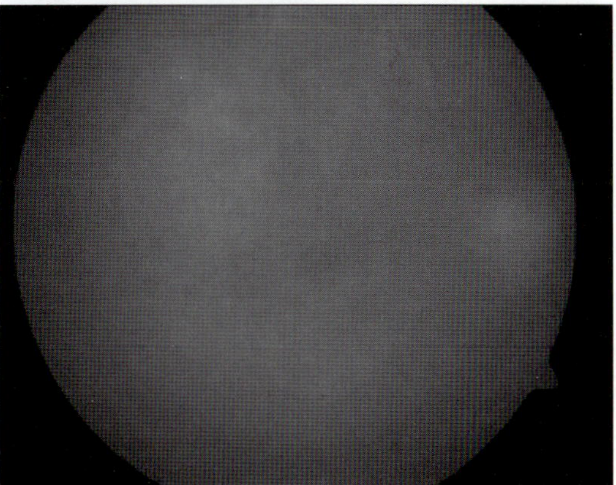

Fig. 61.9 Fundus fluorescein angiogram showed diffuse leakage with cystoid macular edema in late phase.

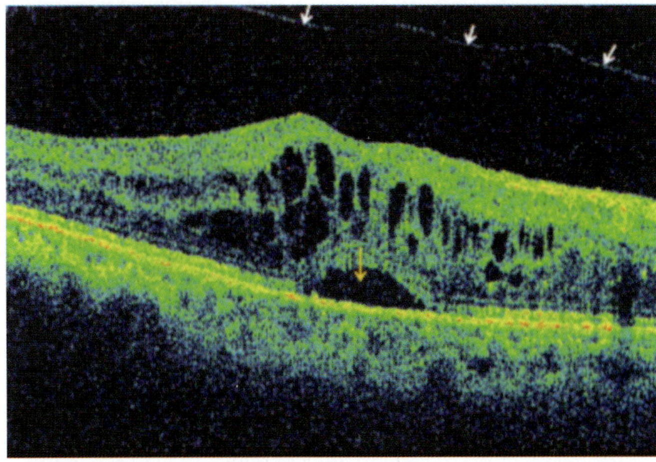

Fig. 61.10 OCT raster line scan shows cystoid spaces with a pocket of subretinal fluid under the fovea (*yellow arrow*). The *white arrows* indicate detached posterior hyaloid.

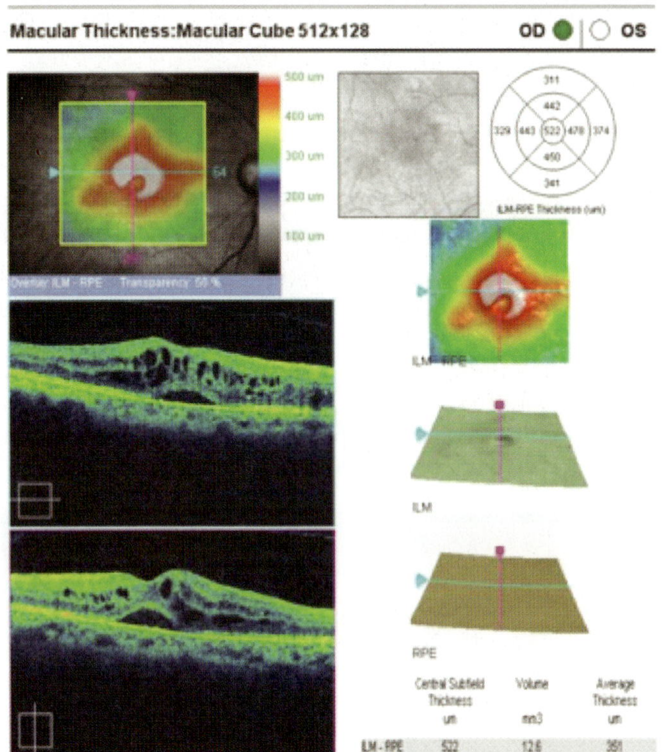

Fig. 61.11 OCT printout shows retinal map indicating retinal thickness in nine quadrants with ILM–RPE map, indicating areas of retinal thickness. The top left picture indicates superimposition of ILM–RPE map on OCT fundus for point-to-point registration. The white color on thickness map indicates retinal thickness of more than 500 microns.

VITREOMACULAR TRACTION

CASE STUDY 4

A 45-year-old man was seen with left-eye diabetic macular edema (**Fig. 61.12**). Fundus fluorescein angiogram showed diffuse leakage with cystoid macular edema (**Fig. 61.13**). OCT line scan showed vitreomacular traction, causing both

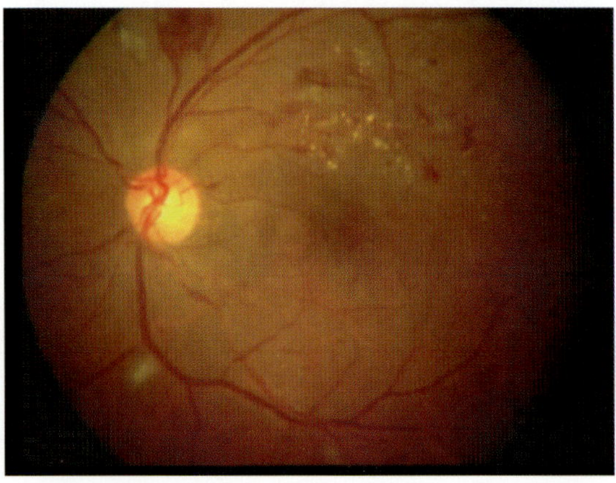

Fig. 61.12 Color fundus photograph of the left eye shows nonproliferative diabetic retinopathy with clinically significant macular edema. No taut hyaloid membrane is seen clinically.

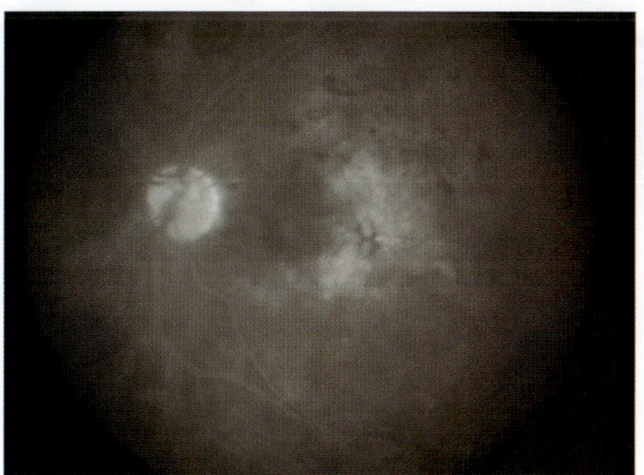

Fig. 61.13 Fundus fluorescein angiogram shows diffuse leakage with cystoid macular edema.

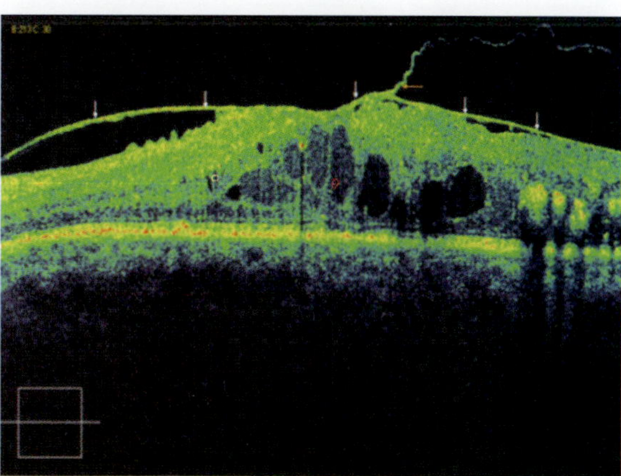

Fig. 61.14 OCT line scan shows vitreomacular traction, causing both anteroposterior (*yellow arrow*) and tangential traction (*white arrows*).

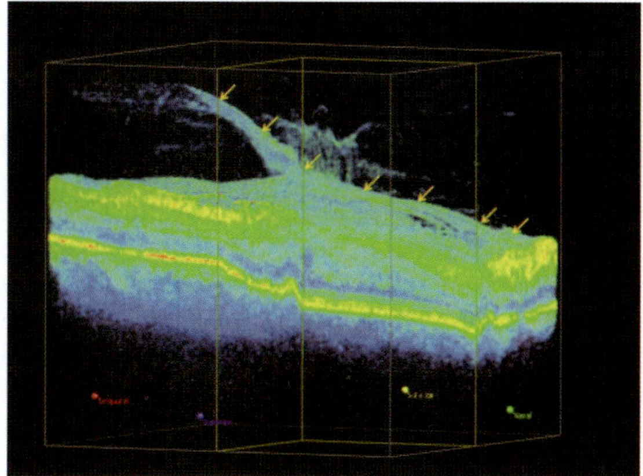

Fig. 61.15 3-D OCT scan confirms vitreomacular traction contributing towards the development of macular edema.

anteroposterior (*yellow arrow*) and tangential traction (*white arrows*) (**Fig. 61.14**), which is confirmed on 3-D scan (**Fig. 61.15**). Such a patient is a candidate for pars plana vitrectomy.

FURTHER READING

Gupta V, Gupta A, Dogra MR, editors: *Atlas Optical Coherence Tomography of Macular Diseases and Glaucoma*, ed 4, Jaypee-Highlights Chap 5, 98–140, 2012.

Diabetic Retinopathy— Macular Edema Subtypes: SPECTRALIS™ SD-OCT

Santosh Gopi Krishna and Naresh Kumar Yadav

Diabetic macular edema (DME) is the main cause of decreased vision in a patient with diabetic retinopathy, especially in nonproliferative diabetic retinopathy (NPDR). Various factors affecting DME include elevated levels of $HbA1_C$, severity of diabetic retinopathy (DR), duration of diabetes mellitus (DM), elevated diastolic blood pressure, gender (more frequent in females), and elevated serum lipid levels. DME is associated with five different morphologic patterns on optical coherence tomography (OCT). These include spongy/diffuse thickening, cystoid macular edema, serous retinal detachment without posterior hyaloid traction (PHT), PHT without tractional retinal detachment (TRD), and PHT with TRD. The different morphological forms may coexist and treatment for each of these entities differs. Clinically significant macular edema (CSME) is another form of DME that is clinically relevant and laser is the standard treatment advocated.

CASE STUDY 1

A 50-year-old diabetic Asian Indian man presented with blurred vision in his left eye. His best-corrected visual acuity (BCVA) was 20/20 in the right eye and 20/50 in the left eye. Anterior segment was normal. Fundus showed both eyes (BE) moderate NPDR with left eye DME (Fig. 62.1).

Spectral-domain optical coherence tomography (SD-OCT) imaging revealed spongy macular edema in the left eye with loss of foveal contour and intact inner segment–outer segment junction (IS–OS) and retinal pigment epithelium (RPE). He underwent modified grid laser in the left eye, following which the macular edema subsided.

CASE STUDY 2

A 57-year-old Asian Indian woman with unremarkable anterior segment and BCVA of 20/25 in the right eye and 20/100 in the left eye presented with blurred vision in the left eye. Fundus showed BE-stable proliferative diabetic retinopathy (PDR), status post-panretinal photocoagulation (PRP) with cystoid macular edema (CME) in the left eye. Fundus fluorescein angiography (FFA) showed diffuse macular leak in the left eye in typical CME pattern (Fig. 62.2). She underwent intravitreal bevacizumab and focal laser, following which the CME resolved and the vision improved to 20/50.

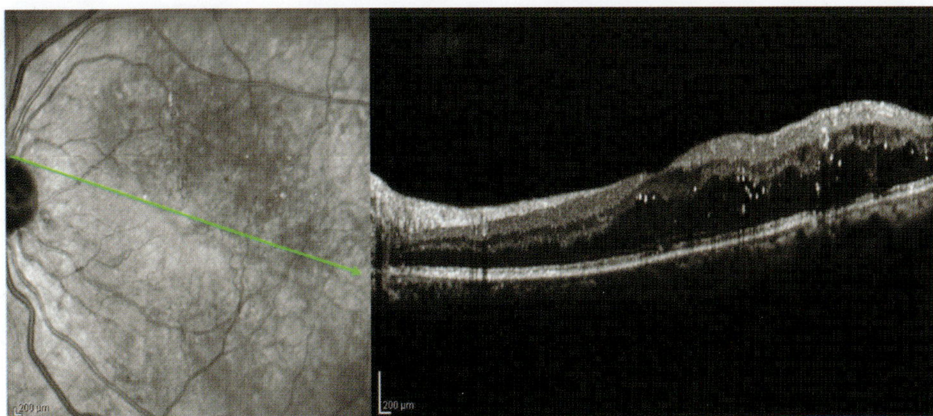

Fig. 62.1 The above SD-OCT scan showed diffuse/spongy thickening of macular retina with intraretinal fluid spaces and loss of foveal architecture. The patient underwent modified grid laser with a resolution of macular edema.

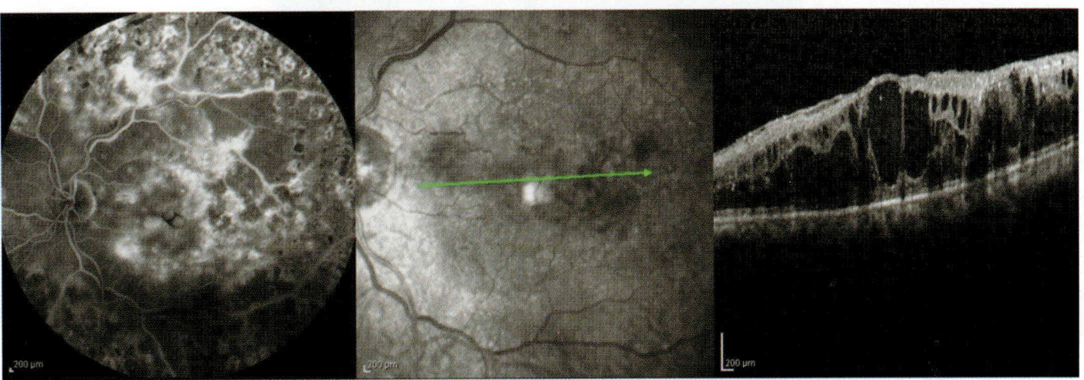

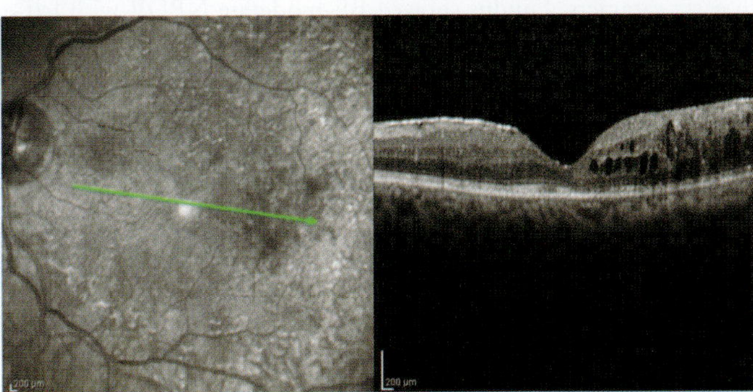

Fig. 62.2 The above FFA image shows diffuse macular leakage in flower petal pattern suggestive of cystoid macular edema. SD-OCT image pretreatment shows gross cystoid macular edema and a post-treatment (*below*) (intravitreal bevacizumab and focal laser) scan shows resolving CME.

CASE STUDY 3

A 62-year-old Asian Indian woman presented with blurred vision in the RE; her BCVA was 20/200 in the right eye and 20/25 in the left with early cataracts. Fundus showed BE-moderate NPDR with DME in the right eye (Fig. 62.3).

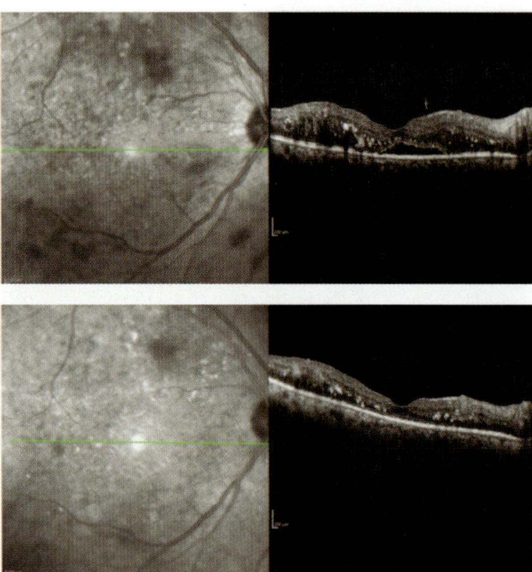

Fig. 62.3 SD-OCT images show macular edema with serous retinal detachment. The patient underwent intravitreal bevacizumab, following which macular edema with serous detachment subsided (*below*).

SD-OCT imaging showed intraretinal edema with subfoveal serous retinal detachment. She underwent right-eye intravitreal bevacizumab and serous detachment subsided with an improvement of BCVA to 20/40.

CASE STUDY 4

A 69-year-old Asian Indian woman presented with blurred vision in her left eye; her BCVA was 20/25 in the right eye and 20/50 in the left with early cataracts. Fundus showed BE-moderate NPDR with left-eye vitreomacular traction (VMT). SD-OCT imaging confirmed presence of VMT with macular edema (**Fig. 62.4**).

She underwent vitrectomy in the left eye with release of the macular traction, following which the foveal contour was restored with a maintained BCVA of 20/50.

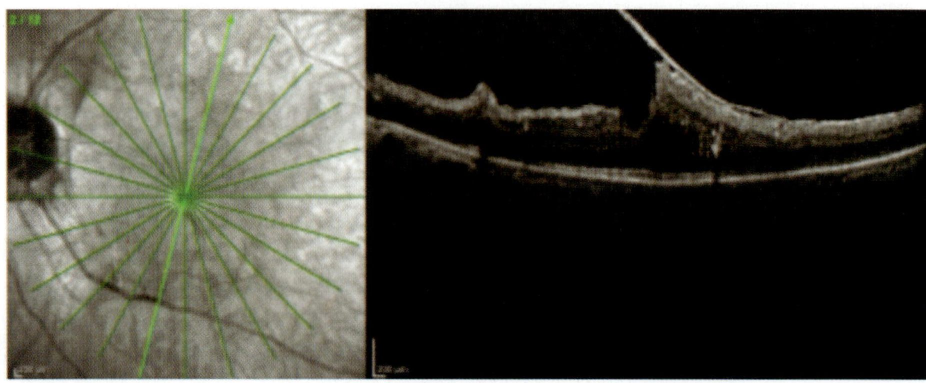

Previtrectomy

Fig. 62.4 (*Continued*)

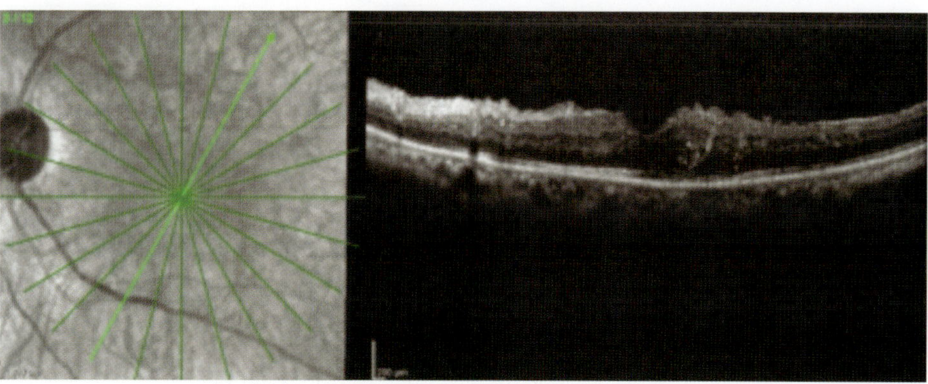

Postvitrectomy

Fig. 62.4 The above SD-OCT images show vitreomacular traction (VMT) without TRD before vitrectomy and restored foveal contour with uneven retinal surface after vitrectomy.

CASE STUDY 5

A 66-year-old Asian Indian woman with unremarkable anterior segment had a BCVA of 20/25 in the right eye and 20/200 in the left eye. Fundus showed right-eye-stable PDR and left-eye-advanced PDR with macular TRD status post-PRP (Fig. 62.5).

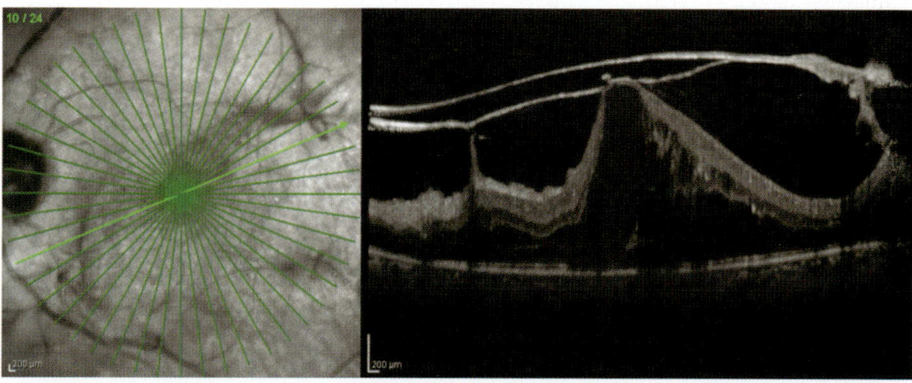

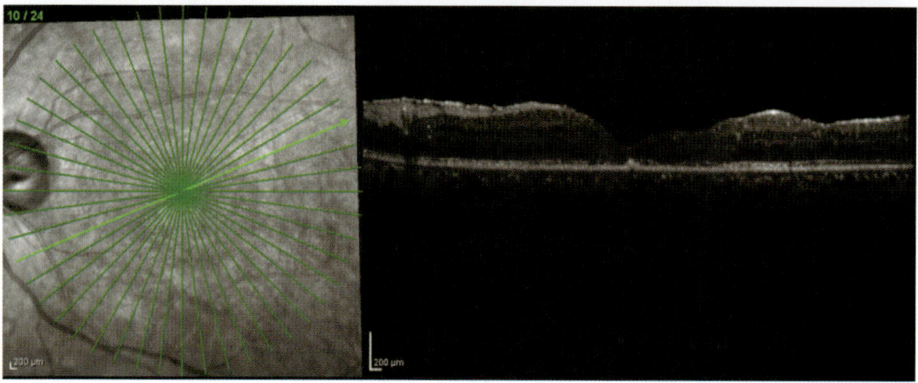

Fig. 62.5 The SD-OCT image shows a case of vitreomacular traction with TRD (*above*), treated surgically by vitrectomy with allied procedures (*below*).

SD-OCT imaging showed taut posterior hyaloid with VMT along with macular TRD. She underwent vitrectomy in the left eye with membrane peeling with fluid–air exchange and silicone oil infusion, followed later by silicone oil removal. Post-treatment her BCVA had improved to 20/100 with an attached macula.

FURTHER READING

1. Kim BY, Smith SD, Kaiser PK. Optical coherence tomographic patterns of diabetic macular edema. *Am J Ophthalmol* 142(3):405–412, 2006.
2. Panozzo G, Parolini B, Gusson E, et al.: Diabetic macular edema: an OCT-based classification. *Semin Ophthalmol* 19(1–2):13–20, 2004.
3. N R Kim, Y J Kim, H S Chin, et al.: Optical coherence tomographic patterns in diabetic macular edema: prediction of visual outcome after focal laser photocoagulation. *Br J Ophthalmol* 93:901–905, 2009. doi:10.1136/bjo.2008.152553.

Diabetic Retinopathy— Pregnancy Related

Adam Muzychuk and Anna Ells

INTRODUCTION

Approximately 1% of pregnancies in the United States occur in the setting of pre-existing diabetes. Type I diabetes is present in 5%–10% of these cases, while 90%–95% of these cases are of type II diabetes. Although gestational diabetes is a major health concern, in the absence of pre-existing diabetes these patients do not seem to be at risk for development of retinopathy and retinal screening is not warranted. Amongst those with pre-existing diabetes, reported rates of progression in pregnancy vary from 5%–70%. Factors that have been linked to the progression of retinopathy in pregnancy include duration of diabetes prior to pregnancy, level of diabetic retinopathy at baseline, coexisting hypertension or pre-eclampsia, and poor glycemic control prior to pregnancy. Macular edema may worsen during pregnancy in a small proportion of patients. Management of the diabetic retinopathy in pregnancy has been much more favorable since the advent of laser photocoagulation, prior to which proliferative diabetic retinopathy was considered a contraindication to conception. We present a case below of worsening diabetic retinopathy in pregnancy leading to a decision to induce labor at 34 weeks gestation.

CASE STUDY

A 38-year-old female with type 1 diabetes was referred at 15 weeks gestation to a retina specialist as her comprehensive ophthalmologist had noted a worsening of her diabetic retinopathy from "mild" to "moderate." She presented to the clinic as an inpatient having been admitted to the hospital the previous day for an uncontrolled blood pressure of 180/130 mmHg, with her most recent hemoglobin A1C being 7.1%.

On examination, her best-corrected visual acuity was $20/50^{-1}$ OD (oculus dexter) and $20/25^{-1}$ OS (oculus sinister). Fundus examination showed hemorrhages, cotton-wool spots, and cystoid macular edema OU (oculus uterque). Optical coherence tomography (OCT) demonstrated cystic intraretinal fluid with central retinal thicknesses of 596 microns OD and 454 microns OS (**Figs 63.1A and B**). No evidence of leaking microaneurysms was evident clinically, and this was felt to be likely due to hypertension. No specific ocular treatments were initiated.

The patient was discharged from hospital 1 week later after adequate blood pressure control was achieved.

On spectral-domain optical coherence tomography (SD-OCT), the intraretinal fluid was stable OD and mild improvement was noted OS (central thickness 599 OD and 393 OS, **Figs 63.3A and B**).

The patient was regularly followed-up during the course of her pregnancy, during which her retinopathy was fairly stable until 30 weeks gestation. Her ocular examination at that time showed severe nonproliferative diabetic retinopathy (SNPDR) with diabetic macular edema in both the eyes. Fluorescein angiography demonstrated an enlarged foveal avascular zone, SNPDR, and marked retinal ischemia (**Fig. 63.2**).

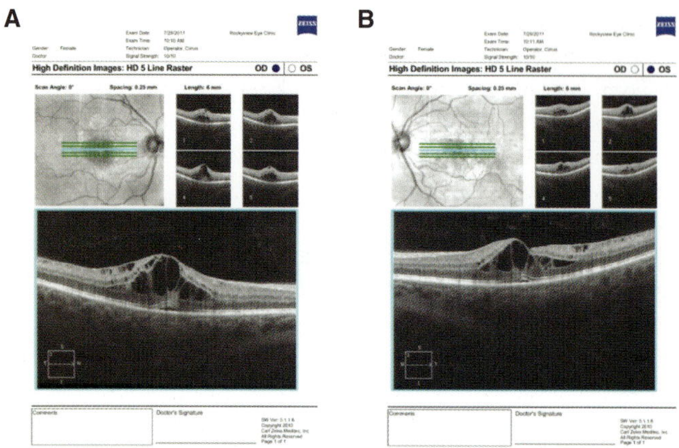

Fig. 63.1 (A) and (B) SD-OCT shows cystic intraretinal fluid OU with central retinal thicknesses of 596 microns OD and 454 microns OS.

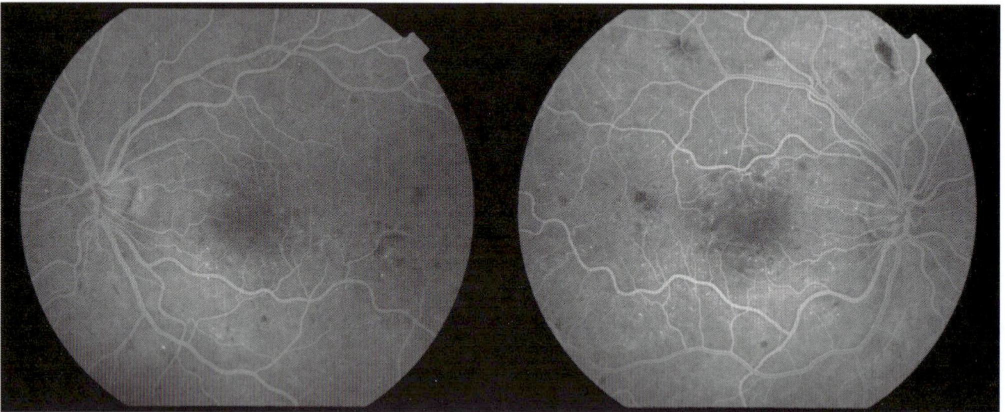

Fig. 63.2 Fluorescein angiography demonstrates an enlarged foveal avascular zone, SNPDR, and marked retinal ischemia.

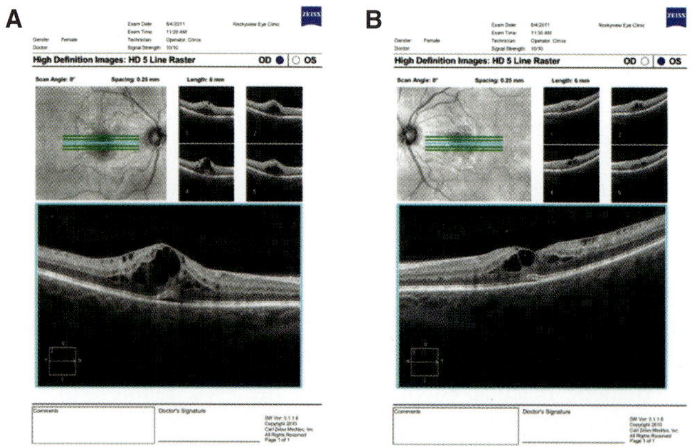

Fig. 63.3 (A) and (B) SD-OCT showed that the cystic intraretinal fluid was stable (central thickness 599 OD and 393 OS).

The best-corrected visual acuity was 20/40 in the right eye and $20/25^{-1}$ in the left eye. The blood pressure was normal. The SD-OCT showed an increase in cystic intraretinal fluid centrally OU (central thickness 638 OD and 535 OS; **Figs 63.3A and B**). Focal laser photocoagulation of leaking microaneurysms was performed.

At 34 weeks of gestation, the patient presented to the clinic with symptoms of blurred vision. The best-corrected visual acuity was $20/30^{-2}$ in the right eye and $20/30^{-1}$ in the left eye. On fundus examination, SNPDR with seemingly worsening macular edema was noted, which was confirmed by the SD-OCT (central thickness 715 in the right eye and 632 in the left eye, **Figs 63.4A and B**).

After consultation with the obstetrician, a decision to induce labor was made based on continued progression of diabetic retinopathy and macular edema resistant to conventional ocular treatments. A healthy male child weighing 3.2 kg was delivered by C-Section after induction of labor was unsuccessful.

The patient was examined 11 days following the delivery. The vision had subjectively improved and the SD-OCT confirmed a reduction in retinal thickness (central thickness 403 OD and 533 OS, **Figs 63.5A and B**).

The patient's OCT showed a significant reduction in the intraretinal fluid and thickness without further specific ocular treatments 6 weeks following the delivery (central thickness 377 OD and 271 OS, **Figs 63.6A and B**).

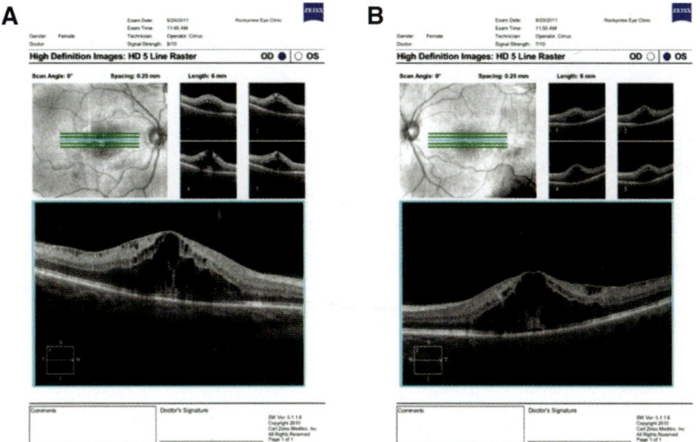

Fig. 63.4 **(A)** and **(B)** Clinical suspicion of worsening macular edema OU was confirmed by SD-OCT (central thickness 715 OD and 632 OS).

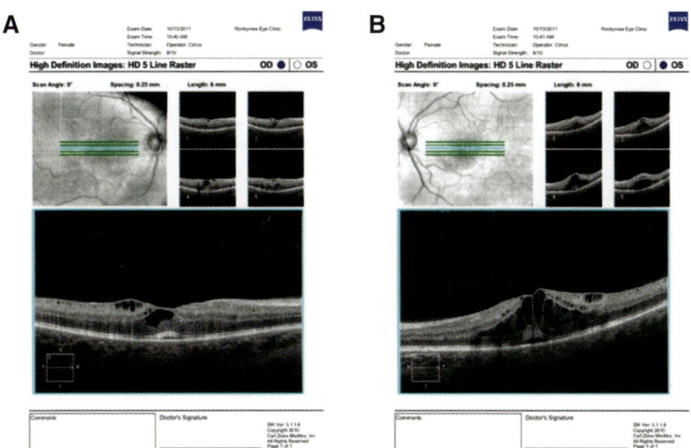

Fig. 63.5 **(A)** and **(B)** Eleven days following delivery of a healthy male child by C-section, SD-OCT confirmed a reduction in cystic intraretinal fluid OU (central thickness 403 OD and 533 OS).

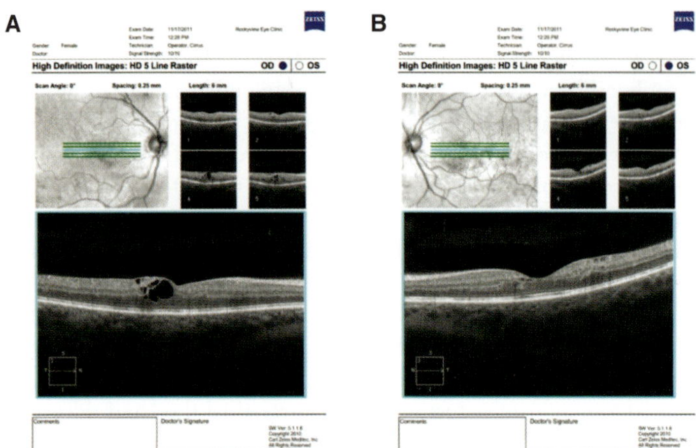

Fig. 63.6 **(A)** and **(B)** Six weeks following delivery there was further improvement in cystic intraretinal fluid seen on SD-OCT without further treatment (central thickness 377 OD and 271 OS).

CONCLUSION

Although diabetic macular edema can often be detected on clinical exam, the OCT provides a clear and objective perspective of subtle improvements or worsening, which may be difficult to differentiate at slit lamp. In this case, the OCT provided a valuable documentation of worsening diabetic macular edema in spite of standard therapy, which contributed significantly to the decision to induce labor.

FURTHER READING

1. Dabelea D, Snell-Bergeon JK, Hartsfield CL, et al.: Increasing prevalence of gestational diabetes mellitus (GDM) over time and by birth cohort: Kaiser Permanente of Colorado GDM Screening Program. *Diabetes Care* 28(3):579–584, 2005.
2. Horvat M, Maclean H, Goldberg L, et al.: Diabetic retinopathy in pregnancy: a 12-year prospective survey. *Br J Ophthalmol* 64(6):398–403, 1980.
3. Bhatnagar A, Ghauri AJ, Hope-Ross M, et al.: Diabetic retinopathy in pregnancy. *Curr Diabetes Rev* 5(3):151–156, 2009.
4. Chew EY, Mills JL, Metzger BE, et al.: Metabolic control and progression of retinopathy. The Diabetes in Early Pregnancy Study. National Institute of Child Health and Human Development Diabetes in Early Pregnancy Study. *Diabetes Care* 18(5):631–637, 1995.
5. Rosenn B, Miodovnik M, Kranias G, et al.: Progression of diabetic retinopathy in pregnancy: association with hypertension in pregnancy. *Am J Obstet Gynecol* 166(4):1214–1218, 1992.
6. Lovestam-Adrian M, Agardh CD, Aberg A, et al.: Pre-eclampsia is a potent risk factor for deterioration of retinopathy during pregnancy in Type 1 diabetic patients. *Diabet Med* 14(12):1059–1065, 1997.
7. Effect of pregnancy on microvascular complications in the diabetes control and complications trial. The Diabetes Control and Complications Trial Research Group. *Diabetes Care* 23(8):1084–1091, 2000.
8. Chan WC, Lim LT, Quinn MJ, et al.: Management and outcome of sight-threatening diabetic retinopathy in pregnancy. *Eye (Lond)* 18(8):826–832, 2004.

Diabetic Retinopathy—Nonproliferative

Santosh Gopi Krishna and Naresh Kumar Yadav

Diabetic retinopathy (DR) is divided into nonproliferative diabetic retinopathy (NPDR) and proliferative diabetic retinopathy (PDR). This division is based on the presence of neovascularization of the disc or elsewhere, vitreous or preretinal hemorrhage, and fibrous proliferation. DR can be further classified by severity. NPDR consists of cotton-wool spots (nerve-fiber-layer infarcts), intraretinal hemorrhages and hard exudates, and microvascular abnormalities (including microaneurysms and dilated or tortuous vessels) primarily in the posterior retina. Visual loss in NPDR occurs mainly due to development of macular edema. The severity can be thus classified.

CLASSIFICATION

- Mild NPDR: microaneurysms (MA) only
- Moderate NPDR: more than just MA but less than severe NPDR
- Severe NPDR: any of the following:
  - Less than twenty intraretinal hemorrhages in each of the four quadrants
  - Definite venous beading in two or more quadrants
  - Prominent intraretinal microvascular abnormalities (IRMA) in one or more quadrants; no PDR
- Very-severe NPDR: any two or more features of severe NPDR

CASE STUDY 1

A 47-year-old Asian Indian diabetic man was screened for DR. His best-corrected visual acuity (BCVA) was 20/20 in both eyes (BE). Anterior segment was normal. Fundus showed microaneurysms in BE with hard exudates in the left eye, suggestive of diabetic macular edema (DME) (**Figs 64.1A and B**). The patient was advised left-eye focal laser, strict diabetes control, and a 6-monthly retinal review.

Mild NPDR

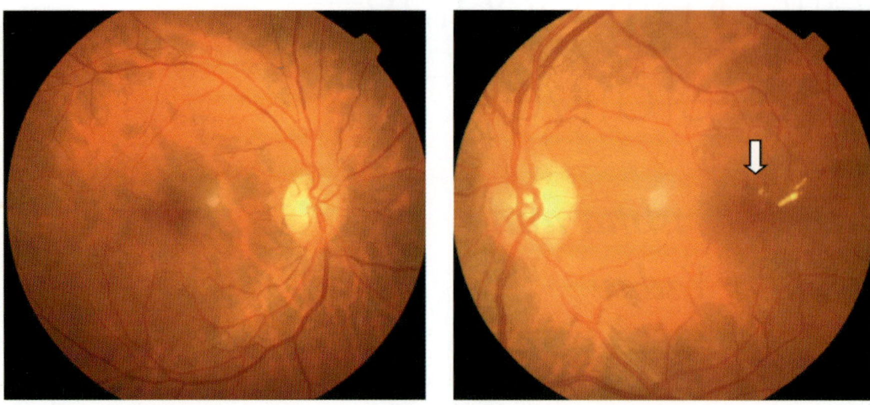

Fig. 64.1 (A) The above fundus image shows the earliest sign of diabetic retinopathy—the microaneurysm (*arrow*). A microaneurysm present at the fovea can remain innocuous or can cause a decrease in vision owing to diabetic macular edema as in the left eye.

SD-OCT images through microaneurysms and hard exudates

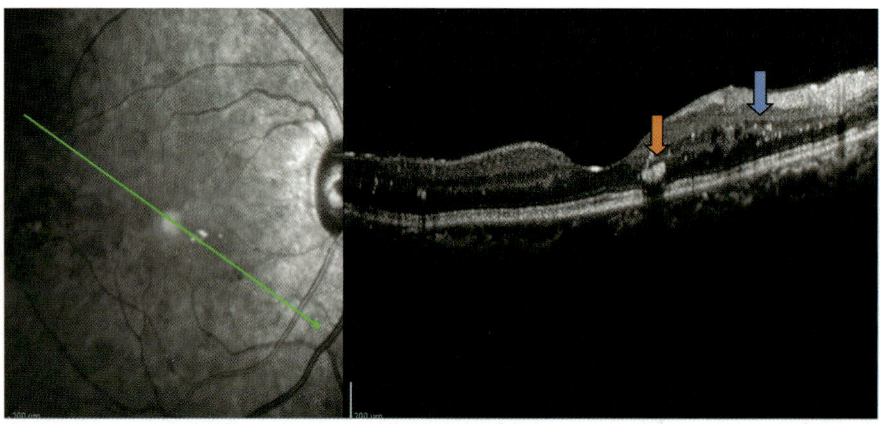

Fig. 64.1 (B) The above SD-OCT image shows a scan section through the microaneurysms (*blue arrow*) and hard exudates (*orange arrow*). The microaneurysms are seen as dot-like hyperreflective echoes in the inner nuclear layer with surrounding hyporeflective spaces suggestive of intraretinal edema and hard exudates are seen as a clump of hyperreflective echoes with backscattering in the outer plexiform layer. The patient was advised focal laser to areas of thickening and aneurysms.

CASE STUDY 2

A 51-year-old Asian Indian woman with a BCVA of 20/30 in the right eye and 20/20 in the left eye, and normal anterior segment was reviewed for diabetic screening. Fundus showed dot hemorrhages, soft exudates, and hard exudates in BE (right eye > left eye) (**Figs 64.2A and B**) suggestive of moderate NPDR with the right eye having clinically significant macular edema (CSME). The patient underwent focal laser in the right eye, and was advised a strict diabetes control and a 6-monthly follow-up.

Moderate NPDR

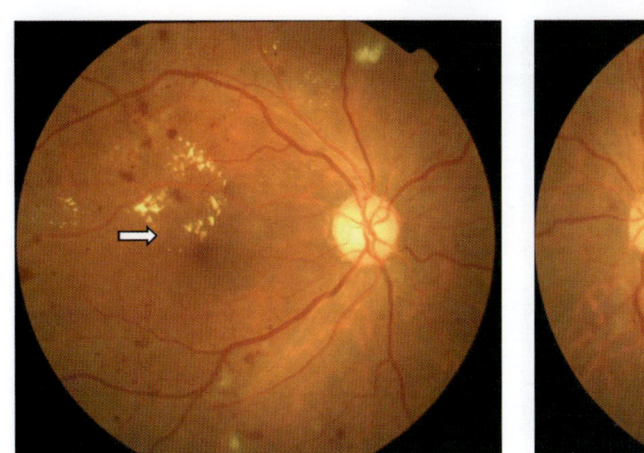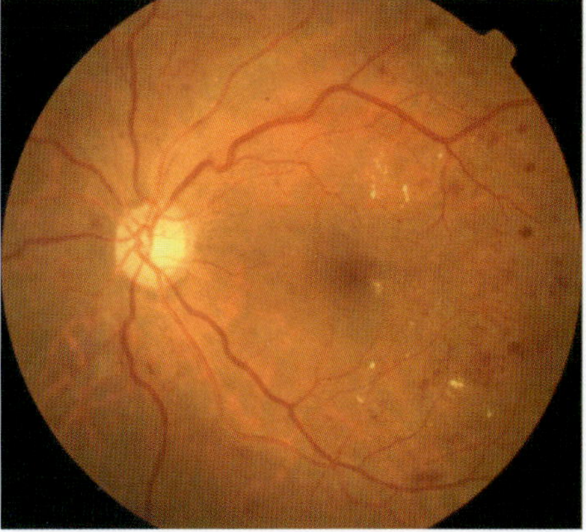

Fig. 64.2 (A) The above figure shows moderate NPDR with right-eye CSME (*arrow*) characterized by the presence of soft exudates with hemorrhages/microaneurysms and hard exudates at the posterior pole (right eye > left eye). The patient underwent focal laser in the right eye, and was advised a strict diabetes control and a 6-monthly follow-up.

SD-OCT images through cotton-wool spots

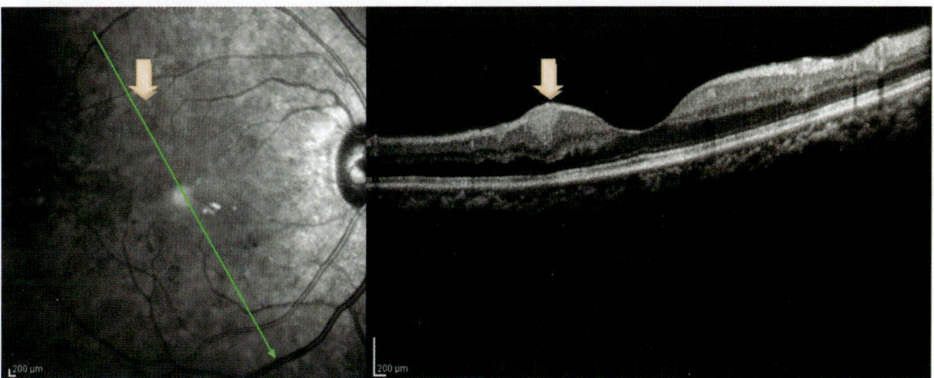

Fig. 64.2 (B) The above figure shows SD-OCT scan through an area of soft exudates/cotton-wool spot, which is seen as a homogenous hyperreflective echo (*orange arrow*) in the inner retinal layer with localized retinal thickening, suggestive of its superficial location.

CASE STUDY 3

A 62-year-old type-2 diabetic Asian Indian man was reviewed for DR. His BCVA was 20/20 in BE and the anterior segment was normal. Fundus showed features of severe NPDR with an ischemic-looking retina (**Figs 64.3A, B, and C**). Fundus fluorescein angiogram (FFA) confirmed microaneurysms/hemorrhages in all quadrants with gross capillary nonperfusion (CNP) areas suggestive of severe NPDR and likelihood of transforming into PDR. As the CNP areas were gross, the patient was advised scatter panretinal photocoagulation (PRP) in BE and a follow-up every 3–4 months.

Severe NPDR

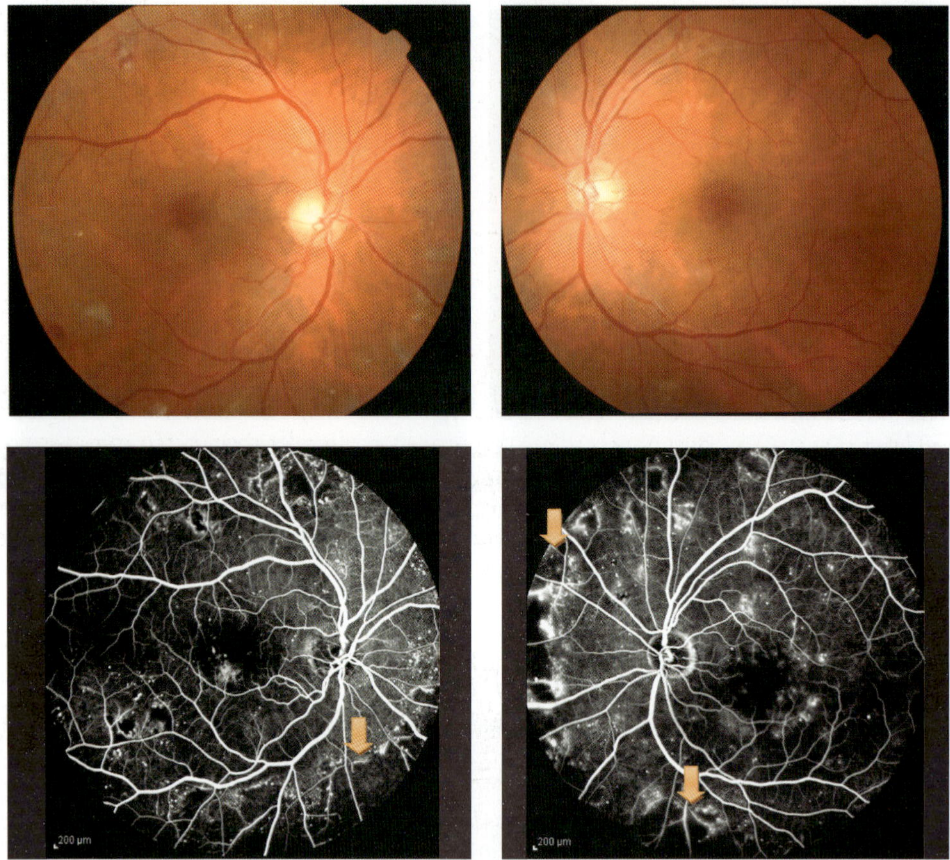

Fig. 64.3 (A) The above fundus image shows hemorrhages/microaneurysms and occasional soft exudates in all quadrants with gross CNP areas (*arrows*) suggestive of severe NPDR and a likelihood of transforming into PDR. As the CNP areas were large, the patient was advised scatter PRP in BE and a follow-up every 3–4 months.

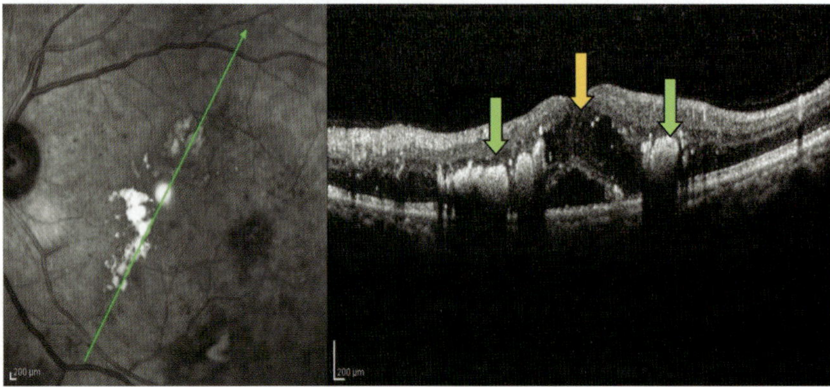

Fig. 64.3 (B) SD-OCT images through exudative maculopathy in a case of severe NPDR.

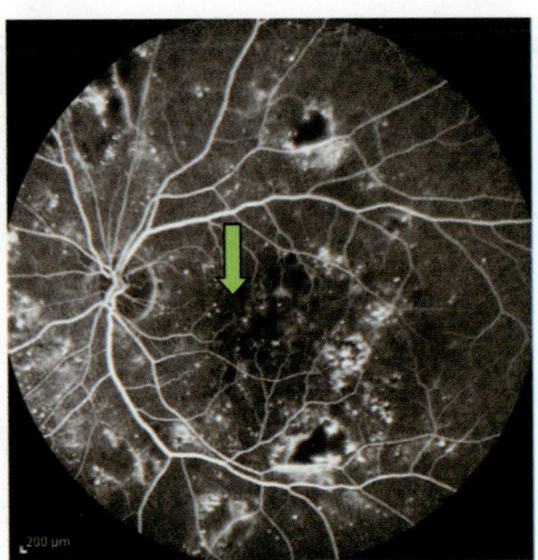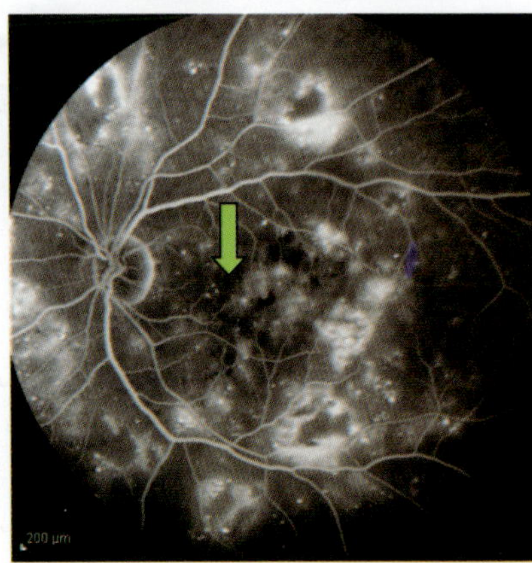

Fig. 64.3 (C) The above SD-OCT (B) and FFA (C) images show areas of early hyperfluorescence, areas of blocked fluorescence, and late leakage at the posterior pole with a distorted foveal avascular zone on FFA corresponding to loss of foveal contour, microaneurysms in the inner nuclear layer, intraretinal edema, hyperreflective clumps in the outer plexiform layer with back scattering and serous retinal detachment on SD-OCT (B). The above patient was advised intravitreal anti-vascular endothelial growth factor injection followed by modified grid laser after resolution of serous retinal detachment. He was also advised a lipid profile besides a strict diabetes and hypertension control.

FURTHER READING

1. Wilkinson CP, Ferris FL, Klein RE, et al.: Proposed international clinical diabetic retinopathy and diabetic macular edema disease severity scales. *Ophthalmology* 110(9):1677–1682, 2003.
2. Stephen J Ryan, David R. Hinton, Andrew P. Schachat, et al.: *Textbook of Retina*, ed 4, 2006.
3. The Diabetic Retinopathy Study Research Group: Design methods and baseline results. Diabetic Retinopathy Study (DRS) Report Number 6. *Invest Ophthalmol Vis Sci* 21:149–209, 1991.

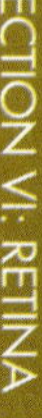

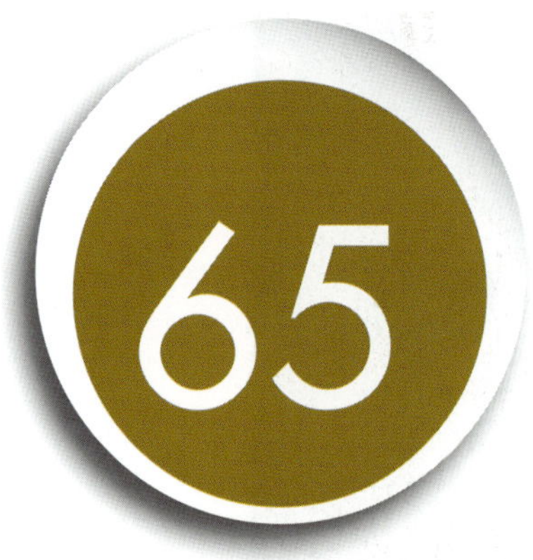

Diabetic Retinopathy— Proliferative

Santosh Gopi Krishna and Naresh Kumar Yadav

Proliferative diabetic retinopathy (PDR) is a severe form of diabetic retinopathy. The risk of PDR is greatest in eyes with severe nonproliferative diabetic retinopathy (NPDR). It is characterized by new vessels on the disc or elsewhere, preretinal or vitreous hemorrhage, and fibrous tissue proliferation. PDR can be classified as:

PDR without high-risk characteristics

New vessels and/or fibrous proliferations, or preretinal and/or vitreous hemorrhage.

PDR with high-risk characteristics

Neovascularization of the disc (NVD)1/3 − 1/2 disc area, less-extensive NVD with vitreous or preretinal hemorrhage, *or* neovascularization elsewhere (NVE) ≥1/2 disc area with vitreous or preretinal hemorrhage.

Advanced PDR

Extensive vitreous hemorrhage precluding grading, retinal detachment involving the macula, phthisis bulbi, or enucleation secondary to a complication of diabetic retinopathy.

The treatment protocol includes prompt laser photocoagulation on the diagnosis of PDR. Other treatment strategies include vitreous surgery for advanced PDR, nonclearing vitreous hemorrhage, and anti-VEGF agents in specific situations.

CASE STUDY 1

A 52-year-old Asian Indian man with uncontrolled diabetes presented for a regular diabetic retinopathy review. He had earlier undergone left eye panretinal photocoagulation (PRP). His BCVA was 20/20 in the right eye and 20/30 in the left eye. Anterior segment was normal. Fundus showed an ischemic-looking retina with NVE in the right eye and left eye status post-PRP with NVD (Fig. 65.1). Fundus fluorescein angiography (FFA) showed PDR with

FFA images

Right eye—early and late frames

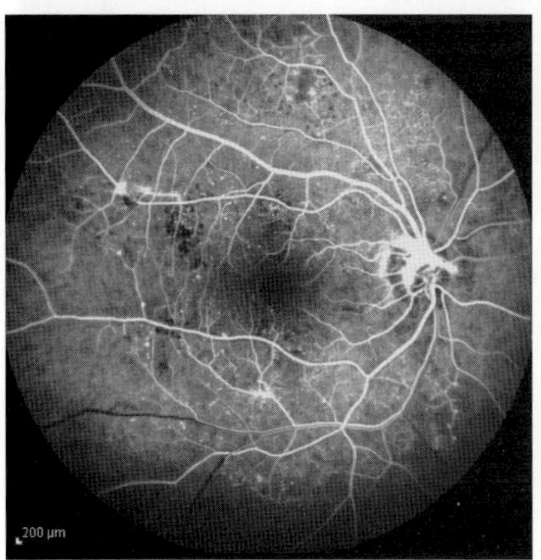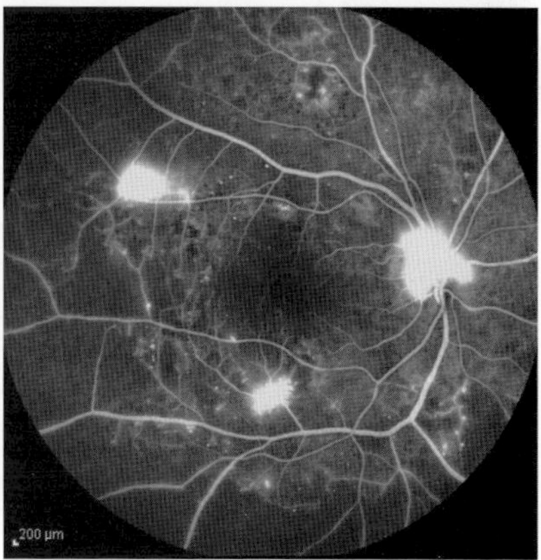

Left eye—early and late frames

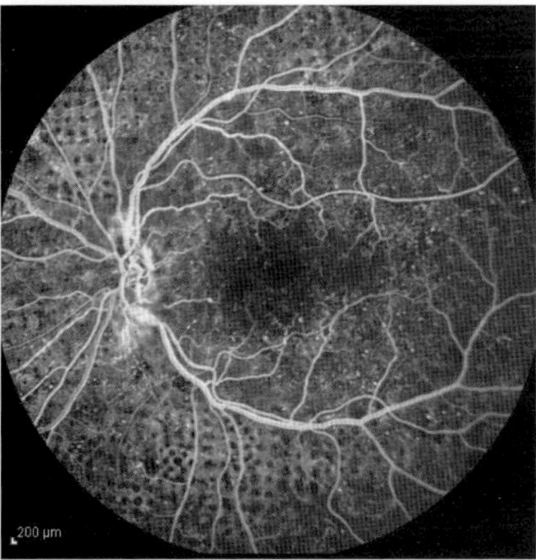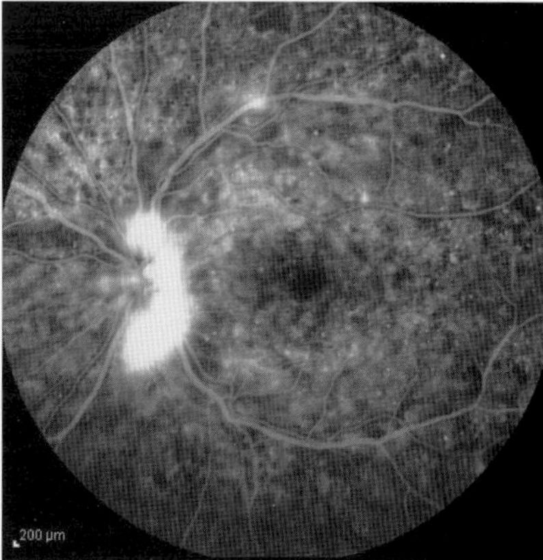

Right eye SD-OCT through the NVE

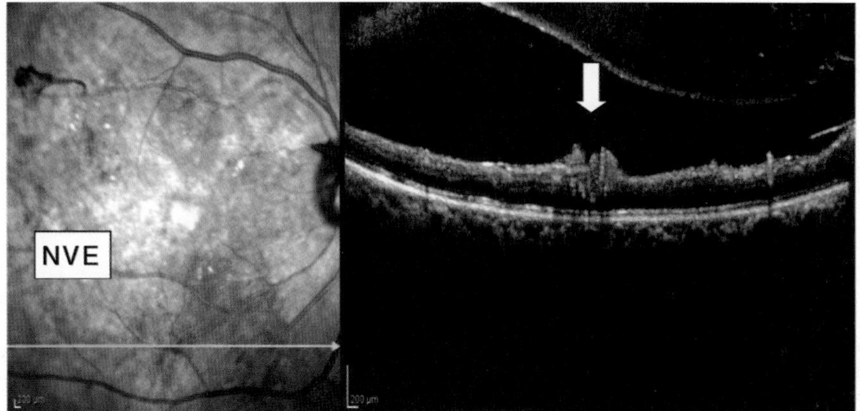

Fig. 65.1 *(Continued)*

Left eye SD-OCT through NVD

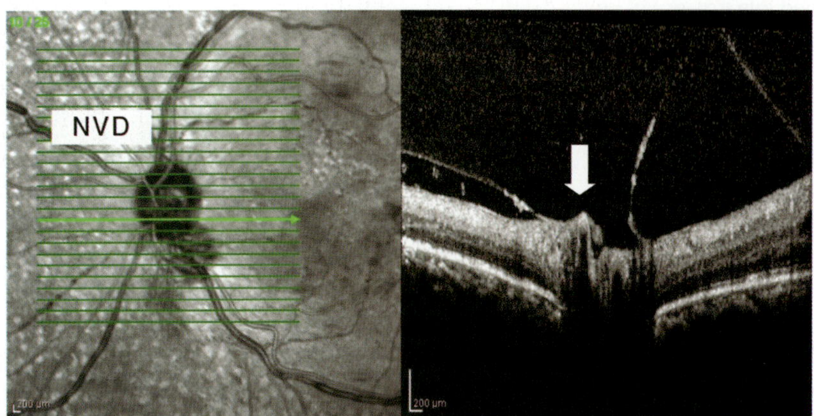

Fig. 65.1 The above figures show FFA confirming PDR with NVD in BE and NVE with CNP in the right eye, left eye status post-PRP. SD-OCT images of the right eye through the NVE show detached posterior hyaloid face (PHF), uneven retinal surface with elevation and hyperreflectivity in the inner retinal layers (*arrow*) and the left eye SD-OCT through NVD shows an attached PHF to disc, obliteration of cup–disc interface with membrane-like elevated and uneven hyper-reflective echoes suggestive of the origin of NVD from the substance of ONH (*arrow*).

NVD, NVE, and capillary nonperfusion (CNP) areas in both right and left eyes. Spectral-domain optical coherence tomography (SD-OCT) images of the right eye through the NVE showed uneven retinal surface with elevation and hyperreflectivity in the inner retinal layers (*arrow*) and left eye SD-OCT showed membrane-like elevated and uneven hyperreflective echoes suggestive of the origin of the NVD from the substance of the optic nerve head (ONH) (*arrow*). He was advised right eye PRP and left eye additional PRP.

CASE STUDY 2

A 48-year-old Asian Indian man with type-1 diabetes presented with complaints of blurred vision in the left eye. His best-corrected visual acuity (BCVA) was 20/20 in the right eye and 20/30 in the left eye. Anterior segment was normal. Fundus showed severe NPDR in the right eye and fibrovascular proliferation in the left eye over the disc with NVE suggestive of PDR (Fig. 65.2). He underwent FFA and SD-OCT. The right eye showed features of severe NPDR

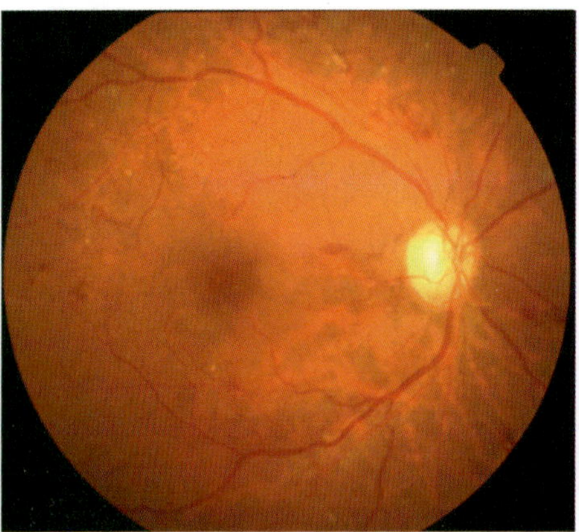
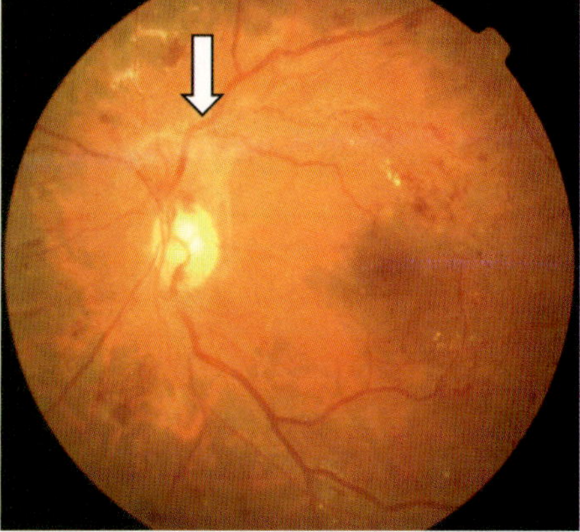

Fig. 65.2 (*Continued*)

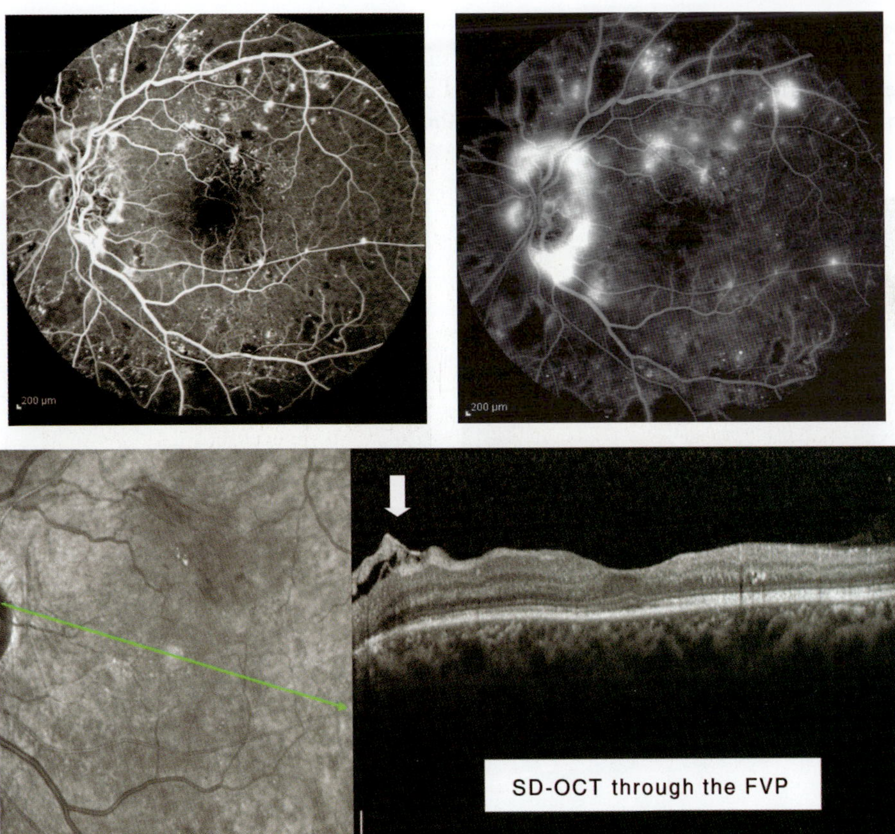

Fig. 65.2 The above figure shows severe NPDR in the right eye and NVD with fibrovascular proliferation (FVP) over the disc suggestive of PDR in the left eye (*arrow*). FFA images show progressive leakage in the left eye around disc and superotemporally suggestive of NVE. SD-OCT imaging through the macula and FVP (*arrow*) shows preretinal membrane-like hyperreflective echoes with uneven surface and minimal traction causing unevenness in the retinal surface and intraretinal edema.

with early NVE and the left eye showed increasing hyperfluorescence around the disc, suggestive of a leak and NVE. Optical coherence tomography (OCT) of the macula and disc show a preretinal membrane-like hyperreflective echo over the disc and extending on to the posterior pole with retinal surface unevenness and mild intraretinal edema. He underwent two sittings of PRP in BE, following which both PDR and visual acuity got stabilized.

CASE STUDY 3

A 58-year-old Asian Indian woman presented with blurred vision BE. She had earlier undergone vitrectomy in the left eye with silicone oil infusion elsewhere. Her BCVA was 20/60 in the right eye and 20/100 in the left eye. Anterior segment showed BE-early cataract. Fundus examination revealed that the right eye had features of advanced PDR with a macula threatening-combined retinal detachment and the left eye features of the advanced PDR, silicone oil-filled eye status post-vitrectomy (Fig. 65.3). An SD-OCT was done to confirm the extent of combined retinal detachment (CRD) and to assess the macula status. SD-OCT showed right eye-attached macula in one of the angled scans; but a vertical scan showed a detached perifoveal retina with an attached fovea. The left eye SD-OCT showed silicone oil–retina interface—an uneven retinal surface with intraretinal edema. The patient was advised vitreous surgery of the right eye with allied procedures and tamponade to maintain vision more so as the detachment was a combined retinal detachment (RD) on fundus examination.

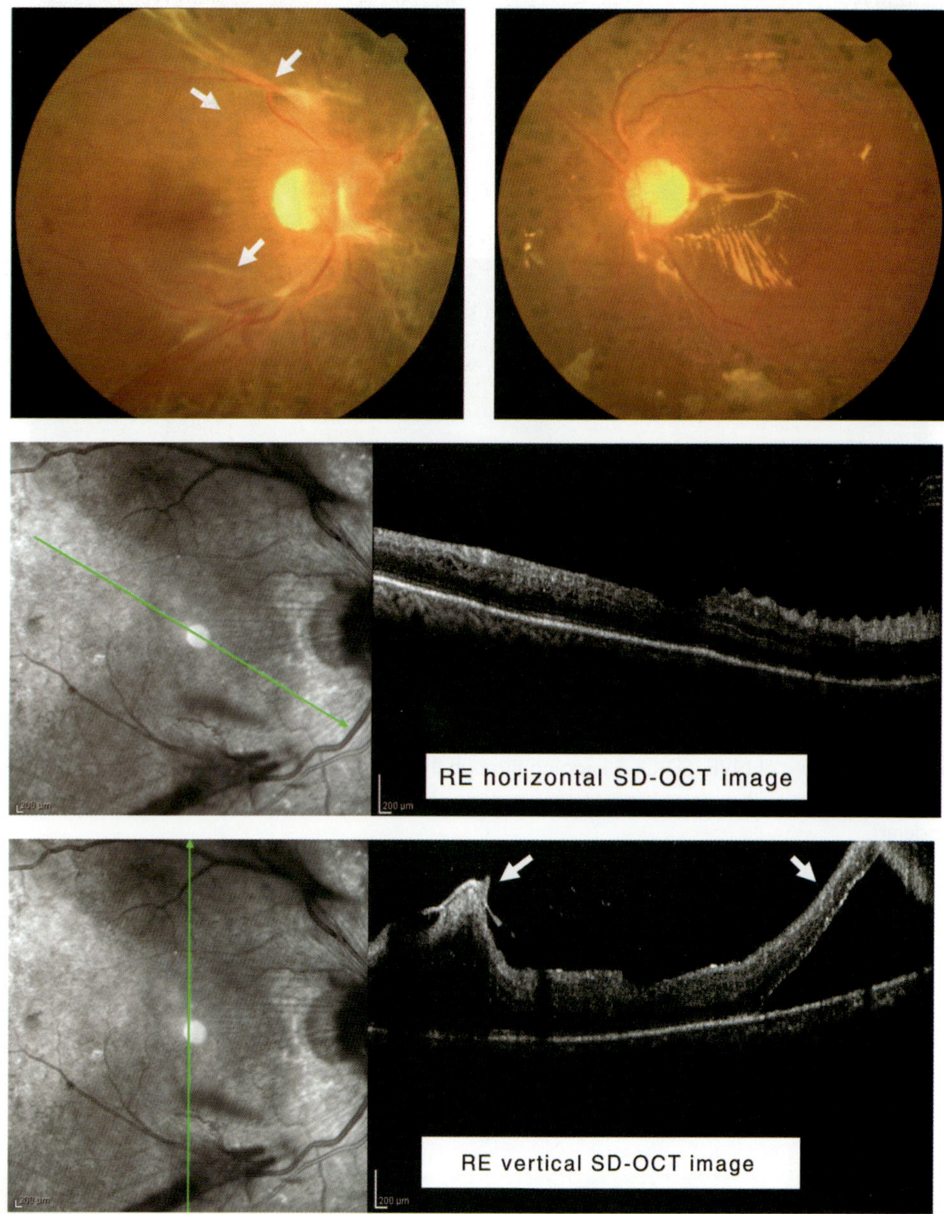

Fig. 65.3 *(Continued)*

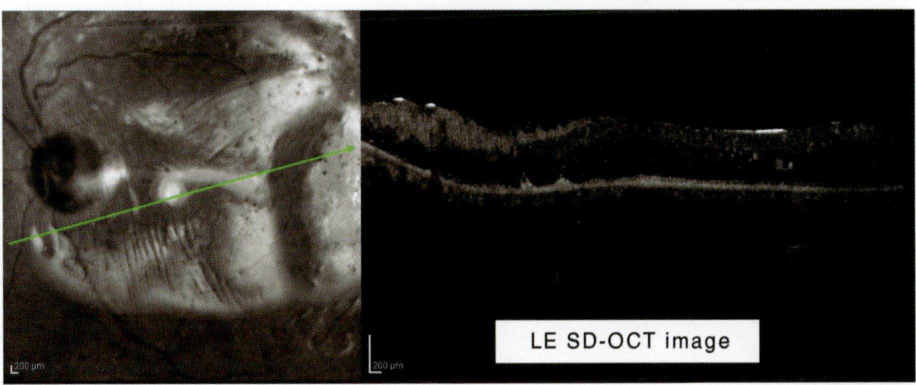

Fig. 65.3 The above figure shows BE-advanced PDR with macula threatening CRD in the right eye (*arrows*) and silicone oil-filled eye status postvitrectomy in the left eye. SD-OCT was done to determine status of the macula. SD-OCT of the right eye showed an attached macula in a horizontal (slightly angled) section, but a perifoveal detachment (*arrows*) with an attached fovea in vertical section concurring with ophthalmoscopy findings. SD-OCT of the left eye shows a hyperreflective membrane echo at the vitreoretinal interface, suggestive of silicone oil with an uneven retinal surface and intraretinal edema.

FURTHER READING

1. Wilkinson CP, Ferris FL, Klein RE, et al.: Proposed international clinical diabetic retinopathy and diabetic macular edema disease severity scales. *Ophthalmology* 110(9):1677–1682, 2003.
2. Ronald E. Klein, et al.: Proposed international clinical diabetic retinopathy and diabetic macular edema disease severity scales. *Ophthalmology* 110(9):1677–1682, 2003.
3. Ryan SJ, Hinton DR, Schachat AP, et al.: *Textbook of Retina*, ed 4, 2006.
4. Diabetic Retinopathy Study Research Group: Design methods and baseline results. DRS report no. 6. *Invest Ophthalmol* 21:149–209, 1991.

Diabetic Retinopathy—Medical Management

Priya BV

Diabetic retinopathy (DR) is a leading cause of blindness worldwide. The main vision-threatening complications of DR are diabetic macular edema (DME) and proliferative diabetic retinopathy (PDR).

Various studies have shown that strict control of glucose and blood pressure significantly decrease the risk of development and the progression of DR.

Lipid lowering may be another approach to reduce DR endpoints, particularly for macular edema and exudation. Statins and fibrates have shown benefits in DR with a reduction in retinal and macular exudation.

CASE STUDY

A 50-year-old Asian Indian female presented with diminution of vision in her right eye for the past 2 months. She was a known diabetic since 5 years on oral hypoglycemic agents and a hypertensive since 2 months on antihypertensive medication.

Visual acuity at presentation was 6/24 in the right eye and 6/6 in the left eye. Anterior segment examination showed pseudophakia in both the eyes.

Fundus examination showed moderate nonproliferative diabetic retinopathy (NPDR) with clinically significant macular edema (CSME) with extensive hard exudates in the posterior pole in the right eye (Fig. 66.1) and moderate NPDR in the left eye (Fig. 66.2).

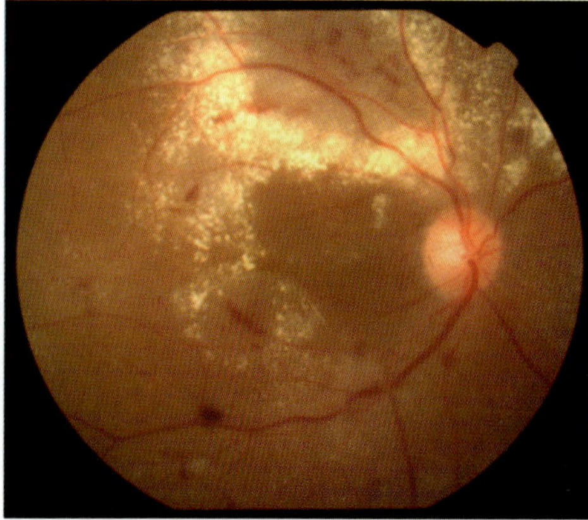

Fig. 66.1 Fundus photograph of the right eye showing extensive hard exudates in the macula.

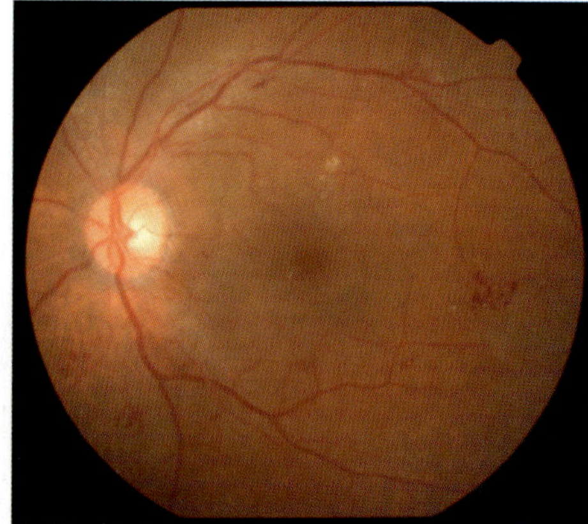

Fig. 66.2 Fundus photograph of the left eye showing moderate NPDR.

Patient underwent fundus fluorescein angiography (FFA) and optical coherence tomography (OCT). FFA revealed macular leaks in the right eye (**Fig. 66.3**) and NPDR in both the eyes (**Figs 66.3 and 66.4**).

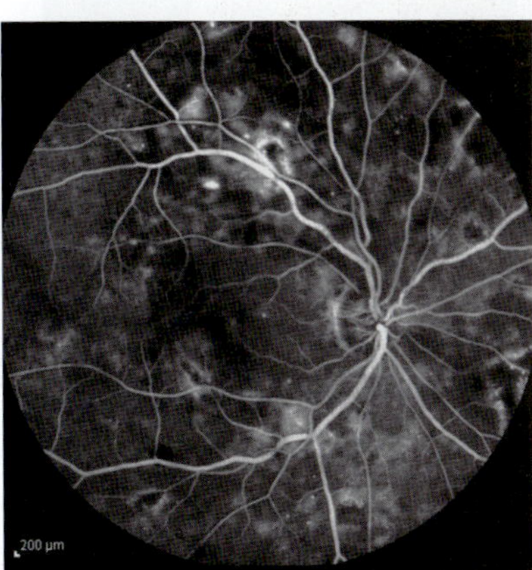

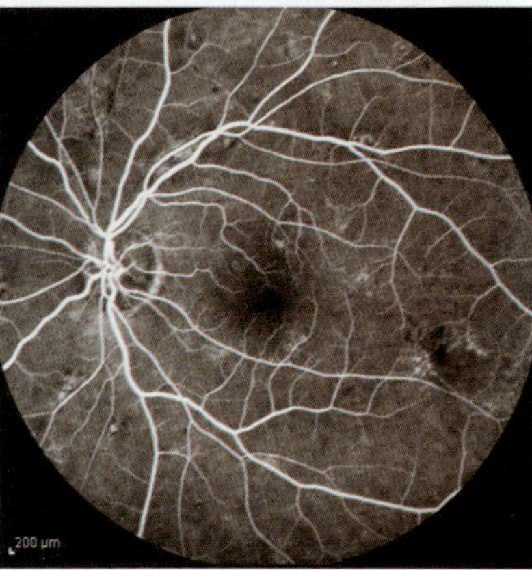

Fig. 66.3 Fundus fluorescein angiogram of the right eye showing dye leakage in the posterior pole with disrupted foveal avascular zone (FAZ).

Fig. 66.4 Fundus fluorescein angiogram of the left eye showing blocked fluorescence corresponding to the retinal hemorrhages with normal FAZ.

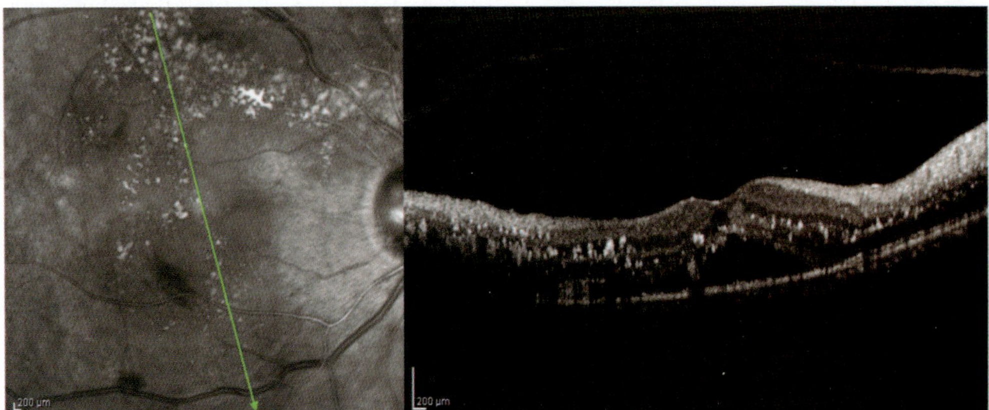

Fig. 66.5 SD-OCT of the right eye showing increased macular thickness with subfoveal hyporeflective area corresponding to serous retinal detachment with multiple hyperreflective dots in the retinal layers corresponding to the hard exudates.

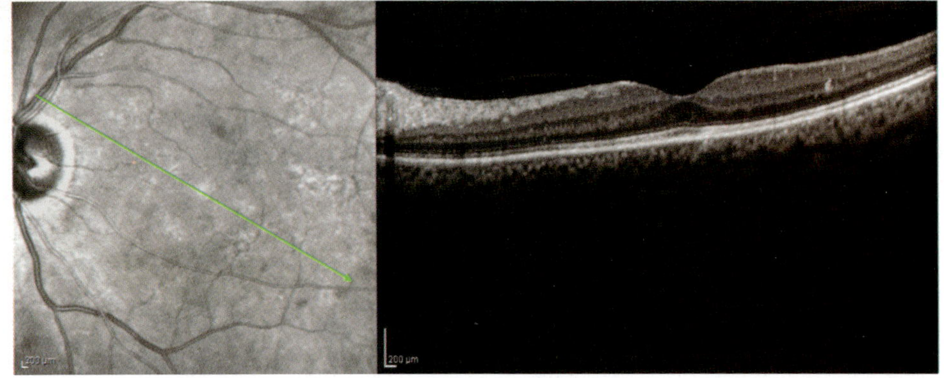

Fig. 66.6 SD-OCT of the left eye showing normal foveal contour.

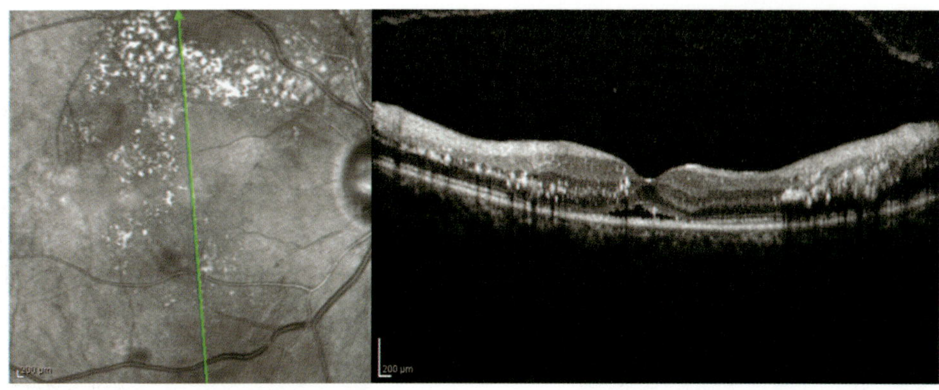

Fig. 66.7 SD-OCT of the right eye done at 1 month after starting the patient on lipid-lowering medications showing decrease in macular thickness with almost complete resolution of subretinal fluid at the fovea.

SD-OCT (SPECTRALIS™; Heidelberg Engineering, Heidelberg, Germany) of the right eye showed increased macular thickness with subretinal fluid at the fovea, with multiple hyperreflective dots in retinal layers corresponding to hard exudates (Fig. 66.5). Central macular thickness (CMT) was 436 microns. OCT of the left eye showed normal foveal contour with CMT of 243 microns (Fig. 66.6).

The patient was advised to get serum lipid profile done, which showed hyperlipidemia with elevated cholesterol, triglyceride, and very-low-density lipoprotein (VLDL) levels. Under physician guidance, the patient was started on a combination of rosuvastatin 10 mg and fenofibrate 160 mg once a day at bedtime.

Follow-up after 1 month showed improvement in her visual acuity in the right eye to 6/9. Fundus examination showed decrease in macular edema. OCT of the right eye showed marked decrease in the macular thickness to 245 microns, with near-complete resolution of subretinal fluid at the fovea (Fig. 66.7).

The patient was advised to continue the lipid-lowering medication and to follow-up regularly.

FURTHER READING

1. ACCORD Study Group; ACCORD Eye Study Group, Chew EY, Ambrosius WT, Davis MD, et al.: Effects of medical therapies on retinopathy progression in type 2 diabetes. *N Engl J Med* 363(3):233–244, 2010.
2. Keech AC, Mitchell P, Summanen PA, et al.: FIELD study investigators. Effect of fenofibrate on the need for laser treatment for diabetic retinopathy (FIELD study): a randomized controlled trial. *Lancet* 370(9600):1687–1697, 2007.
3. Simó R, Hernández C. Advances in the Medical Treatment of Diabetic Retinopathy. *Diabetes Care* 32(8):1556–1562, 2009.

Diabetic Retinopathy—Pharmacological Treatment of Diabetic Macular Edema

Subhashchandra HD,
Naresh Kumar Yadav, and
Supriya Dabir

CASE STUDY 1

A 57-year-old lady with 8-years history of diabetes mellitus had decreased vision in both eyes. Her best-corrected visual acuity (BCVA) was 6/24, N6 in the right eye and 6/6p, N6 in the left eye. Fundus examination revealed moderate

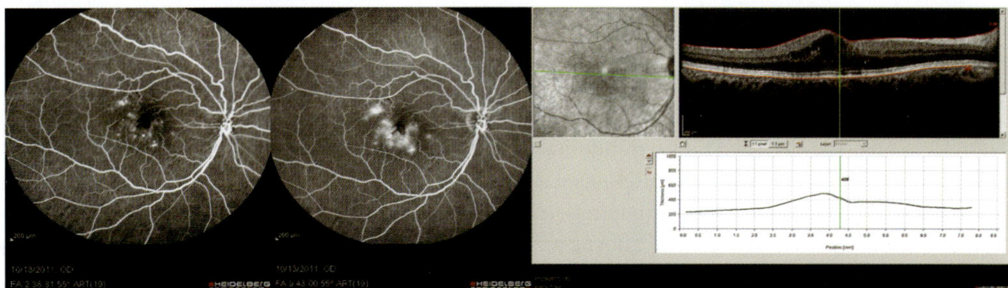

Pretreatment right eye

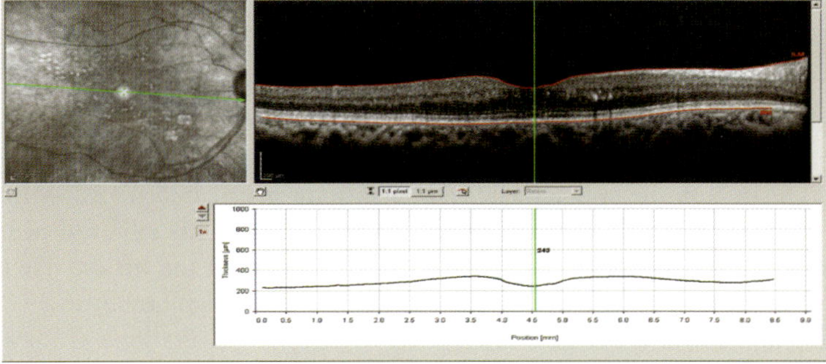

Post-treatment right eye

Fig. 67.1 Pretreatment-FFA of right eye showing features of moderate NPDR with macular edema. SD-OCT shows cystoid spaces with a CMT of 425 microns. Post-IVTA treatment, SD-OCT (*below*) shows reduction in the cystoid edema with persistent disruption of the IS–OS junction.

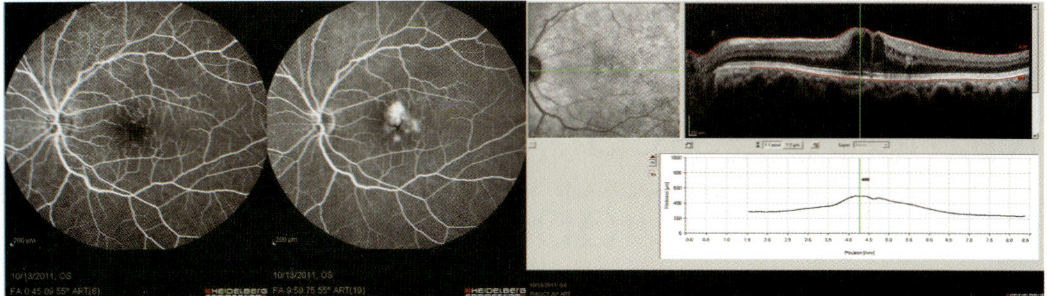

Pretreatment left eye

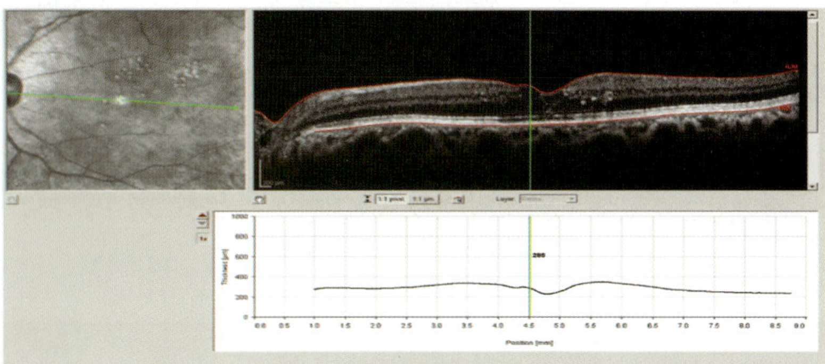

Post-treatment left eye

Fig. 67.2 Pretreatment FFA of left eye showing features of moderate NPDR with cystoid macular edema. SD-OCT shows cystoid spaces with a CMT of 488 microns. Post-IVTA treatment, SD-OCT (*below*) shows reduction in the cystoid edema.

nonproliferative diabetic retinopathy (NPDR) with diabetic macular edema in both eyes, which was confirmed on fundus fluorescein angiography (FFA). Spectral-domain optical coherence tomography (SD-OCT) revealed cystoid macular edema in both the eyes with a central macular thickness (CMT) of 425 microns in the right eye and 488 microns in the left eye. She underwent intravitreal triamcinolone injection (IVTA) in both the eyes followed by focal laser after 4 weeks. Her BCVA post-treatment was 6/18, N6 in the right eye and 6/9, N6 in the left eye. Post-treatment OCT showed a CMT of 224 microns with disruption of inner segment–outer segment junction (IS–OS) in the right eye and CMT of 285 microns with small intraretinal cystic space in the left eye (**Figs 67.1 and 67.2**).

CASE STUDY 2

A 65-year-old man with a known history of diabetes mellitus, hypertension, and renal disease had gradually decreasing vision in the right eye. His BCVA in the right eye was 6/36, N36 and 6/6p, N6p in the left eye. Fundus examination showed severe NPDR in both the eyes and clinically significant macular edema (CSME) in the right eye. FFA confirmed the above findings. SD-OCT showed cystoid macular edema with subfoveal neurosensory detachment and CMT of 550 microns in the right eye, and a CMT of 220 microns in the left eye. He underwent intravitreal injection of ranibizumab in the right eye. Central macular thickness reduced significantly to 297 microns with minimal subfoveal fluid persisting in the right eye (**Fig. 67.3**).

As fluid was persisting on optical coherence tomography (OCT), he underwent repeat injection of intravitreal ranibizumab in the right eye after 2 months. Post-treatment, there was no fluid on OCT. Three months after repeat injection, he had a best-corrected visual acuity of 6/24, N10 in the right eye and 6/6, N6p in the left eye, with disruption of IS–OS junction and absence of fluid on right-eye OCT (**Fig. 67.4**).

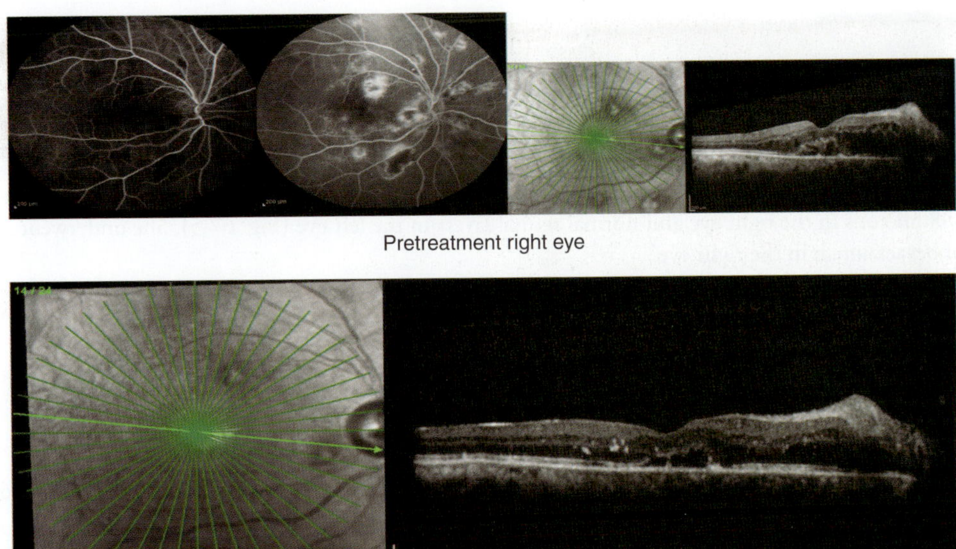

Pretreatment right eye

Post-treatment right eye

Fig. 67.3 FFA of the right eye showing features of severe NPDR with macular edema. SD-OCT of the right eye showing cystoid macular edema with subfoveal sensory detachment. Postranibizumab treatment, the CMT reduced significantly with persistence of subfoveal fluid.

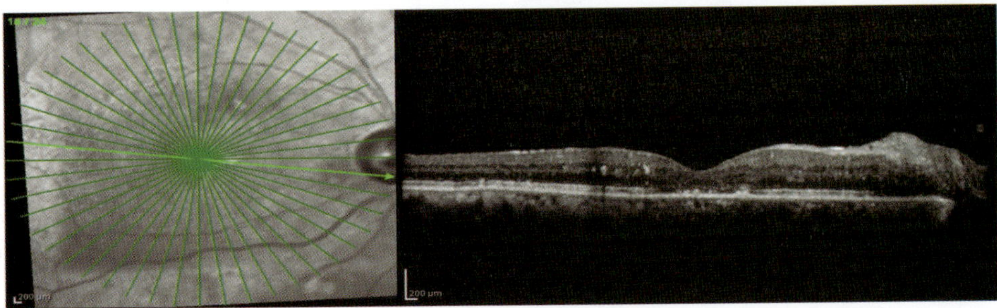

Postrepeat intravitreal injection

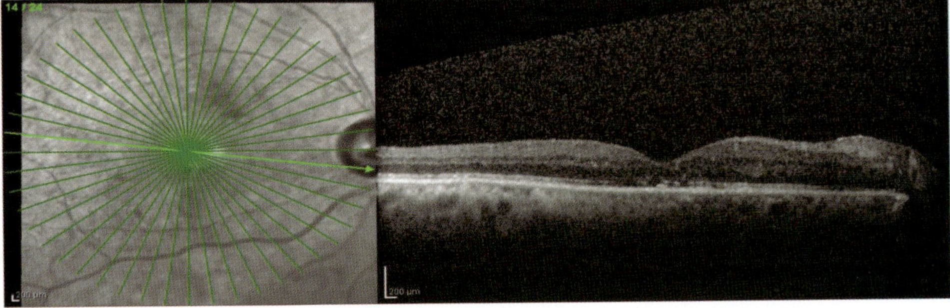

Last visit

Fig. 67.4 Postrepeat intravitreal ranibizumab injection, SD-OCT of the right eye showing complete resorption of the fluid at the macula with an irregular IS–OS junction.

CASE STUDY 3

A 37-year-old woman with diabetes and hypertension had decreased vision in the right eye since 2 months. Her BCVA was 6/18p, N18 in the right eye and 6/6p and N6p in the left eye. Fundus examination revealed high-risk proliferative diabetic retinopathy (PDR) in both the eyes, with diabetic macular edema in the right eye. FFA confirmed the above findings. SD-OCT showed cystoid macular edema with subfoveal neurosensory detachment and CMT of 888 microns in the right eye and normal retinal layers in the left eye (Fig. 67.5). She underwent intravitreal injection of bevacizumab in the right eye.

Her BCVA in the right eye was 6/18, N18 and 6/9, N6p in the left eye and the CMT had reduced to 189 microns after 1 month of intravitreal injection in the right eye (Figs 67.6 and 67.7).

DISCUSSION

Laser photocoagulation used to be the standard treatment for diabetic macular edema until the advent of steroids and anti-vascular endothelial growth factors (anti-VEGF). Recently there has been an interest in other treatment modalities like oral protein kinase C β-inhibitors, pars plana vitrectomy, and intravitreal aptamers or antibodies directed against vascular endothelial growth factors (VEGF).

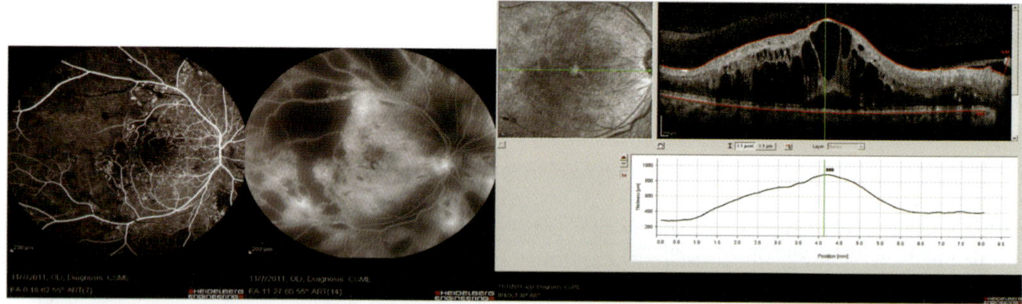

Fig. 67.5 FFA of the right eye showing significant areas of nonperfusion with features of PDR and diffuse macular edema. SD-OCT shows severe cystoid edema with subfoveal neurosensory detachment and CMT of 888 microns.

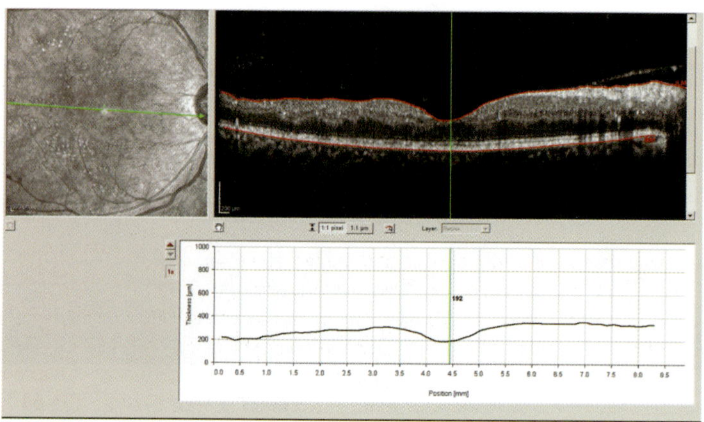

Fig. 67.6 SD-OCT post-treatment with intravitreal injection of bevacizumab. The foveal contour was restored with reduction in the fluid and CMT.

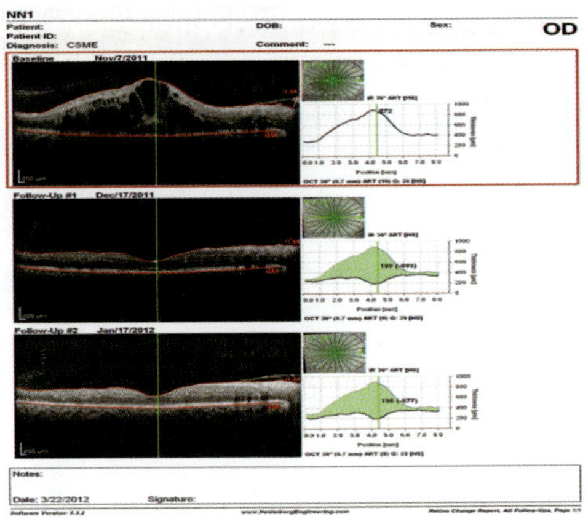

Fig. 67.7 SD-OCT serial follow-up images of Case Study 3 showing macular edema pre- and post-treatment.

VEGF leads to a breakdown in the blood–retina barrier and an increase in retinal vascular permeability leading to retinal edema. VEGF levels are upregulated in several conditions including diabetic retinopathy. Three currently available anti-VEGF agents are pegaptanib sodium, ranibizumab, and bevacizumab.

- *Intravitreal triamcinolone acetonide (IVTA)* reduces macular edema, with its peak action a week following the injection; although its effect lasts for 3–6 months. IVTA has been used both as a primary modality of treatment and an adjunct to photocoagulation.
- *POSURDEX*—Currently the phase 3 trial of Posurdex biodegradable implant (sustained delivery formulation of dexamethasone) for treatment of diabetic macular edema is ongoing.
  - *Pegaptanib sodium* is a pegylated aptamer directed against the VEGF-A$_{165}$ isoform.
  - A phase 2 prospective clinical trial showed improvement in the anatomic and visual outcome in patients with diabetic macular edema.
  - *Ranibizumab* is a recombinant humanized antibody fragment that acts against all isoforms of VEGF-A.
  - Multiple phase 3, randomized controlled clinical trials are on-going to study the effect of ranibizumab in diabetic macular edema like RESOLVE study, READ-2 study, RESTORE study. The Diabetic Retinopathy Clinical Research Network phase 3 randomized multicenter trial has shown favorable results.
  - *Bevacizumab* is a full-length recombinant humanized antibody that acts against all isoforms of VEGF-A. The intravitreal bevacizumab or laser therapy (BOLT) in the management of diabetic macular edema study has shown favorable results for management of diabetic macular edema with intravitreal bevacizumab.

FURTHER READING

1. PKC-DRS Study Group. The effect of ruboxistaurin on visual loss in patients with moderately severe to very-severe non-proliferative diabetic retinopathy: Initial results of the protein kinase C β-inhibitor diabetic retinopathy study (PKC-DRS) multicenter randomized clinical trial. *Diabetes* 54:2188–2197, 2005.
2. Diabetic Retinopathy Clinical Research Network, A randomized trial comparing intravitreal triamcinolone acetonide and focal/grid photocoagulation for diabetic macular edema. *Ophthalmology* 115:1447–1449, 2008.
3. Haller JA, Kuppermann BD, Blumenkranz MS, et al.: Randomized controlled trial of an intravitreous dexamethasone drug delivery system in patients with diabetic macular edema. *Arch Ophthalmol* 128(3):289–296, 2010.
4. Sultan MB, Zhou D, Loftus J, et al.: A phase 2/3, multicenter, randomized, double-masked, 2-year trial of pegaptanib sodium for the treatment of diabetic macular edema. *Ophthalmology* 118(6):1107–1118, 2011.
5. Elman MJ, Bressler NM, Qin H, et al.: Expanded 2-year follow-up of ranibizumab plus prompt or deferred laser or triamcinolone plus prompt laser for diabetic macular edema. *Ophthalmology* 118(4):609–614, 2011.
6. Michaelides M, Kaines A, Hamilton RD, et al.: A prospective randomized trial of intravitreal bevacizumab or laser therapy in the management of diabetic macular edema (BOLT study). 12-month data: Report 2. *Ophthalmology* 117(6): 1078–1086, 2010.

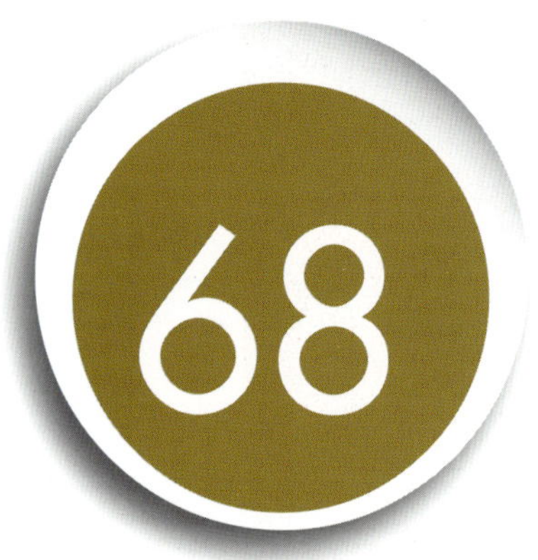

Drusen—Dry Age-related Macular Degeneration

Rajani Battu

Drusen are one of the earliest signs of age-related macular degeneration (AMD). Drusen are characterized as hard or soft as well as small (<63 μm), intermediate (>63 μm but <125 μm), or large (>125 μm). The number of drusen, their size, and pigmentary changes in the macula are important in staging disease severity and predicting likelihood of disease progression and vision loss.

CASE STUDY

An 85-year-old man presented with decreased vision in both eyes since 6 months. Ocular examination showed a vision of 6/6, N6 in the right eye and 6/18, N18 in the left eye. He had significant cataracts in both the eyes. Fundus examination in the right eye showed multiple hard drusen in the right eye, and multiple hard and soft drusen in the left eye. There was no evidence of choroidal neovascular membrane (Fig. 68.1). Fundus fluorescein

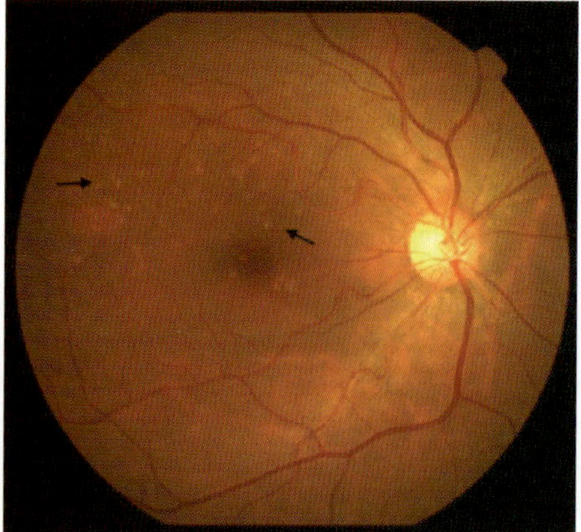
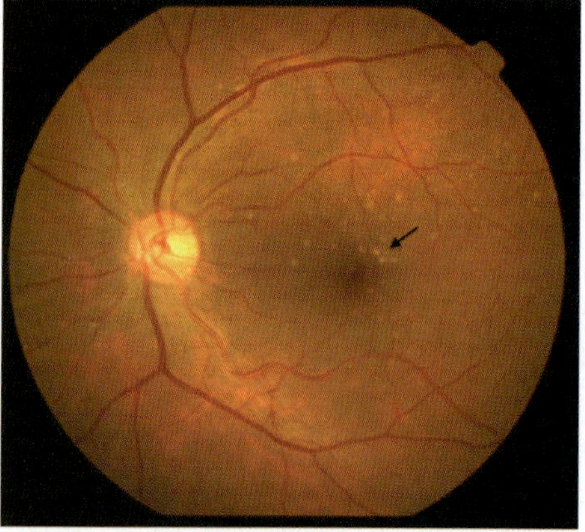

Fig. 68.1 Fundus picture of the right and left eye showing multiple hard drusen (*black arrows*).

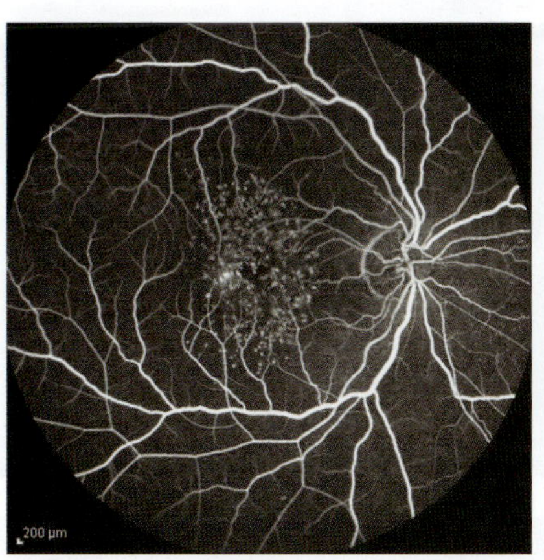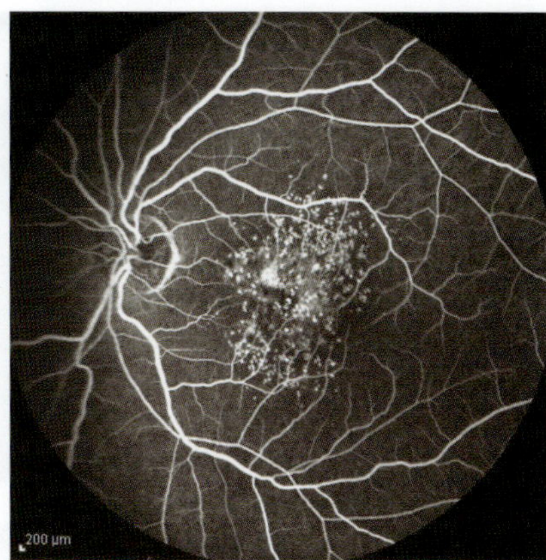

Fig. 68.2 Fundus fluorescein angiogram (arteriovenous phase) of a 56-year-old woman showing multiple areas of hyperfluorescence corresponding to drusen. The hyperfluorescence is mostly due to loss of retinal pigment epithelium (RPE) overlying the drusen (window defects).

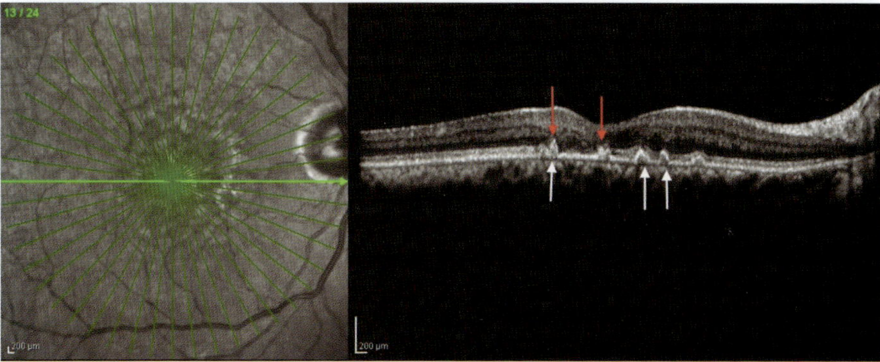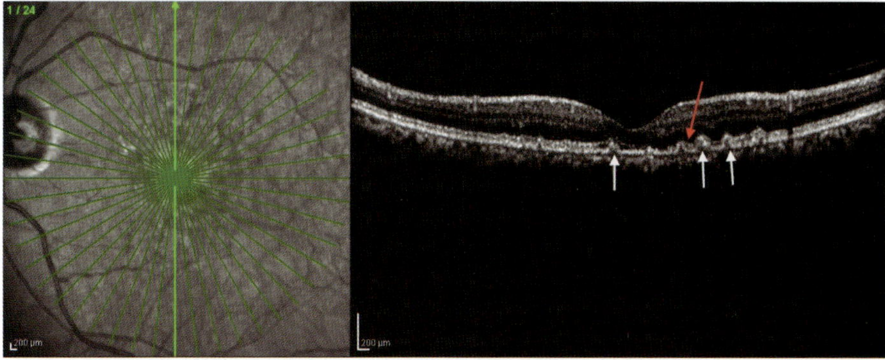

Fig. 68.3 Infrared optical coherence tomography (IR-OCT) of the right and left eye (of the same patient as in Fig. 68.2). The *white arrows* represent areas of RPE excrescences (drusen) while the *red arrows* depict disruption of inner segment–outer segment (IS–OS) junction corresponding to the drusen.

angiogram (FFA) showed multiple window defects corresponding to the drusen (Fig. 68.2). Spectral-domain optical coherence tomography (SD-OCT) showed retinal pigment epithelial (RPE) excrescences corresponding to the drusen (Fig. 68.3). In patients with geographic atrophy, SD-OCT shows areas of RPE loss and thinning of retina (Figs 68.4 and 68.5).

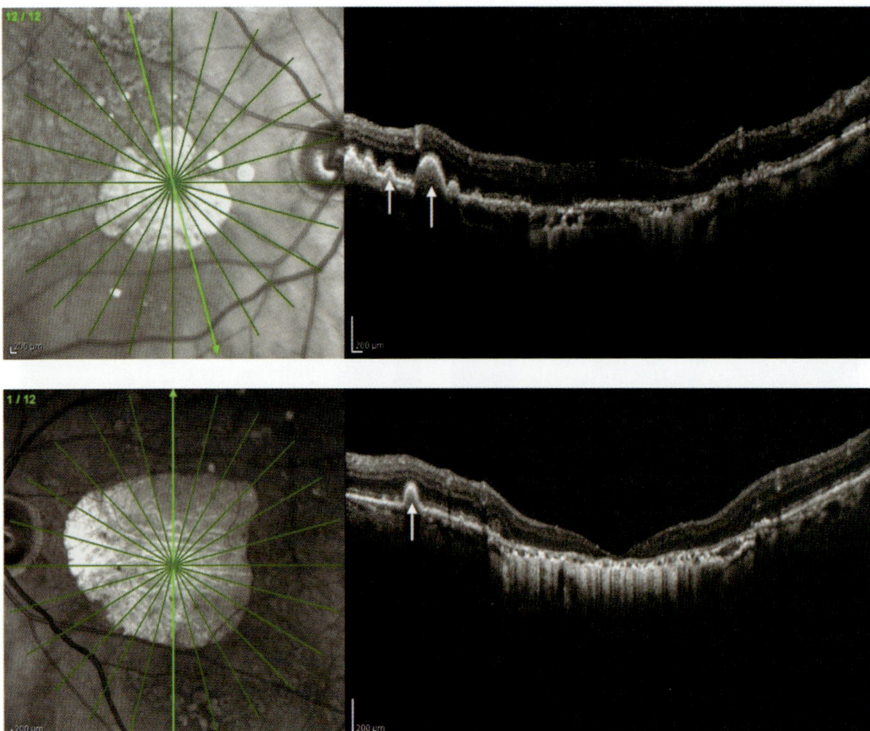

Fig. 68.4 IR-OCT of the right and left eye of a patient with geographic atrophy along with multiple areas of RPE excrescences corresponding to areas of drusen. Note the large area of loss of RPE and significant thinning of retina corresponding to area of geographic atrophy, more prominent in the left eye.

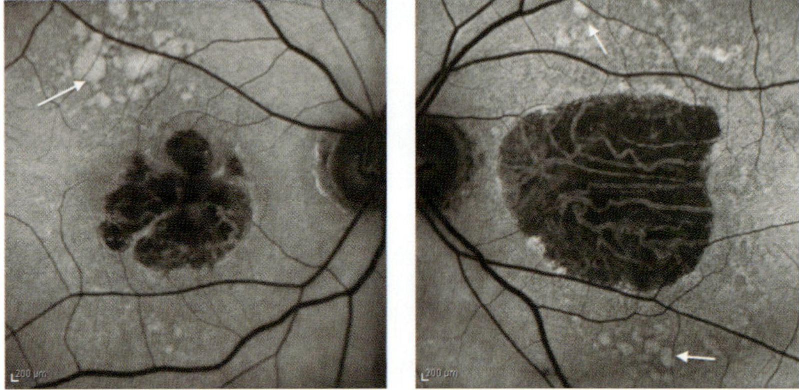

Fig. 68.5 Fundus autofluorescence (FAF) of the same patient showing hyperautofluorescence (*white arrows*) corresponding to areas of drusen. Note the hypoautofluorescence corresponding to the areas of geographic atrophy (due to the RPE loss).

DISCUSSION

Drusen are the hallmark of AMD, and the amount of drusen and their effect on retinal pigment epithelium is a strong predictor of progression of AMD and vision loss. Information obtained from optical coherence tomography (OCT) may help us understand pathogenesis of disease better and aid in its management. Algorithms may be created for qualitative and quantitative assessment of drusen. It is also possible to assess drusen volume that can help grade severity of the eyes with dry AMD. Various patterns of abnormal fundus autofluorescence (FAF) may be useful in monitoring progression of nonexudative AMD, reflecting different stages of the disease. OCT has become an increasingly useful tool for differentiating drusen morphologic parameters such as shape, internal reflectivity, homogeneity, and presence of overlying hyperreflective foci.

CONCLUSION

Optical coherence tomography (OCT) provides in vivo imaging of drusen in cross-section. Periodic observation of drusen with SD-OCT and FAF examination is of great clinical value in management of patients with AMD.

FURTHER READING

1. Mitchell P, Foran S: Age-related eye disease study severity scale and simplified severity scale for age-related macular degeneration. *Arch Ophthalmol* 123(11):1598–1599, 2005.
2. Freeman SR, Mueller A, Maniotis A, et al.: Optical coherence tomography-raster scanning and manual segmentation in determining drusen volume in age-related macular degeneration. *Retina* 30(3):431–435, 2010.
3. Gregori G, Wang F, Rosenfeld PJ, et al.: Spectral domain optical coherence tomography imaging of drusen in nonexudative age-related macular degeneration. *Ophthalmology* 118(7):1373–1379, 2011.
4. Xuan Y, PQ Zho, Q Peng: Fundus autofluorescence patterns of drusen in age-related macular degeneration. *Zhonghua Yan Ke Za Zhi*, 46(8):708–713, 2010.
5. Landa G, Rosen RB, Patel A, et al.: Qualitative spectral OCT/SLO analysis of drusen change in dry age-related macular degeneration patients treated with Copaxone. *J Ocul Pharmacol Ther* 27(1):77–82, 2011.

Epiretinal Membrane

*Naresh Kumar Yadav and
Santosh Gopi Krishna*

Epiretinal membrane (ERM) is an avascular, fibrocellular membrane that grows on the inner surface of the retina and can cause visual disturbance. ERM may be found in association with intraocular inflammation, retinal detachments, ocular trauma, and following procedures like retinal cryopexy, laser photocoagulation, and intraocular surgery. Without any of these, it may occur in an idiopathic manner in people over the age of 50. When thin and immature, the membrane may appear as a glistening light reflex, while it may be more obvious as the membrane thickens. Various changes associated with an ERM include surface wrinkling, vascular distortion, cystoid macular edema, and pseudohole. The Watzke–Allen test may help differentiate a pseudohole thus formed from a true macular hole. Optical coherence tomography (OCT) not only helps differentiate the two, but can also predict clinical macular function through measurements of retinal base thickness. If the retinal base is abnormally thick, thin, or irregular, visual acuity of the eye is significantly lower. Most cases of ERM are asymptomatic, unless they involve the macular or perimacular area. The common presenting symptoms include decreased visual acuity, metamorphopsia, micropsia, macropsia, and monocular diplopia.

Eyes with an idiopathic ERM predominantly have good vision; careful selection of cases for surgical removal of the membrane therefore becomes imperative, especially since the surgical indications for its removal have not been standardized.

CASE STUDY

A 65-year-old lady visited our clinic with complaints of diminution of vision in the left eye since the last 5–6 months. On examination, her best-corrected visual acuity (BCVA) was 6/6, N6 and 6/18, N10 in the right and left eyes, respectively. She had undergone cataract surgery in both the eyes 1 year back. She was diagnosed to have idiopathic ERM in the left eye.

Spectral-domain optical coherence tomography (SD-OCT) imaging (Fig. 69.1) showed a thick ERM with cystoid macular edema and loss of foveal contour. She underwent vitrectomy with ERM removal. Postsurgery the visual acuity improved to 6/9 and a repeat SD-OCT (Fig. 69.2) showed a clear preretinal surface devoid of ERM with restoration of normal foveal contour and grossly decreased cystoid macular edema (CME).

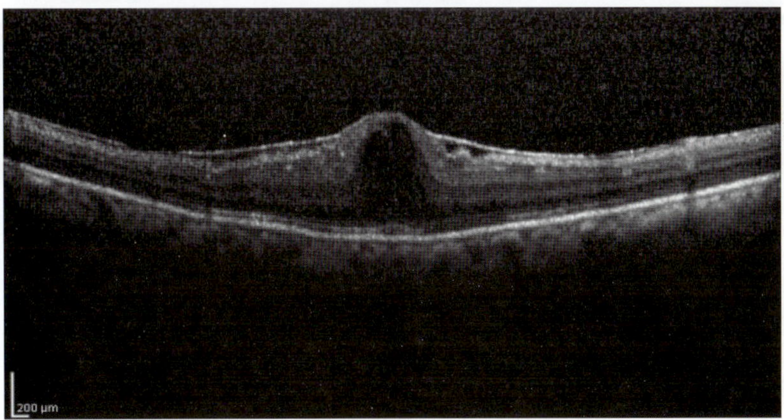

Fig. 69.1 SD-OCT of the left eye macula showing ERM, cystoid macular edema, and increased central retinal thickness.

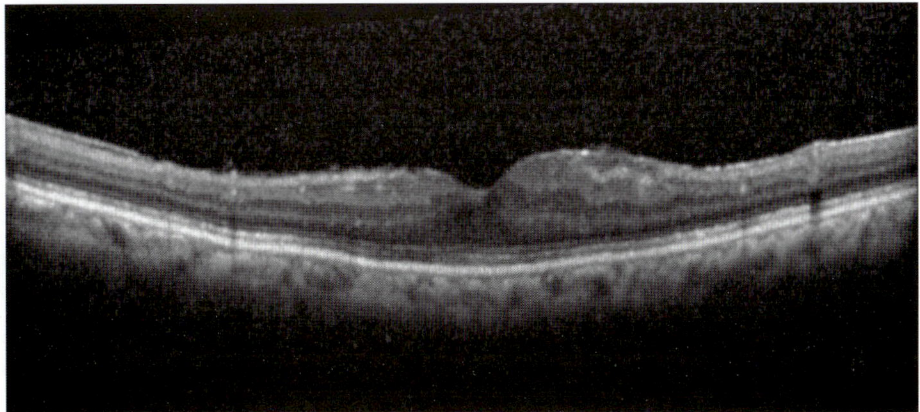

Fig. 69.2 The SD-OCT image, 2 months after ERM removal—the foveal contour is almost normal with significant reduction in cystoid macular edema.

FURTHER READING

1. Klein R, Klein BE, Wang Q, et al.: The epidemiology of epiretinal membranes. *Trans Am Ophthalmol Soc* 92: 403–430,1994.
2. Trese MT, Chandler DB, Machemer R: Macular pucker. I. Prognostic criteria. *Graefes Arch Clin Exp Ophthalmol* 221:12–15, 1983.
3. Michels RG: A clinical and histopathologic study of epiretinal membranes affecting the macula and removed by vitreous surgery. *Trans Am Ophthalmol Soc* 80:580–656, 1982.
4. Mitchell P, Smith W, Chey T, et al.: Prevalence and association of epiretinal membranes—The Blue Mountains Eye Study, Australia. *Ophthalmology* 104:1033–1044, 1997.
5. Park DW, Dugel PU, Garda J, et al.: Macular pucker removal with and without internal limiting membrane peeling: pilot study. *Ophthalmology* 110:62–64, 2003.

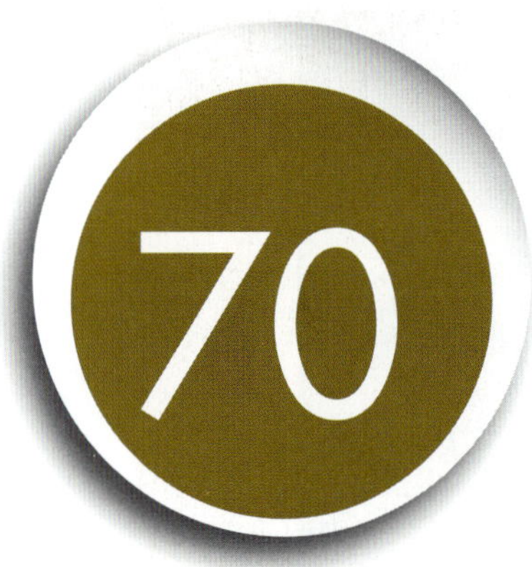

Fundus Albipunctatus

Ajay Shalwala and Anita Agarwal

Fundus albipunctatus is an autosomal recessive disorder characterized by congenital stationary night blindness. The classically nonprogressive difficulty with scotopic vision is punctuated by difficulty with visual adaptation to darkness after exposure to bright environments. The characteristic features on funduscopy are numerous whitish-yellow subretinal spots scattered in the midperiphery and macula, but sparing fovea. These spots may vary with age.

A Caucasian female at age 37 first presented with a chief complaint of night blindness in both eyes. This symptom was ongoing for as long as she could remember and she had been given a diagnosis of a retinal disorder in the first year of her life. She had no difficulty seeing in well-lit areas and her vision had not changed. She had one sister with night blindness and another with no visual problem. She was followed over the next 7 years, during which time fundus photography (Figs 70.1–70.5) and spectral-domain optical coherence tomography (SD-OCT) (Fig. 70.6) were performed.

DISCUSSION

Fundus albipunctatus is a rare disease classically thought to result in stationary night blindness since birth. However, Querques et al. suggest that some of these patients may eventually develop cone dystrophy, and fundus appearance has been reported by several authors to change over course of the disease.

The pathophysiology of the disease relates to a deficiency in regeneration of rod chromophore, 11-*cis*-retinal. When light impinges on visual pigment in the retina, 11-*cis*-retinal isomerizes to an all-trans configuration and dissociates from the associated opsin protein. Regeneration of the *cis* isomer in retinal pigment epithelium (RPE) cells involves dehydrogenase enzymes including *RDH*5 which is abundantly present as a transmembrane protein in RPE cells. RDH5 is mutated in most cases of fundus albipunctatus, resulting in poor turnover of chromophores and a low threshold for bleaching of photoreceptors. Thus one of the primary symptoms of fundus albipunctatus is delayed dark adaptation. While 18 mutations in RDH5 have been shown to segregate with fundus albipunctatus, some reported cases are associated with mutations in other genes involved in chromophore turnover including *RLB*P1 and *RPE*65.

The underlying mechanism behind accumulation of white spots is not well understood. The disrupted process of 11-*cis*-retinal regeneration leads to presumed production of *cis*-retinol and *cis*-retinyl esters, whose accumulation is

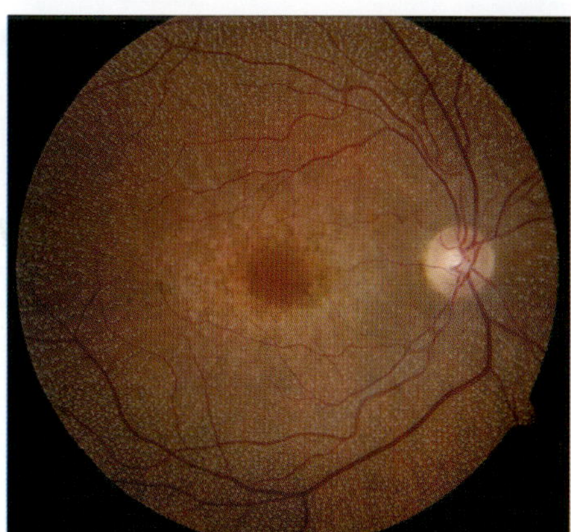

Fig. 70.1 Fundus picture of the right eye showing multiple white dots throughout the posterior pole. The central macula is spared with a bull's-eye appearance. (Photo courtesy: Gass Atlas of Macular Diseases by Anita Agarwal, 5th edition, Vol. I, Fig. 5.38 (E), p. 327, Elsevier, 2012.)

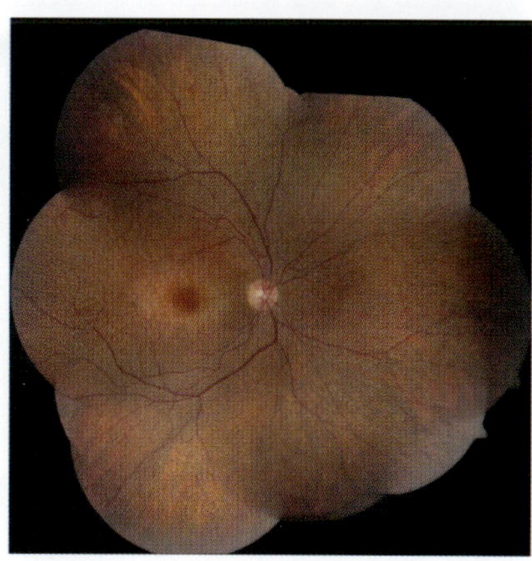

Fig. 70.2 Color montage of the right eye shows white–yellow spots extending up to the periphery. (Photo courtesy: Gass Atlas of Macular Diseases by Anita Agarwal, 5th edition, Vol. I, Fig. 5.38 (J), p. 327, Elsevier, 2012.)

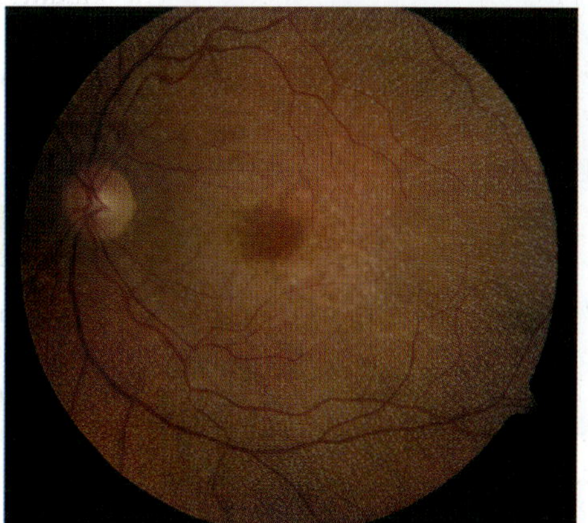

Fig. 70.3 Fundus picture of the left eye showing a similar appearance as the right eye. There is also a "bulls-eye" appearance to the central macula. The patient maintained a visual acuity of 20/25 or better at all office visits. (Photo courtesy: Gass Atlas of Macular Diseases by Anita Agarwal, 5th edition, Vol. I, Fig. 5.38 (H), p. 327, Elsevier, 2012.)

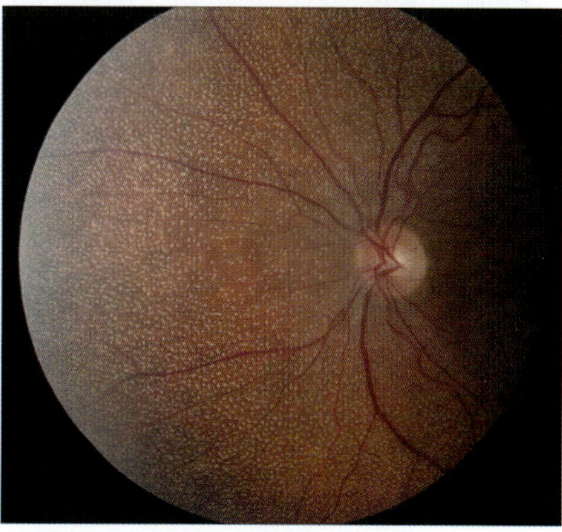

Fig. 70.4 The nasal retina showing the punctate dots. (Photo courtesy: Gass Atlas of Macular Diseases by Anita Agarwal, 5th edition, Vol. I, Fig. 5.38 (F), p. 327, Elsevier, 2012.)

thought to create the characteristic fundus appearance. There is no well-established hypothesis at present explaining why punctate deposition occurs rather than diffuse deposition.

This condition has to be differentiated from retinitis punctata albescens, which has a similar fundus appearance. However, natural history of retinitis punctata albescens is a severe and progressive retinal dystrophy.

No known treatment exists for fundus albipunctatus. A mouse model of the disease recently showed some benefit of 9-*cis*-retinal oral therapy on electroretinography, which led to a phase I study in humans of oral administration of 9-*cis*-β-carotene. There was some benefit shown on electroretinography and automated perimetry in those patients; further studies are underway to evaluate potential benefit of 9-*cis*-β-carotene.

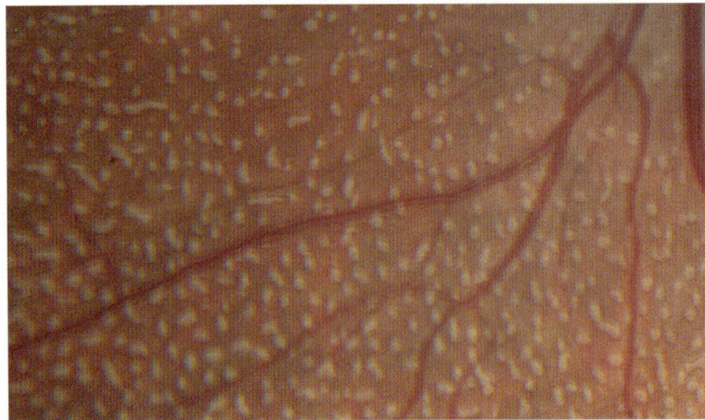

Fig. 70.5 This magnified photograph demonstrates minor variability in the shape of the deposits as well as their sharply demarcated borders. (Photo courtesy: Gass Atlas of Macular Diseases by Anita Agarwal, 5th edition, Vol. I, Fig. 5.38 (I), p. 327, Elsevier, 2012.)

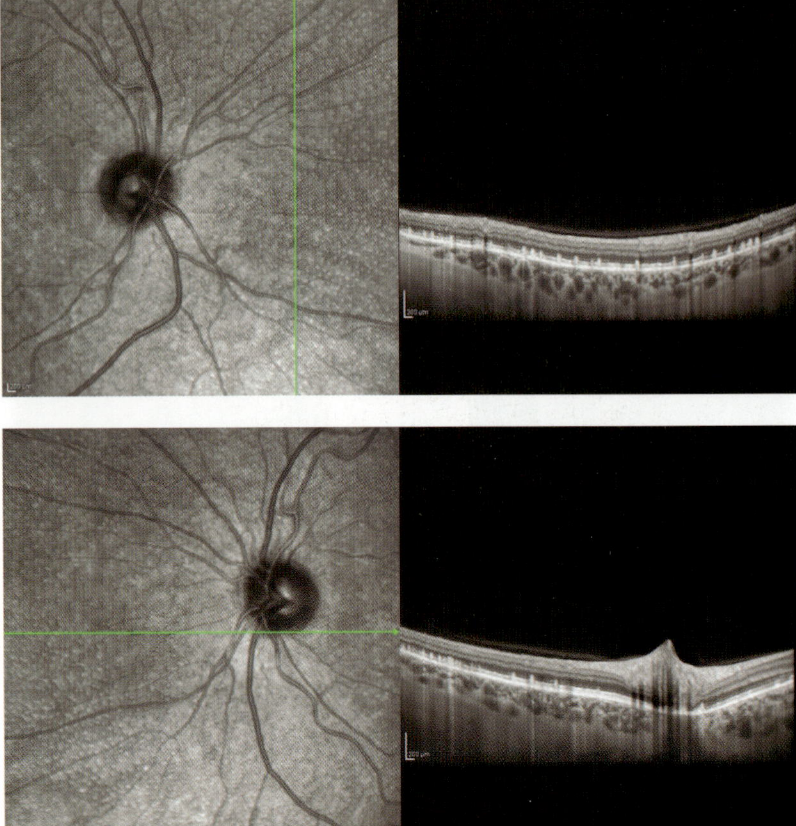

Fig. 70.6 The SD-OCT scan imaged using the SPECTRALIS™ (Heidelberg Engineering), cutting through areas containing white–yellow spots, shows location of these lesions in outer retina in both eyes. These hyperreflective lesions occur between areas of apparently normal retina and retinal pigment epithelium (RPE). The lesions appear to be centered on the photoreceptor outer segments extending inwardly towards the outer limiting membrane and extending outwardly towards the RPE. The lesions show uniform reflectivity across their heights.

FURTHER READING

1. Genead MA, Fishman GA, Lindeman M: Spectral-domain optical coherence tomography and fundus autofluorescence characteristics in patients with fundus albipunctatus and retinitis punctata albescens. *Ophthalmic Genet* 31(2):66–72, 2010.

2. Maeda A, Maeda T, Palczewski K: Improvement in rod and cone function in mouse model of Fundus albipunctatus after pharmacologic treatment with 9-*cis*-retinal. *Invest Ophthalmol Vis Sci* 47(10):4540–4546, 2006.

3. Naz S, Ali S, Riazuddin SA, et al.: Mutations in *RLBP1* associated with fundus albipunctatus in consanguineous Pakistani families. *Br J Ophthalmol* 95(7):1019–1024, 2011.

4. Querques G, Carrillo P, Querques L, et al.: High-definition optical coherence tomographic visualization of photoreceptor layer and retinal flecks in fundus albipunctatus associated with cone dystrophy. *Arch Ophthalmol* 127(5):703–706, 2009.

5. Rotenstreich Y, Harats D, Shaish A, et al.: Treatment of a retinal dystrophy, fundus albipunctatus, with oral 9-*cis*-β-carotene. *Br J Ophthalmol* 94(5):616–621, 2010.

6. Schatz P, Preising M, Lorenz B, et al.: Fundus albipunctatus associated with compound heterozygous mutations in RPE65. *Ophthalmology* 118(5):888–894, 2011.

7. Schatz P, Preising M, Lorenz B, et al.: Lack of autofluorescence in fundus albipunctatus associated with mutations in RDH5. *Retina* 30(10):1704–1713, 2010.

8. Sergouniotis PI, Sohn EH, Li Z, et al.: Phenotypic variability in RDH5 retinopathy (Fundus Albipunctatus). *Ophthalmology.* 118(8):1661–1670, 2011.

Hypertensive Retinopathy

Supriya Dabir

Retinal blood circulation acts as a window to view the condition of the systemic circulation. Systemic hypertension is associated with visible changes in retinal microvasculature including choroidopathy, and optic neuropathy. There is also an increased risk of vascular occlusive disease and retinal arteriolar macroaneurysm formation in uncontrolled hypertension.

CASE STUDY

A 45-year-old man came with history of sudden drop in vision in both his eyes. He was a known hypertensive on alternate (native) medication. On examination, his best-corrected visual acuity was 6/60, N24 in both eyes. Intraocular pressure was 16 and 14 mmHg in right and left eye, respectively. Anterior segment was normal, pupils were brisk, and on fundus examination, there was arteriolar attenuation, arteriovenous crossing changes, perivascular multiple cotton-wool spots, and flame-shaped hemorrhages in both eyes. The foveal reflex was obliterated with the presence of submacular subretinal fluid, as seen in **Figure 71.1**.

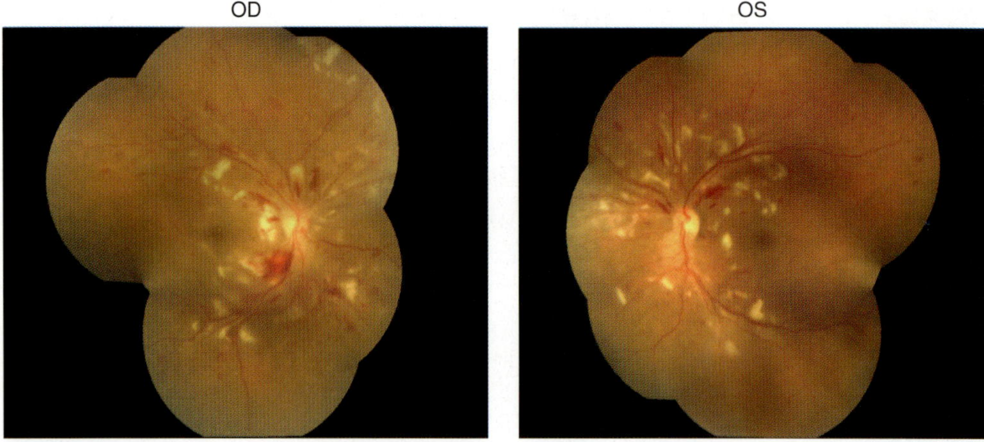

Fig. 71.1 Montage fundus photograph showing arteriolar attenuation, arteriovenous crossing changes, perivascular multiple cotton-wool spots, and flame-shaped hemorrhages. The foveal reflex was obliterated with the presence of submacular subretinal fluid.

The patient subsequently underwent a fluorescein angiography (Fig. 71.2), which showed multiple foci of hyperfluorescence due to pooling secondary to choroidal leakage into the subretinal space. Blocked fluorescence due to superficial retinal hemorrhages was seen.

Radial spectral-domain optical coherence tomography sections through the macula showed intraretinal edema and subretinal fluid with disrupted inner segment–outer segment (IS-OS) junction in both eyes, as seen in Figure 71.3.

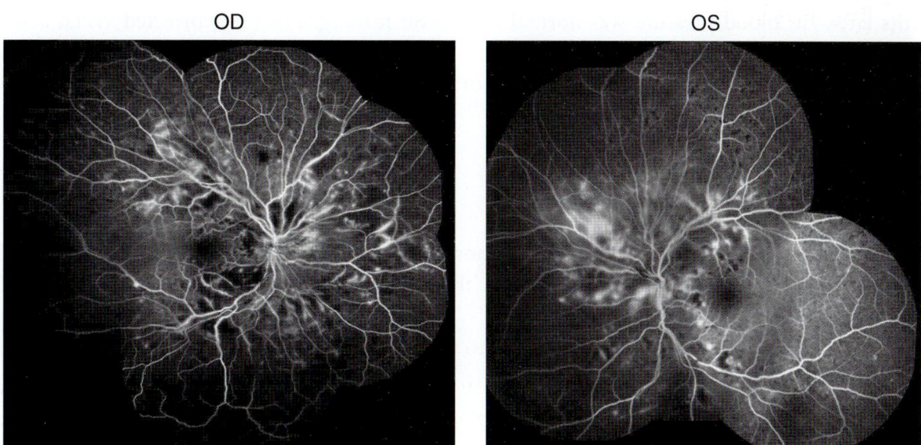

Fig. 71.2 Fluorescein angiography, shows multiple foci of hyperfluorescence due to pooling secondary to choroidal leakage into the subretinal space. Blocked fluorescence due to superficial retinal hemorrhages was seen.

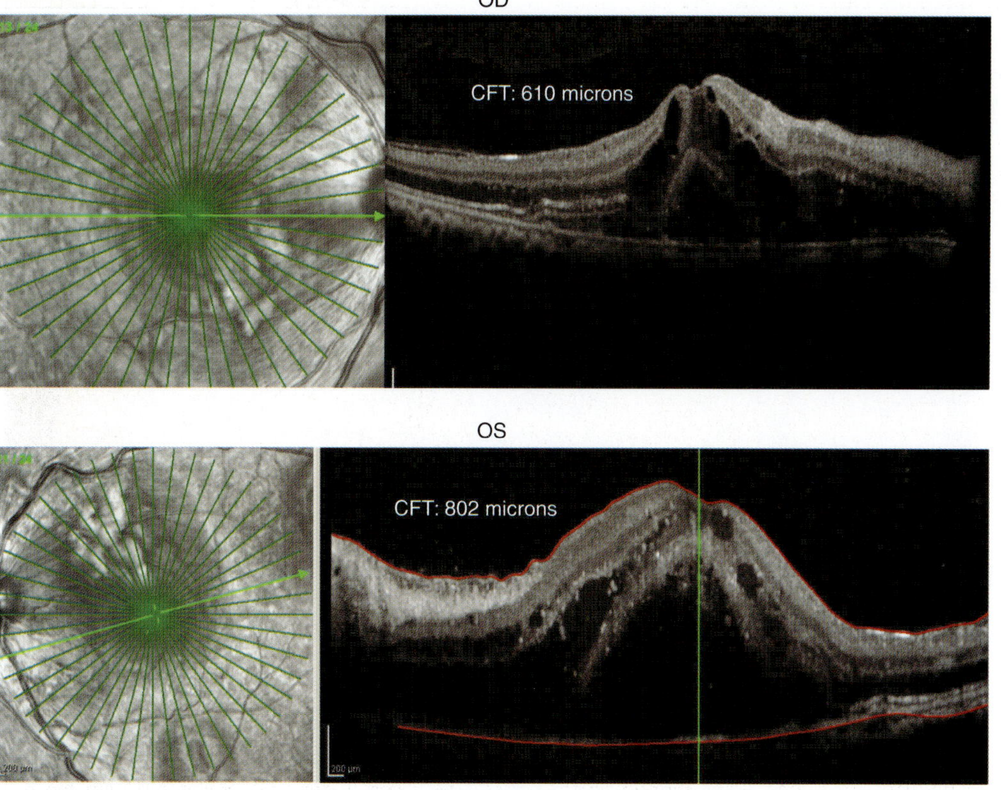

Fig. 71.3 SD-OCT showing subfoveal subretinal fluid and intraretinal cystoid spaces, more in OS than in OD.

Uncontrolled hypertension leads to sustained ischemic damage to retinal pigment epithelium, causing fluid to leak from choroid into subretinal space. Without the presence of barriers or tight cell junctions in the neural retina, the fluid moves easily through retinal tissue and accumulates in it, thereby producing retinal edema.

The patient's blood pressure was uncontrolled at 220/124 mmHg. Laboratory tests revealed renal dysfunction with elevated levels of serum creatinine (3.5 mg/dL) and blood urea nitrogen (45 g/dL). He was referred to an internist for systemic management of his uncontrolled blood pressure.

Two months later, his blood pressure was normal at 126/80 mmHg. His best-corrected visual acuity was 6/12, N8 in both eyes. Fundus examination showed resolution of serous detachment with retinal pigment epithelial changes at fovea, decreased hemorrhages, and cotton-wool spots.

DISCUSSION

The presence of retinopathy acts as an indication for more aggressive management of the associated cardiovascular risk factors and hence plays a role in decision making by the internist (for example, antihypertensive and antiplatelet aggregation).

Along with routine fundus photographs, it is useful to document resolution of macular serous detachments with serial optical coherence tomography (OCT) scans. This allows the ophthalmologist to guide the internist in his management and follow-up.

FURTHER READING

1. Hayreh SS, Servais GE, Virdi PM: Macular lesions in malignant arterial hypertension. *Ophthalmologica* 198:230–246, 1989.
2. Wong TY, Mitchell P: Hypertensive retinopathy. *N Engl J Med* 351:2310–2317, 2004.
3. Rogers AH: Hypertensive retinopathy. In Yanoff M, Duker JS, editors. *Ophthalmology*, ed 2, St. Louis: Mosby: 849–853, 2004.
4. Gallasch G, Ritz E: The fundus in malignant hypertension. *Nephrol Dial Transplant* 12:1518–1519, 1997.
5. Suzuki M, Minamoto A, Yamane K, et al.: Malignant hypertensive retinopathy studied with optical coherence tomography. *Retina* 25:383–384, 2005.

Idiopathic Polypoidal Choroidal Vasculopathy

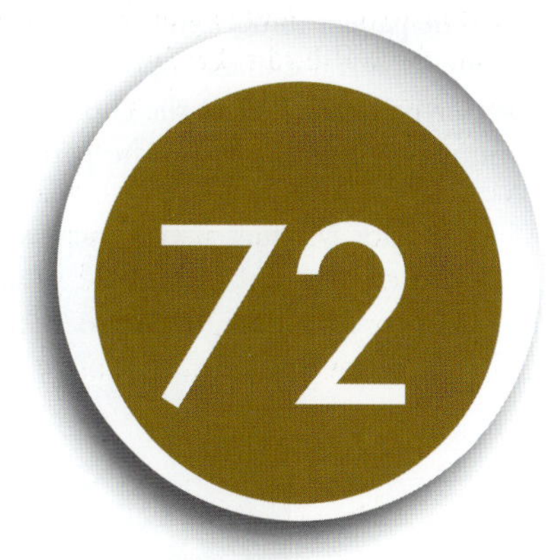

Naresh Kumar Yadav and VP Poonkodi

Idiopathic polypoidal choroidal vasculopathy (IPCV) was first described in 1982 as a cause of recurrent hemorrhagic and exudative pigment epithelial and neurosensory retinal detachments. IPCV is characterized by an abnormal vascular branching network originating from the inner choroidal plexus, which terminates in a spheroidal polyp-like lesion. These polyps are clinically described as reddish-orange subretinal nodules with a preponderance to the temporal juxtapapillary region.

Typical IPCV fundus fluorescein angiography (FFA) reveals a stippled hyperfluorescence in the region of the polyps in the early stage of the angiogram, which increases in intensity and may become fuzzy in the late films. Indocyanine green (ICG) angiogram is essential for detecting the choroidal network of vessels and polyps. Polyps may not be seen in the early phase of ICG. In the midphase they are seen to appear usually in clusters at the termination of the choroidal network of vessels. Late-phase angiogram shows either a washout of dye from the polyp with staining of its walls or may show retention of dye within the polyp with leakage into surrounding tissue.

Optical coherence tomography (OCT) through the IPCV lesions shows a characteristic hyperreflectivity in the choroidal layers. Using the OCT, Lijima et al. reported that the polyps had their own distinct patterns distinct from that of choroidal neovascular membrane (CNM), protruding anteriorly, and raising the overlying neurosensory retina.

Laser photocoagulation of polyps, surrounding areas of leakage, and retinal pigment epithelial detachments (RPED) leads to rapid resorption of the fluid. IPCV can lead to significant visual loss, particularly when blood is subfoveal. Treatment for predominantly hemorrhagic lesions (IPCV) include photodynamic therapy (PDT), pneumatic displacement of subretinal blood, vitrectomy, and subretinal drainage with fluid–gas exchange, and antivascular endothelial growth factor (anti-VEGF), either alone or in combination with the above mentioned.

CASE STUDY

A 67-year-old lady presented with complaints of sudden decrease in vision since 2 weeks in the right eye. She gave history of poor vision in the left eye since 2 years. On examination, her best-corrected visual acuity (BCVA) was 6/12 and 6/36 in the right and left eyes, respectively. The fundus examination of the right eye showed hemorrhagic pigment epithelial detachment superior to the fovea and subretinal fluid involving the center of the fovea. The left eye showed a scar involving the macula.

The patient underwent FFA, ICG, and OCT. The ICG showed polyps underneath the pigment epithelial detachment. Spectral-domain optical coherence tomography (SD-OCT) showed RPEDs with subretinal fluid (SRF) and hyperreflectivity of the choroidal layers (**Fig. 72.1**). The patient was advised photodynamic therapy (PDT) and intravitreal ranibizumab. The patient responded well to one sitting of PDT and three injections of ranibizumab.

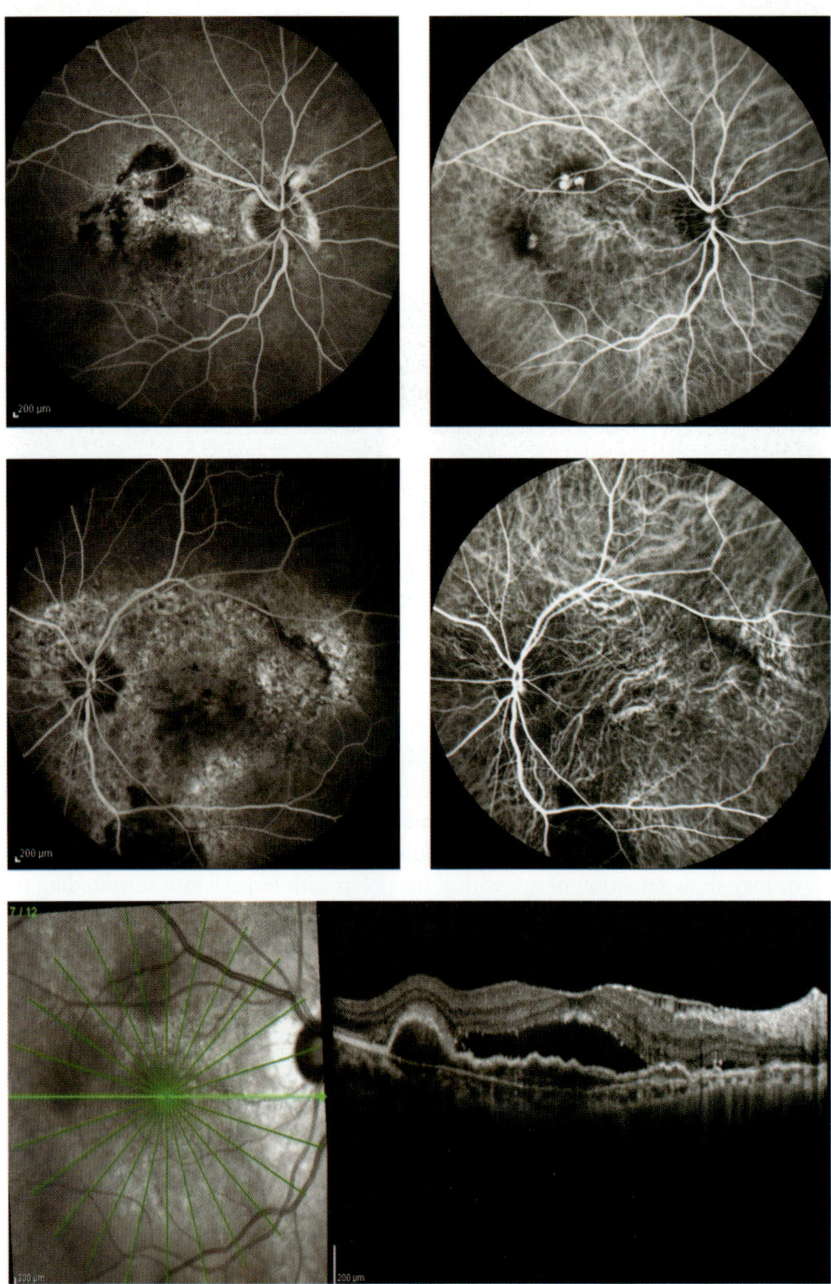

Fig. 72.1 Pretreatment FFA and ICG: OD—The FFA (*top*) showing stippled hyperfluorescence with areas of blocked fluorescence corresponding to the RPED and subretinal blood. The ICG picture shows a group of polyps temporal and superior to the center of the fovea. OS—The FFA (*middle*) showing diffuse retinal pigment epithelial changes and central scarring. The ICG shows baring of the large choroidal vessels. SD-OCT: OD (*bottom*) shows loss of foveal contour, RPEDs, choroidal hyperreflectivity suggestive of polyps, subretinal fluid, and epiretinal membrane.

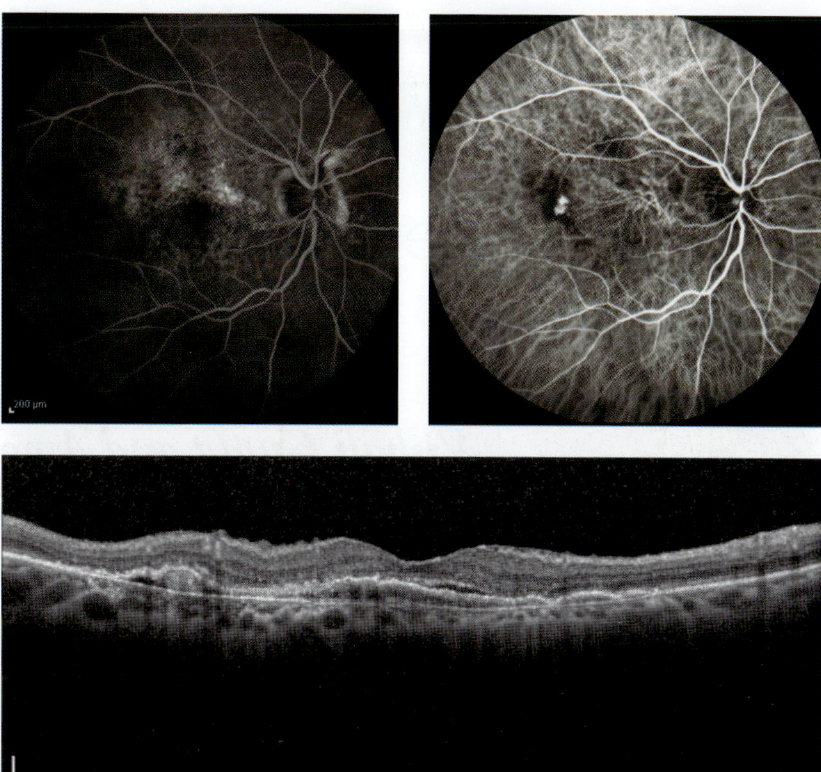

Fig. 72.2 Post-treatment: FFA and ICG: OD—The FFA and ICG (*above*) after 3 months of PDT and three injections of Ranibizumab showing resolution of one group of PCV that was located superior to the foveal center. SD-OCT (Post-treatment): OD—The SD-OCT (*below*) showing marked reduction in the subretinal fluid and RPED. The foveal contour has also improved.

Post-treatment FFA/ICG and SD-OCT showed resolution of leaks superior to the fovea and a marked reduction of pigment epithelial detachments (PEDs) with subretinal fluid (**Fig. 72.2**) with an improvement in vision.

FURTHER READING

1. Yannuzzi LA, Sorenson J, Spaide RF, et al.: Idiopathic polypoidal choroidal vasculopathy (IPCV). *Retina* 10(1)–8.81-8:1990.
2. Yannuzzi LA, Ciardella A, Spaide RF, et al.: The expanding clinical spectrum of idiopathic polypoidal choroidal vasculopathy. *Arch Ophthalmol* 115478–115485, 1997.
3. Yannuzzi LA, Wong DWK, Sforzolini BS, et al.: Polypoidal choroidal vasculopathy and neovascularized age-related macular degeneration. *Arch Ophthalmol* 1171503–1171510, 1999.
4. Spaide RF, Yannuzzi LA, Slakter JS, et al.: Indocyanine green videoangiography of idiopathic polypoidal choroidal vasculopathy. *Retina* 15100–15110, 1995.
5. Iijima H, Imai M, Gohdo T, et al: Optical coherence tomography of idiopathic polypoidal choroidal vasculopathy. *Am J Ophthalmol* 127301–127305, 1999.
6. Iijima H, Iida T, Imai M, et al.: Optical coherence tomography of orange-red subretinal lesions in eyes with idiopathic polypoidal choroidal vasculopathy. *Am J Ophthalmol* 12921–12926, 2000.

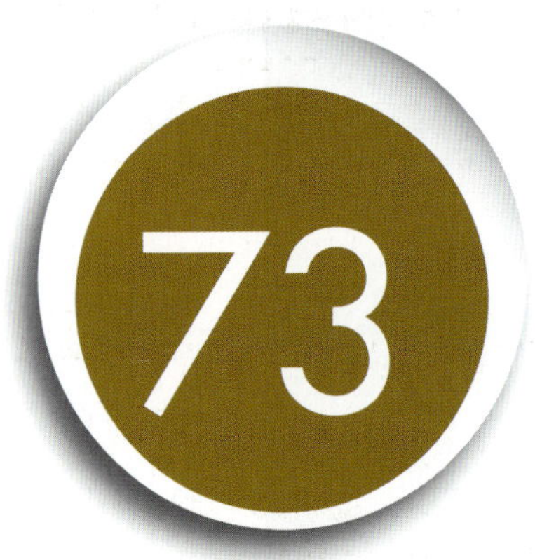

Juxtafoveal Telangiectasia: Retinal Angiomatous Proliferation

Vishali Gupta and Amod Gupta

Juxtafoveal telangiectasia (JFT) is further subgrouped as:

Group 1A: Unilateral congenital parafoveal telangiectasis: These patients suffer from a localized mild form of focal telangiectasia with the presence of yellow, lipid-rich exudation at the outer margin of the area of telangiectasis.

Group 1B: Unilateral, idiopathic, focal juxtafoveal telangiectasis: These are middle-aged men having exudation from a minute area of capillary telangiectasis, generally within 2 clock hours or less at the edge of the foveal avascular zone.

Group 2A: Bilateral, idiopathic, acquired parafoveal telangiectasis: This is seen in the fifth–sixth decade of life and involves both the sexes equally. It has five stages:

Stage 1: No biomicroscopic abnormality. Fluorescein angiography shows minimal or no capillary dilatation in the early phase and mild staining in the late phase.

Stage 2: Slight retinal graying with minimal or absent telangiectatic vessels. Fluorescein angiography shows mild capillary telangiectasis.

Stage 3: Clinically shows parafoveolar dilated and blunted retinal venules and refractile deposits. Fluorescein angiography shows capillary dilation with leak in the outer retina.

Stage 4: In this stage, stellate foci of black retinal pigment epithelium (RPE) hypertrophy are seen at the posterior end of retinal venules.

Stage 5: In this stage subretinal neovascularization occurs in the parafoveal area. Cystoid edema and yellow exudates are seen only in subretinal neovascularization.

It is believed that telangiectasia in the capillary wall causes reduced metabolic exchange, which, in turn, causes nutritional deficiencies to retinal cells including Müller cells. This is seen as diffuse staining of fluorescein into damaged cells. Changes in the capillary bed may induce altered pattern of venous flow, resulting clinically in the formation of right-angled venules. This further leads to degeneration and atrophy of these cells with overlying photoreceptors resembling a lamellar macular hole. This causes RPE cells to migrate along right-angled venules and form hyperplastic black plaques. Finally new vessels proliferate in the subretinal space and form type-II choroidal neovascular membrane. These new vessels are believed to be retinal rather than choroidal; thus are also termed retinal angiomatous proliferation (RAP).

Group 2B: Juvenile occult familial idiopathic JFT.

Groups 3A and 3B are rare and thus not discussed here.

The diagnosis of JFT is essentially based on fluorescein angiography that helps in the grouping and staging of the disease. Optical coherence tomography (OCT) showed following features in JFT:

1. OCT shows hyporeflective spaces in the inner or outer retina in stages 2 and 3 of Group 2A JFT. These spaces probably represent atrophy of Müller's cells. Loss of tissue may result in internal limiting membrane draping across the foveola due to loss of underlying tissue.
2. There maybe loss or disruption of photoreceptor layer.
3. There maybe intraretinal deposits of plaques/pigment.
4. OCT is helpful in depicting cystoid spaces and neovascular membranes in the retina. The neovascularization in JFT is believed to be due to proliferation of retinal new vessels called RAP.

CASE STUDY

A 32-year-old woman was seen with complaints of decreased vision in both eyes. Fundoscopy of the right eye showed type 2A, stage 3 JFT with parafoveal discoloration of the retina (Fig. 73.1). Fluorescein angiogram showed capillary telangiectasia (Fig. 73.2) with extravasation of dye in the late phase (Fig. 73.3). Raster line scan passing through the fovea showed small hyporeflective spaces within the neurosensory retina with ILM draping over the foveola (Fig. 73.4).

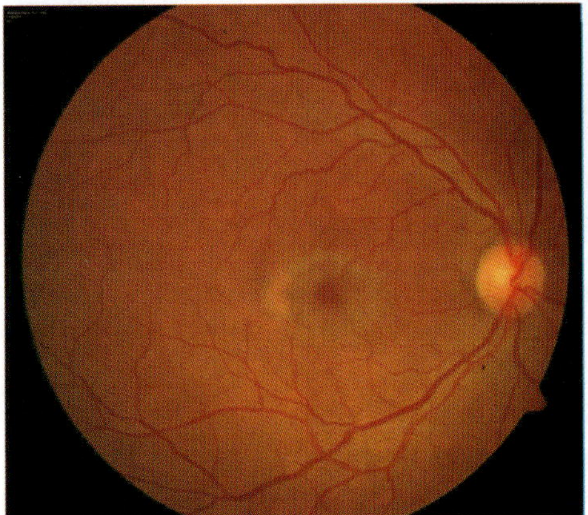

Fig. 73.1 Color fundus photograph of the right eye shows type 2A, stage 3 JFT with parafoveal discoloration of retina.

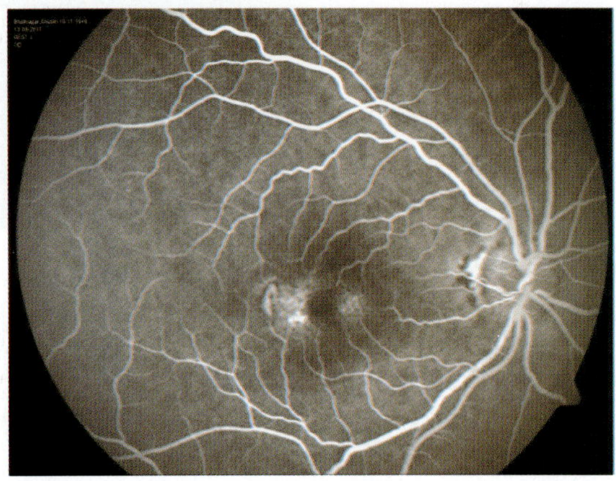

Fig. 73.2 Fluorescein angiogram of the right eye shows parafoveal capillary telangiectasia during dye transit.

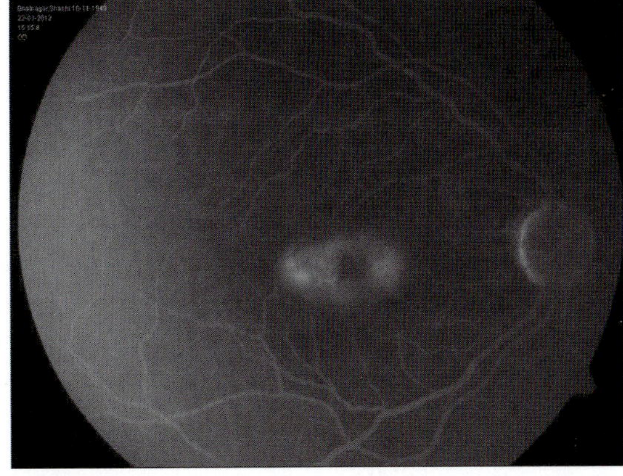

Fig. 73.3 Late phase fluorescein angiogram of the right eye shows extravasation of the dye.

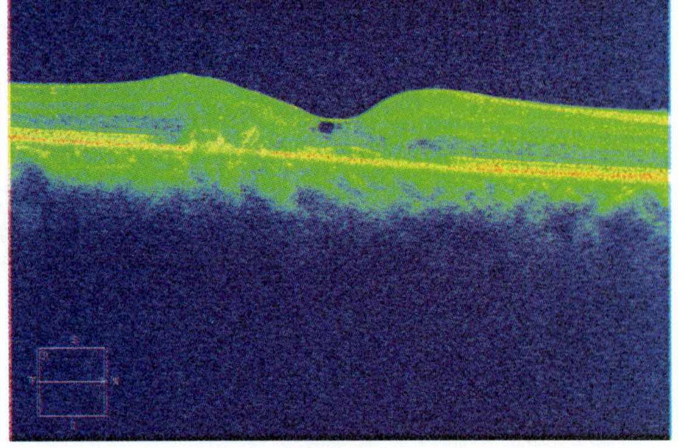

Fig. 73.4 Raster line scan passing through the fovea in the right eye shows small hyporeflective spaces within neurosensory retina with ILM draping over the foveola.

Another line scan passing just above the fovea too showed these hyporeflective spaces (Fig. 73.5). OCT thickness map did not show any increase in thickness (Fig. 73.6).

The patient was kept under follow-up. She complained of blurred vision in this eye 4 months later. Fundoscopy now showed retinal hemorrhage nasal to the fovea, suggesting development of RAP (stage 5) (Fig. 73.7).

Fundus fluorescein angiogram of the right eye showed blocked fluorescence corresponding to retinal hemorrhage (Fig. 73.8), with extravasation of dye from telangiectatic vessels seen temporal to the fovea in the late phase (Fig. 73.9). Repeat raster line scan showed increased retinal thickening with intraretinal fluid accumulation nasal to the fovea (Fig. 73.10), and disrupted retinal pigment epithelium layer with irregular inner segment–outer segment

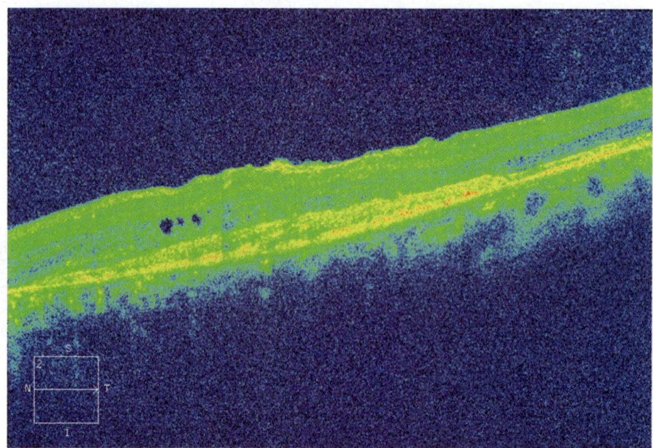

Fig. 73.5 Raster line scan of the right eye passing just above the fovea shows hyporeflective spaces.

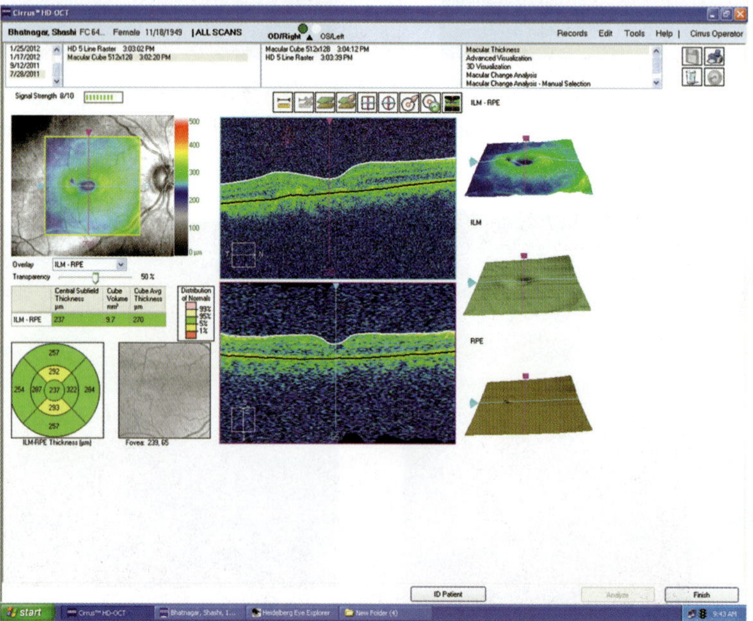

Fig. 73.6 Optical coherence tomography thickness map of the right eye does not show any increase in thickness.

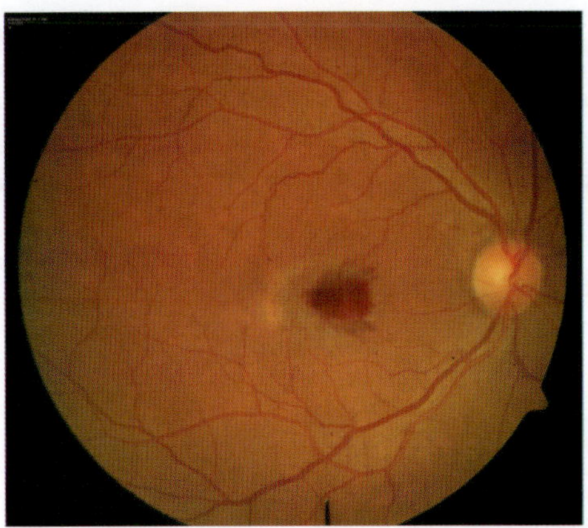

Fig. 73.7 Color fundus photograph of the right eye shows retinal hemorrhage nasal to the fovea suggesting development of retinal angiomatous proliferans.

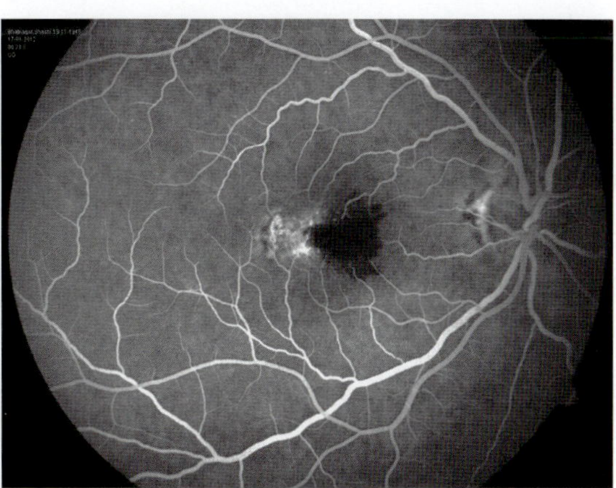

Fig. 73.8 Fundus fluorescein angiogram of the right eye shows blocked fluorescence corresponding to retinal hemorrhage.

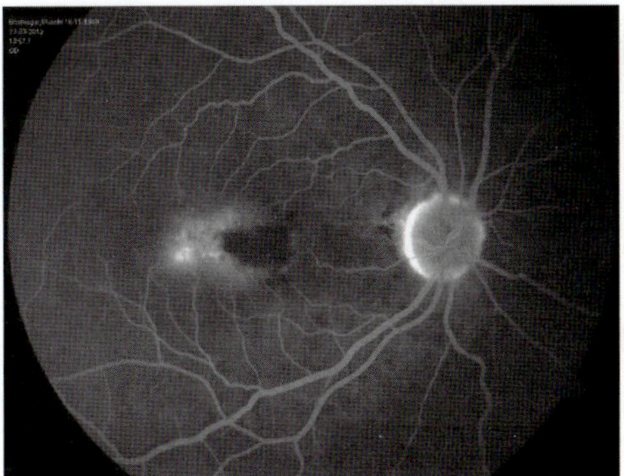

Fig. 73.9 Late phase fluorescein angiogram of the right eye shows extravasation of dye from telangiectatic vessels seen temporal to the fovea.

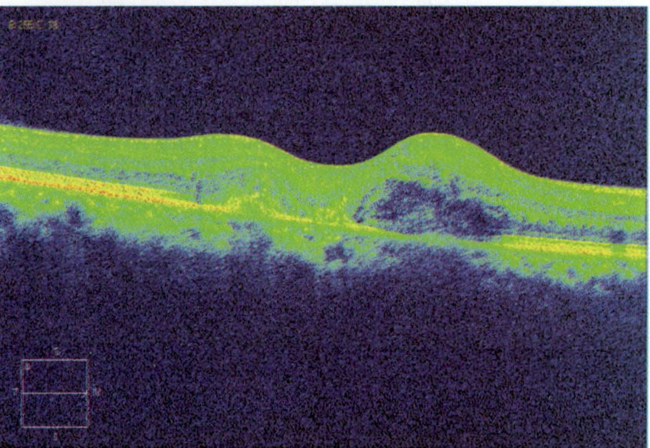

Fig. 73.10 Repeat raster line scan of the right eye shows increased retinal thickening with intraretinal fluid accumulation nasal to the fovea.

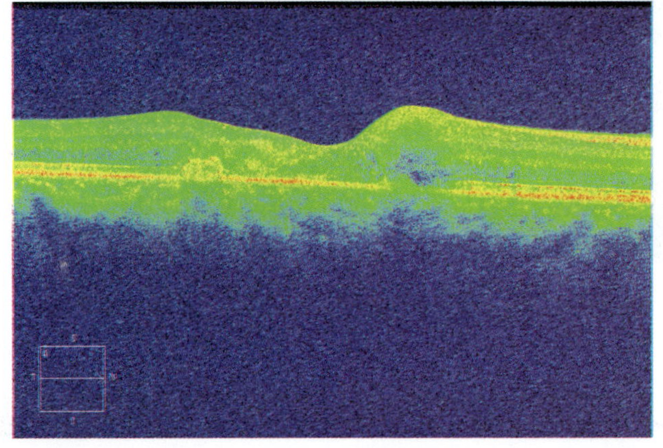

Fig. 73.11 Optical coherence tomography raster line scan of the right eye shows disrupted IS–OS junction.

(IS–OS) junction (**Fig. 73.11**). The retinal thickness map now showed an increased retinal thickness in the nasal quadrant (**Fig. 73.12**). Macular-thickness-change analysis showed an increase in retinal thickness compared to the previous visit (**Fig. 73.13**).

Her best-corrected visual acuity was 20/400 in the left eye that showed stage-5 JFT with development of neovascular membrane scar most likely due to development of RAP (**Fig. 73.14**) that was confirmed on fluorescein angiography

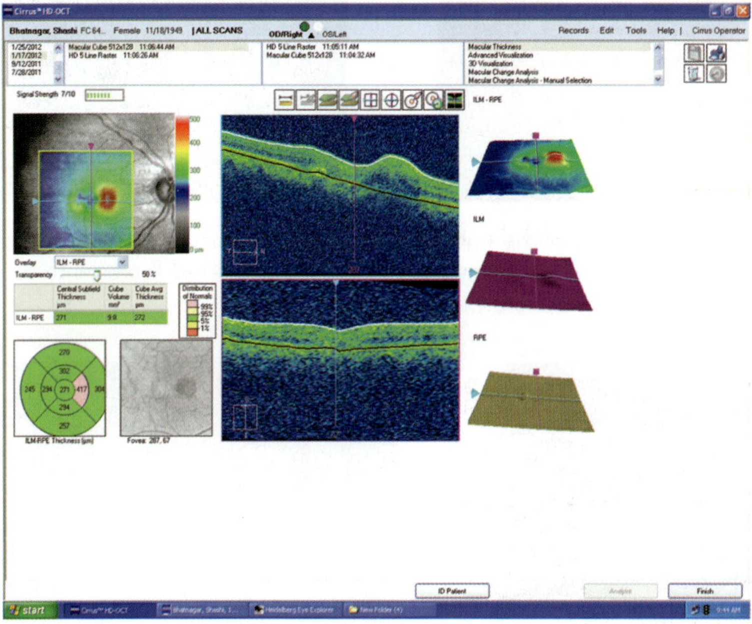

Fig. 73.12 The retinal thickness map of the right eye now shows an increased retinal thickness in the nasal quadrant.

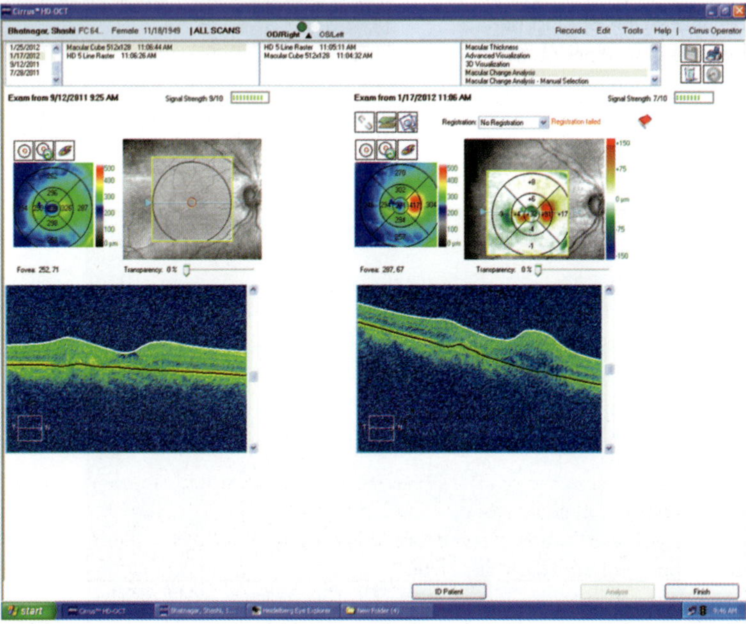

Fig. 73.13 Macular-thickness-change analysis shows an increase in retinal thickness compared to the previous visit.

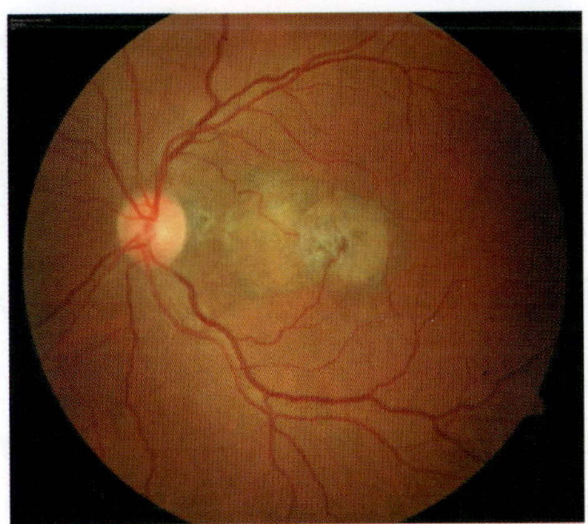

Fig. 73.14 Color fundus photograph of the left eye shows stage-5 JFT with development of neovascular membrane scar most likely due to development of RAP.

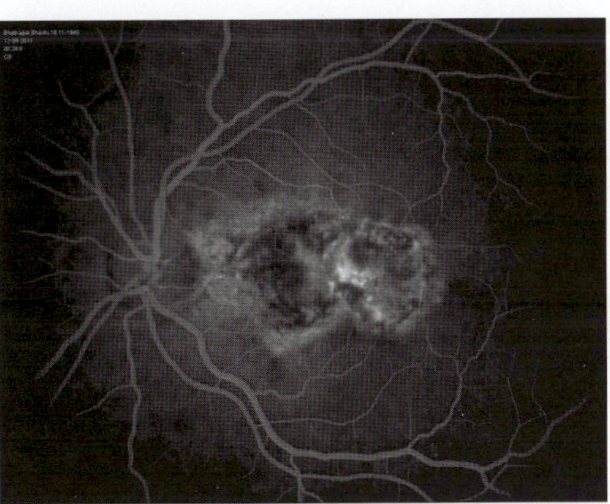

Fig. 73.15 Fundus fluorescein angiogram of the left eye during dye transit shows a window defect.

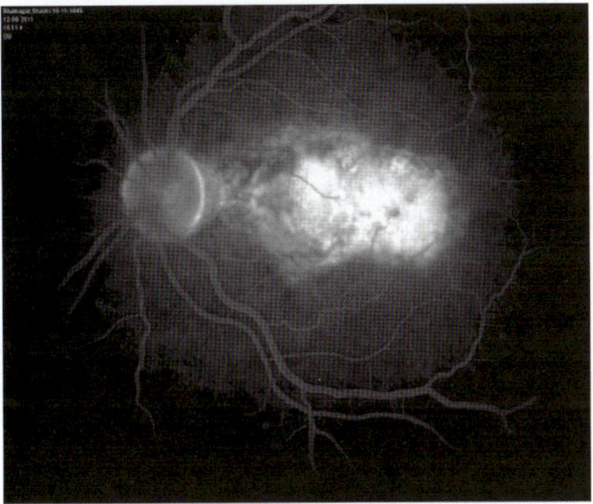

Fig. 73.16 Late phase fluorescein angiogram of the left eye shows staining of the scar.

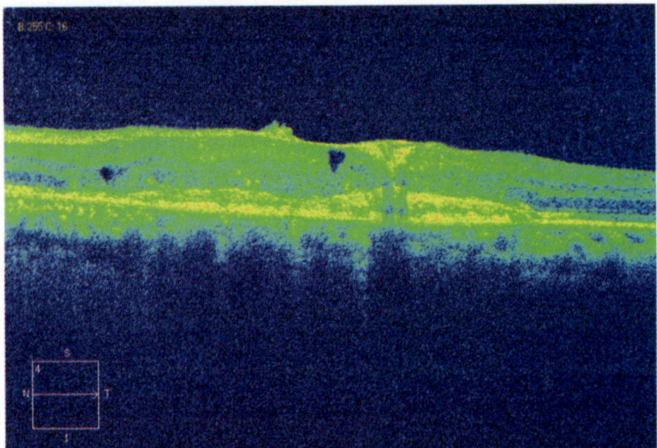

Fig. 73.17 The OCT line scan of the left eye shows moderately reflective spindle-shaped scar with no fluid and pigment migration into the inner layers of retina. Additionally, small hyporeflective spaces too are seen.

(**Figs 73.15 and 73.16**). The OCT line scan showed moderately reflective spindle-shaped scar with no fluid and pigment migration into the inner layers of retina. Additionally, small hyporeflective spaces too were seen (**Fig. 73.17**).

FURTHER READING

1. Paunescu LA, Ko TH, Duker JS, et al.: Idiopathic juxtafoveal retinal telangiectasis: new findings by ultrahigh-resolution optical coherence tomography. *Ophthalmology* 113:48–57, 2006.
2. Gupta V, Gupta A, Dogra MR, et al.: Optical coherence tomography in Group 2A idiopathic juxtafoveolar telangiectasis. *Ophthalmic Surg Lasers Imaging* 36:482–486, 2005.
3. Agarwal A (ed) Gass' Atlas of Macular diseases, ed 5, Elsevier Saunders, 522–532.
4. Gupta V, Gupta A, Dogra MR: Atlas Optical Coherence Tomography of Macular Diseases and Glaucoma, ed 4. JP Medical Publishers 360–381.

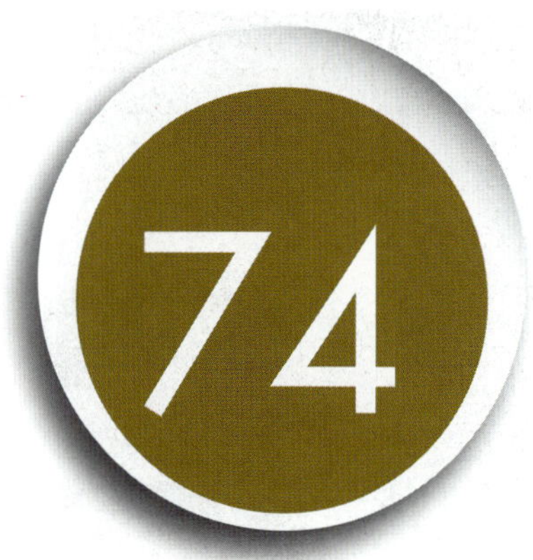

Juxtafoveal Telangiectasia: Type 2A

*Santosh Gopi Krishna and
Naresh Kumar Yadav*

Idiopathic juxtafoveolar telangiectasis [idiopathic parafoveal, perifoveal, or macular telangiectasia or telangiectasis (IJFT)] is characterized by the presence of an area of ectatic and incompetent retinal capillaries in the foveolar region in the absence of other known causes for retinal telangiectasis. *Reese* first defined the term *retinal telangiectasis* in 1956. In 1982, *Gass and Oyakawa* defined idiopathic juxtafoveal telangiectasis (IJFT). Classification and staging of IJFT was based on clinical and fluorescein angiographic findings. In 1993, *Gass and Blodi* examined 140 such cases seen at the Bascom Palmer Eye Institute, Miami, over a 28-year period and further classified these entities into three distinct groups I, II, and III with two subgroups in each (A and B) and five stages in group IIA. Group I was unilateral, congenital, and predominantly in males with telangiectasis and macular edema. Group II was commonest with acquired bilateral telangiectasis along with neovascular membrane and atrophy of the fovea. Group III was extremely rare and characterized by progressive obliteration of perifoveal capillary network. In 2006, Yannuzzi, et al. proposed a simplified classification of IJFT based on the Gass–Blodi model. They proposed the term *"idiopathic macular telangiectasia"* with two distinct types: type 1 or "aneurysmal telangiectasia" and type 2 or "perifoveal telangiectasia" equivalent to IJFT Group IIA. The remaining types described by Gass and Blodi (Groups IIB, IIIA, and IIIB) were omitted due to rarity. Various treatment modalities have been described for treatment of macular edema and associated neovascular membrane (NVM).

CASE STUDY

A 51-year-old Asian Indian woman presented with blurred vision in the left eye and a best-corrected visual acuity (BCVA) of 20/25 in the right eye and 20/50 in the left eye. Ocular examination showed a normal anterior segment. Fundus examination showed graying of the parafoveal area in the right eye and in the left-eye a grayish membrane with foveal hemorrhages, and right-angled deflection of venules suggestive of NVM. A diagnosis of Group IIA IJFT with left-eye NVM was made. A fundus fluorescein angiography (FFA) revealed aneurysmal hyperfluorescence in the right eye and progressive leakage in the left eye, suggestive of NVM in the left eye (Fig. 74.1).

Spectral-domain optical coherence tomography (SD-OCT) imaging revealed right-eye focal retinal thickening with inner segment–outer segment (IS–OS) disruption and retinal pigment epithelium (RPE) clumping with no evidence of fluid/active NVM and left-eye retinal thickening with loss of foveal contour, intra and subretinal fluid suggestive of an active NVM. The patient received three injections of intravitreal bevacizumab in the left eye, following which lesion scarred and vision was maintained at 20/50.

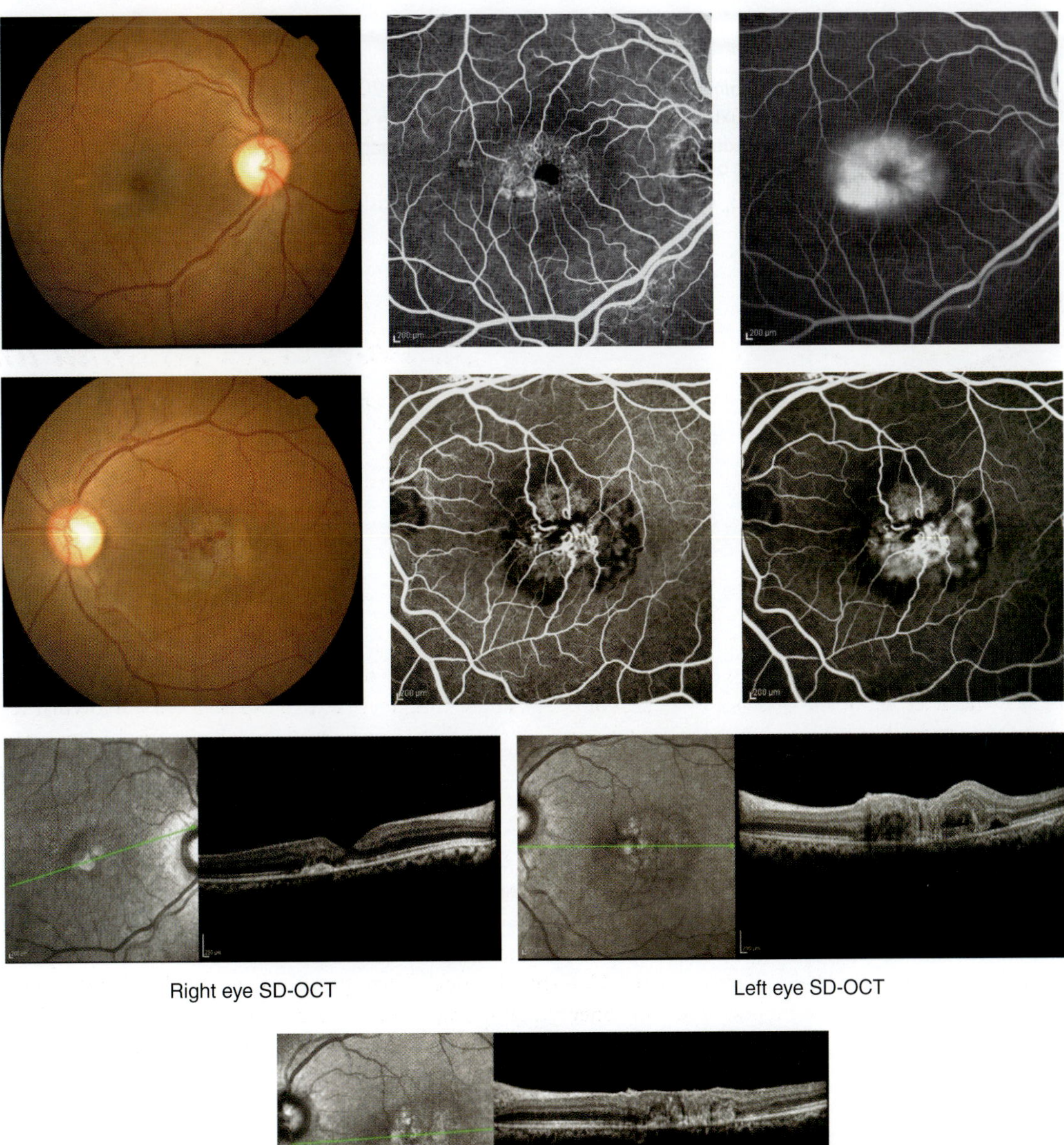

Fig. 74.1 Fundus photographs show both eyes JFT with left-eye NVM with hemorrhages. FFA-early and -late frames suggestive of right-eye aneurysmal hyperfluorescence and left-eye aneurysmal and telangiectatic dilatation and progressive leakage suggestive of NVM. SD-OCT images show right-eye RPE clumping with IS–OS disruption, foveal atrophy, and loss of foveal contour with intra- and subretinal fluid in the left eye, suggestive of NVM. A repeat SD-OCT image shows a scarred NVM after a course of intravitreal bevacizumab.

FURTHER READING

1. Yanoff M, Duker JS, Editors: *Ophthalmology* St. Louis: Mosby; 196–203, 2004.
2. Gass JD, Oyakawa RT: Idiopathic juxtafoveolar retinal telangiectasis. *Arch Ophthalmol* 100:769–780, 1982.
3. Gass JD, Blodi BA: Idiopathic juxtafoveolar retinal telangiectasis. Update of classification and follow-up study. *Ophthalmology* 100:1536–1546, 1993.
4. Yannuzzi LA, Bardal AM, Freund KB, et al.: Idiopathic macular telangiectasia. *Arch Ophthalmol* 124:450–460, 2006.

Macroaneurysm

Manish Nagpal and Navneet Mehrotra

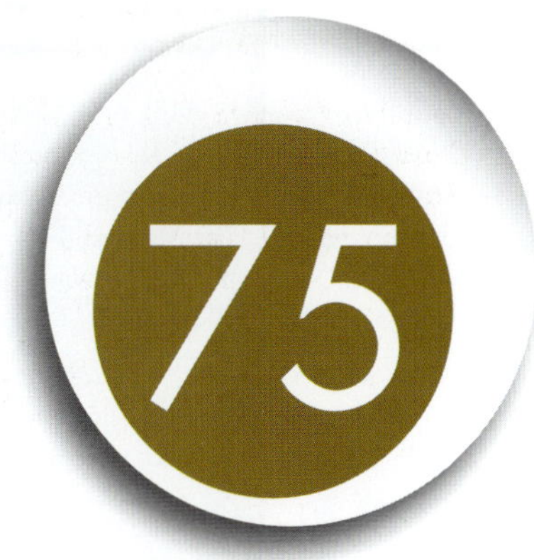

Retinal arterial macroaneurysm is a localized fusiform or saccular dilatation of a retinal arterial vessel within the first three orders of bifurcation. Diameter of a macroaneurysm exceeds 100 microns. Multiple aneurysms are common, occurring in approximately 20% of affected eyes. These are associated with exudation and hemorrhage, which may result in decreased visual acuity if it involves the central macula.

CASE STUDY

A 64-year-old Asian Indian male came with a hemorrhage of around 3 disc diameter at the posterior pole of the right eye with asteroid hyalosis (Fig. 75.1). Best-corrected vision in the right eye was counting fingers 2 meters. Patient

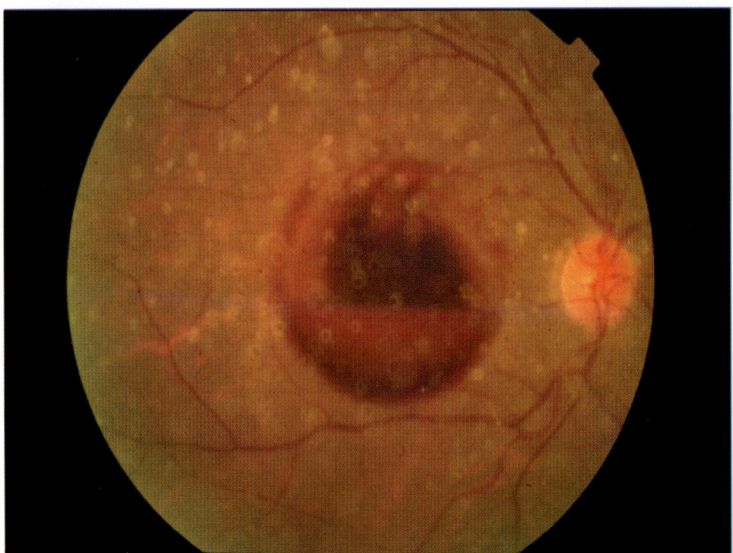

Fig. 75.1 Right eye fundus photograph imaged on TOPCON TRC-50DX showing bright-red blood settled in the inferior half of the lesion and dark-red blood in the center with asteroid hyalosis.

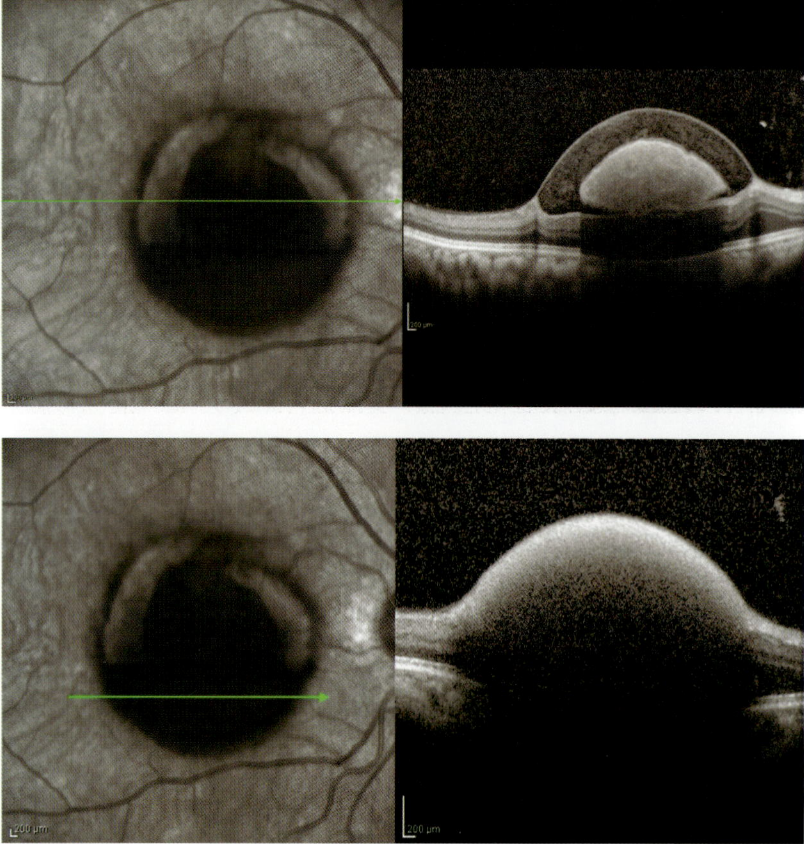

Fig. 75.2 Horizontal SD-OCT scan imaged using the SPECTRALIS™ (Heidelberg Engineering) showing sub-internal limiting membrane (ILM) hemorrhage in the scan passing through the upper part of the hemorrhage and boat-shaped subhyaloid hemorrhage in the lower part.

had no systemic illness. Patient underwent spectral-domain optical coherence tomography (SD-OCT) (**Fig. 75.2**), fundus fluorescein angiography (FFA), and indocyanine green (ICG) angiography (**Fig. 75.3**).

The patient had a boat-shaped subhyaloid hemorrhage and subinternal limiting membrane hemorrhage measuring approximately 2 disc diameters at the macula. Fluorescein angiography showed two saccular lesions along the superior arcade suggestive of macroaneurysm. We treated the patient with focal laser photocoagulation to the lesions and intravitreal gas to displace blood.

Retinal macroaneurysm occurs most commonly in the sixth to seventh decade. It is rare before the age of 60 years. Females are three times more commonly affected than males.

Two classical types of aneurysm—saccular and fusiform—affect retinal arteries. Systemic hypertension, atherosclerotic disease, and serum lipid abnormalities may contribute to formation of retinal macroaneurysms. Defects in the vessel wall, which may be sites-at-risk for the aneurysm formation, may occur in patients with focal arterial wall atheromas. Exudation and hemorrhage occur due to leakage from the aneurysm; following an acute hemorrhage, spontaneous thrombosis may lead to closure of the aneurysm. The retinal macroaneurysms may lead to vitreous hemorrhage, retinal detachment, macular holes, and choroidal neovascular membrane formation. Treatment of macroaneurysm involves direct photocoagulation to the lesion.

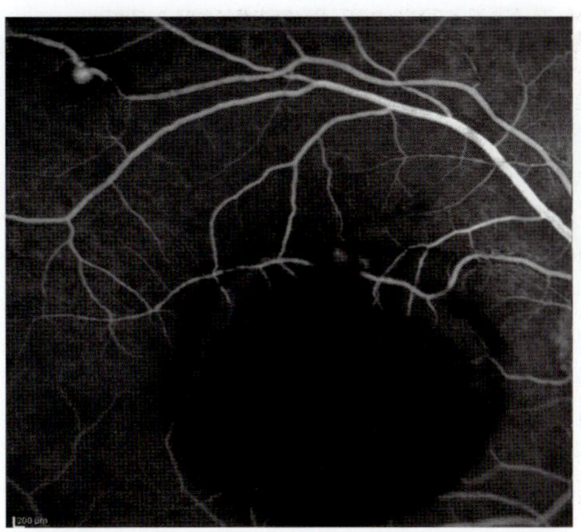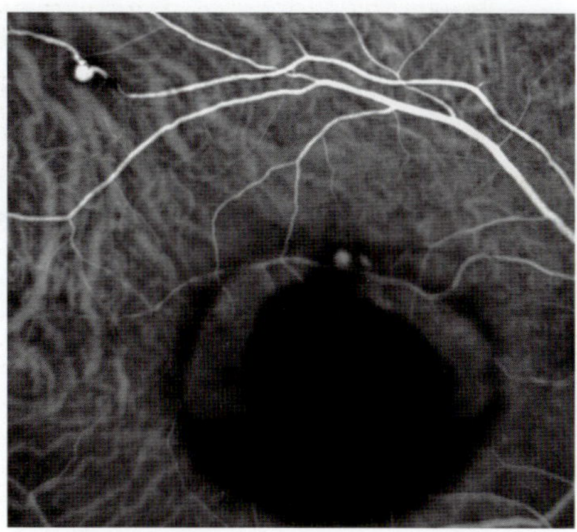

Fig. 75.3 Simultaneous FA and ICG of the patient showing blocked fluorescence corresponding to the hemorrhage and hyperfluorescent saccular lesion along the superior arcade suggestive of macroaneurysm; another similar lesion is seen in the superotemporal region.

FURTHER READING

1. Murthy K, Puri P, Talbot JF.: Retinal macroaneurysm with macular hole and subretinal neovascular membrane. *Eye* 19(4):488–489, Apr 2005.
2. Das-Bhaumik RG, Lindfield D, Quinn S, et al.: Optic disc macroaneurysm in evolution: from incidental finding to branch retinal artery occlusion and spontaneous resolution. *Br J Ophthalmol* doi: 10.1136/bjo.2008.151928, May 2009.
3. DellaCroce JT, Vitale AT.: Hypertension and the eye. *Curr Opin Ophthalmol* 19(6):493–498, Nov 2008.
4. Mitamura Y, Miyano N, Suzuki Y, et al:. Branch retinal artery occlusion associated with rupture of retinal arteriolar macroaneurysm on the optic disc. *Jpn J Ophthalmol* 49(5):428–429, Sep–Oct 2005.
5. Sato R, Yasukawa T, Hirano Y, et al.: Early-onset macular holes following ruptured retinal arterial macroaneurysms. *Graefes Arch Clin Exp Ophthalmol* 246(12):1779–1782, Dec 2008.
6. Chaum E, Greenwald MA.: Retinochoroidal anastomoses and a choroidal neovascular membrane in a macular exudate following treatment for retinal macroaneurysms. *Retina* 22(3):363–366, Jun 2002.
7. Chanana B, Azad RV.: Intravitreal bevacizumab for macular edema secondary to retinal macroaneurysm. *Eye* 23(2):493–494, Feb 2009.
8. Abdel-Khalek MN, Richardson J.: Retinal macroaneurysm: natural history and guidelines for treatment. *Br J Ophthalmol* 70(1):2–11, Jan 1986.

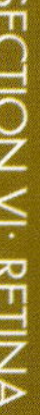

Macular Hole

Vishali Gupta and Amod Gupta

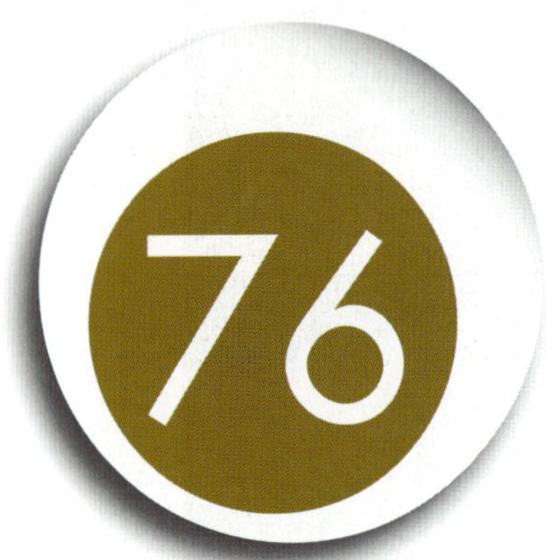

Optical coherence tomography (OCT) is useful in diagnosis and management of macular holes. It helps in differentiating full thickness from lamellar holes, macular cysts, foveal detachments of retinal pigment epithelium or neurosensory retina, and epiretinal membrane with pseudoholes. OCT helps in diagnosing vitreofoveal traction as well as progression in fellow eyes of patients with macular holes. OCT has also improved our understanding of the pathoanatomy of macular holes and has led to a revised classification of staging.

OCT has now provided evidence that presence of a localized perifoveal vitreous detachment is seen in the earliest stages of macular hole formation. Forces that initiate the formation of macular hole are currently believed to be resulting from the direct tractional effect [during development of posterior vitreous detachment (PVD)] by the vitreous on the fovea that leads to the mechanical breakdown of the integrity of the fovea. OCT has led to a new classification of macular holes as follows:

Stage 1A: Foveal pseudocyst
Stage 1B: Impending macular hole characterized by disruption of outer retina
Stage 2: Lamellar macular hole
Stage 3: Full-thickness macular hole without PVD
Stage 4: Full-thickness macular hole with PVD

OCT is also useful in following-up patients following pars plana vitrectomy (PPV). Two patterns of hole closure are seen on OCT following pars plana vitrectomy (PPV):

Type 1 closure: Close without neurosensory deficit
Type 2 closure: Close with neurosensory deficit

Alternatively, u-, v-, and w-shaped patterns of hole closure have also been described.
The smaller sized holes tend to show type 1 closure pattern, and thus have a better prognosis.

FOVEAL PSEUDOCYST

CASE STUDY 1

A 56-year-old woman was seen with full-thickness macular hole in her right eye (**Fig. 76.1**). Her left eye was showing an apparently normal-looking fundus (**Fig. 76.2**).

A horizontal OCT line scan passing through the fovea showed a perifoveal detachment of the posterior hyaloid that was still attached to the center of the foveola. An intraretinal pseudocyst was seen in the inner part of the

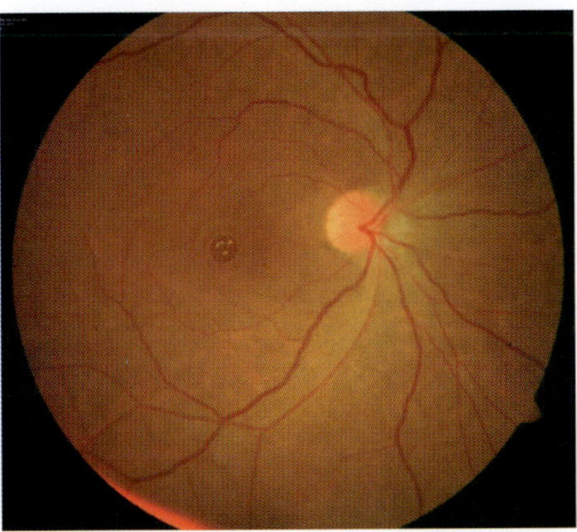

Fig. 76.1 Fundus of the right eye showing a full-thickness macular hole with a cuff of subretinal fluid.

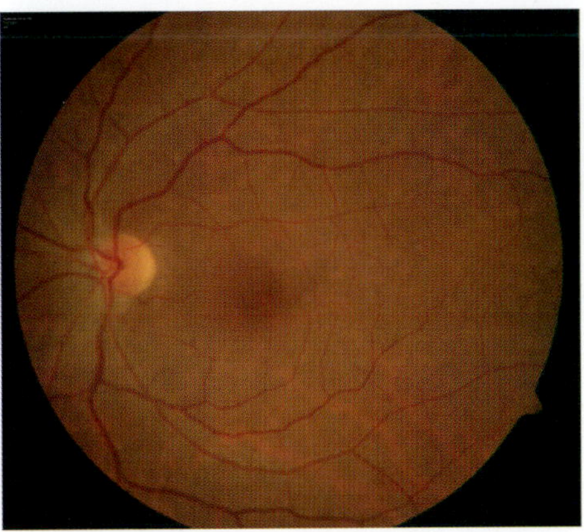

Fig. 76.2 Normal-appearing fundus of the left eye.

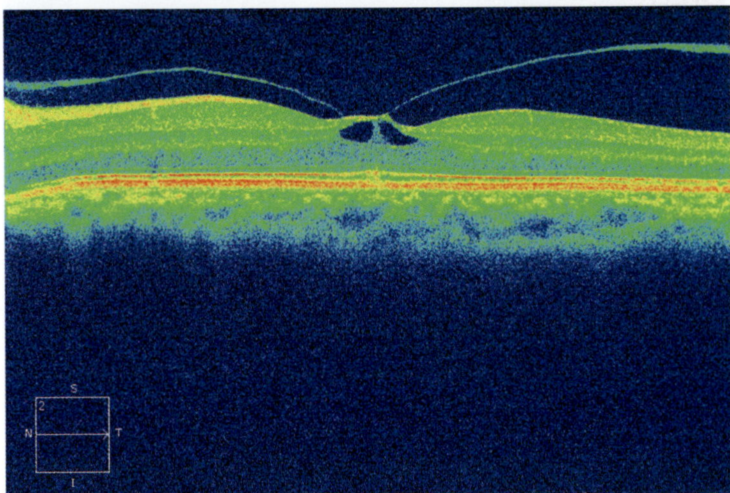

Fig. 76.3 OCT of the right eye showing perifoveal detachment of the posterior hyaloid with persistent attachment to foveola.

foveola. Focal adhesion of the vitreous to the macula leads to mechanical deformation of the fovea with pseudocyst formation (Fig. 76.3).

IMPENDING MACULAR HOLE/VITREOMACULAR TRACTION

CASE STUDY 2

A 43-year-old man complained of metamorphopsia in the right eye. Fundoscopy showed a dull foveal reflex. OCT line scan through fixation showed loss of foveal contour (Fig. 76.4). The posterior hyaloid membrane was attached to the center of the foveola. The foveal traction had resulted in disruption of the foveal pit and hyporeflectivity in the inner retinal layers with a small pocket of fluid under the fovea (Fig. 76.5). The patient underwent pars plana vitrectomy. Forty-eight hours postoperatively, the fundus (Fig. 76.6) and OCT (Fig. 76.7) showed relieved traction.

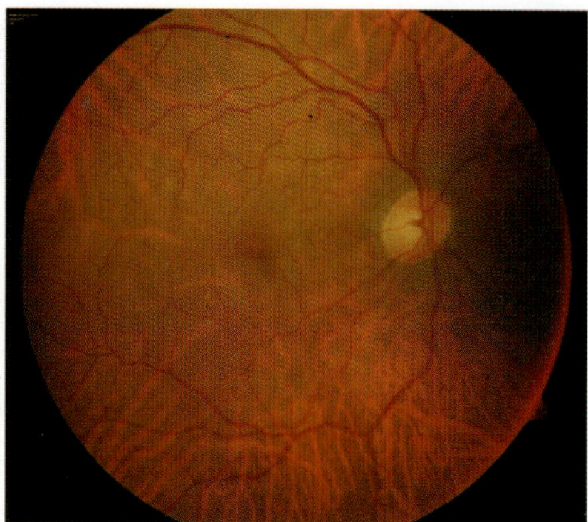

Fig. 76.4 Fundus of the right eye showing a dull foveal reflex.

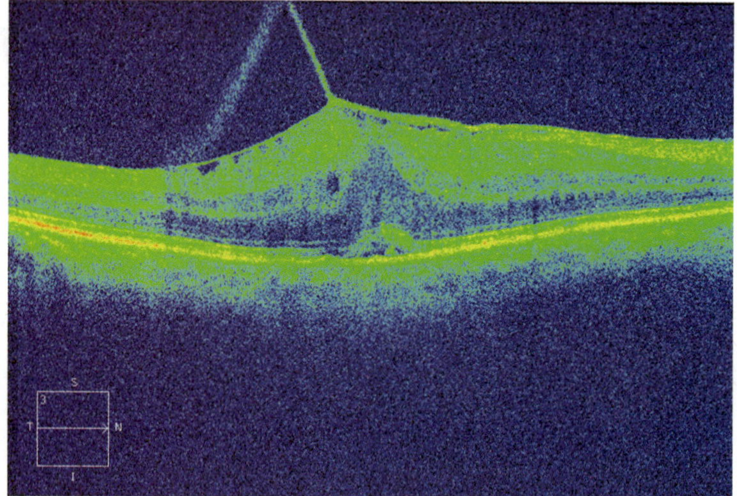

Fig. 76.5 OCT of the right eye showing foveal traction and a small pocket of subretinal fluid.

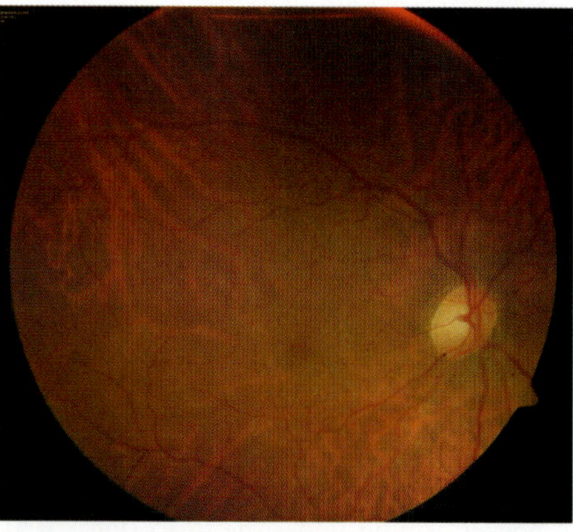

Fig. 76.6 Fundus of the right eye following pars plana vitrectomy.

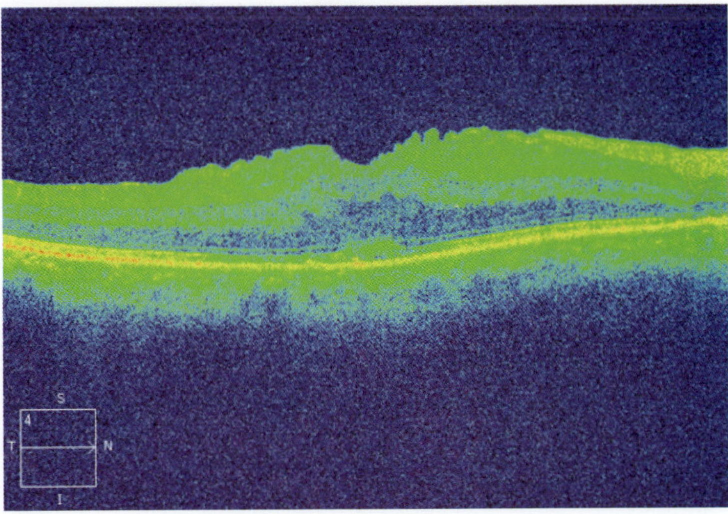

Fig. 76.7 OCT of the right eye after PPV showing complete removal of foveal traction and restoration of foveal contour.

LAMELLAR MACULAR HOLE WITH EPIRETINAL MEMBRANE

CASE STUDY 3

A 56-year-old woman was seen with epiretinal membrane and macular hole (**Fig. 76.8**). OCT line scan showed lamellar-thickness macular hole (**Fig. 76.9**). Single-layer internal limiting membrane (ILM) surface map showed wrinkling on the ILM surface with a lamellar hole in the center (**Fig. 76.10**). Three-dimensional map showed traction on the surface resulting in the development of macular hole (**Fig. 76.11**).

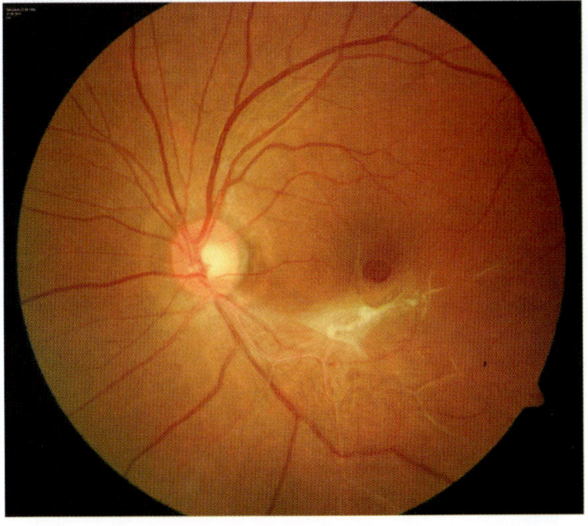

Fig. 76.8 Fundus of the left eye showing epiretinal membrane and macular hole.

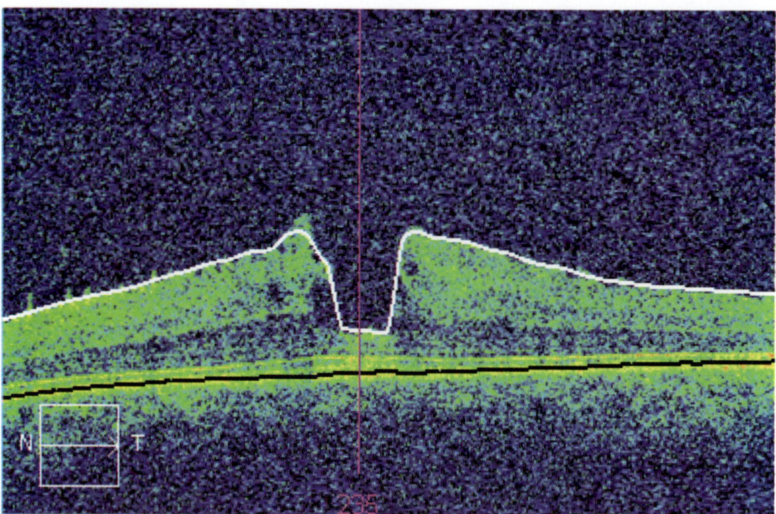

Fig. 76.9 OCT of the left eye showing lamellar macular hole.

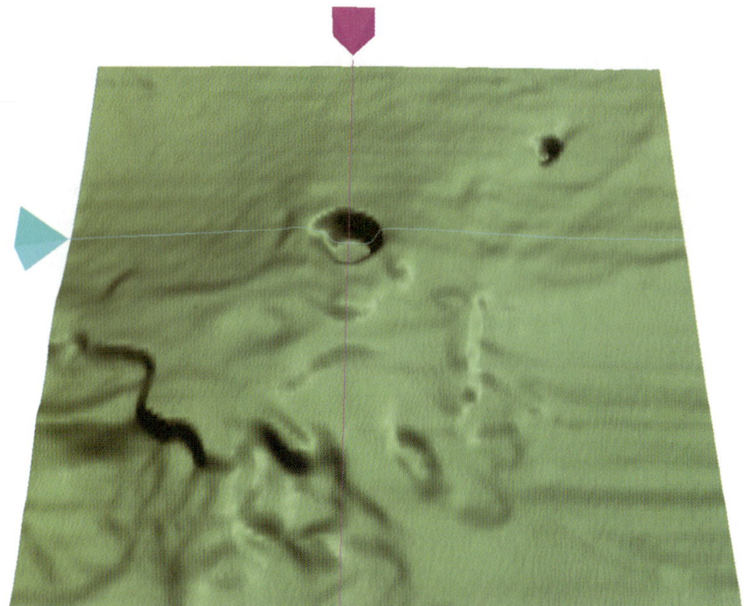

Fig. 76.10 ILM surface map showing a wrinkled ILM with a lamellar macular hole.

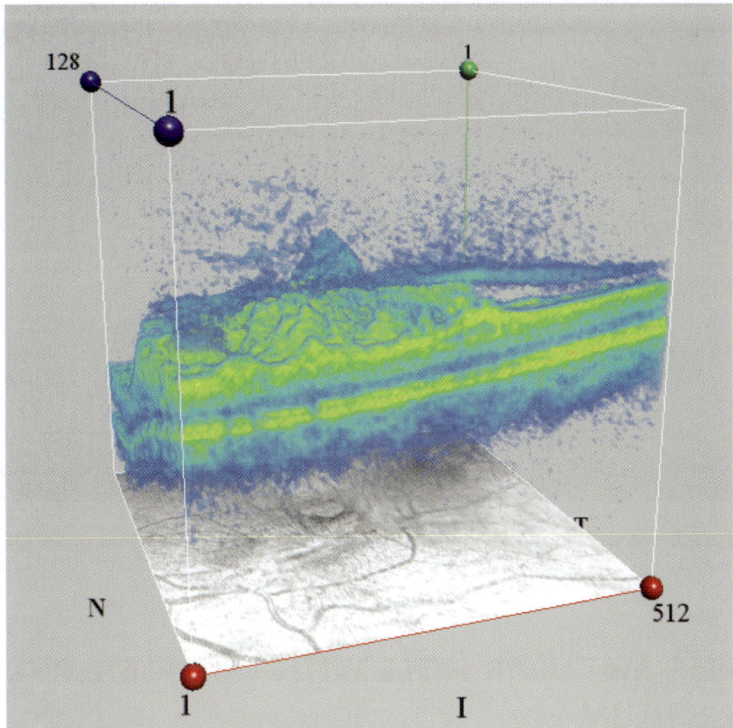

Fig. 76.11 Three-dimensional map showing surface traction.

FULL-THICKNESS MACULAR HOLE

CASE STUDY 4

A 51-year-old woman was seen with left-eye–full-thickness macular hole (**Fig. 76.12**). OCT line scan showed the full-thickness macular hole with cystoid changes at the edges of the hole. Posterior vitreous was completely detached and was seen anteriorly as a hyperreflective line (**Fig. 76.13**).

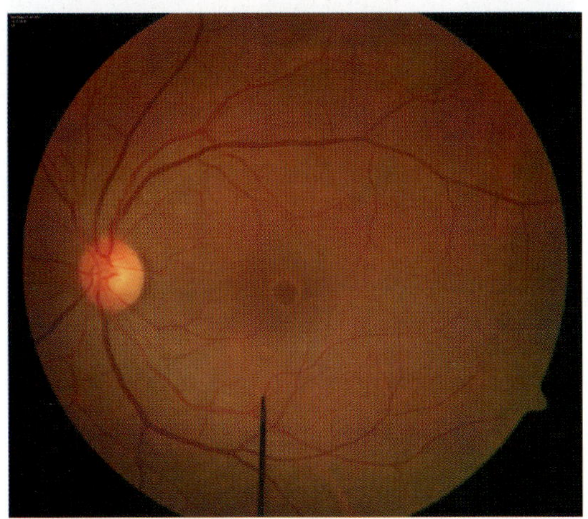

Fig. 76.12 Fundus of the left eye showing a full-thickness macular hole with a cuff of subretinal fluid.

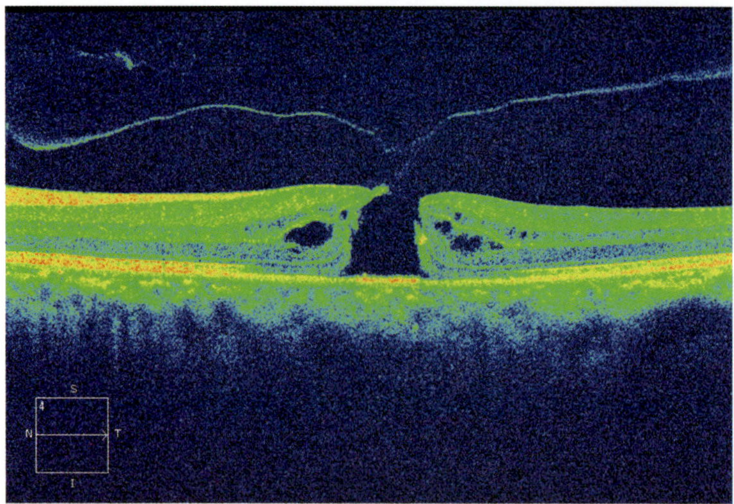

Fig. 76.13 OCT of the left eye showing the full-thickness macular hole and detached posterior hyaloid. Note cystoid changes at the edge of the hole.

FULL-THICKNESS MACULAR HOLE WITH COMPLETE PVD AND PSEUDO-OPERCULUM

CASE STUDY 5

A 78-year-old woman was seen with a full-thickness macular hole (**Fig. 76.14**). OCT raster line scan showed full-thickness large macular hole with cystoid degenerative changes at the edges of the hole. Additionally, complete PVD with a central condensed tissue was seen lying anterior to the hole (**Figs 76.15 and 76.16**).

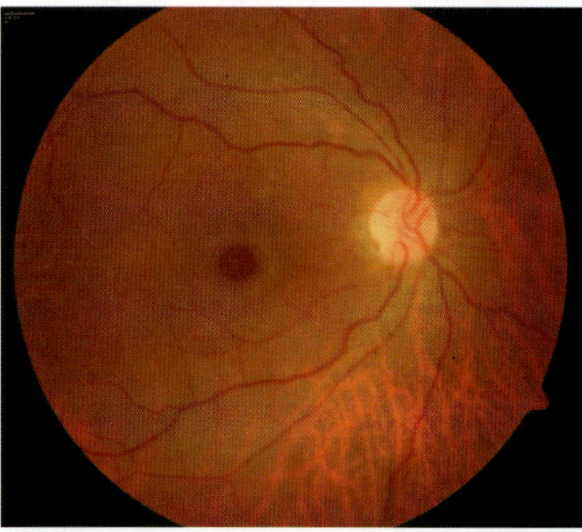

Fig. 76.14 Fundus of the right eye showing a full-thickness macular hole and a cuff of subretinal fluid.

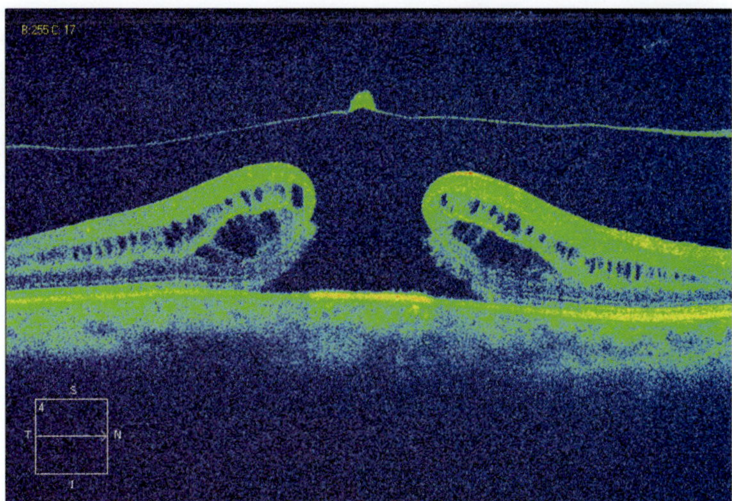

Fig. 76.15 OCT of the right eye showing the full-thickness macular hole with extensive cystoid changes at the edge. The detached posterior hyaloid is noted anterior to the hole.

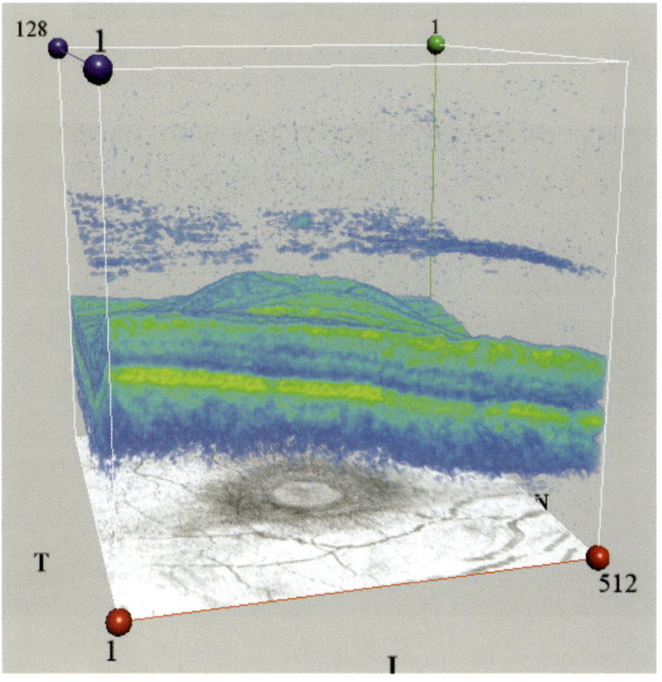

Fig. 76.16 Three-dimensional map showing PVD and macular hole.

POST-PARS PLANA VITRECTOMY HOLE CLOSURE

CASE STUDY 6

A 53-year-old man was seen with full-thickness macular hole in the left eye (Figs 76.17 and 76.18). The patient was advised surgery, but he came back 3 months later with an increase in the size of the hole as well as development of intraretinal cystoid changes at the edges of the hole (Fig. 76.19). He underwent pars plana vitrectomy with SF6 gas tamponade. Four weeks postoperatively, the hole was closed (Fig. 76.20) with restoration of the photoreceptor layer (Fig. 76.21).

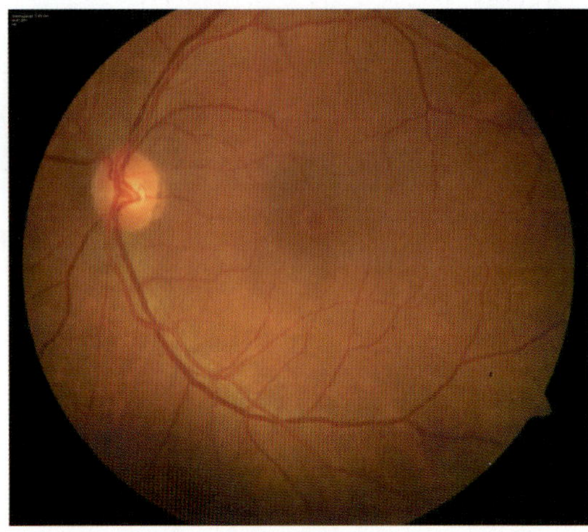

Fig. 76.17 Fundus of the left eye showing full-thickness macular hole.

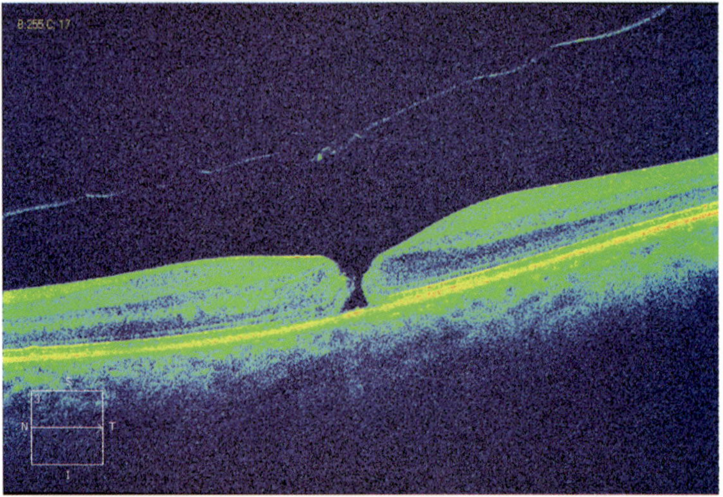

Fig. 76.18 OCT of the left eye showing the macular hole.

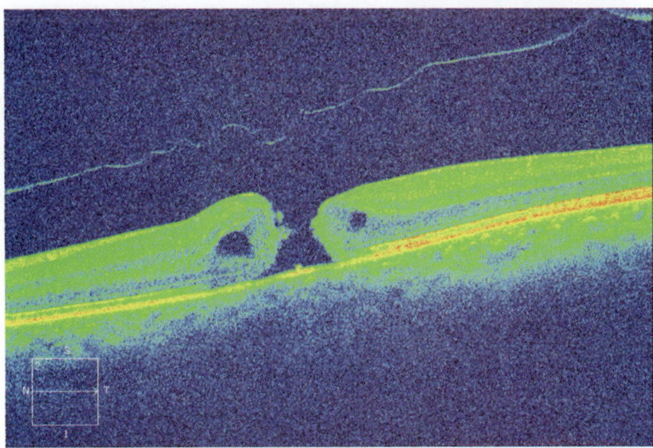

Fig. 76.19 OCT 3-months later showing an enlarged macular hole and cystoid changes at its edges.

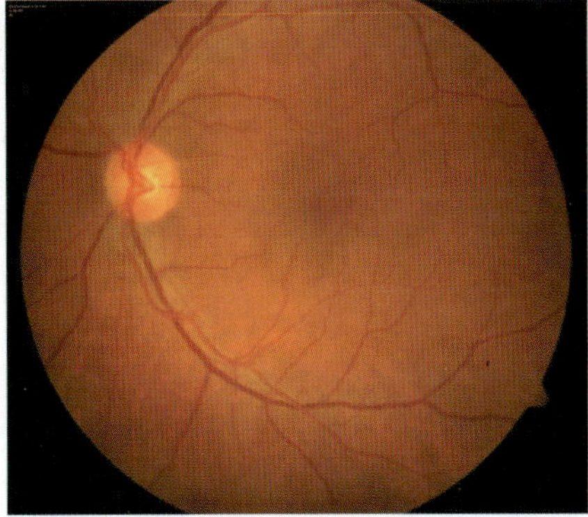

Fig. 76.20 Fundus of the left eye showing closure of macular hole following PPV.

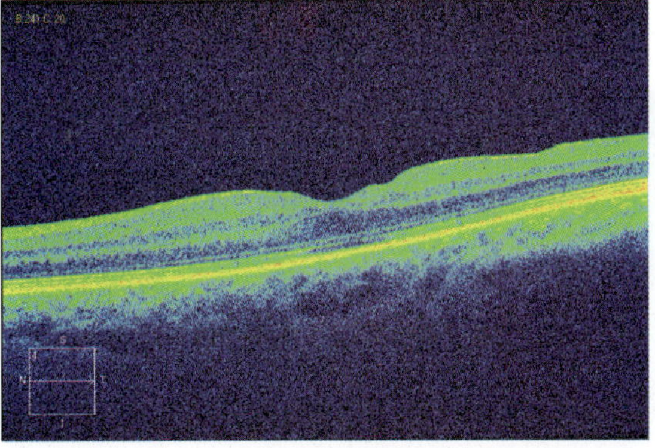

Fig. 76.21 OCT of the same eye showing type-1 closure of the macular hole.

FURTHER READING

Gupta V, Gupta A, Dogra MR, editors: Atlas Optical Coherence Tomography of Macular Diseases and Glaucoma. Fourth edition. *Jaypee-Highlights*, chap 8, 182–227.

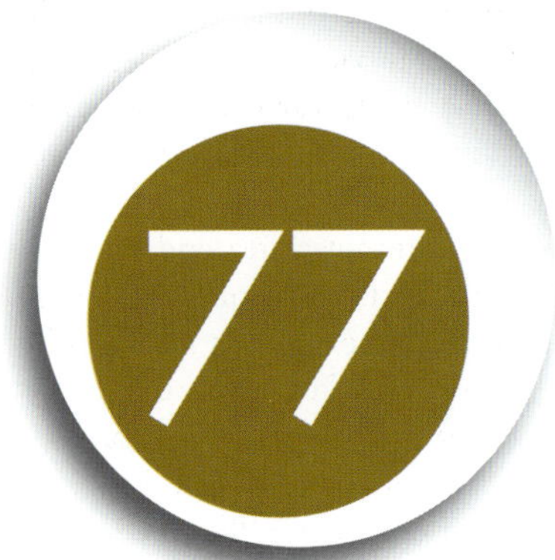

Malattia Leventinese

Anita Agarwal

A dominantly inherited disorder characterized by a radial pattern of innumerable, small, elongated basal laminar drusen was initially reported in a family from the Levantine valley in Switzerland. Doyne had described a similar clinical appearance as dominantly inherited honeycomb retinal dystrophy in 1899.

A 64-year-old female became symptomatic around age 40 with a visual acuity of 20/200 in each eye. Central macular atrophy surrounded by nodular cuticular drusen that extended nasal to the disc with radial distribution of the drusen was seen temporally in both eyes (**Figs 77.1 and 77.2**). Nodular drusen are highly autofluorescent and the central atrophic area is hypo-autofluorescent (**Figs 77.3 and 77.4**). Spectral-domain optical coherence tomography demonstrated nodular and confluent retinal pigment epithelial/epithelium (RPE) accumulations corresponding to the drusen in

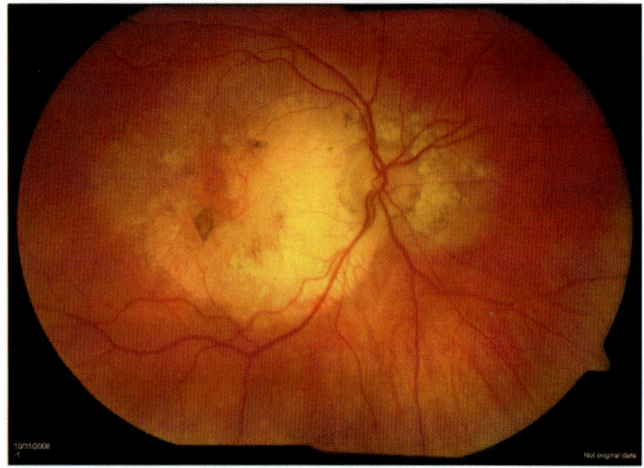

Fig. 77.1 The right eye with typical nodular drusen filling the entire macula and the region nasal to the disc. The fovea is atrophic with visible choroidal vessels and pigment clumps. (Photo courtesy: Gass Atlas of Macular Diseases by Anita Agarwal, 5th edition, Vol. I, Fig. 5.26 (C), p. 294, Elsevier, 2012.)

both eyes (**Figs 77.5A and B**). Her 66-year-old sister had a visual acuity of 20/40 in each eye and showed a much milder phenotype (**Figs 77.6 and 77.7**) comprising of small drusen, arranged in a radial pattern in the left eye, resembling cuticular drusen of North Carolina macular dystrophy. Their maternal uncle carried a diagnosis of Doyne's honeycomb dystrophy; their mother was relatively asymptomatic by history till she died at age 80. A daughter and son of the two sisters examined at age 32 and 34 were unaffected.

Radiating pattern in Malattia Leventinese (ML) is most prominent in the temporal macular area and is often accompanied by larger nodular or papillary drusen and variable amounts of irregular subretinal fibrous metaplasia and hyperplasia of the RPE (**Figs 77.1 and 77.2**). The visual acuity is often good in spite of fibrous metaplastic changes. The radial drusen demonstrate early discrete fluorescence similar to that of basal laminar drusen. On indocyanine green angiography, the lesions mask fluorescence early, and the central part of the drusen stains late with hypofluorescence of its edge. The drusen are brilliantly autofluorescent, while the fibrous metaplasia is hypo-autofluorescent (**Figs 77.3 and 77.4**). High-resolution OCT shows conical deposits between the RPE and Bruch's membrane, and secondary disruption of the outer nuclear layer in the late stages (**Figs 77.5A and B**). Choroidal neovascularization is known to occur and responds to photodynamic therapy and antivascular endothelial growth

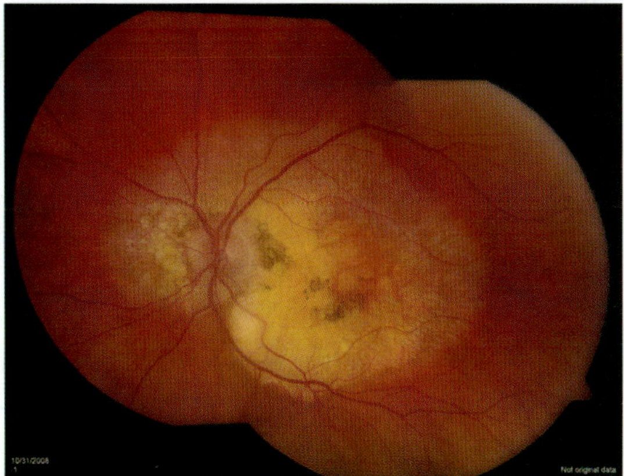

Fig. 77.2 The left eye with similar appearance as the right eye. (Photo courtesy: Gass Atlas of Macular Diseases by Anita Agarwal, 5th edition, Vol. I, Fig. 5.26 (D), p. 294, Elsevier, 2012.)

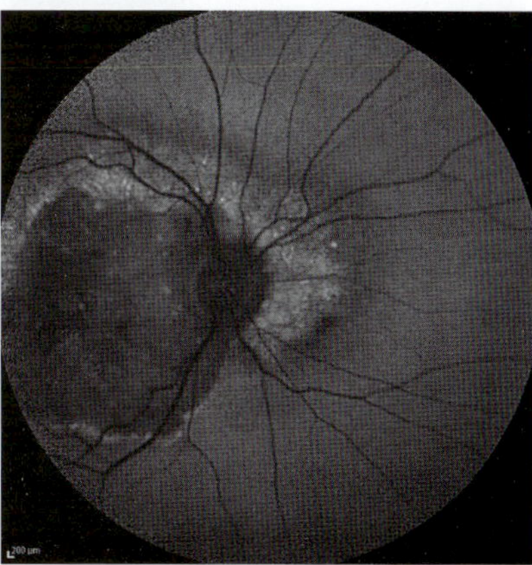

Fig. 77.3 The nodular drusen are hyper-autofluorescent while the atrophic areas are hypo-autofluorescent in the right eye. (Photo courtesy: Gass Atlas of Macular Diseases by Anita Agarwal, 5th edition, Vol. I, Fig. 5.26 (E), p. 295, Elsevier, 2012.)

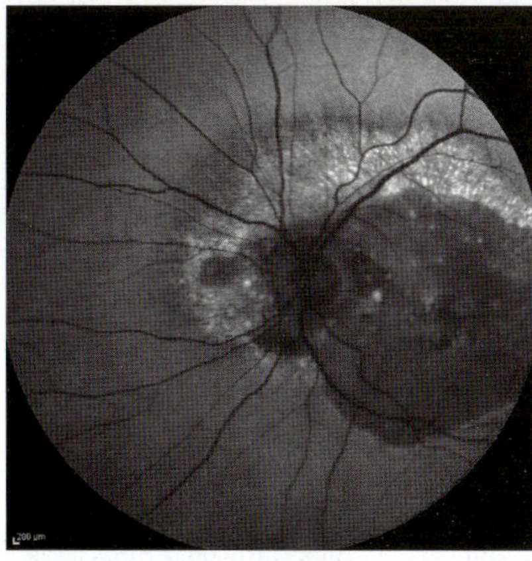

Fig. 77.4 The left eye has a similar appearance on autofluorescence imaging. (Photo courtesy: Gass Atlas of Macular Diseases by Anita Agarwal, 5th edition, Vol. I, Fig. 5.26 (F), p. 295, Elsevier, 2012.)

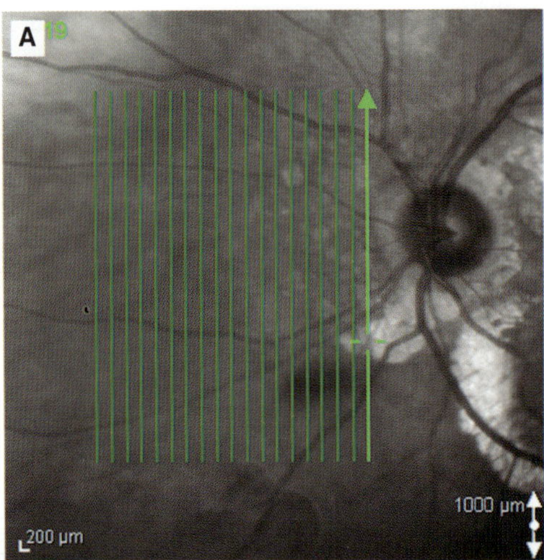

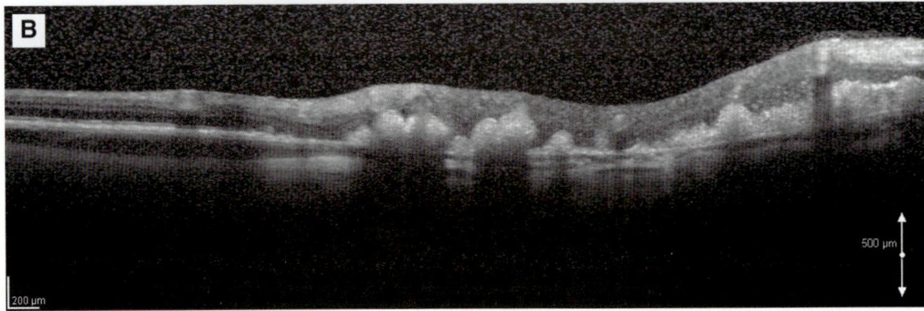

Fig. 77.5 Spectral domain OCT demonstrates nodular and confluent accumulations within the RPE. (Photo courtesy: Gass Atlas of Macular Diseases by Anita Agarwal, 5th edition, Vol. I, Figs 5.26 (I) and (J), p. 295, Elsevier, 2012.)

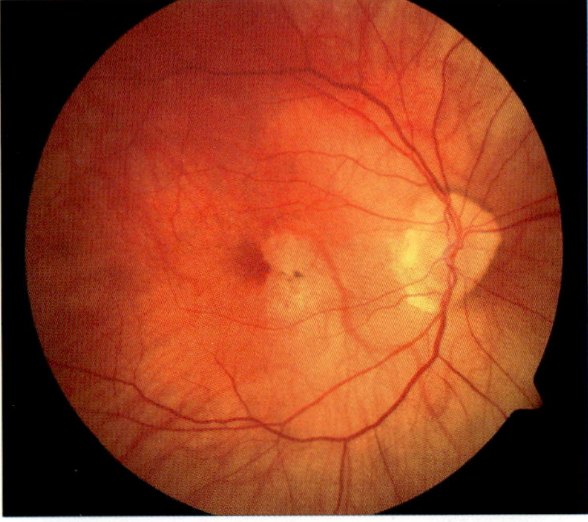

Fig. 77.6 The right fundus of a 66-year-old sister with compactly arranged small drusen in the fovea. (Photo courtesy: Gass Atlas of Macular Diseases by Anita Agarwal, 5th edition, Vol. I, Fig. 5.26 (K), p. 295, Elsevier, 2012.)

factor antibodies. Even though typical appearance is of nodular drusen that fill the macula and often the area nasal to the disc, phenotypic heterogeneity is seen in some families, showing less-extensive drusen or predominant fibrous change rather than drusen (Figs 77.6 and 77.7). Mutation in *EFE*MP1 gene (*Arg*345Trp) is responsible for the condition. Light and electron microscopic findings in one patient demonstrated evidence that these drusen are caused by thickening of basement membrane of the RPE.

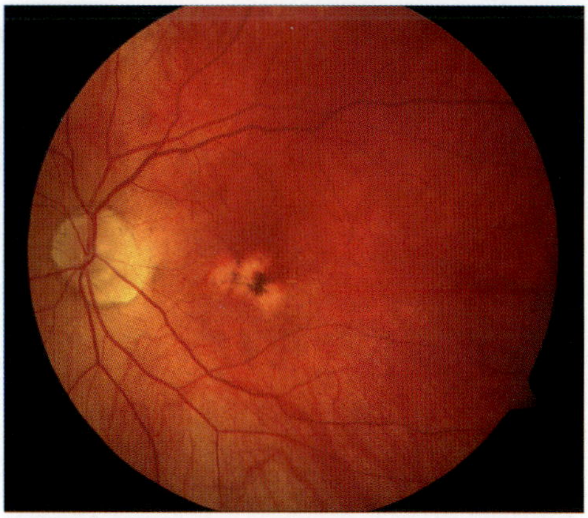

Fig. 77.7 Similar appearance in the left fovea with the temporal ones arranged in a radial pattern. (Photo courtesy: Gass Atlas of Macular Diseases by Anita Agarwal, 5th edition, Vol. I, Fig. 5.26 (L), p. 295, Elsevier, 2012.)

FURTHER READING

1. Forni S, Babel J: Etude clinique et histologique de la malattia leventinese; affection appartenant au groupe de dégénérescences hyalines du pôle postérieur. *Ophthalmologica* 143:313–322, 1962.
2. Souied EH, Leveziel N, Querques G, et al.: Indocyanine green angiography features of malattia leventinese. *Br J Ophthalmol* 90:296–300, 2006.
3. Gerth C, Zawadzki RJ, Werner JS, et al.: Retinal microstructure in patients with *EFEMP1* retinal dystrophy evaluated by Fourier domain OCT. *Eye* 23:4 80–83, 2009.
4. Souied EH, Leveziel N, Letien V, et al.: Optical coherent tomography features of Malattia Leventinese . *Am J Ophthalmol* 141:404–407, 2006.
5. Stone EM, Lotery AJ, Munier FL, et al.: A single *EFEMP1* mutation associated with both malattia leventinese and Doyne honeycomb retinal dystrophy. *Nat Genet* 22:199–202, 1999.
6. Fu L, Garland D, Yang Z, et al.: The R345W mutation in *EFEMP1* is pathogenic and causes AMD-like deposits in mice. *Hum Mol Genet* 16:2411–2422, 2007.
7. Matsumoto M, Traboulsi EL: Dominant radial drusen and Arg345Trp EFEMP1 mutation. *Am J Ophthalmol* 131: 810–812, 2001.

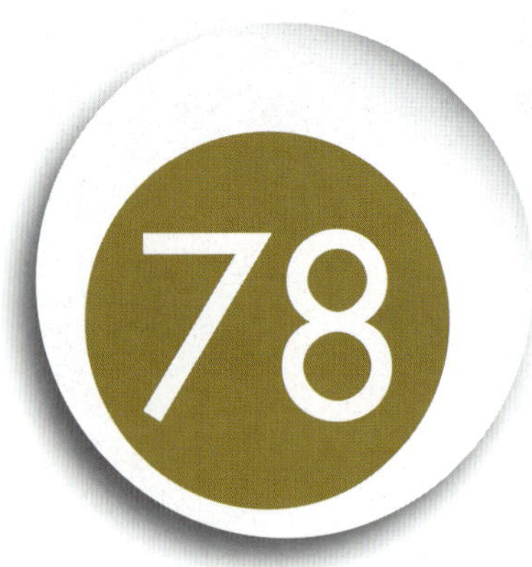

North Carolina Macular Dystrophy

Anita Agarwal

North Carolina Macular Dystrophy (NCMD) is an autosomal dominant inherited disorder with complete penetrance. Its onset is in infancy with a generally stable course and a highly variable phenotype that includes drusen-like changes, disciform lesions with choroidal neovascularization, macular staphyloma, and peripheral drusen. Electroretinography, electrooculography, and color vision are normal.

CASE STUDY 1

A 13-year-old girl was found to have compact small drusen with temporal radial arrangement in both eyes typical of NCMD, on a routine examination for glasses (**Figs 78.1A and B**). Four years later the lesions were unchanged, demonstrating stability and very slow progression. Autofluorescence was nonspecific with some lesions showing punctate hyperautofluorescence (**Figs 78.2A and B**). Her 45-year-old father was asymptomatic and had small compact drusen in the fovea also. A brother was known to have similar changes when examined elsewhere.

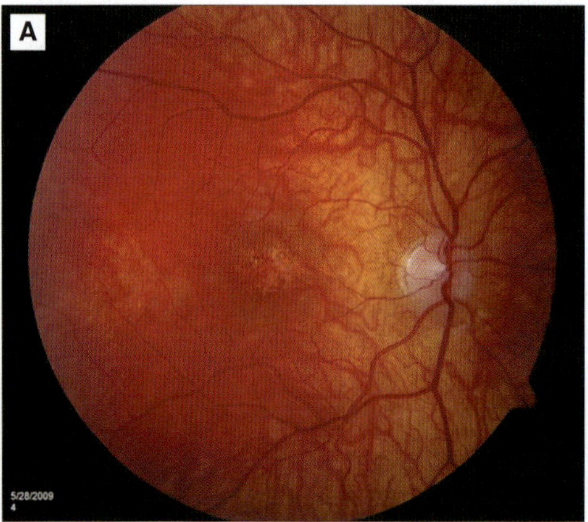
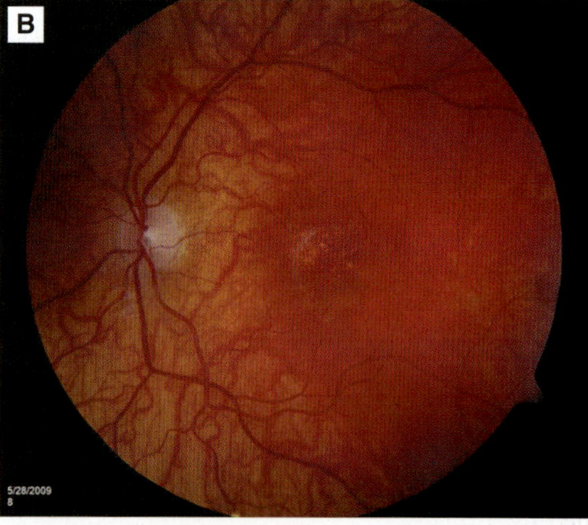

Fig. 78.1 **(A)** and **(B)** Fine drusen arranged in a compact manner in the right and left fovea of an asymptomatic 13-year-old girl. (Photo courtesy: Gass Atlas of Macular Diseases by Anita Agarwal, 5th edition, Vol. I, Figs 5.28 (I) and (J), p. 299, Elsevier, 2012.)

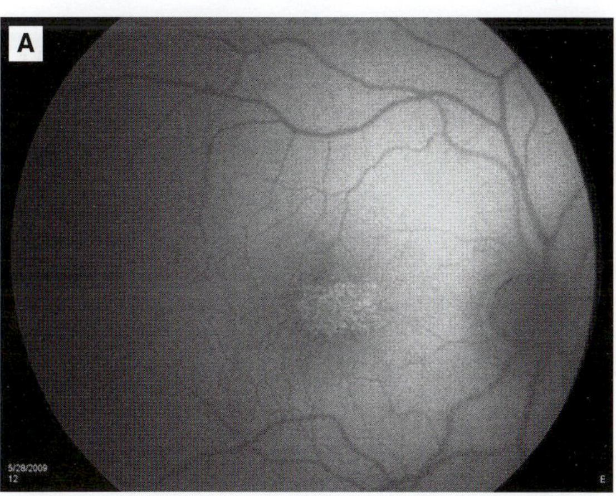 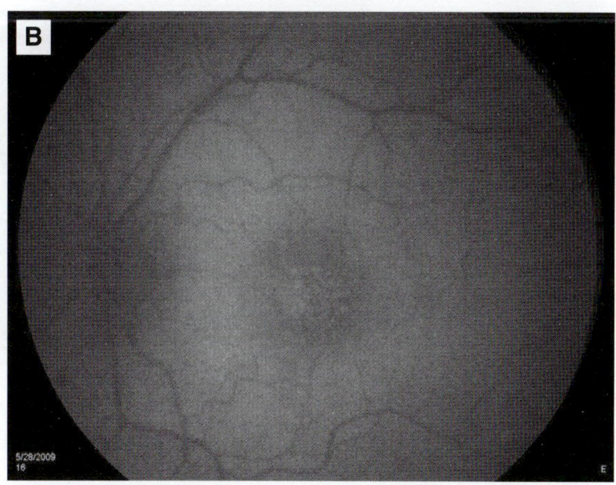

Fig. 78.2 **(A)** and **(B)** Mottled hyper-autofluorescence of the right and left fovea corresponding to the drusen in both eyes.

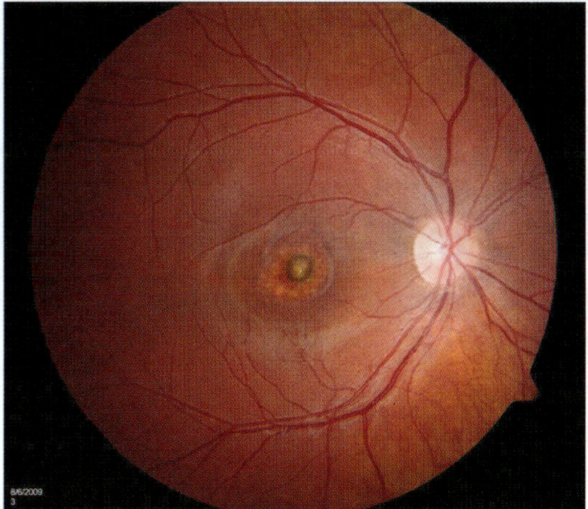 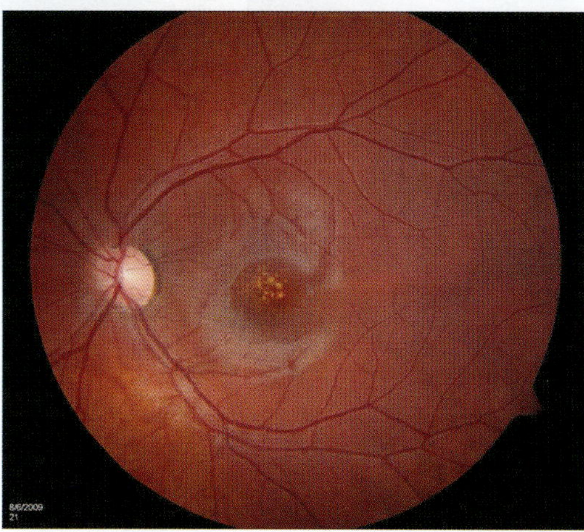

Fig. 78.3 The right fundus with central hyperpigmented lesion corresponding to a regressed-type choroidal neovascular membrane, surrounded by hypopigmented RPE. (Photo courtesy: Gass Atlas of Macular Diseases by Anita Agarwal, 5th edition, Vol. I, Fig. 5.28 (A), p. 299, Elsevier, 2012.)

Fig. 78.4 Distinct drusen arranged in a compact manner in the left fovea. (Photo courtesy: Gass Atlas of Macular Diseases by Anita Agarwal, 5th edition, Vol. I, Fig. 5.28 (B), p. 299, Elsevier, 2012.)

CASE STUDY 2

A 16-year-old girl noted central metamorphopsia and distortion in her right eye for 2 months, which gradually improved over the next month. Her vision was 20/25 in the right eye and 20/20 in the left eye. A hyperpigmented raised central lesion surrounded by a ring of mottled retinal pigment epithelium (RPE) with a few punctate drusen within it was seen in the right eye (Fig. 78.3). Small and intermediate punctate drusen distributed within the fovea was seen in the left eye (Fig. 78.4). Findings suggest a spontaneously regressed type-2 choroidal neovascular membrane in a patient with NCMD. Autofluorescence imaging showed a ring of increased autofluorescence (AF) surrounded by a ring of decreased AF corresponding to the ring of mottled RPE (not shown). An optical coherence tomography (OCT) showed no activity on the right, and the drusen could not be seen by OCT (Figs 78.5A and B and 78.6A and B). Her 40-year-old asymptomatic mother with a corrected visual acuity of 20/20 showed similar small compact drusen within the fovea in both eyes.

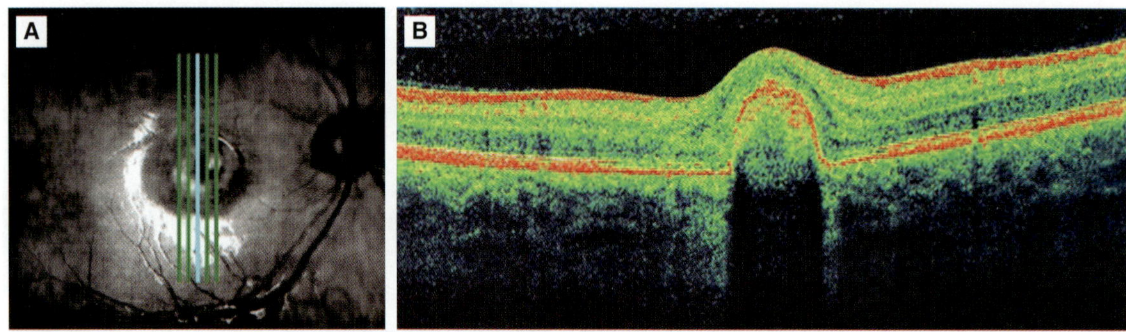

Fig. 78.5 Section through the regressed choroidal neovascular membrane shows no subretinal or intraretinal fluid. (Photo courtesy: Gass Atlas of Macular Diseases by Anita Agarwal, 5th edition, Vol. I, Fig. 5.28 (D1), p. 299, Elsevier, 2012.)

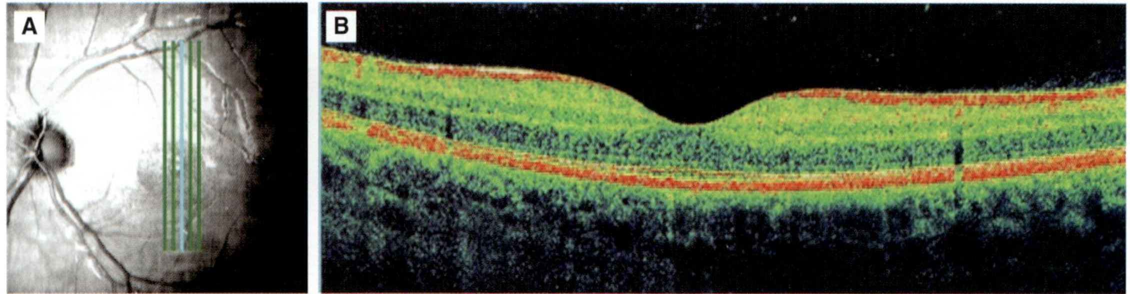

Fig. 78.6 Optical coherence tomography through the drusen in the left fovea shows no abnormality. (Photo courtesy: Anita Agarwal: Gass Atlas of Macular Diseases by Anita Agarwal, 5th edition, Vol. I, Fig. 5.28 (D2), p. 299, Elsevier, 2012.)

Scattered lesions with drusen and pigmentary changes in the macula with normal visual acuity are the earliest fundus findings (stage 1) (**Figs 78.1A and B**). As the vision declines to the 20/50 range, there is an increase in number, as well as confluence of the drusen-like changes (stage 2). In many patients, the fundus changes do not progress beyond the drusen stage and visual acuity may remain normal. Other family members may show a progressive decrease in the acuity to the 20/200 level concomitant with development of almost total atrophy of the choroid, RPE, and retina in the macular area (stage 3). Peripheral drusen-like changes and evidence of choroidal neovascularization and disciform detachment can develop.

The NCMD gene (*MCD*R1) is mapped to the 6q14–q16.2 region; though the disease-causing gene is yet to be identified. Though initially described in inhabitants of North Carolina, with their descendancy traced to three Irish brothers, the phenotype has been found in Caucasian patients outside North Carolina and the United States, in African–American, Belize, and Korean patients. An African–American family from Chicago with involvement of three generations has been described.

FURTHER READING

1. Lefler WH, Wadsworth JAC, Sidbury JB Jr: Hereditary macular degeneration and amino-aciduria. *Am J Ophthalmol* 71:224–230, 1971.
2. Frank HR, Landers MB III, Williams RJ, et al.: A new dominant progressive foveal dystrophy. *Am J Ophthalmol* 78:903–916, 1974.
3. Gass JDM: Stereoscopic atlas of macular diseases: diagnosis and treatment, ed 2, St. Louis: CV Mosby 74; 1977.
4. Rohrschneider K, Blankenagel A, Kruse FE, et al.: Volcker HE. Macular function testing in a German pedigree with North Carolina macular dystrophy. *Retina* 18(5):453–459, 1998.

5. Reichel MB, Kelsell RE, Fan J, et al.: Phenotype of a British North Carolina macular dystrophy family linked to chromosome 6q. *Br J Ophthalmol* 82(10):1162–1168, 1998.
6. Small KW, Puech B, Mullen L, et al.: North Carolina macular dystrophy phenotype in France maps to the MCDR1 locus. *Mol Vis* 2;3:1, 1997.
7. Rabb MF, Mullen L, Yelchits S, et al.: A North Carolina macular dystrophy phenotype in a Belizean family maps to the MCDR1 locus. *Am J Ophthalmol* 125(4):502–508, 1998.
8. Kim SJ, Woo SJ, Yu HG: A Korean family with an early-onset autosomal dominant macular dystrophy resembling North Carolina macular dystrophy. *Korean J Ophthalmol* 20(4):220–224, 2006.

Optic Pit

Priya BV

Optic pits are congenital excavations of the optic nerve head. They result from an imperfect closure of embryonic fissure. Incidence of optic pit is about 1 in 10,000. Optic pits are most commonly located on the temporal side of the optic disc. They may also be situated centrally or anywhere along the margin of the optic disc.

Optic pits along the margin of the optic disc are most likely to lead to serous detachments of the retina. Other findings that may be present include full-thickness or laminar retinal holes, retinal pigment epithelium mottling, and cystic changes.

CASE STUDY

An 18-year-old Asian Indian woman presented with complaints of painless blurring of vision in her left eye for the past 2 years. Visual acuity at presentation was 6/6 in the right eye and 3/60 in the left eye.

Ophthalmoscopic examination showed a temporally located optic disc pit with prominent peripapillary retinal pigment epithelial changes (Fig. 79.1) and serous macular detachment in the left eye (Fig. 79.2).

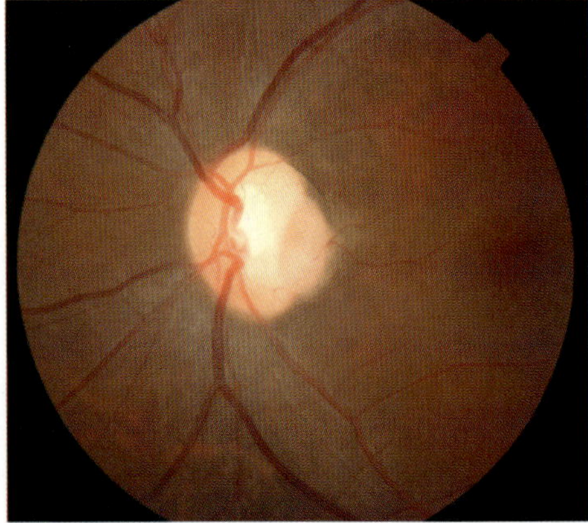

Fig. 79.1 Fundus photograph of the left eye centered around the optic disc showing the temporally located optic pit.

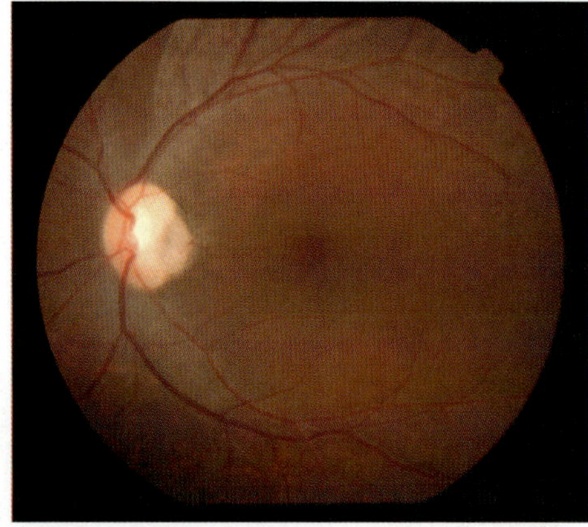

Fig. 79.2 Fundus photograph of the left eye showing the serous detachment of the macula.

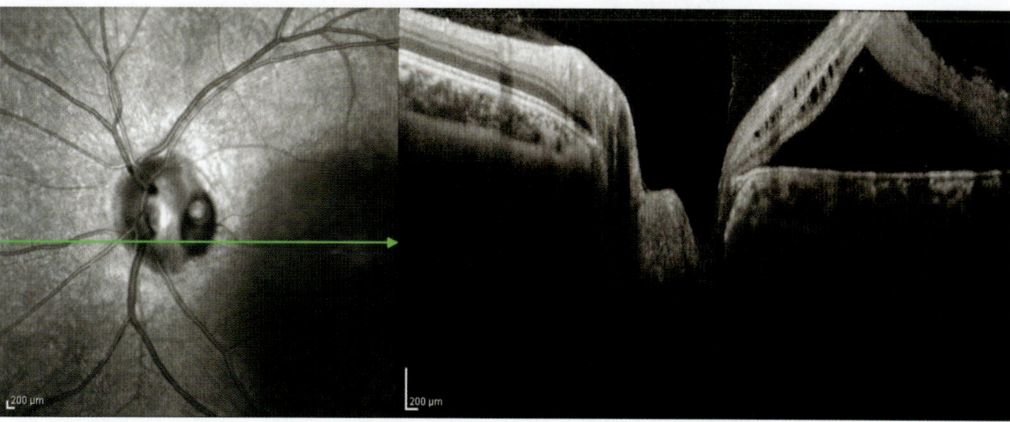

Fig. 79.3 SD-OCT section through the optic pit showing the excavation in the optic nerve.

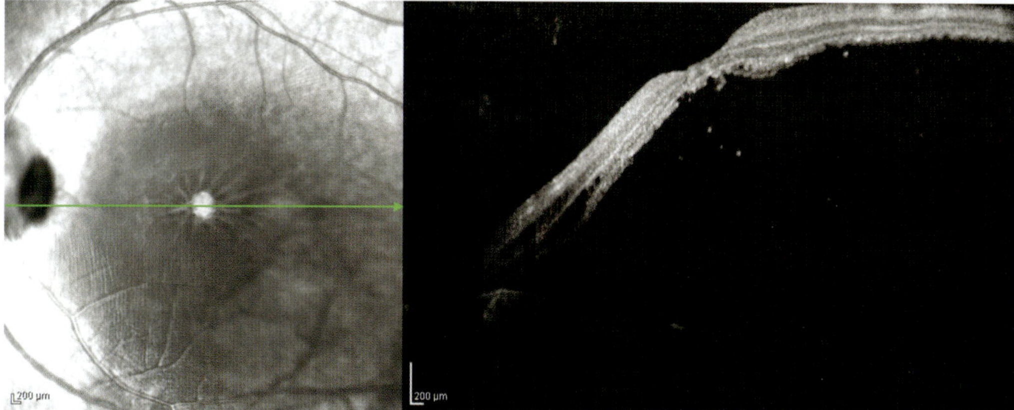

Fig. 79.4 SD-OCT section passing through the retina adjacent to the optic pit showing intraretinal cystic spaces nasal to the fovea and the large serous macular detachment.

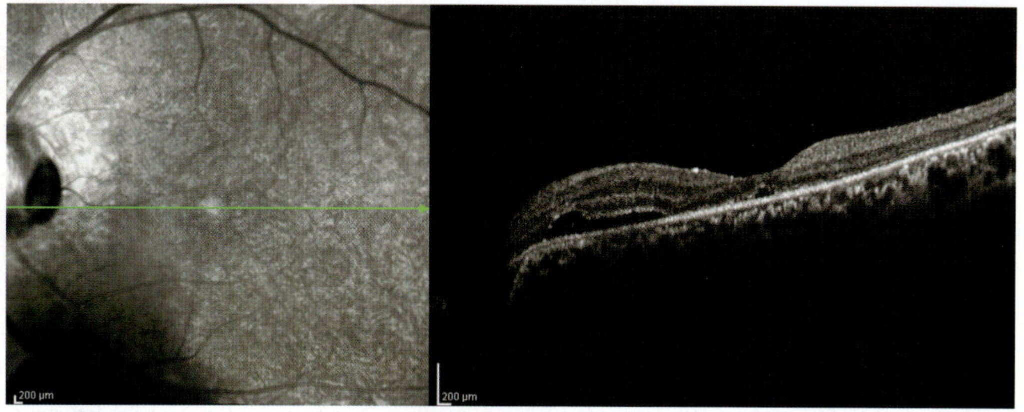

Fig. 79.5 SD-OCT section through the same area as in Figure 79.4 done at 1 month following the peripapillary laser treatment showing the decreased subretinal fluid at the macula.

Spectral-domain optical coherence tomography (SD-OCT) (SPECTRALIS™; Heidelberg Engineering, Heidelberg, Germany) sections through the pit showed excavation in the optic nerve (Fig. 79.3). There was no communication noted between the pit and adjacent subretinal space on high-resolution scanning.

Optical coherence tomography (OCT) also showed cystic spaces in retinal layers nasal to the fovea and a large serous macular detachment (Fig. 79.4).

The patient underwent peripapillary laser treatment in the left eye. Follow-up after 1 month revealed decreased subretinal fluid at the macula (Fig. 79.5), though her vision had not improved. (This could be due to the retinal-pigment-epithelial alterations and possible outer retinal damage associated with chronic serous macular detachment.)

Serous macular detachment associated with optic pit was earlier thought to be due to direct communication between the optic pit and the subretinal space. However, Lincoff, et al. suggested that fluid from the optic pit may primarily move into the retina leading to a schisis-like separation of the inner and outer layers. The neurosensory serous retinal detachment occurred secondary to this schisis.

FURTHER READING

1. Brar VS, Murthy RK, Chalam KV: Functional microperimetry and SD-OCT confirm consecutive retinal atrophy from optic nerve pit. *Clin Ophthalmol* 3:625–628, 2009.
2. Lincoff H, Kreissig I: Optical coherence tomography of pneumatic displacement of optic disc pit maculopathy. *Br J Ophthalmol* 82(4):367–372, 1998.

Optic Neuritis

Rajani Battu and
Anupama Kiran Kumar

Demyelinating optic neuritis (ON) is the most common cause of acute unilateral visual loss in young adults between ages of 15 and 49; women are more often affected. Approximately, 50% of patients with isolated ON and asymptomatic lesions in the central nervous system develop definite multiple sclerosis (MS) within 15 years.

Optical coherence tomography (OCT) is used to measure the peripapillary retinal nerve fiber layer (RNFL) thickness in patients. In normal subjects, the thickness of the RNFL is higher in superior and inferior portions of the optic disc than in the nasal and temporal portions. The OCT software automatically compares results obtained in each quadrant with a normative database, in order to identify overall thinning of the layer, as well as focal defects. Macular volume can be measured with OCT in addition to RNFL thickness. Since macula consists of mostly ganglion cell bodies, assessment of macular volume provides an opportunity to determine whether axonal loss (measured by the RNFL thickness) is associated with neuronal degeneration itself.

Several studies have confirmed thinning of the RNFL after ON with or without multiple sclerosis (MS). There is an average 33% reduction in RNFL thickness in affected eyes of patients with previous ON compared with eyes of matched controls. Retrobulbar neuritis with no apparent disc swelling may show a mild disc edema on OCT. RNFL thinning occurs mostly between months 3 and 6 in 85% of patients. However, RNFL thinning correlates mostly with the severity of ON and visual loss, and may not help predict subsequent risk of MS.

CASE STUDY

A 39-year-old female presented with rapid decrease in vision in the left eye for 10 days. She had mild pain on moving the eye. She also complained of numbness in both hands for 2 weeks. There was no history of recent viral illness or vaccination.

Her best-corrected visual acuity was 6/6 in the right eye and 6/6(p) in the left eye. Color vision was normal in the right eye and defective in the left eye. Brightness perception was reduced in the left eye. Confrontation fields in both eyes were normal. The left pupil showed a relative afferent pupillary defect. Fundus of both eyes was normal.

A diagnosis of left retrobulbar neuritis was made. A visual evoked potential (VEP) testing of both eyes showed a delayed P100 response in the left eye (**Fig. 80.1**).

An OCT of the left eye was done (**Fig. 80.2**).

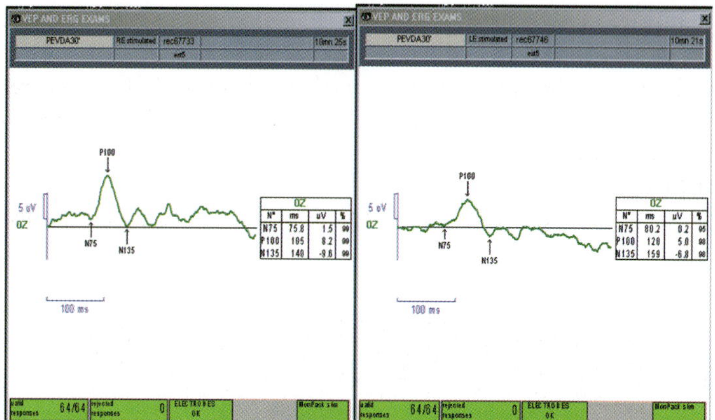

Fig. 80.1 Pattern VEP of the right and left eye showing a delay in the P100 response and decreased amplitude of the waveforms in the left eye.

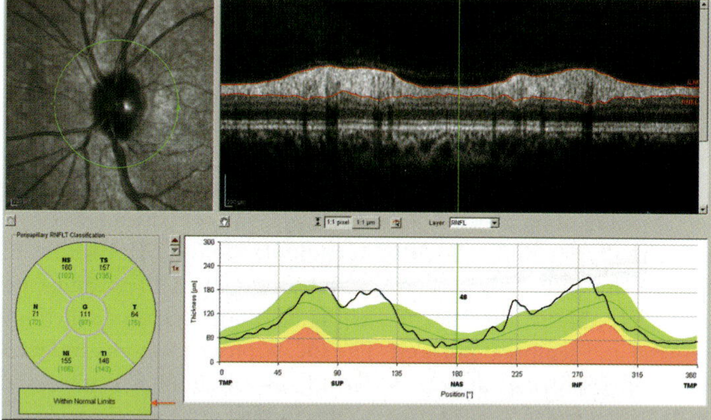

Fig. 80.2 OCT–RNFL analysis of the left eye showing normal thickness in all the quadrants. The *red arrow* points to the report generated in RNFL scan.

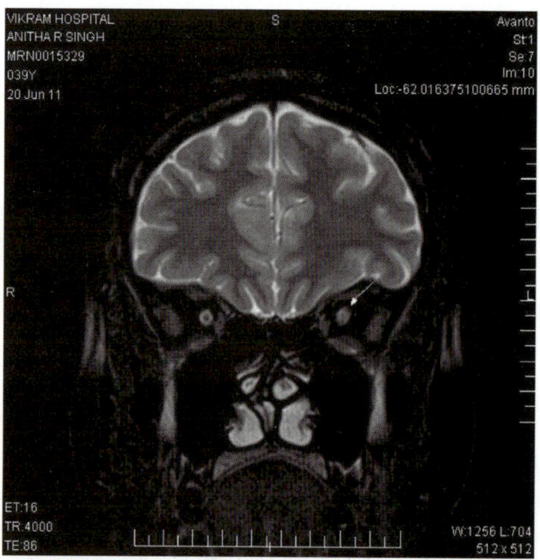

Fig. 80.3 T2-weighted–fat-saturated image with 3-mm slice thickness through both orbits showing hyperintense left optic nerve (*white arrow*).

All routine blood investigations were normal. Neurological examination was essentially normal. An MRI of brain was done (Figs 80.3–80.5).

The patient was started on pulse therapy intravenous methyl prednisolone by the neurologist. Patient recovered vision in the left eye to 6/6; there was complete recovery of color vision. She subsequently developed a recurrent attack of ON and was treated for the same.

An OCT done during follow-up is shown in **Figures 80.6** and **80.7**.

RNFL thinning has been associated with optic neuritis, and is increasingly being used as a surrogate for the severity of MS.

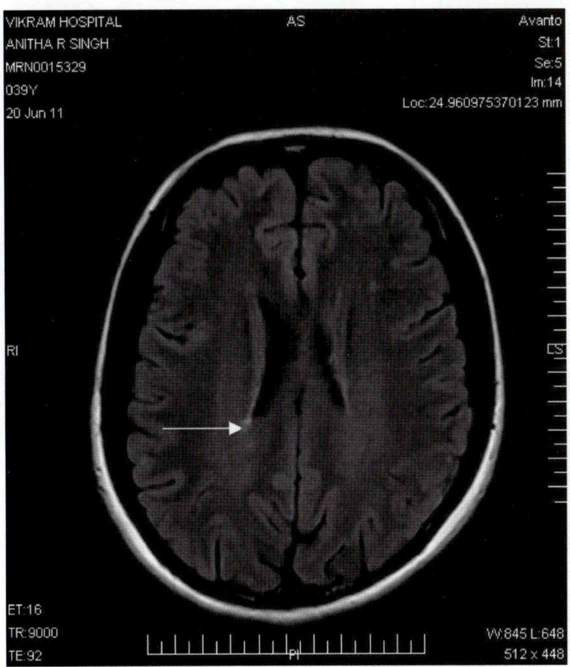

Fig. 80.4 Axial FLAIR sequence showing small right periventricular plaque (*white arrow*).

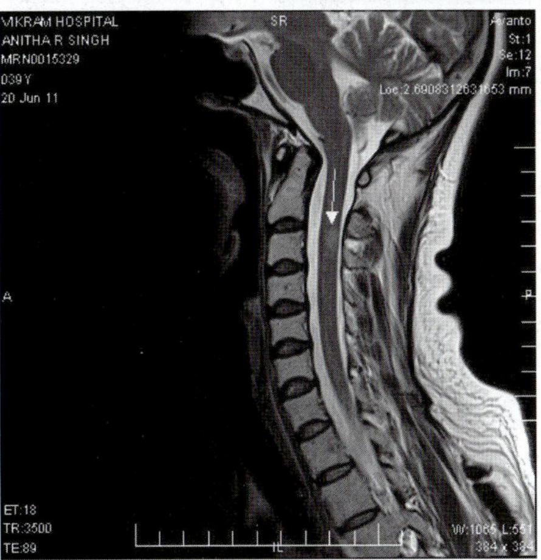

Fig. 80.5 T2-weighted sagittal image for cervical spine shows vertical intramedullary small hyperintense plaque opposite to C3 vertebra (*white arrow*).

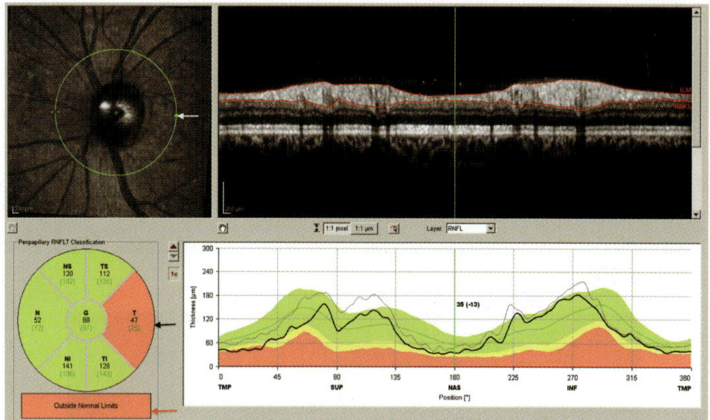

Fig. 80.6 OCT–RNFL analysis of the left eye showing retinal thinning in temporal quadrant (*white and black arrows*). The *red arrow* points to report generated in RNFL scan, which indicates that the scan is outside normal limits.

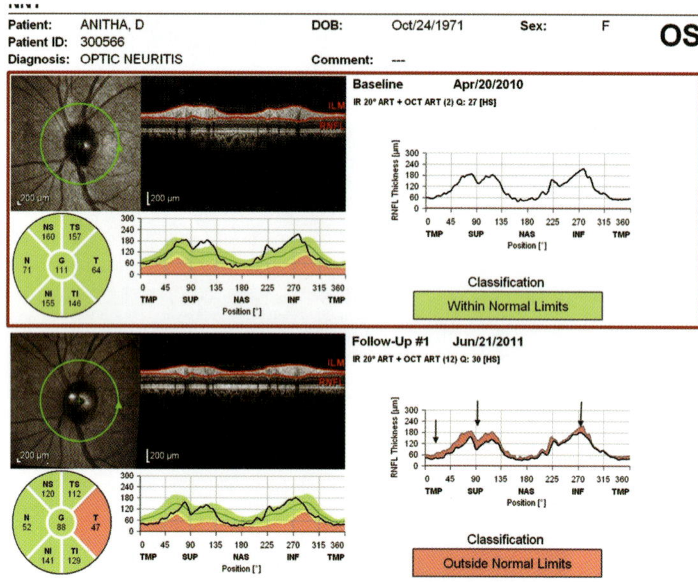

Fig. 80.7 Follow-up scans of the left eye that compares the RNFL thickness in the same eye at two different time frames of examination. The area in red shows the amount of RNFL loss between the two examinations (*black arrows*).

FURTHER READING

1. Voss E, Raab P, Trebst C, et al.: Clinical approach to optic neuritis: pitfalls, red flags and differential diagnosis. *Ther Adv Neurol Disord* 4(2):123–134, 2011.
2. Group ONS: Multiple sclerosis risk after optic neuritis: final optic neuritis treatment trial follow-up. *Arch Neurol* 65(6):727–732, 2008.
3. Lamirel C, Newman NJ, Biousse V: Optical coherence tomography (OCT) in optic neuritis and multiple sclerosis. *Rev Neurol (Paris)* 166(12):978–986, 2010.

4. Jindahra P, Hedges TR, Mendoza-Santiesteban CE, et al.: Optical coherence tomography of the retina: applications in neurology. *Curr Opin Neurol* 23(1):16–23, 2010.
5. Khanifar AA, Parlitsis GJ, Ehrlich JR, et al.: Retinal nerve fiber layer evaluation in multiple sclerosis with spectral domain optical coherence tomography. *Clin Ophthalmol* 4:1007–1013, 2010.
6. Trip SA, Schlottmann PG, Jones SJ, et al.: Retinal nerve fiber layer axonal loss and visual dysfunction in optic neuritis. *Ann Neurol* 58(3):383–391, 2005.
7. Pro MJ, Pons ME, Liebmann JM, et al.: Imaging of the optic disc and retinal nerve fiber layer in acute optic neuritis. *J Neurol Sci* 250(1–2):114–119, 2006.
8. Costello F, Coupland S, Hodge W, et al.: Quantifying axonal loss after optic neuritis with optical coherence tomography. *Ann Nerol* 59(6):963–969, 2006.
9. Costello F, Hodge W, Pan YI, et al.: Retinal nerve fiber layer and future risk of multiple sclerosis. *Can J Neurol Sci* 35(4):482–487, 2008.

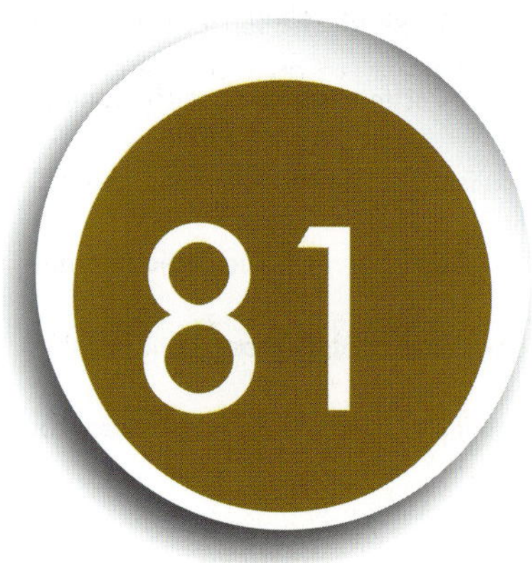

Purtscher's Retinopathy

Naresh Kumar Yadav and Kanav Gupta

Purtscher's retinopathy was first described in 1910 by Otmar Purtscher in a middle-aged man who fell from a tree onto his head and suffered a brief loss of consciousness. It has also been described in a variety of conditions, including acute pancreatitis, fat embolism syndrome, renal failure, childbirth, and connective tissue disorders.

Patients with Purtscher's retinopathy present with loss of acuity in one or both eyes, ranging from minimal impairment to hand movements visual acuity. Loss of acuity may be accompanied by field loss in the form of central, paracentral, or arcuate scotoma. Peripheral visual function is usually preserved.

Fundus findings in acute Purtscher's retinopathy include disc edema, Purtscher's flecken, cotton-wool spots, and retinal hemorrhages. The characteristic Purtscher's flecken corresponds to areas of multiple, discrete areas of retinal whitening in the inner retina between the vessels. These are usually polygonal with size varying from a quarter to several disk areas. The retinal whitening may extend to the edge of an adjacent venule, but a clear zone usually exists between affected retina and an adjacent arteriole. Abnormalities in Purtscher's retinopathy is usually confined to the posterior pole, and may be unilateral or bilateral.

Pathogenesis: The mechanism of Purtscher's retinopathy is as follows:

1. Increased intracranial pressure and extravasation of lymph.
2. Increased intrathoracic pressure and venous dilatation.
3. Vasculitis due to free fatty acids.
4. Vascular occlusion by emboli, e.g., fat, air, leucocytes, fibrin, platelets, and complement activation.

There is no definite treatment for Purtscher's retinopathy. Systemic steroids have been tried; although there is no hard evidence supporting its use. However, majority of the patients recover some visual function without treatment.

CASE STUDY

A 45-year-old man was referred with complaints Purf blurring of vision in the right eye more than the left eye since 1 week. There was a history of road traffic accident 1 week back. Patient had a head-on collision with a four wheeler while driving his car. He was not wearing a seat belt; and sustained chest injuries with difficulty in breathing. He was taken to an ophthalmologist following the accident and was given intravenous methyl prednisolone for 4 days.

Ocular examination revealed vision of counting fingers 2 meters in the right eye and 6/6 in the left eye. Anterior segment examination was normal in both the eyes. Fundus of both eyes showed multiple cotton-wool spots with preretinal and subhyaloid hemorrhages (Fig. 81.1).

Fundus fluorescein angiography (FFA) findings correlated with the fundus findings (Fig. 81.2).

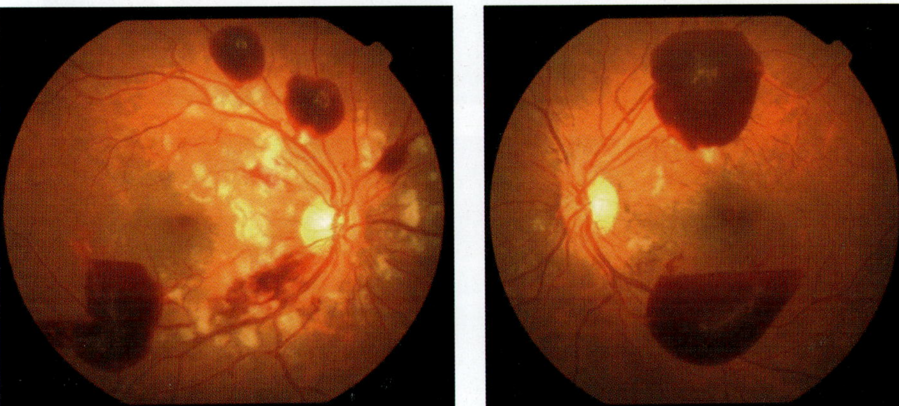

Fig. 81.1 Preretinal and flame-shaped hemorrhages with multiple cotton-wool spots posteriorly and around the arcade with normal periphery.

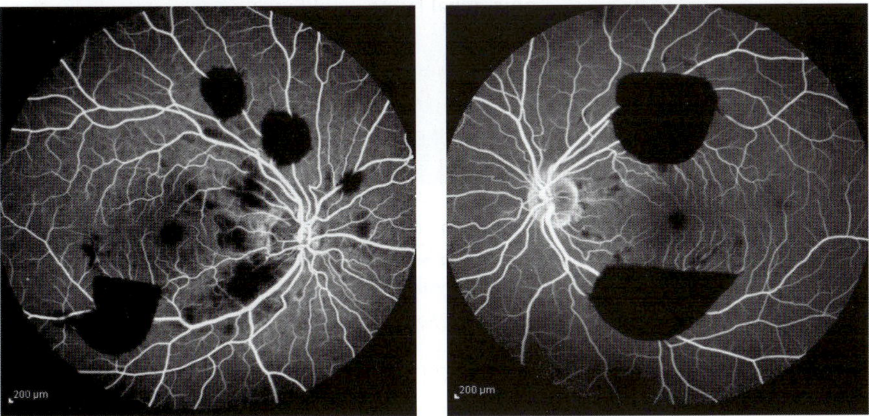

Fig. 81.2 FFA showing blocked fluorescence corresponding to preretinal hemorrhages and cotton-wool spots. No area of leakage is noted.

Spectral-domain optical coherence tomography (SD-OCT) showed intraretinal edema, inner segment–outer segment (IS–OS) junction disruption, and preretinal and subhyaloid hemorrhages (Figs 81.3 and 81.4).

Patient was not a hypertensive or diabetic.

MRI of brain and orbit, X-ray of chest (PA), and CT of head were normal. CT of thorax plain and contrast revealed pulmonary edema. Visual evoked potential revealed poor optic nerve conduction in the right eye more than the left eye.

He was started on oral steroids 1 mg/kg/day in a tapering dose.

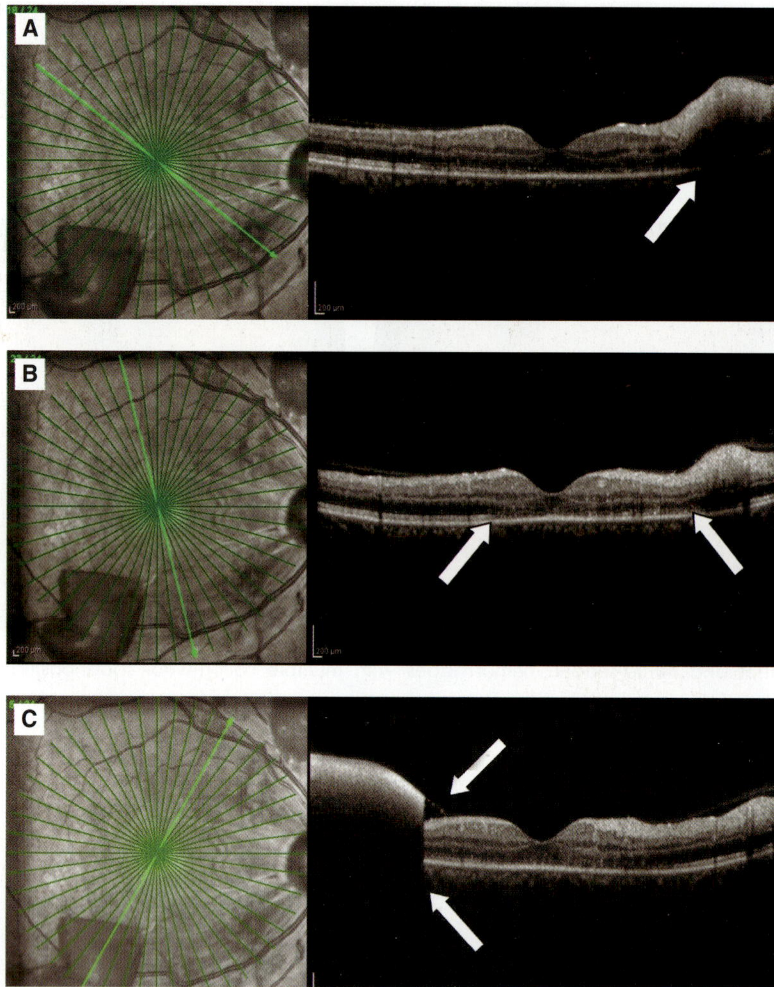

Fig. 81.3 (A) Section through flame-shaped hemorrhage showing characteristic intraretinal edema with hemorrhage obscuring posterior retinal layers by backscattering. (B) IS–OS disruption. (C) Section through subhyaloid hemorrhage obscuring retinal layers by backscattering, and posterior hyaloid interface seen between the normal retina and elevated retina by subhyaloid hemorrhage.

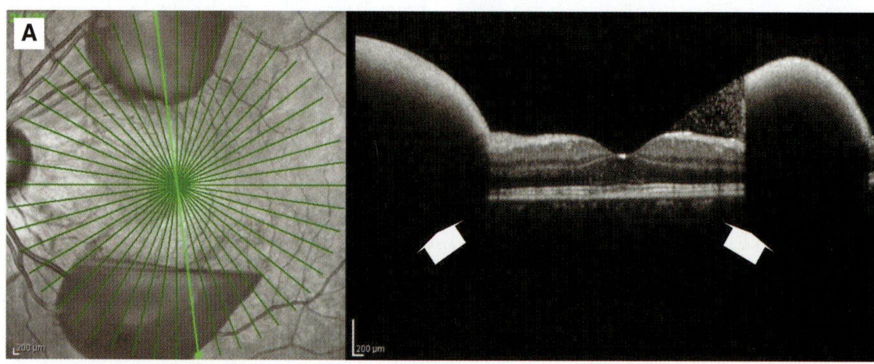

Fig. 81.4 (A) Vertical section through massive preretinal hemorrhages with backscattering obscuring retinal layers.

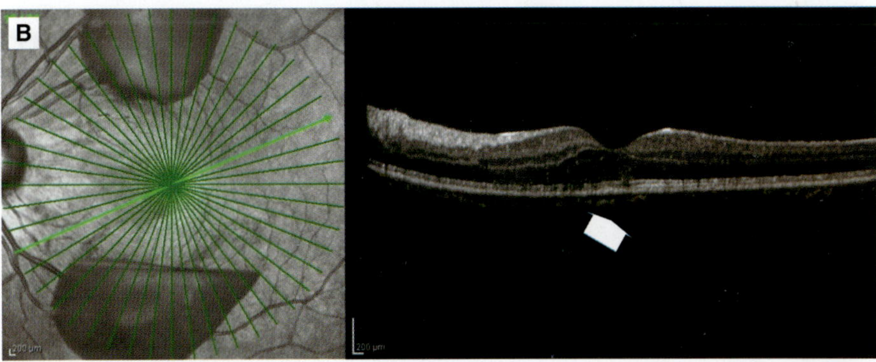

Fig. 81.4 **(B)** Mild disruption of IS–OS junction with edema of inner retinal layers and some cystic spaces.

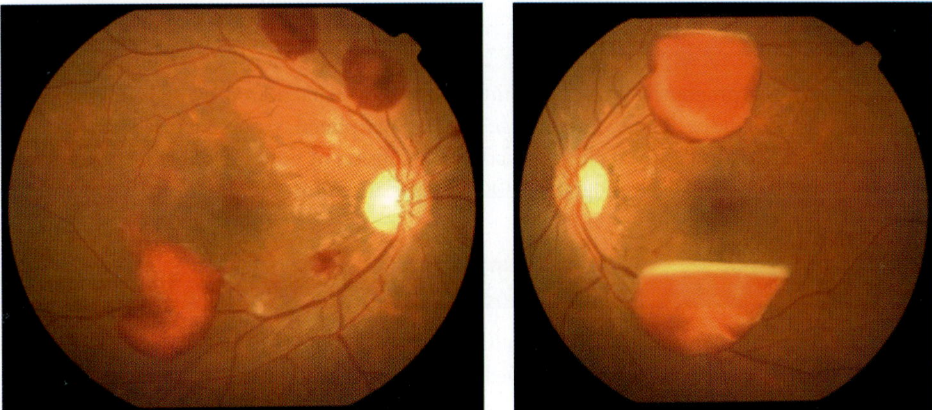

Fig. 81.5 Cotton-wool spots have reduced with resolving preretinal hemorrhages.

FOLLOW-UP

Fundus examination showed decreasing hemorrhages and cotton-wool spots, but without any improvement in the visual acuity, 3 weeks later (Fig. 81.5).

In this case, the patient presented with diminution of vision and a history of road traffic accident with chest compression history. Characteristically, the changes are confined to posterior pole and around arcades only. Findings were confirmed clinically, and by fundus fluorescein angiography (FFA) and SD-OCT. The patient was treated with oral steroids, and fundus in the follow-up visit showed resolving preretinal hemorrhages with no improvement in vision, suggestive of an ischemic event.

FURTHER READING

1. Agrawal A, McKibbin MA: Purtscher's and Purtscher-like retinopathies: a review. *Surv Ophthalmol* 51(2):129–136, 2006.
2. Oh J, Jung JH, Moon SW, et al.: Commotio retinae with spectral-domain optical coherence tomography. *Retina* 31:2044–2049, 2011.
3. Agrawal A, McKibbin MA: Purtscher's retinopathy: epidemiology, clinical features, and outcome. *Br J Ophthalmol* 91:1456–1459, 2007.

Retinitis Pigmentosa

Rajani Battu

Retinitis pigmentosa (RP) is a progressive inherited retinal dystrophy characterized by night blindness, bone-spicule-like pigmentary changes in midperiphery, progressive loss of peripheral vision, and decreased or undetectable responses on an electroretinogram. Classical clinical triad of RP consists of bone corpuscles, attenuated blood vessels, and a waxy pale disc. Optical coherence tomography (OCT) plays an important role in management of the disease.

CASE STUDY

A 40-year-old businessman presented with night blindness since childhood. None of his family members suffered from a similar complaint. Ocular examination showed a vision of 6/18, N8 in both eyes. Fundus examination showed normal discs in both eyes, attenuated arterioles, and multiple bony spicules in midperiphery. Fundus features were consistent with a diagnosis of RP (Fig. 82.1). Visual fields showed significant constriction of peripheral fields. Electroretinography (ERG) showed a rod–cone dysfunction (Fig. 82.2). Spectral-domain optical coherence tomography (SD-OCT) showed loss of the inner segment–outer segment (IS–OS) layer and the external limiting membrane (ELM) (Figs 82.3 and 82.5). Fundus autofluorescence (FAF) showed an increase in the autofluorescence (AF) (Fig. 82.4).

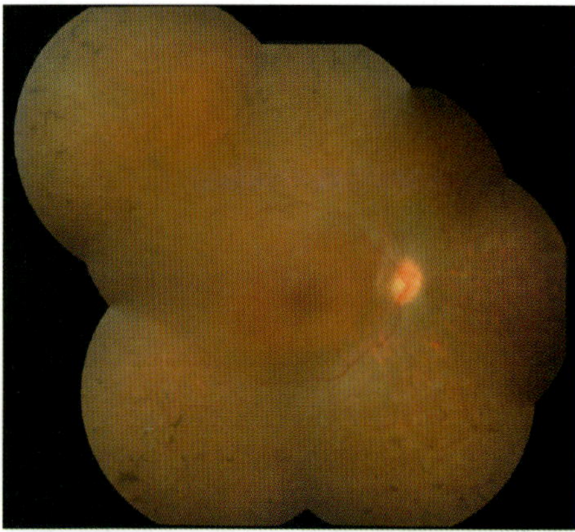
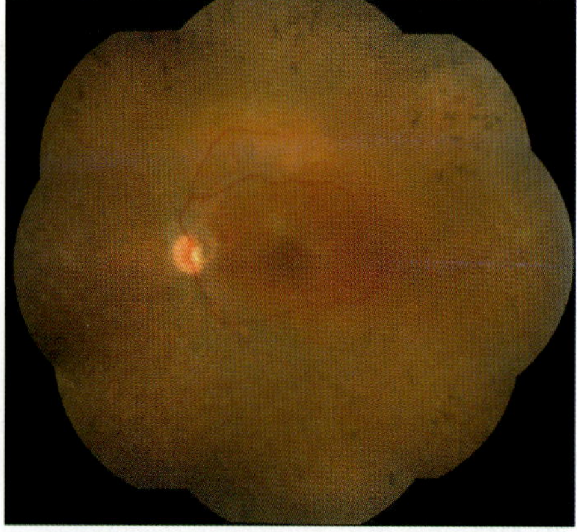

Fig. 82.1 Fundus picture of both eyes showing features of retinitis pigmentosa.

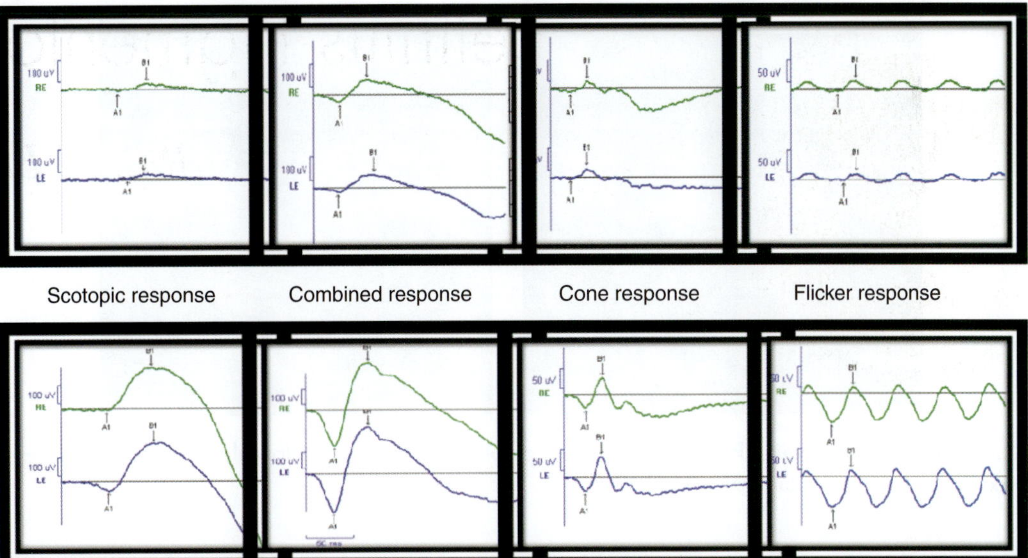

Fig. 82.2 An electroretinogram recording performed according to ISCEV standards showed total absence of scotopic responses and significant attenuation of cone responses suggestive of rod–cone dysfunction. Upper panel is the patient recording while lower is normal control.

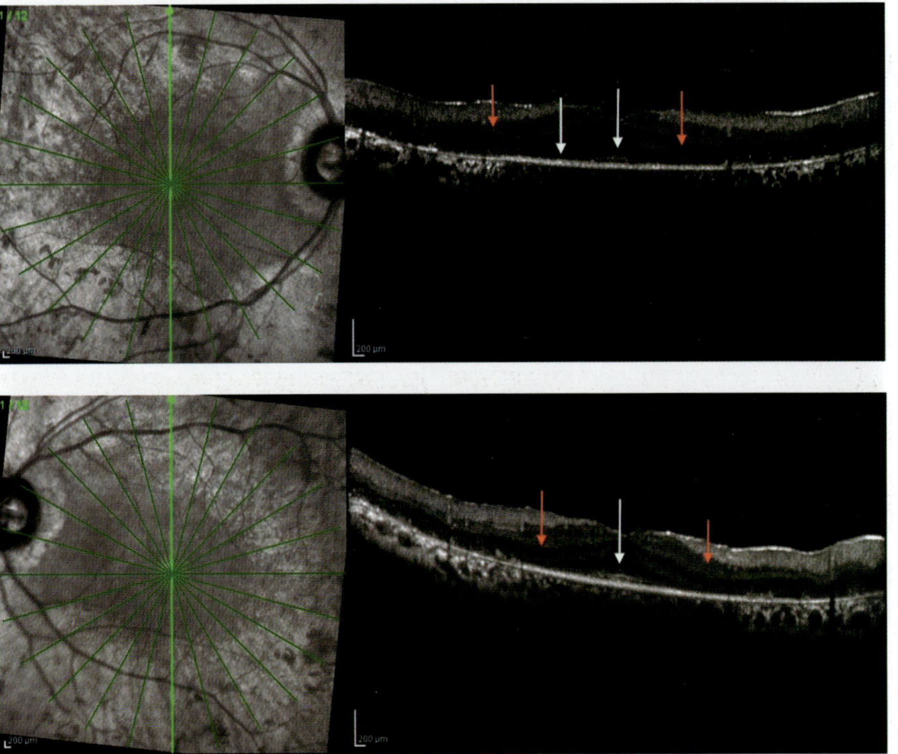

Fig. 82.3 SD-OCT of both eyes showing significant loss of IS–OS junction and the ELM layers (*white arrows*). There is also an early loss of inner retinal layers in both the eyes (*red arrows*).

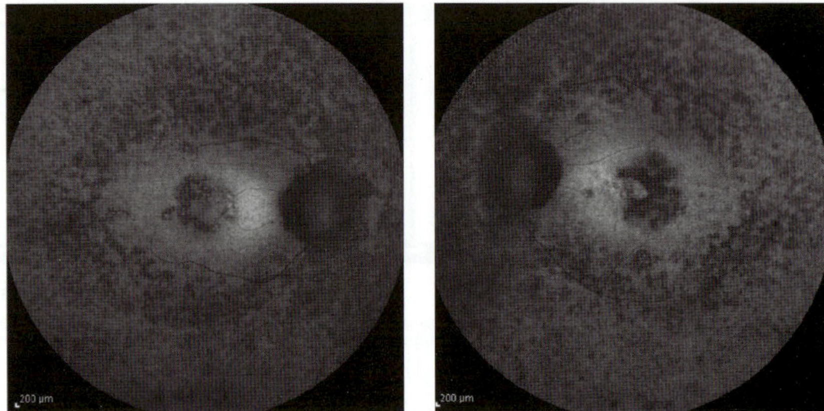

Fig. 82.4 FAF of a patient with RP showing increased autofluorescence in parafoveal area probably corresponding to the area of functioning retinal pigment epithelium.

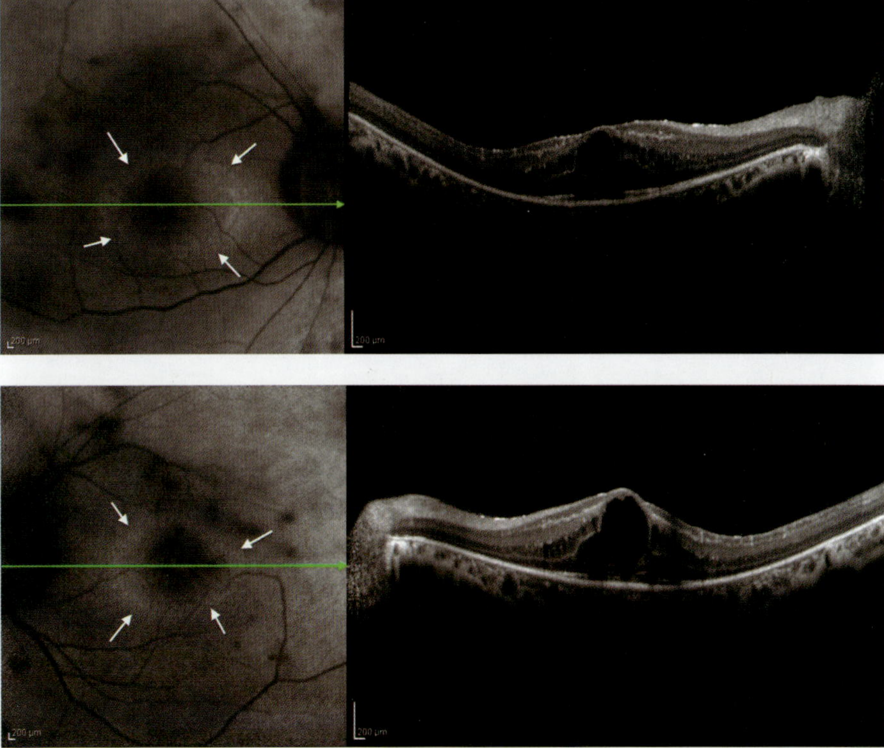

Fig. 82.5 SD-OCT of another patient with RP showing cystoid macular edema in both the eyes. Also note areas of increased hyper-autofluorescence (*white arrows*) in both the eyes. Monitoring the size of this hyper-autofluorescent ring is useful in monitoring the progression of the disease.

DISCUSSION

OCT is increasingly being used in studying and monitoring progression of macular changes in RP. Significant thinning of various layers at macula is commonly noted in RP. It is also used to assess the photoreceptor layer at the macula and changes in IS–OS junction may provide an insight into progressive loss of cones and rods. FAF is used to assess areas in the macula with preserved retinal pigment epithelium (RPE). A ring of increased FAF within this area may correspond to remaining cone function. OCT is also used to diagnose and monitor efficacy of treatment of the patients who develop cystoid macular edema. Lately, there are several studies that are analyzing the IS–OS junction with OCT and amplitudes of multifocal electroretinogram that may be helpful for monitoring RP patients in addition to time-tested visual acuity and visual fields.

CONCLUSION

OCT is an extremely useful tool in studying various changes that occur at the macula in the patients with RP, and is increasingly being used to monitor the progression of the disease.

FURTHER READING

1. Hamada S, Yoshida K, Chihara E: Optical coherence tomography images of retinitis pigmentosa. *Ophthalmic Surg Lasers* 31(3):253–256, 2000.
2. Kellner U, Kellner S, Weber BH, et al.: Lipofuscin- and melanin-related fundus autofluorescence visualize different retinal pigment epithelial alterations in patients with retinitis pigmentosa. *Eye (Lond)* 23(6):1349–1359, 2009.
3. Chung H, Hwang JU, Kim JG, et al.: Optical coherence tomography in the diagnosis and monitoring of cystoid macular edema in patients with retinitis pigmentosa. *Retina* 26(8):922–927, 2006.
4. Hajali M, GA Fishman, RJ Anderson: The prevalence of cystoid macular oedema in retinitis pigmentosa patients determined by optical coherence tomography. *Br J Ophthalmol* 92(8):1065–1068, 2008.
5. Oishi A, Nakamura H, Tatsumi I, et al.: Optical coherence tomographic pattern and focal electroretinogram in patients with retinitis pigmentosa. *Eye (Lond)* 23(2):299–303, 2009.

Solar Retinopathy

Supriya Dabir

Solar retinopathy is characterized by macular damage that results from intense and unprotected sun exposure. Sometimes the patient may give positive history either of eclipse viewing or as a professional hazard (e.g., aviation, astronomy); but more commonly the patient has no history at all and this pathology is picked up on routine retinal examination. Prolonged sun gazing is commonly observed among psychiatric patients.

CASE STUDY

A 20-year-old male presented with complaints of sudden-onset decrease in vision, central scotoma, and metamorphopsia since 1 week.

On examination best-corrected visual acuity (BCVA) was 20/40 in the right eye and 20/60 in the left eye. Amsler's grid showed distortion in both the eyes. Anterior segment was normal. Fundus showed a yellow cystic lesion at the fovea in both the eyes, as seen in **Figure 83.1**.

Fundus fluorescein angiography (FFA) showed a hyperfluorescent spot, not increasing in size or intensity at the fovea, suggesting a window defect. On spectral-domain optical coherence tomography (SD-OCT) imaging, radial scan showed irregular hyperreflectivity and discontinuity of inner segment–outer segment (IS–OS) junctional layer, as seen in **Figure 83.2**.

The patient was given antioxidants, counseled, and asked to review again.

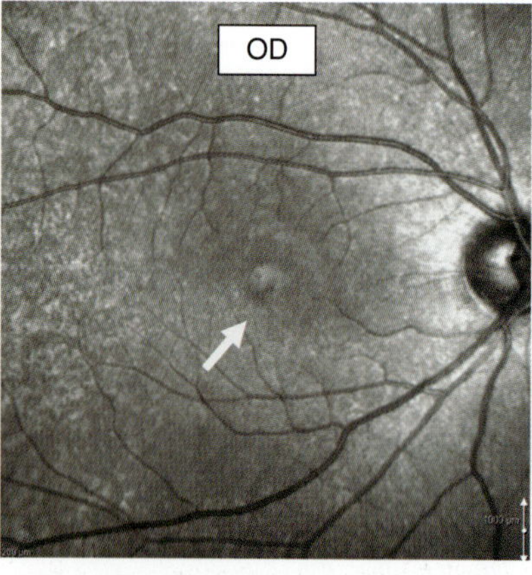

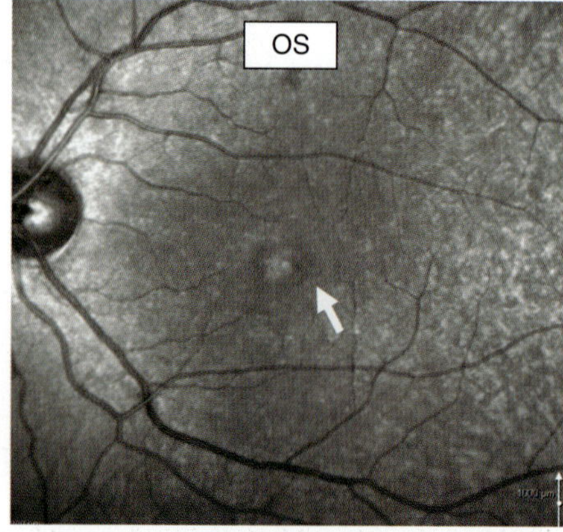

Fig. 83.1 Red free photographs show pigment epithelial cystic change in perifoveal zone in both the eyes.

When he came back for a review visit 2 months later, his symptoms had resolved. His BCVA was 20/20 in both the eyes with a normal Amsler's grid chart. On fundus examination, there was a resolution of the cystic lesion at the macula.

A repeat SD-OCT showed resolution of irregularity of the IS–OS junction. Foveal contour remained normal. Comparison scan showed difference between the two visits, as seen in **Figure 83.3**.

DISCUSSION

SD-OCT is a very useful investigative tool in solar retinopathy, especially in those cases where patient is symptomatic and the fundus appears clinically normal.

In acute cases (within a few days of exposure) of solar retinopathy, an intense amount of irradiation is absorbed preferentially by melanosomes of the retinal pigment epithelium (RPE), leading to loss of melanin granules and sloughing of necrotic RPE. This leads to outer retinal defects. Since the RPE can regenerate itself within weeks, this defect recovers. This is what was seen in our patient. But with, prolonged exposure the damage may further progress to involve photoreceptor outer segments. RPE is capable of regeneration, but the photoreceptors are incapable of it. This explains the outer lamellar hole seen in few patients.

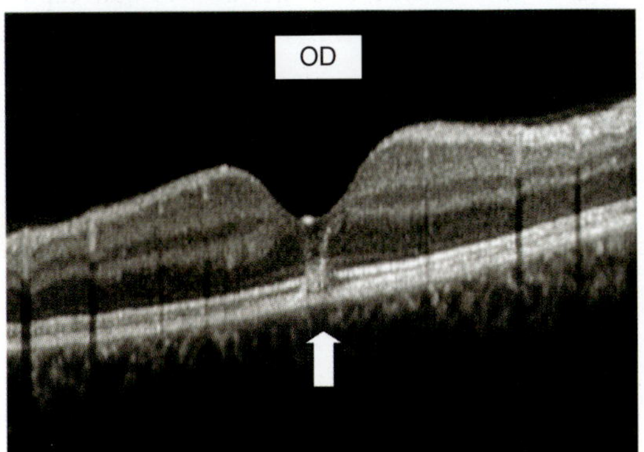
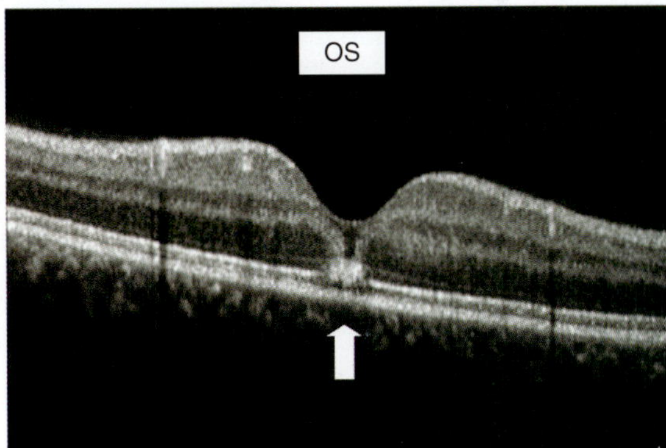

Fig. 83.2 Spectral-domain optical coherence tomography (SD-OCT) imaging, radial scan of both eyes shows irregular hyperreflectivity and discontinuity of inner segment–outer segment (IS–OS) junctional layer as shown by the white arrows.

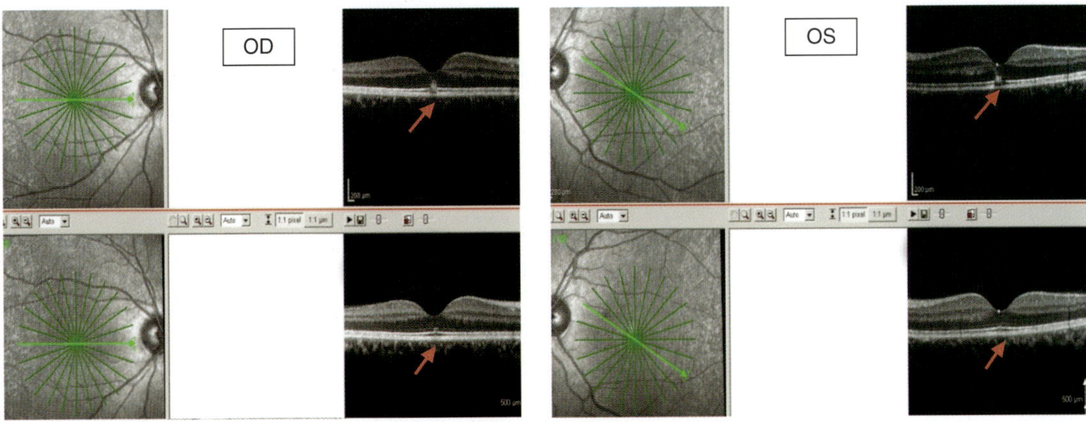

Fig. 83.3 Comparison scans of both eyes shows resolution of the irregularity in the outer layers as shown by the red arrows.

FURTHER READING

1. Yannuzzi LA, Fisher YL, Krueger A, et al.: Solar retinopathy: a photobiological and geophysical analysis. *Trans Am Ophthalmol Soc* 85:120–158, 1987.
2. Huang SJ, Gross NE, Costa DL, et al.: Optical coherence tomography findings in photic maculopathy. *Retina* 23:863–866, 2003.
3. Devadason DS, Mahmood S, Stanga PE, et al.: Solar retinopathy in a patient with bipolar affective disorder. *Br J Ophthalmol* 90:247, 2006.
4. Jain A, Desai RU, Charalel RA, et al.: Solar retinopathy: comparison of optical coherence tomography (OCT) and fluorescein angiography (FA). *Retina* 29:1340–1345, 2009.
5. Jiangmei W, Seregard S, Algvere PV: Photochemical damage of the retina. *Surv Ophthalmol* 51:461–481, 2006.

Sorsby's Fundus Dystrophy

Scott Schoenberger and Anita Agarwal

Sorsby's fundus dystrophy (also known as Sorsby's pseudoinflammatory macular dystrophy) is an autosomal dominantly inherited condition characterized by early-onset choroidal neovascularization, subretinal hemorrhage, atrophy, and disciform scarring in the macula. Peripheral changes may include atrophy, pigment clumping, and drusen-like deposits at the level of the retinal pigment epithelium. The following case highlights many of these abnormalities, including bilateral choroidal neovascularization, disciform scarring and atrophy, peripheral yellow deposits, and pigment clumping.

As in the following case, visual loss may be severe due to geographic atrophy or disciform scarring in the macula. Nyctalopia, prolonged dark adaptation, and peripheral visual field loss may also occur. Bilateral, multifocal choroidal neovascular membranes often develop. The genetic defect is in the *TIMP-3* gene (tissue inhibitor of metalloproteinase-3), which encodes a protein that is secreted by the retinal pigment epithelium and incorporated into Bruch's membrane. Symptoms typically develop in the third to fifth decade of life. A strong family history of early-onset macular degeneration with vision loss is usually present.

CASE STUDY

A 50-year-old female presented with decreased vision in her right eye. She carried a diagnosis of "juvenile macular degeneration" and had undergone previous laser photocoagulation and photodynamic therapy for recurrent choroidal neovascularization in her left eye over 5 years. She had a visual acuity of 20/25 oculus dexter (OD) and 3/200 oculus sinister (OS). She had a strong family history of early-onset macular degeneration. Genetic testing confirmed a mutation in the TIMP-3 gene, confirming Sorsby's macular dystrophy.

The dilated funduscopic examination at presentation showed numerous drusen-like deposits in both eyes with a disciform scar in the left eye (**Fig. 84.1**). The temporal macula of the right eye had a small area of discrete subretinal hemorrhage with subretinal fluid. Fluorescein angiography showed early, well-defined hyperfluorescence with surrounding blockage and late leakage, consistent with a classic choroidal neovascular membrane (**Fig. 84.2**). Three years later, a new, raised gray lesion was present inferonasal to the fovea (**Fig. 84.3**). Fluorescein angiography was consistent with a classic choroidal neovascular membrane. The patient received monthly intravitreal antivascular endothelial growth factor injections with involution of the neovascular membrane. Two years later, new, multifocal areas of subretinal hemorrhage were present in the left eye, consistent with recurrent choroidal neovascularization (**Fig. 84.4**). The previous neovascular sites in the right eye were replaced by chorioretinal scars. Spectral-domain optical coherence tomography revealed subretinal hyperreflectivity and choroidal thickening, consistent with a hyperpigmented scar (**Fig. 84.5**, *white arrows*), subretinal pigment epithelial drusen-like deposits (*black arrows*) and subretinal deposits.

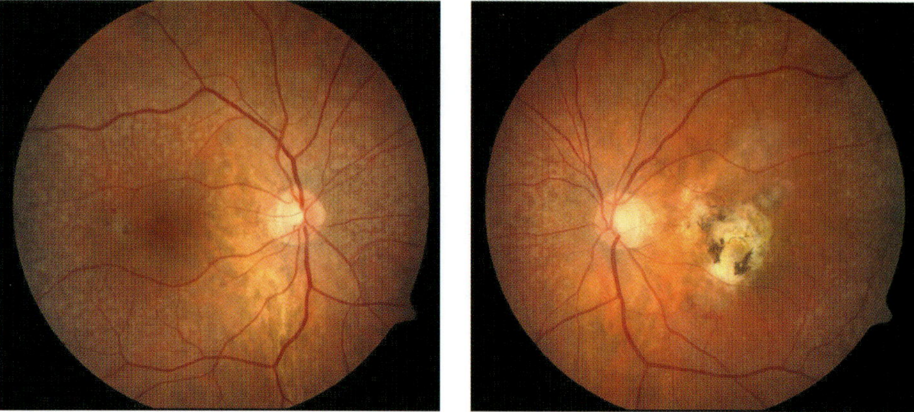

Fig. 84.1 Fundus photography of both eyes show extensive drusen-like deposits. The right eye has a small area in the temporal macula with discrete subretinal hemorrhage and subretinal fluid. The left eye has a disciform scar.

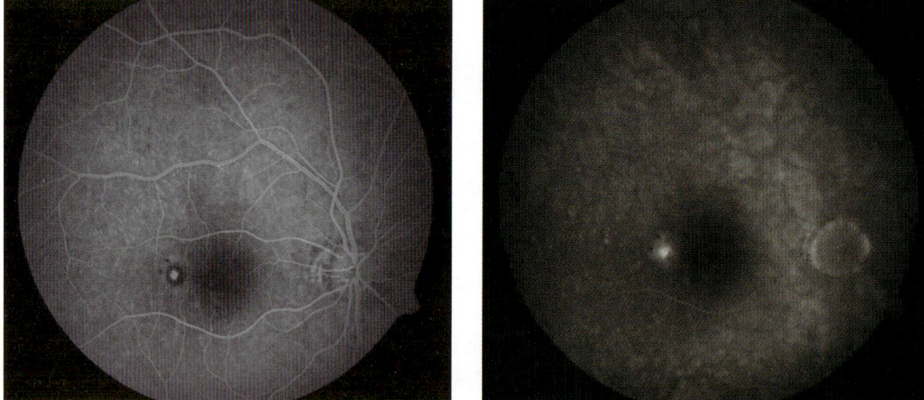

Fig. 84.2 Fluorescein angiography of the right eye shows early well-defined hyperfluorescence with surrounding blockage and late leakage, consistent with a classic choroidal neovascular membrane.

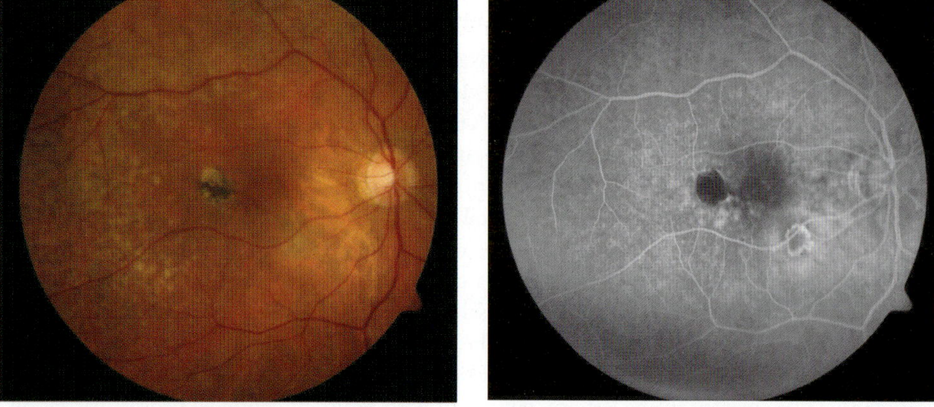

Fig. 84.3 Repeat fundus photography 3 years later shows an increase in the drusen-like deposits, a chorioretinal scar in the temporal macula corresponding to prior focal laser, and a new ill-defined, raised gray lesion inferonasal to the fovea. On fluorescein angiography, early well-defined hyperfluorescence is present, consistent with a classic choroidal neovascular membrane.

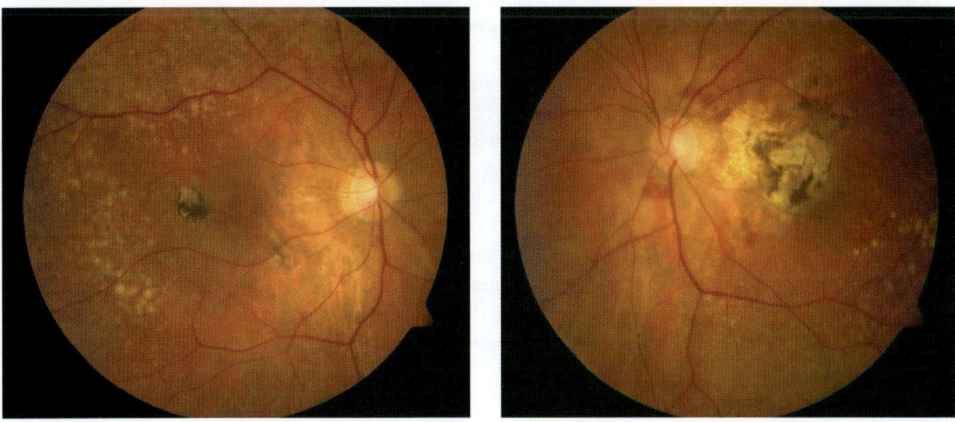

Fig. 84.4 Two years later, fundus photographs show extensive drusen-like deposits and chorioretinal scars corresponding to previous neovascular sites. The left eye demonstrates drusen-like deposits, a disciform scar, and new, multifocal areas of subretinal hemorrhage consistent with recurrent choroidal neovascularization.

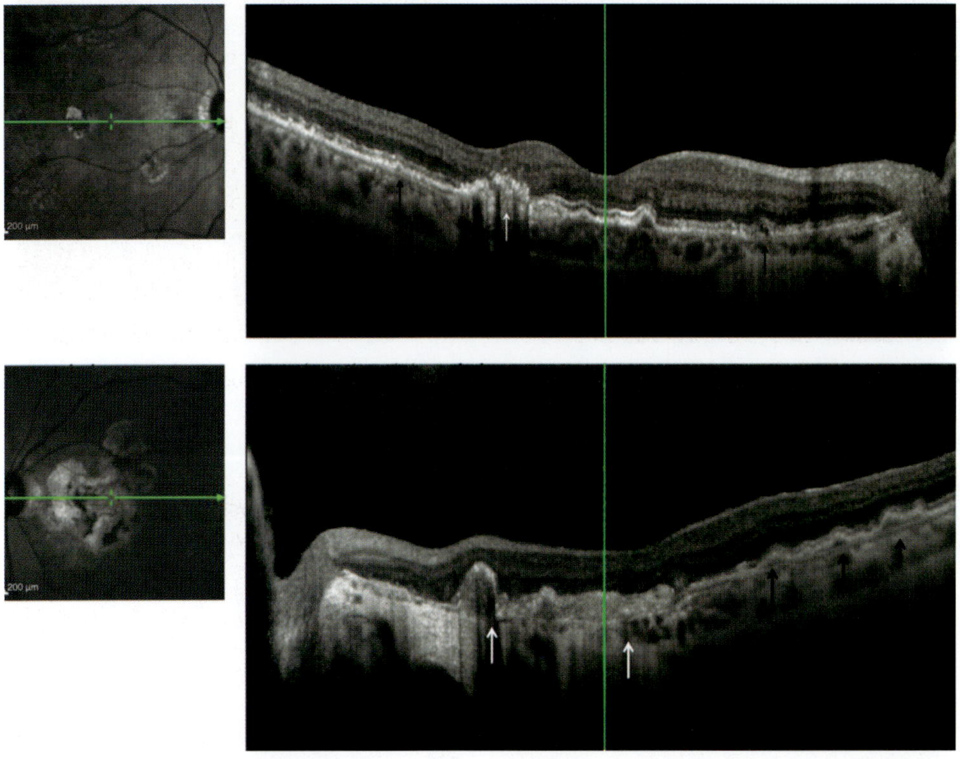

Fig. 84.5 Infrared imaging and spectral-domain optical coherence tomography of the right eye (*top*) and left eye (*bottom*). Findings include subretinal hyper-reflectivity and choroidal shadowing, consistent with a hyperpigmented scar (*white arrows*). Also present are numerous subretinal pigment epithelial drusen-like deposits (*black arrows*) and subretinal deposits, corresponding to the deposits seen on fundus photography.

FURTHER READING

1. Sivaprasad S, Webster AR, Egan CA, et al.: Clinical course and treatment outcomes of Sorsby fundus dystrophy. *Am J Ophthalmol* 146:228–234, 2008.
2. Weber BH, Vogt C, Pruett RC, et al.: Mutations in the tissue inhibitor of metalloproteinases-3 (*TIMP3*) in patients with Sorsby's fundus dystrophy. *Nat Genet* 8:352–356, 1994.
3. Polkinghorne PJ, Capon MR, Berninger T, et al.: Sorsby's fundus dystrophy: a clinical study. *Ophthalmology* 96:1763–1768, 1989.
4. Sorsby A, Mason ME: A fundus dystrophy with unusual features. *Br J Ophthalmol* 33:67–97, 1949.
5. Ashton N, Sorsby A: Fundus dystrophy with unusual features: a histological study. *Br J Ophthalmol* 35:751–764, 1951.
6. Hamilton WK, Ewing CC, Ives EJ, et al.: Sorsby's fundus dystrophy. *Ophthalmology* 96:1755–1762, 1989.
7. Peters AL, Young MJ, Miller JK: Optical coherence tomography for assessing disease progression in Sorsby fundus dystrophy. *Retina* 26:1082–1084, 2006.

Stargardt's Disease

Rajani Battu

Stargardt's disease is the most common cause of juvenile macular dystrophy that can cause progressive central visual loss. Autosomal recessive inheritance is the commonest one; although an autosomal dominant Stargardt's has also been described. The disease affects retinal pigment epithelium (RPE) and photoreceptor layer, and typically has an onset in childhood or young adulthood. The disease is caused by mutations in gene encoding photoreceptor cell-specific–ATP-binding cassette transporter *ABC*A4 that leads to an abnormal accumulation of lipofuscin in the RPE and the photoreceptors causing degenerative changes. Based on the electrophysiology findings, the disease has been classified into three groups. Group 1 disease is normal except for abnormalities in pattern electroretinography (ERG). Group 2 disease shows additional loss of photopic ERG, while Group 3 shows abnormalities in both photopic and scotopic ERGs.

CASE STUDY

A 32-year-old man presented with blurred vision for distance. His younger brother had a similar complaint. Ocular examination showed a vision of 6/36, N10 in both eyes. Fundus examination of both the eyes showed normal discs, normal vessels, and atrophic changes at the macula suggestive of Stargardt's disease (Fig. 85.1). Classically, the disease

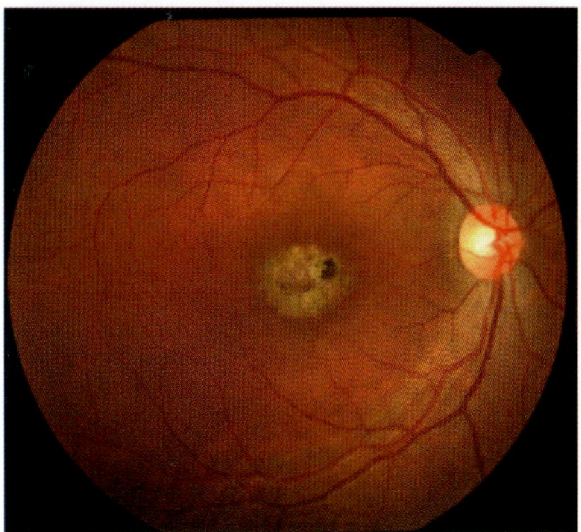
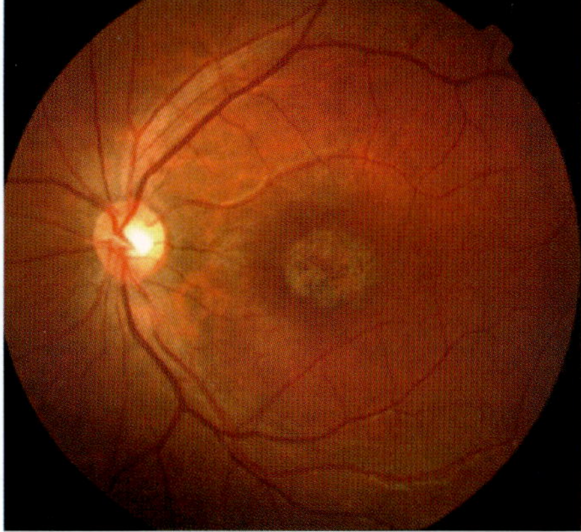

Fig. 85.1 Fundus picture of both eyes showing beaten-metal appearance at the macula with early atrophic changes. Disease is confined to the macula.

shows multiple flecks, which is sometimes referred to as "fundus flavimaculatus" (**Figs 85.2 and 85.3**). Fundus fluorescein angiogram in Stargardt's disease shows the typical "dark choroid" due to masking of the choroidal fluorescence by the accumulated lipofuscin (**Fig. 85.4**). Spectral-domain optical coherence tomography (SD-OCT) shows thinning of the macular area corresponding to the macular atrophy (**Fig. 85.5**).

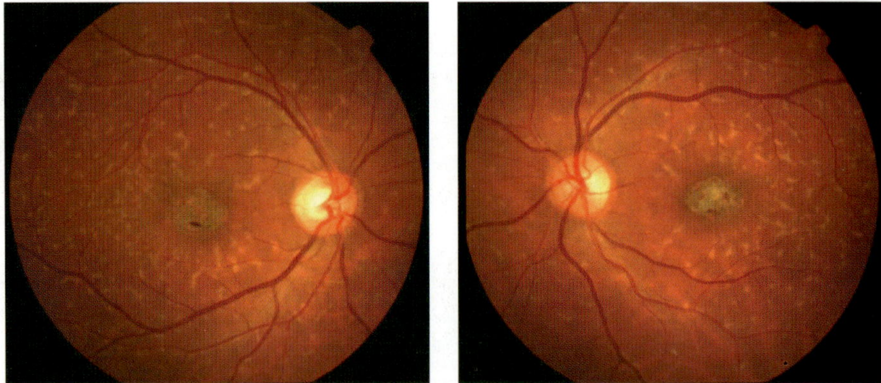

Fig. 85.2 Fundus picture of another patient with Stargardt's disease showing typical flecks and macular atrophy.

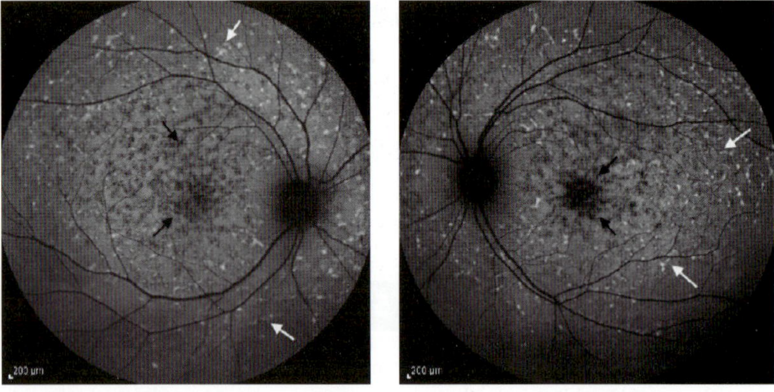

Fig. 85.3 Fundus autofluorescence of the same patient as in Figure 85.2. The flecks appear hyperautofluorescent (*white arrows*) corresponding to areas of increased lipofuscin, while macula shows hypoautofluorescence (*black arrows*) corresponding to the areas of RPE loss and atrophy.

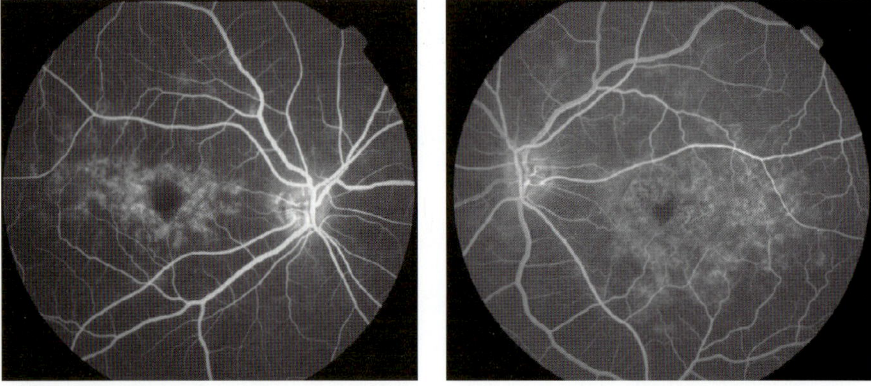

Fig. 85.4 Midphase fundus fluorescein angiogram of a patient showing lack of choroidal fluorescence. The "silent choroid" is typically due to excessive accumulation of lipofuscin.

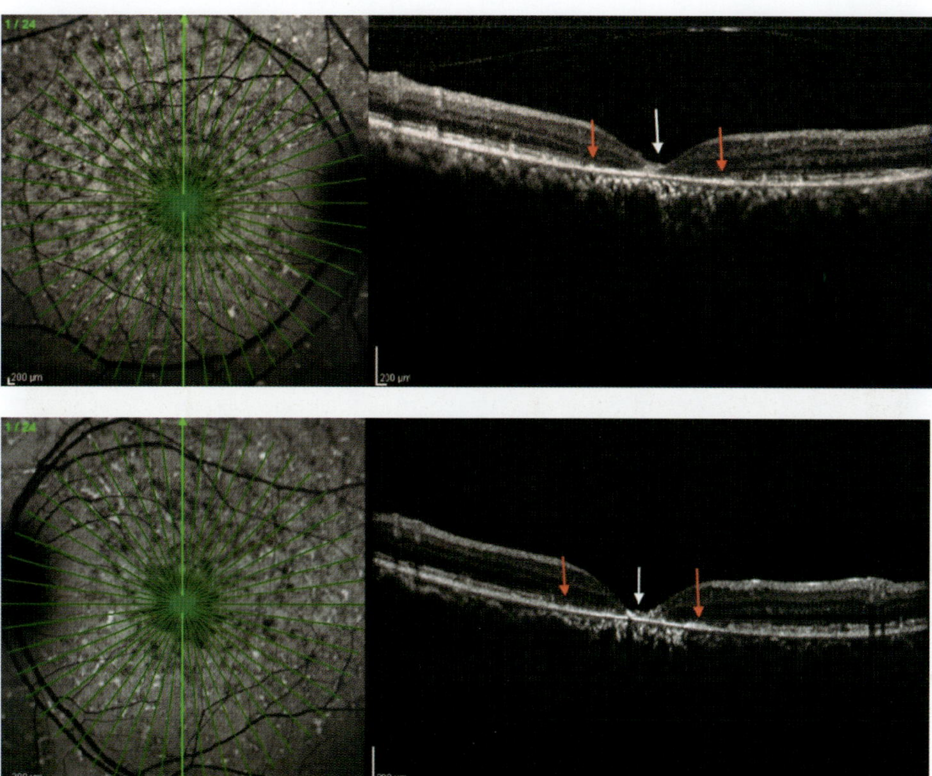

Fig. 85.5 SD-OCT of both eyes of the same patient as in Figure 85.2. The *white arrows* point to severe thinning of central retina corresponding to areas of central macular atrophy. The *red arrows* show the areas of significant inner segment–outer segment (IS–OS) disruption, probably corresponding to the areas of loss of photoreceptors.

DISCUSSION

Optical coherence tomography (OCT) imaging has enabled in-vivo–cross-sectional analysis of retinal pathology in various retinal degenerative diseases. Atrophy of the photoreceptors and RPE layer is characteristic of Stargardt's disease. Fundus autofluorescence enables visualization of lipofuscin in the retinal pigment epithelium and may be useful in evaluating extent of the disease. Studies using SD-OCT in patients with Stargardt's disease have demonstrated IS–OS junctional loss and photoreceptor thinning, as well as atrophy of choriocapillaries. OCT may also facilitate measurements of thickness of retinal sublayers, allowing precise mapping of their loss in retinal degeneration. It has also been possible to study the flecks on the OCT and characterize different types of flecks seen in Stargardt's disease.

CONCLUSION

SD-OCT helps in better understanding of the morphology of the retina in Stargardt's disease, facilitating earlier diagnosis and monitoring of the disease progression.

FURTHER READING

1. Vasireddy V, Wong P, Ayyagari R: Genetics and molecular pathology of Stargardt-like macular degeneration. *Prog Retin Eye Res* 29(3):191–207, 2010.

2. Rozet JM, Gerber S, Ducroq D, et al.: Hereditary macular dystrophies. *J Fr Ophtalmol* 28(1):113–124, 2005.
3. Koenekoop RK: The gene for Stargardt disease, *ABCA4*, is a major retinal gene: a mini review. *Ophthalmic Genet* 24(2): 75–80, 2003.
4. Fishman G: Fundus flavimaculatus. *A clinical classification. Arch Ophthalmol* 94:2061–2067, 1976.
5. Chen Y, Roorda A, Duncan JL: Advances in imaging of Stargardt disease. *Adv Exp Med Biol* 664:333–340, 2010.
6. Lim JI, Tan O, Fawzi AA, et al.: A pilot study of fourier domain optical coherence tomography of retinal dystrophy patients. *Am J Ophthalmol* 146(3):417–426, 2008.
7. Querques G, Leveziel N, Benhamou N, et al.: Analysis of retinal flecks in fundus flavimaculatus using optical coherence tomography. *Br J Ophthalmol* 90(9):1157–1162, 2006.

Traumatic Choroidal Rupture

Kavitha Avadhani, Anand Vinekar,
and Padmamalini Mahendradas

Chorioretinal rupture is a relatively common posterior segment manifestation of ocular trauma, especially of blunt force injuries. They are often the result of compressive forces that occur in blunt trauma and generally occur concentric to the optic disc. Visual loss occurs in acute cases only if the rupture involves the macula. Delayed visual loss is often seen due to development of a choroidal neovascular membrane, which then requires appropriate management.

CASE STUDY

A 16-year-old male presented to the outpatient department with a history of blunt trauma to the left eye following a fall at home. His best-corrected visual acuity was 20/60 in the left eye. Anterior segment examination of the left eye showed anterior chamber flare. There were no other anterior segment manifestations of the blunt trauma. Fundus examination of the left eye showed two linear choroidal ruptures—one large passing right through the macula just temporal to the center of the fovea and another inferotemporal to the macula (Fig. 86.1A).

Spectral-domain optical coherence tomography (SD-OCT) scan showed the rupture clearly as a hyperreflective area/disruption involving retinal pigment epithelium (RPE), outer retina, and inner choroid. There was

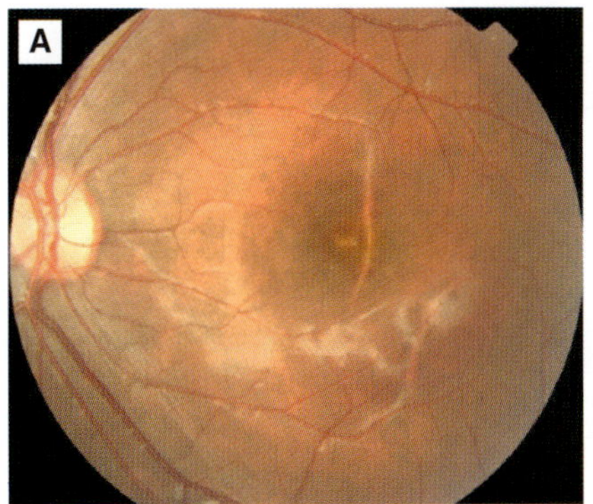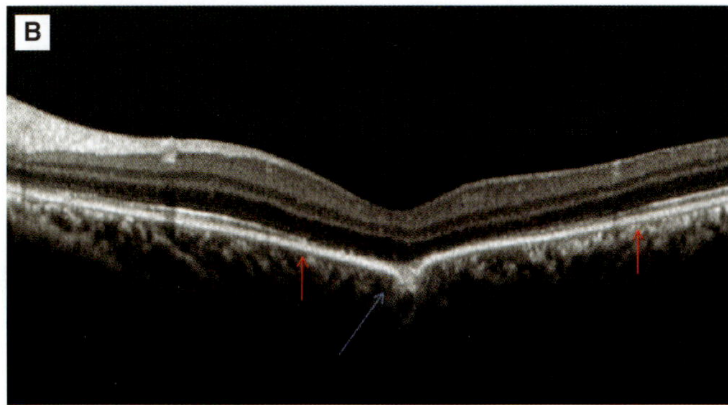

Fig. 86.1 (A) Fundus photograph of left eye showing two chorioretinal ruptures. (B) SD-OCT scan through rupture showing area of the rupture as a hyperreflective area involving the RPE, outer retina, and the inner choroid (*blue arrow*). The limit marked by two red arrows shows the area adjacent to the rupture where there is a loss of outer photoreceptor layer (IS–OS junctions).

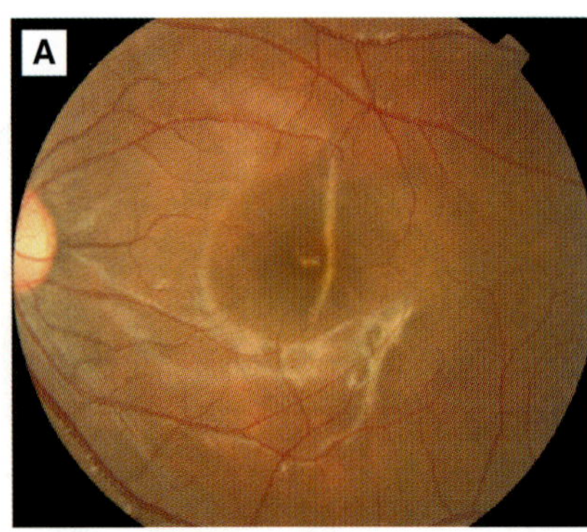 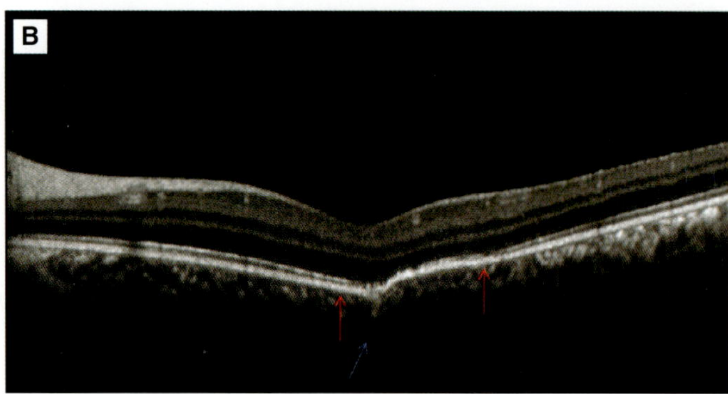

Fig. 86.2 (A) Fundus photograph of left eye showing same choroidal ruptures as seen in Fig. 86.1 (A) 3 months after initial presentation. **(B)** SD-OCT scan through the same area seen in Fig. 86.1 (B) showing a decrease in hyperreflectivity corresponding to healed rupture (*blue arrow*). Limit marked by *red arrows* delineates area of loss of the outer photoreceptor layer. It can be easily seen that area of photoreceptor loss is significantly reduced when compared with Fig. 86.1 (B), suggesting a regeneration of photoreceptor layer in the 3 months following initial trauma.

also loss of the IS–OS (inner segment–outer segment) portion of photoreceptor layer on either side of the rupture (more loss temporal to the rupture than nasal to it) (**Fig. 86.1B**). The patient was seen after 3 months following the trauma. His best-corrected visual acuity in the left eye was 20/40. SD-OCT done at this visit showed that there was a decrease in area/size of hyperreflectivity corresponding to the rupture. Also, there was a regeneration of the IS–OS portion of the photoreceptor layer on either side of the rupture (**Figs 86.2A and B**). This optical coherence tomography (OCT) finding of regeneration of photoreceptor layer may be of prognostic significance in patients with traumatic choroidal rupture.

FURTHER READING

1. Lavinsky D, Martins EN, Cardillo JA, et al.: Fundus autofluorescence in patients with blunt ocular trauma. *Acta Ophthalmol* 89(1):e89–94, 2011.
2. Williams DF, Mieler WF, Williams GA: Posterior segment manifestations of ocular trauma. *Retina* 10 Suppl 1:S35–S44. 1990.
3. Ament CS, Zacks DN, Lane AM, et al.: Predictors of visual outcome and choroidal neovascular membrane formation after traumatic choroidal rupture. *Arch Ophthalmol* 124(7):957–966, 2006.
4. Abri A, Binder S, Pavelka M, et al.: Choroidal neovascularization in a child with traumatic choroidal rupture: clinical and ultrastructural findings. *Clin Experiment Ophthalmol* 34(5):460–463, 2006.

Vitreomacular Traction Syndrome

Naresh Kumar Yadav and Kanav Gupta

Vitreomacular traction syndrome (VMT) was described first by Reese, et al. as a condition characterized by persistent vitreous attachment in the center of macula, causing a cystoid configuration and decreased vision. Cause could be macular traction impending completion of posterior vitreous separation or aborted posterior vitreous separation stimulating preretinal tissue proliferation. Most of the reported studies suggest that the incidence of VMT is about 65% in the age group of 26–85 years.

Optical coherence tomography (OCT) also demonstrates pathognomonic vitreoretinal attachment. Idiopathic macular pucker is the most commonly encountered condition that may mimic VMT. With macular pucker, however, Weiss' ring usually is present, which indicates complete posterior vitreous detachment. Most cases do not require treatment.

The surgical treatment involves three-port pars plana vitrectomy and induction of PVD.

CASE STUDY

A 76-year-old female patient presented to us with complaints of blurred central vision in the left eye since 1 year. She gave a history of undergoing cataract surgery in both the eyes 5-years back.

Fundus examination showed preretinal membrane with a pseudohole configuration. Spectral-domain OCT was done, which showed vitreomacular traction with loss of foveal contour and cystoid spaces (Fig. 87.1A). She underwent pars plana vitrectomy with posterior vitreous detachment (PVD) induction. Intraoperatively hand-held spectral domain OCT (Bioptigen) was used to ensure the complete removal of the traction (Fig. 87.1B). Post vitrectomy again SD-OCT was done, which showed normalization of the foveal contour (Fig. 87.1C).

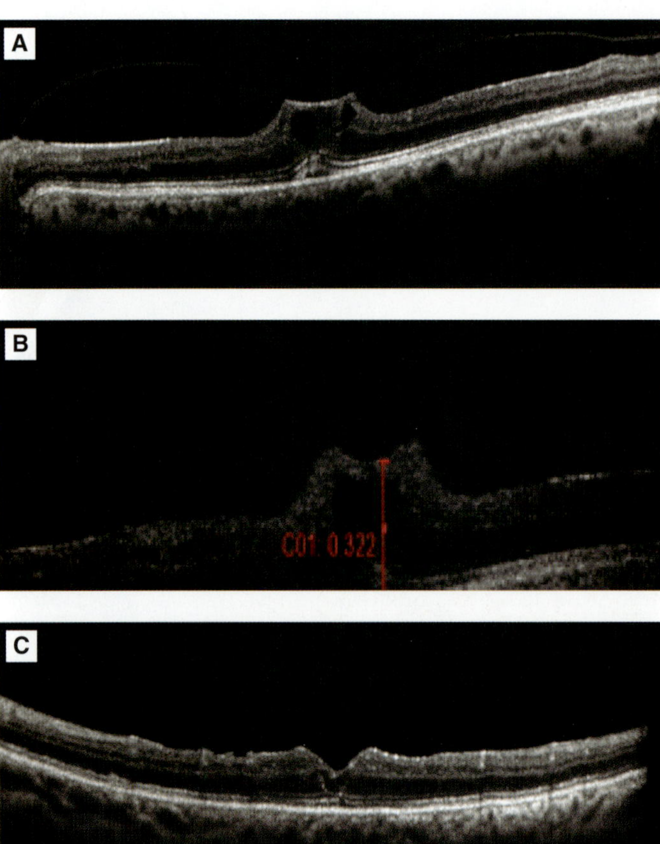

Fig. 87.1 (A) SPECTRALIS™ spectral-domain optical coherence tomography (SD-OCT) shows vitreomacular traction and loss of foveal contour. Hyporeflective cystoid cavities are seen (cystoid edema). (B) The intraoperative hand-held SD-OCT (Bioptigen) of the same patient performed immediately after induction of posterior vitreous detachment and ILM peeling shows release of the traction at the fovea. The central retinal thickness is 322 microns. The ILM edge is also visible. (C) The SPECTRALIS™ SD-OCT of the same patient after pars plana vitrectomy and ILM peeling shows normalization of the foveal contour.

FURTHER READING

1. Reese AB, Jones IR, Cooper WC: Macular changes secondary to vitreous traction. *Am J Ophthalmol* 51:544–549, 1967.
2. Smiddy WE, Michels RG, Glaser BM: Vitrectomy for macular traction caused by incomplete vitreous separation. *Arch Ophthalmol* 106:624–628, 1988.
3. Margherio RR, Trese MT, Margherio AR, et al.: Surgical management of vitreomacular traction syndromes. *Ophthalmology* 96:1437–1445, 1989.
4. MacDonald HR, Johnson RN, Schatz H: Surgical results in the vitreomacular traction syndrome. *Ophthalmology* 101:1397–1403, 1994.
5. Melberg N, Williams DF, Balles MW, et al.: Vitrectomy for vitreomacular traction syndrome with macular detachment. *Retina* 15:192–197, 1995.

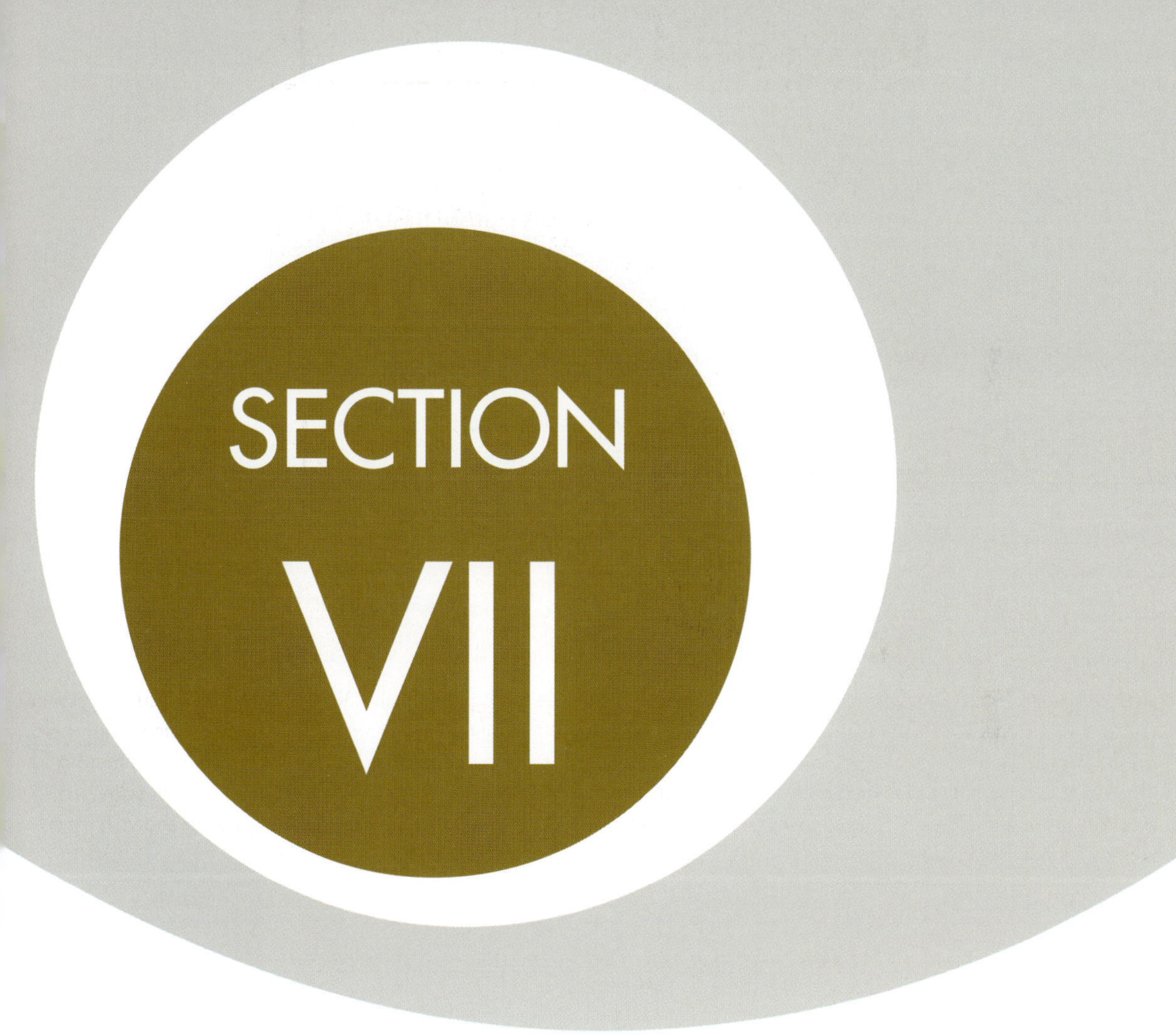

Pediatric Retina

Imaging an Infant on Optical Coherence Tomography

Anand Vinekar

Despite becoming a commonly used imaging modality in adult ophthalmic practice, particularly in posterior segment evaluation, pediatric OCT imaging has not become very popular. This is chiefly because of limited options in available equipment design that disallow easy acquisition of images, especially in the unanesthetized, preverbal, and uncooperative child.

Pediatric patients must therefore be sedated or anesthetized, necessitating the procedure to be completed in the operating room, with a full-fledged team comprising of a pediatric nurse and an anesthetist (Fig. 88.1).

To circumvent general anesthesia, several modifications have been described. The "flying baby" position described in the time-domain optical coherence tomography (TD-OCT) era allows the nonsedated infant to be horizontally held at the chin rest of the device (Fig. 88.2). Images are oriented as in an adult and lateral inversion is not a problem.

More recently, SPECTRALIS™ has been modified converting the tabletop device into a hand-held optical coherence tomography (OCT) device to successfully image premature infants. This is a two-step disassembly and frees the camera, allowing the user to align the axis in any plane for capture (Fig. 88.3). The infant is supine and needs no sedation or anesthesia; although monitoring by an anesthetist is advisable, especially if angiography is to be performed.

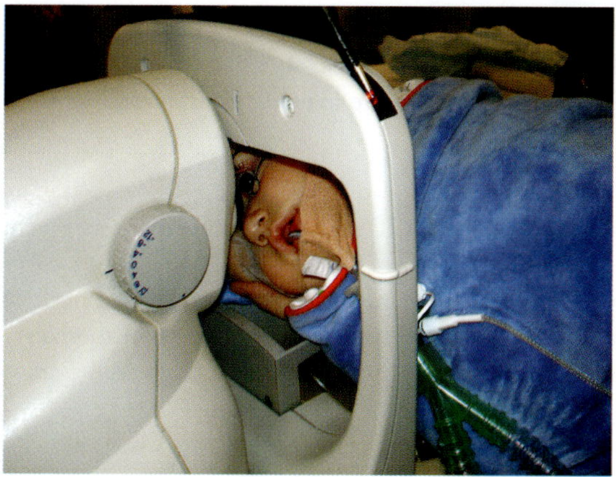

Fig. 88.1 A child is intubated for an imaging procedure. Such procedures are often combined with a complete examination under anesthesia or even definitive surgery. [Photo courtesy: CK Patel, Andrew Farmery, and Paul Harris (Oxford University Hospital, UK).]

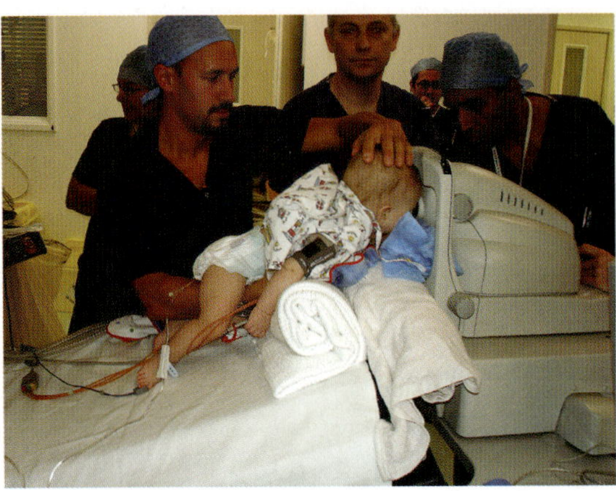

Fig. 88.2 Child is held in the horizontal position on a tilted table to maintain face and eyes in the straight axis of the OCT camera. [Photo courtesy: CK Patel, Andrew Farmery, and Paul Harris (Oxford University Hospital, UK).]

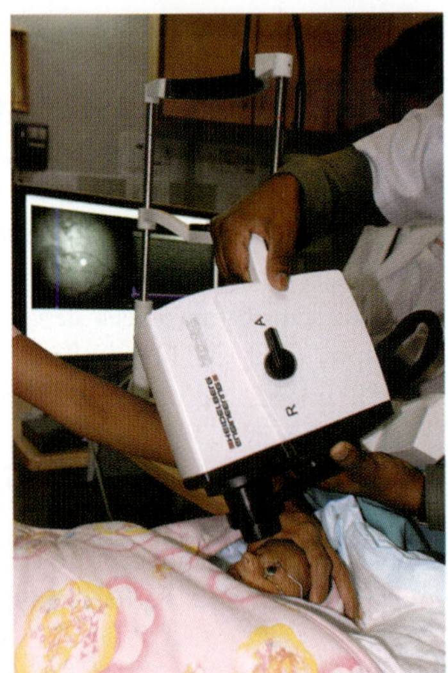

Fig. 88.3 Freed camera is aligned for image capture. The child is sans sedation or anesthesia in this noncontact procedure. The images are captured in the office. As the infant's head is closer to the camera and the technician stands at the head end of the infant, the resulting images are laterally inverted and must be kept in mind while interpreting localization.

Advantage of the SPECTRALIS™ is that the OCT may be combined with other procedures including fluorescein and indocyanine green angiography.

Another method, especially in a slightly older infant who has established neck control, would be to swaddle the infant in tight, enclosing wraps within linen sheets (Fig. 88.4) and prop the baby against the chin rest. Synthetic material must be avoided as they are more uncomfortable to the child as well as allows more "wriggly" movement of the infant inside the sheets.

More recently, with the commercial availability of the hand-held OCT device, Bioptigen, NC, USA, imaging children and infants has become much simpler. Modifications to the tabletop devices are not necessary (Fig. 88.5). The infant is conveniently imaged in the office or the operating room, depending on the clinical situation. The reference arm has to be changed for anterior or posterior segment imaging, and the distance and focus are adjusted manually using the noncontact camera of the device.

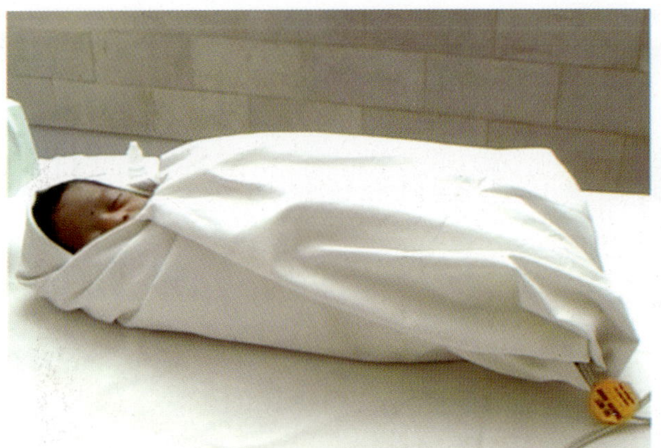

Fig. 88.4 Linen wrap is secure and tight enough to reduce movement of limbs, but is loose enough to allow easy respiration. The last fold of the sheet may cover the head, which allows the assistant to hold the head more easily. Often two assistants are necessary to prop and stabilize the infant in front of the device.

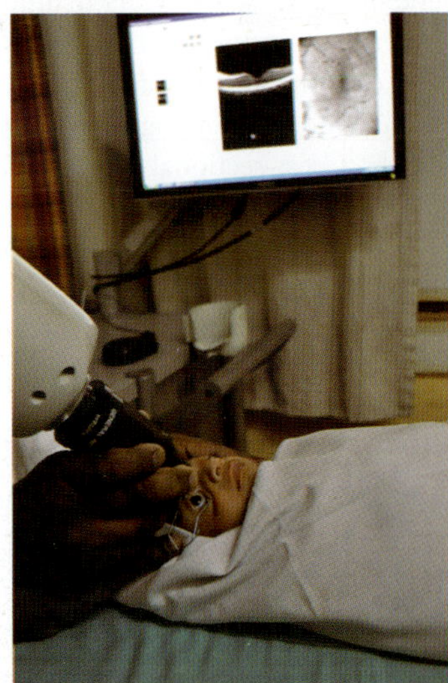

Fig. 88.5 The hand-held OCT by Bioptigen (Bioptigen NC, USA) is useful in pediatric imaging, as it allows both supine and sitting positions (in an older child) and produces upright, noninverted images.

With continual improvement in availability and capabilities of OCT devices, especially for pediatric cases, we are probably going to witness an increasing use of OCT imaging in children in the near future.

FURTHER READING

1. Patel CK: Optical coherence tomography in the management of acute retinopathy of prematurity. *Am J Ophthalmol* 141(3):582–584, 2006.
2. Maldonado RS, Izatt JA, Sarin N, et al.: Optimizing hand-held spectral domain optical coherence tomography imaging for neonates, infants, and children. *Invest Ophthalmol Vis Sci* 51(5):2678–2685, 2010.
3. Vinekar A, Sivakumar M, Shetty R, et al.: A novel technique using spectral-domain optical coherence tomography (Spectralis, SD-OCT + HRA) to image supine non-anaesthetized infants: utility demonstrated in aggressive posterior retinopathy of prematurity. *Eye (Lond)* 24(2):379–382, 2010.

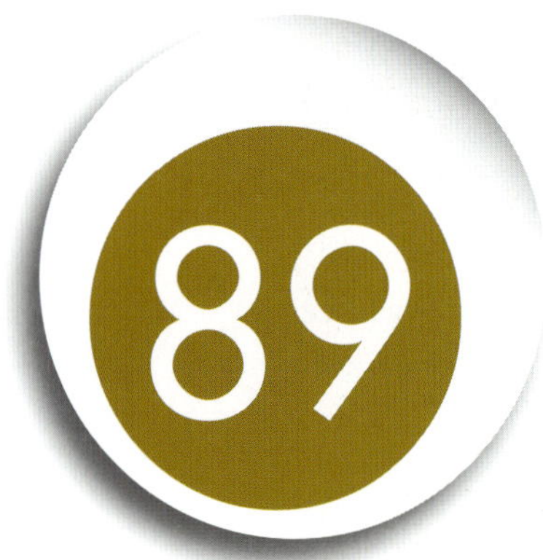

Foveal Layers in an Infant

Anand Vinekar, Ramiro Maldonado, and Cynthia Toth

Spectral-domain optical coherence tomography (SD-OCT) offers a unique in vivo opportunity to study infant retina. At birth, fovea is immature; and understanding the layers of a developing and maturing fovea allows us to evaluate the first important component of the evolving visual system.

Owing to differences in reflectivity properties among adjoining retinal layers, substructure differentiation, and layer identification is possible and even quantifiable. Cross-sectional images oriented within a 3-D (three-dimensional) stack of scans can reconstruct microanatomy.

Study of retinal layers from premature infants significantly contributes to the understanding of dynamic substructure changes during this critical time in visual development.

TERMINOLOGIES

1 Central foveal thickness: Thickness of the entire retina extending from the inner aspect of inner limiting membrane (ILM) to the inner aspect of retinal pigment epithelium (RPE) at the foveal center.

2 Inner retina: Inner retinal layer (IRL) includes all the retinal layers from the inner aspect of the ILM to the outer border of the inner nuclear layer (INL).

3 Outer retina: The outer retinal layer extends from the inner aspect of the outer plexiform layer (OPL) to the inner border of the RPE.

4 Photoreceptor layer: The photoreceptor layer (PRL) extends from the outer aspect of the OPL to the inner border of the RPE.

Compared to an older child or adult, the premature eye has several differences including: (1) a shallower foveal depression; (2) presence of one to many IRLs at the foveal center; (3) thinner retinal layers overall; and (4) attenuation of the PRL with absence of photoreceptor sublayers relative to the adult.

The most immature foveas are characterized by the presence of ganglion cell layer (GCL), inner plexiform layer (IPL), and INL as distinctly measurable at the foveal center. As the infant grows older, the IPL and the INL condense into a single thin hyperreflective band.

Blue lines denote the IRLs and comprise of the nerve fiber layer, ganglion cell layer, inner plexiform layer, and the INL. Due to reflectivity properties, the nuclear layers appear as more hyporeflective layers compared to the plexiform layers (**Fig. 89.1**).

Red lines denote the outer retinal layers and include the outer plexiform, the outer nuclear, the external limiting membrane, the inner segment and outer segment, and the RPE layer (**Fig. 89.1**).

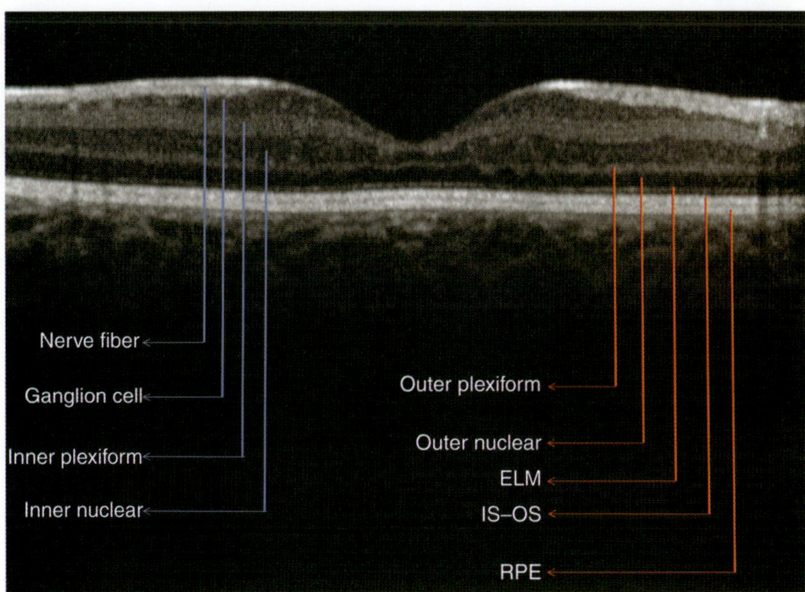

Fig. 89.1 SD-OCT image of the foveal center of a 36-weeks postmenstrual age male infant born with a birth weight of 1250 gm and 31 weeks of gestation.

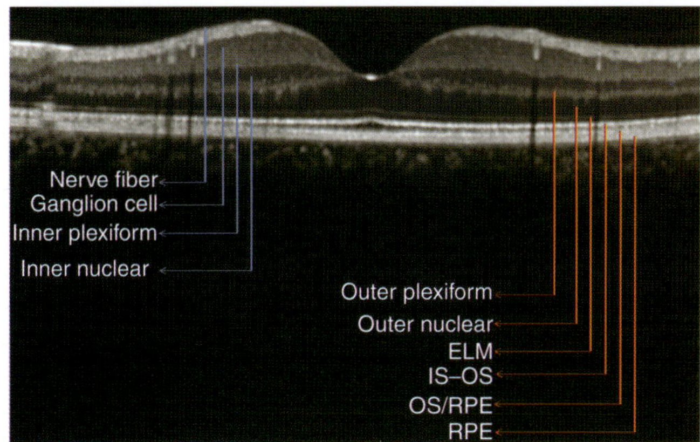

Fig. 89.2 SD-OCT image of the foveal center of a 37-year-old male.

It is noteworthy that, as our understanding of these layers continues to advance, some researchers believe that the hyperreflective band believed to be the "inner segment–outer segment (IS–OS)" layer should more appropriately be called the "inner segment ellipsoid band" (ISe band).

The foveal center of a healthy adult is shown alongside (Fig. 89.2) and shows that with increasing age the IRLs underwent a centrifugal migration of tissue and condensation into a single hyperrefective band at the foveal center. The outer retinal layers, on the other hand, are much thicker at the foveal center in an adult with further differentiation and increased thickness in photoreceptor nuclei and inner and outer segments.

FURTHER READING

1. Maldonado RS, O'Connell RV, Sarin N, et al.: Dynamics of human foveal development after premature birth. *Ophthalmology* 118:2315–2325, 2011.
2. Vinekar A, Avadhani K, Sivakumar M, et al.: Understanding clinically undetected macular changes in early retinopathy of prematurity on spectral domain optical coherence tomography. *Invest Ophthalmol Vis Sci* 52(8):5183–5188, 2011.
3. Vinekar A, Avadhani K, Sivakumar M, et al.: Macular edema in premature infants. *Ophthalmology* 119(6):1288–1289.e1, 2012; author reply 1289–1290.e1.
4. Vajzovic L, Hendrickson AE, O'Connell RV, et al.: Maturation of the human fovea: correlation of spectral-domain optical coherence tomography findings with histology. *Am J Ophthalmol* 154(5):779–789.e2, 2012.

Foveal Maturation in Infants

Anand Vinekar, Ramiro Maldonado, and Cynthia Toth

Retinal layers in an immature fovea have been detailed in Chapter 89, Foveal Layers in an Infant. In this chapter, the photoreceptor layer (PRL) in a developing infant with particular reference to progressive differentiation of substructures and critical differences with an adult has been described.

The inner retinal layer (IRL) migration at foveal center occurs over time in a premature infant eye. This results in deepening of the foveal pit to resemble that of an adult.

There is evidence to suggest that progressive centrifugal migration of these layers at the fovea begins as early as 26–28 weeks postmenstrual age (PMA) and has been observed by optical coherence tomography (OCT) at 31 weeks PMA and continues to a variable endpoint beyond 45 weeks (**Fig. 90.1**).

As central foveal IRL thickness decreases, parafoveal IRL thickness increases, resulting in a decrease in the foveal to parafoveal thickness (parafoveal annulus) ratio with increasing age. In contrast, PRL increases centrally to a lesser height and over a longer period.

The PRL in an infant is thinner compared to an adult and thinnest in the foveal center. This thickens centrally with age, especially after 38th week postmenstrual age, and continues until young adulthood. This PRL axial growth is maximum in the cone-dense fovea.

In a very premature infant, the photoreceptor subcellular structures have not developed to a level to be visible yet on OCT. These include external limiting membrane (ELM) and inner segment–outer segment (IS–OS) junction.

The IS–OS layer progressively approaches the foveal center in a pattern of centripetal growth between the 33rd and 48th weeks (**Figs 90.2–90.6**). The ELM has been reported to be visible on spectral-domain optical coherence tomography (SD-OCT) as early as 40.3 weeks PMA in Asian Indian eyes.

The IS–OS band first appears as a poorly defined reflective band, just visible above retinal pigment epithelium (RPE) and is seen outside the foveal center at approximately 33rd week of PMA. Thereafter, the thickness increases and together with the outer segments begins to appear both in the periphery and the center of the foveal zone to reach the foveal center by 43rd–48th week PMA (**Figs 90.2–90.6**).

It is noteworthy that as our understanding of these layers continues to advance, some researchers believe that the hyperreflective band believed to be "inner segment–outer segment (IS–OS)" layer should be more appropriately called "inner segment ellipsoid band (ISe band) (**Fig. 90.1**)."

The RPE reflex is a well-defined hyperreflective band that is easily imaged and serves as an anatomical landmark on OCT images of an infant. Most infants demonstrate this layer from 31 weeks PMA up to adulthood.

There is a second very subtle hyperreflective band between the RPE and the IS–OS, and is believed to be the interface between photoreceptor outer segments and the RPE microvilli. This is often referred to as the OS–RPE layer. There is considerable ambiguity as to when this layer matures to form a more well-defined "third layer," but certainly occurs later than the IS–OS fusion at the center. This is consistent with the growth of apical microvilli of the RPE.

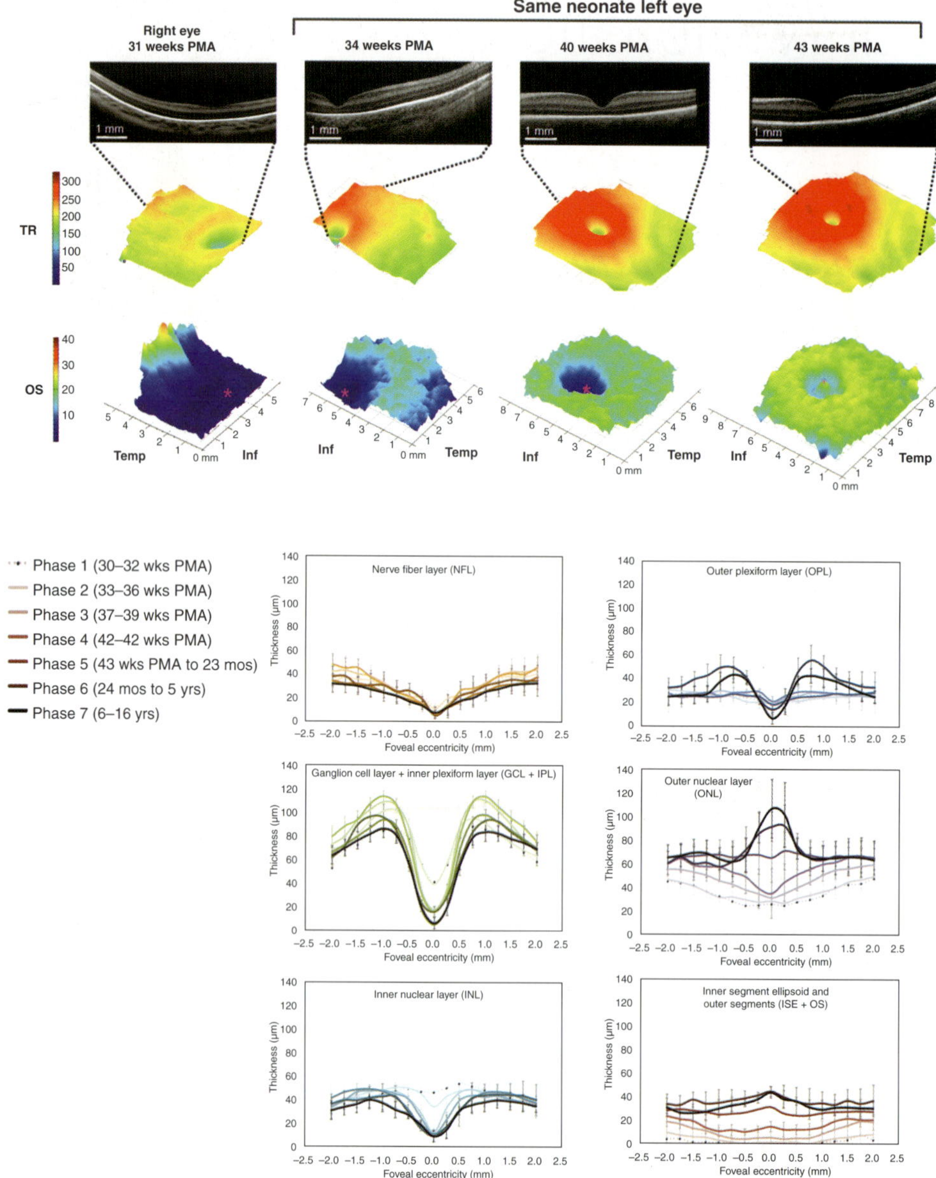

Fig. 90.1 Three dimensional map of retinal layers and their dynamic changes with age in a neonate. The lower portion of the image has a segment on ISe. (Photo courtesy: *For the top portion of the figure (color maps)*: Taken from Figure 2A, Page 2320. Maldonado RS, O'Connell RV, Sarin N, et al.: Dynamics of human foveal development after premature birth. *Ophthalmology* 118(12):2315–2325, Dec 2011. doi: 10.1016/j. ophtha. 2011.05.028. Epub Sep 21, 2011. *For the bottom portion of the figure (graphs)*: Taken from Figure 2, Page 782. Vajzovic L, Hendrickson AE, O'Connell RV, et al.: Maturation of the human fovea: correlation of spectral-domain optical coherence tomography findings with histology. *Am J Ophthalmol* 154(5):779–789, Nov 2012. e2. doi: 10.1016/j.ajo.2012.05.004. Epub Aug 13, 2012.)

The sloping "tent" of the IS–OS at the foveal center also accentuates with age and corresponds to longer outer segments of cones that are most densely packed in the foveal center.

The timing of appearance and the pattern of these layers in health and disease and its correlation with visual acuity will be useful in future research and clinical care.

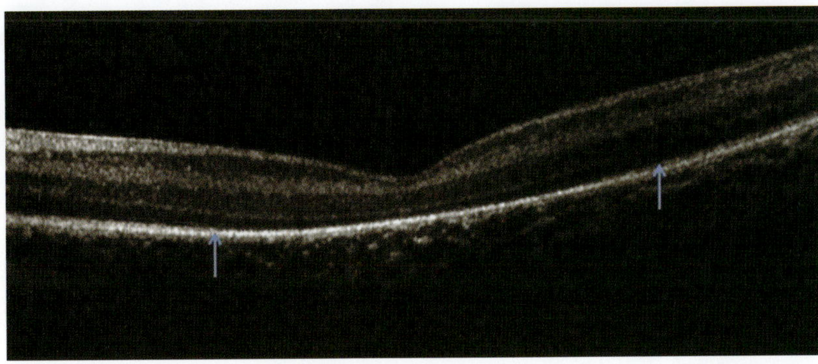

Fig. 90.2 The IS–OS band appears as a distinct hyperreflective band that first appears above the RPE band and converges towards the center from the periphery (centripetal). At 38 weeks PMA, in this example, two faint "shadow-like" lines (*blue arrows*) are seen at the two ends of the image.

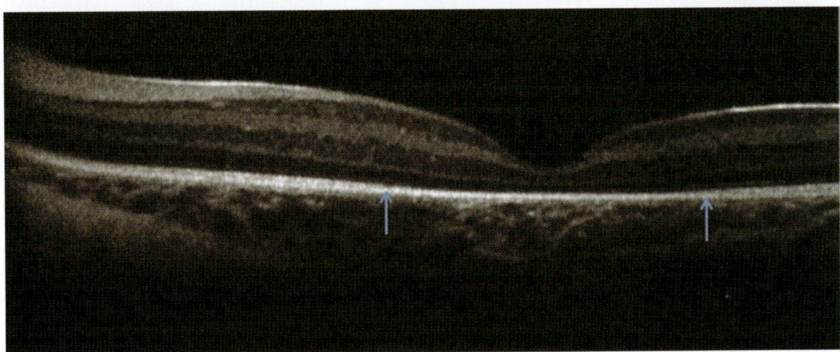

Fig. 90.3 The same infant and same eye imaged after 4 weeks (42 weeks PMA), now shows a more clearly visible second layer at the periphery (*blue arrows*) above the RPE.

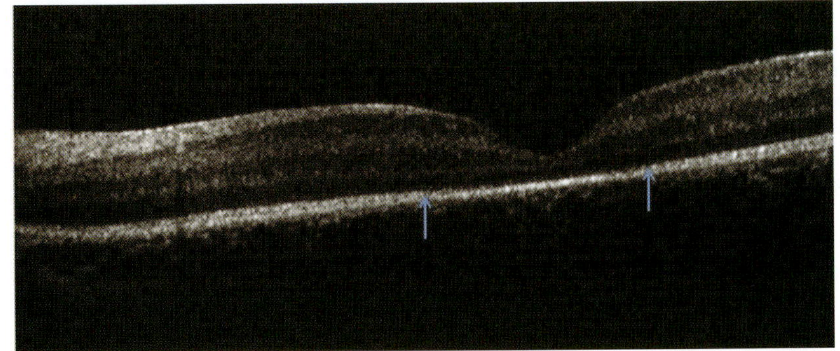

Fig. 90.4 At 46 weeks PMA, the two bands (IS–OS) are seen coming closer to each other (*blue arrows*) towards the foveal center.

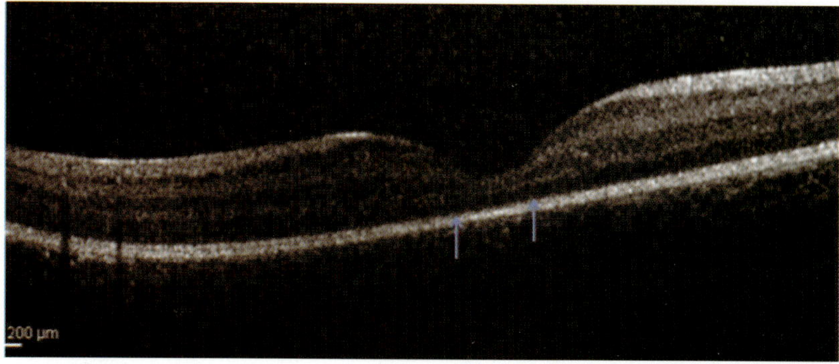

Fig. 90.5 At 47 weeks PMA, the IS–OS from either side almost touch (*blue arrows*) at the foveal center.

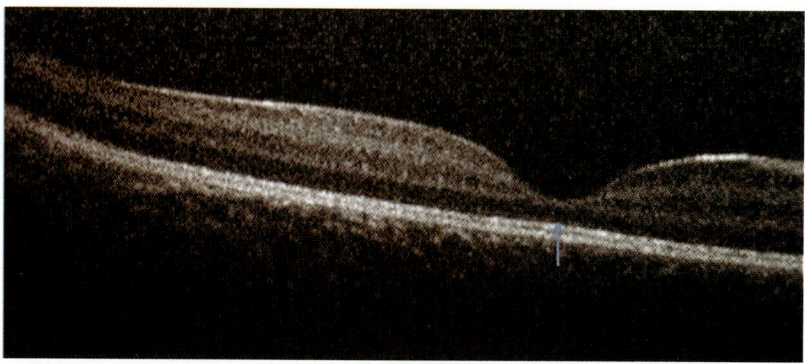

Fig. 90.6 At 48 weeks PMA, both layers are joined at the foveal center and appears as a distinct layer (*blue arrow*).

FURTHER READING

1. Maldonado RS, O'Connell RV, Sarin N, et al.: Dynamics of human foveal development after premature birth. *Ophthalmology* 118:2315–2325, 2011.
2. Vinekar A, Avadhani K, Sivakumar M, et al.: Understanding clinically undetected macular changes in early retinopathy of prematurity on spectral domain optical coherence tomography. *Invest Ophthalmol Vis Sci* 52:5183–5188, 2011.
3. Vinekar A, Avadhani K, Sivakumar M, et al.: Macular edema in premature infants. *Ophthalmology* 119(6):1288–1289.e1, 2012; author reply 1289–1290.e1.
4. Vajzovic L, Hendrickson AE, O'Connell RV, et al.: Maturation of the human fovea: correlation of spectral-domain optical coherence tomography findings with histology. *Am J Ophthalmol* 154(5):779–789.e2, 2012.

Albinism

Anand Vinekar

Ocular albinism (OA) is a genetic disorder of melanin production limited to eyes and differs from oculocutaneous albinism (OCA), which also involves skin and hair in addition.

Visual acuity in children with OA may vary and ranges often from 20/25 to 20/200. Nystagmus often presents at 2–3 months of age and is usually due to foveal hypoplasia or aberrant visual pathways. Additionally, refractive errors, strabismus, and amblyopia contribute to visual problems of these young patients.

CASE STUDY

A 3-year-old male child with OA presented with nystagmus and a best-corrected visual acuity of 20/100 in both eyes. Skin and hair had normal pigmentation. Iris pigmentation was lighter, but did not demonstrate definite transillumination examined on a slit lamp in a dark room prior to dilatation. The child presented with significant nystagmus. The fundus photograph demonstrates classical hypopigmentation due to a reduction in retinal pigment and with a greater visibility of choroidal vasculature (Fig. 91.1).

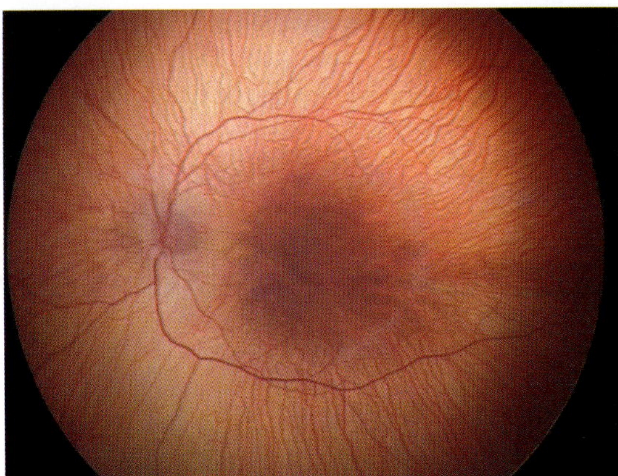
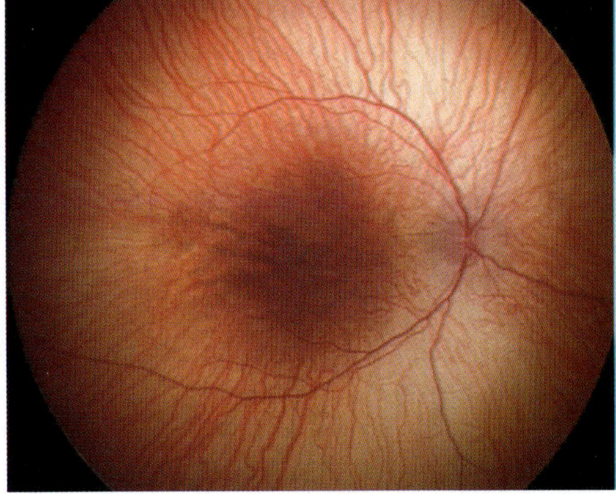

Fig. 91.1 This fundus image belongs to a 3-year-old boy with OA demonstrating hypopigmented retina, prominence of choroidal vessels, and absence of foveal reflex.

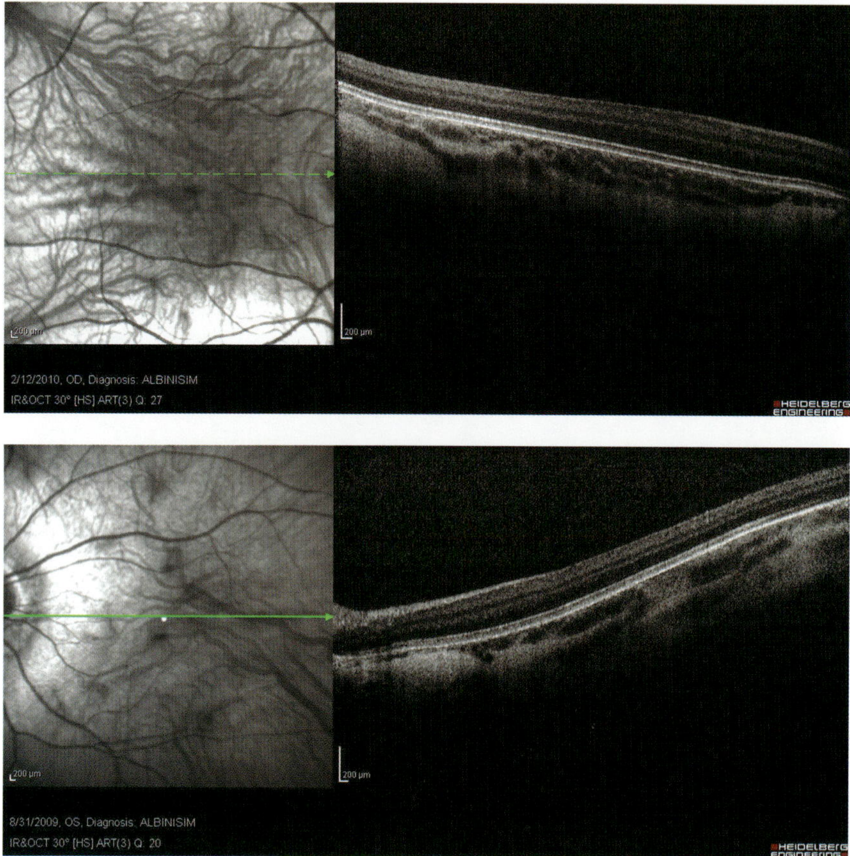

Fig. 91.2 SD-OCT images obtained on the SPECTRALIS™ in office without anesthesia. The persistence of the inner retinal layers in the foveal center, nonfusion at foveal dip, absence of foveal tent in the outer retina and prominence of choroidal layers are key features.

Optical coherence tomography (OCT) images were obtained on Heidelberg SPECTRALIS™ spectral-domain optical coherence tomography (SD-OCT) device (Heidelberg Engineering, Germany). Despite the nystagmus, the relatively quick acquisition of scans allowed details of the posterior pole to be captured as well. The infrared (IR) images show a fair consistency with the center of the macula, which show correlation with the OCT image alongside it (**Fig. 91.2**).

Typical features of the OA foveae with hypoplasia on the OCT are relative persistence of inner retinal layers (IRLs) across the foveal center. These are normally absent or thinned out at the foveal dip. In OA, there is persistence and nonfusion of the IRLs at the fovea due to incomplete centrifugal migration of this layer. The layers are differentiated but not mature. The absence of the foveal pit on the OCT correlates clinically with a poorly discernible foveal reflex.

Outer retinal layers are more readily discernible with visibility of external limiting membrane (ELM) and photoreceptor inner and outer segment layers (IS–OS). However, a classical foveal tent is absent or attenuated, as seen in **Figure 91.2**. This tent is believed to be due to longer outer cone segments in the fovea, which are absent or attenuated in albinism. A short or shallow tent would suggest that the cones are spaced more apart. True ultrastructure of the foveal photoreceptors in albinism is still not fully understood.

SD–OCT findings similar to this case have also been reported in cases of suspected OA as well as OCA. High-resolution OCT imaging is therefore a very important tool in the study of foveal hypoplasia and albinism.

FURTHER READING

1. Chong GT, Farsiu S, Freedman SF, et al.: Abnormal foveal morphology in ocular albinism imaged with spectral-domain optical coherence tomography. *Arch Ophthalmol* 127(1):37–44, 2009.
2. Seo JH, Yu YS, Kim JH, et al.: Correlation of visual acuity with foveal hypoplasia grading by optical coherence tomography in albinism. *Ophthalmology* 114(8):1547–1551, 2007.

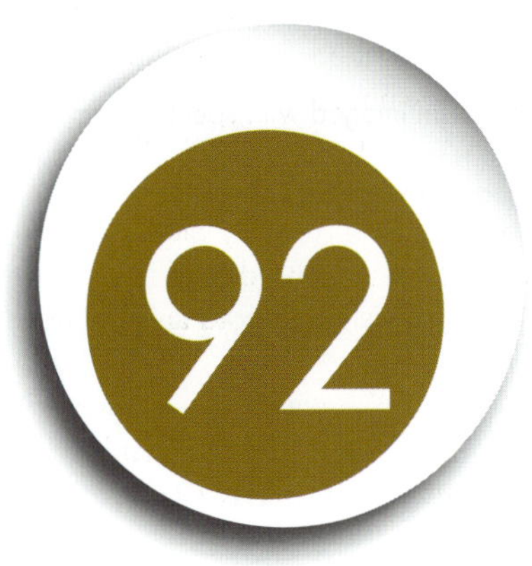

Combined Hamartoma of the Retina and Retinal Epithelium

Anand Vinekar and Kavitha Avadhani

Combined hamartoma of the retina and retinal pigment epithelium (CHR–RPE) is a rare benign tumor involving sensory retina, the RPE, retinal vasculature, and overlying vitreous. Most commonly seen unilaterally, these lesions are characterized by proliferation of the RPE and glial tissue, causing epiretinal membranes (ERM), retinal distortion, and even tractional retinal detachment leading to visual loss.

Optical coherence tomography (OCT), fundus fluorescein angiography (FFA), and indocyanine green angiography (ICGA) have been shown to be useful in diagnosis of this entity at this late stage. Early features of this lesion on spectral-domain optical coherence tomography (SD-OCT) are unknown.

In this case, we describe FFA, ICGA, and SD-OCT findings in a 4-week-old infant with CHR–RPE. Early lesions such as the one described could resemble a retinal astrocytoma.

CASE STUDY

A male baby of birth weight 1600 gm born at 34 weeks of gestation was detected to have a yellow–orange retinal lesion during retinopathy of prematurity (ROP) screening on Retcam™ (Fig. 92.1).

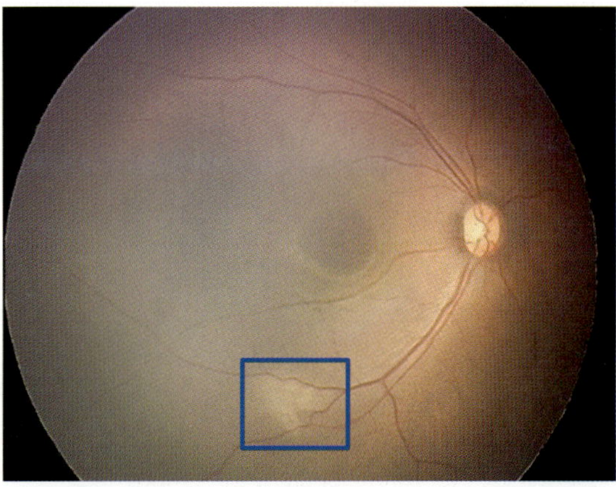

Fig. 92.1 Combined hamartoma of the retina and retinal pigment epithelium (CHR–RPE) (*blue box*).

Ultrasound B-scan showed a lesion at the retinal level, 3.08 mm × 3.00 mm with a thickness of 1.14 mm, with high surface reflectivity and regular internal architecture. There was no fluid, choroidal excavation, or after shadowing. The vitreous cavity was clear. The surrounding retina, underlying choroid and sclera were normal.

A bedside-combined OCT, FFA, and ICGA procedure was performed using the SPECTRALIS™ by modifying the tabletop unit into a hand-held device, as described in Chapter 88.

The FFA and ICGA revealed a triangular hyperfluorescent lesion with intrinsic vascularity (early lacy pattern) in the arteriovenous (AV) phase, becoming more hyperfluorescent in late phases with distinct borders (**Fig. 92.2**). There was no increase in the size of the leak, which persisted in the late phases. The underlying choroid and the rest of the retina were normal.

The horizontal SD-OCT scan showed a hyperreflective lesion with homogenous reflectivity and no internal cystic alteration, with greatest linear length of 293 microns and 228 microns in thickness seen in inner retinal layers. At the same spot, retinal thickness was 423 microns. At the edge of the lesion the retinal thickness was 193 microns; deeper retinal layers appeared intact (**Fig. 92.3**).

The enhanced depth image (EDI) scan showed early discontinuity in the RPE layer that was consistent across radial scans of the underlying lesion (**Fig. 92.4**). The SD-OCT scan of the lesion was also obtained using the hand-held Bioptigen with the baby supine (**Fig. 92.5**).

The child underwent serial ROP screening weekly, until the retina was fully mature. During this period of 7 weeks, there was no change in either the size or composition of the lesion.

CHR & RPE lesions are rare entities that produce visual complaints in early childhood, especially owing to the formation of epiretinal membrane.

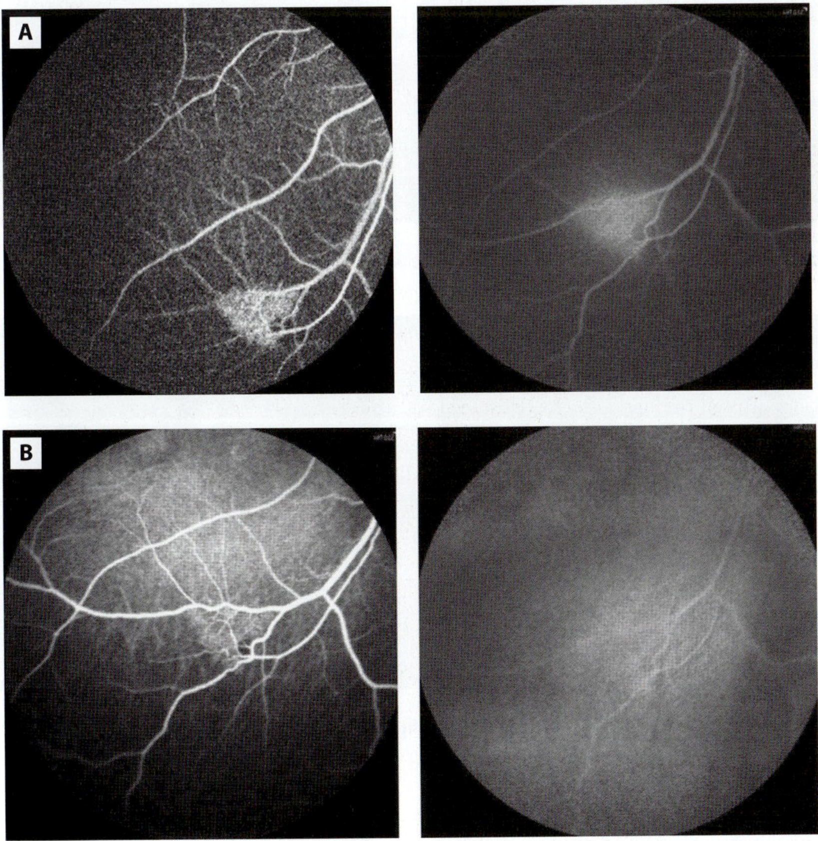

Fig. 92.2 (A) Fundus fluorescein angiograph (FFA) of the lesion in early and late phase showing triangular-shaped hyperfluorescence with a lacy pattern. **(B)** Indocyanine green angiography (ICGA) of the lesion showing similar hyperfluorescence with normal choroidal vasculature.

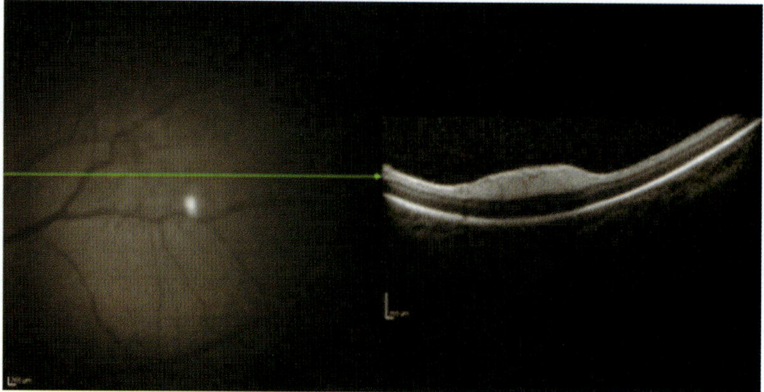

Fig. 92.3 SD-OCT image of the lesion on the SPECTRALIS™ showing inner retinal involvement, homogeneous reflectivity, and smooth contours.

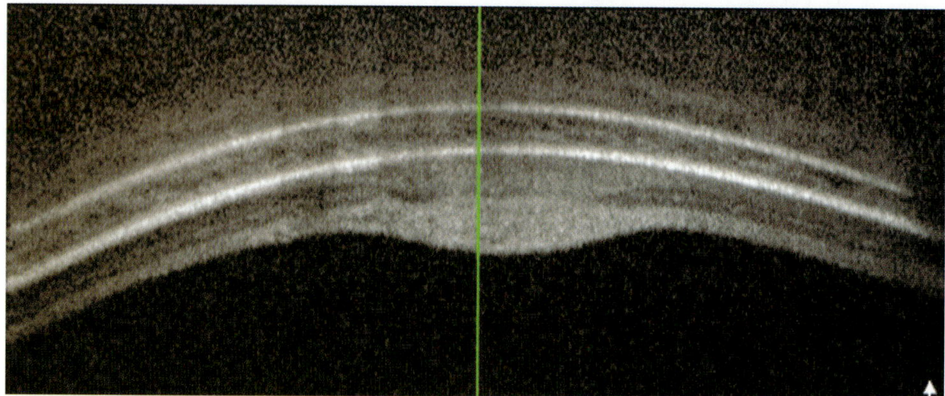

Fig. 92.4 Enhanced depth imaging (EDI) of the lesion showing the deeper retinal layers and the choroid.

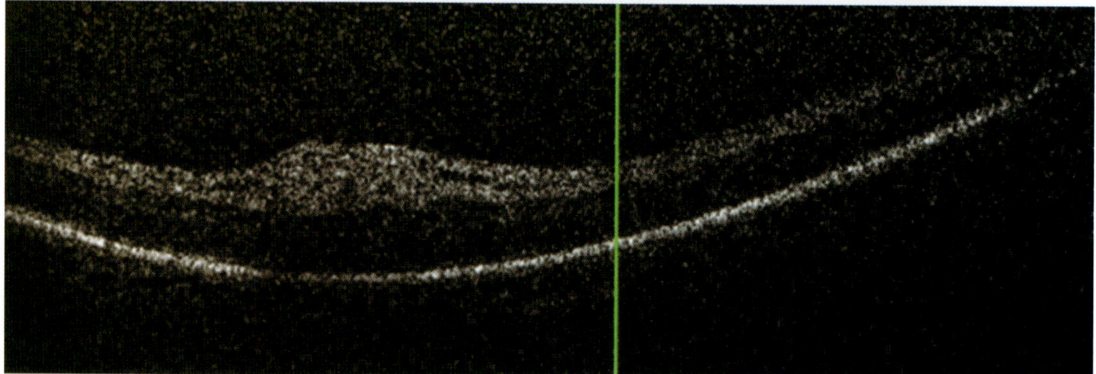

Fig. 92.5 This scan is obtained using the hand-held Bioptigen SD-OCT device with the baby supine.

Wide-field retinal imaging has been proved to be very useful in ROP screening. This case report highlights the fact that imaging of the retina can serendipitously detect other lesions as well.

In addition, this report demonstrates the utility of multimodality imaging performed in an infant in the office without anesthesia. Early detection of this lesion (in this case study at 4 weeks of life) has allowed us to appreciate epiretinal alterations even before the classical ERMs or tractional detachments have formed.

FURTHER READING

1. Vinekar A, Quiram P, Sund N, et al.: Plasmin-assisted vitrectomy for bilateral combined hamartoma of the retina and retinal pigment epithelium: histopathology, immunohistochemistry and optical coherence tomography. *Retinal Cases and Brief Reports* 3:186–189, 2009.
2. Palmer ML, Carney MD, Combs JL: Combined hamartomas of the retinal pigment epithelium and retina. *Retina* 10(1): 33–36, 1990.
3. Shields CL, Mashakevi A, Dai VV, et al.: Optical coherence tomographic findings of combined hamartoma of the retina and retinal pigment epithelium in 11 patients. *Arch Ophthalmol* 123:1746–1750, 2005.
4. Moschos M, Ladas ID, Zafirakis PK, et al.: Recurrent vitreous hemorrhages due to combined pigment epithelial and retinal hamartoma: natural course and indocyanine green angiographic findings. *Ophthalmologica* 215(1):66–69, 2001.
5. Vinekar A, Sivakumar M, Shetty R, et al.: A novel technique using spectral-domain optical coherence tomography (Spectralis, SD-OCT + HRA) to image supine non-anaesthetized infants: utility demonstrated in aggressive posterior retinopathy of prematurity. *Eye* 24:379–382, 2010.

Cone–Rod Dystrophy

Yoshihiro Yonekawa,
Demetrios G Vavvas, and
RV Paul Chan

Cone–rod dystrophies are a heterogeneous group of disorders characterized by full-field electroretinogram (ERG) patterns where the cone-isolated ERG is affected more than the rod-isolated ERG. Patients present with progressive central visual loss, deterioration of light/dark adaptation, mild photophobia, and myopia. Fundus findings can vary significantly from bull's eye maculopathy, macular atrophy, peripheral retinal degeneration, retinal pigment epithelium (RPE) mottling to findings associated with myopia. Cone–rod dystrophies may also present with bone spicules, arteriolar narrowing, and temporal disc pallor, in which case differentiation from retinitis pigmentosa may be challenging. Gene mutations have been linked to cone–rod dystrophies, including *GUCA1A, GUCY2D, AIPL1, CRX, RIMS1, Sema4A, UNC119, CORD4, CORD8, CORD9, RPGR (CORDX1), CORDX2, CORDX3, ABCA4,* and *COD*4. Most cases are inherited in an autosomal recessive manner, although autosomal dominant and X-linked variants occur in approximately 10% of cases. A recent study of 83 patients with cone–rod dystrophy noted that early age of onset and *ABCA*4 gene mutations were independent indicators for poorer visual prognosis.

While spectral-domain optical coherence tomography (SD-OCT) alone cannot diagnose cone–rod dystrophies, it has emerged as a useful adjunctive imaging modality to better characterize the lesions. In 2008, Lim, et al. described a patient with cone–rod dystrophy that showed choriocapillaries attenuation and central macular thinning. Sergouniotis et al. recently reported on 12 patients with KCNV2 retinopathy ("cone dystrophy with supernormal rod ERG") and found that disruption of IS–OS junction was the predominant feature. RPE/Bruch's membrane thinning was also seen in several patients. A case report of cone–rod dystrophy 6 (*CORD6*) also described abnormalities at the IS–OS junction and outer segment layer, and a case report of a 5-year-old boy with cone–rod dystrophy associated with Alström syndrome showed a single layer of short, thick cones and rods, and immature outer segments. Further studies are indicated to better understand this group of dystrophies.

CASE STUDY

A 42-year-old man was referred for declining visual acuity and RPE changes in both eyes. He had a history of keratoconus, myopia, pigment dispersion syndrome, and ocular hypertension. Blue–purple–green color vision started to decline 25 years ago, and visual acuity started to deteriorate 6 years ago, particularly in daylight. He also noted occasional flashes and floaters. Family history was noncontributory. Best-corrected visual acuity was 20/60 OD and 20/120 OS. Color vision testing with pseudoisochromatic plates showed that he could only identify the control plates in both eyes. Numerous errors were made on the D-15 panel (Farnsworth Dichotomous Test), some of which were along a tritan axis.

Dilated fundus examination revealed RPE atrophy centrally in both eyes, with attenuated retinal arteries (Fig. 93.1). Fluorescein angiography (FA) showed annular window defects around the fovea, as well as peripapillary window defects, and along the inferior temporal arcade (not shown). Autofluorescence also showed an annular

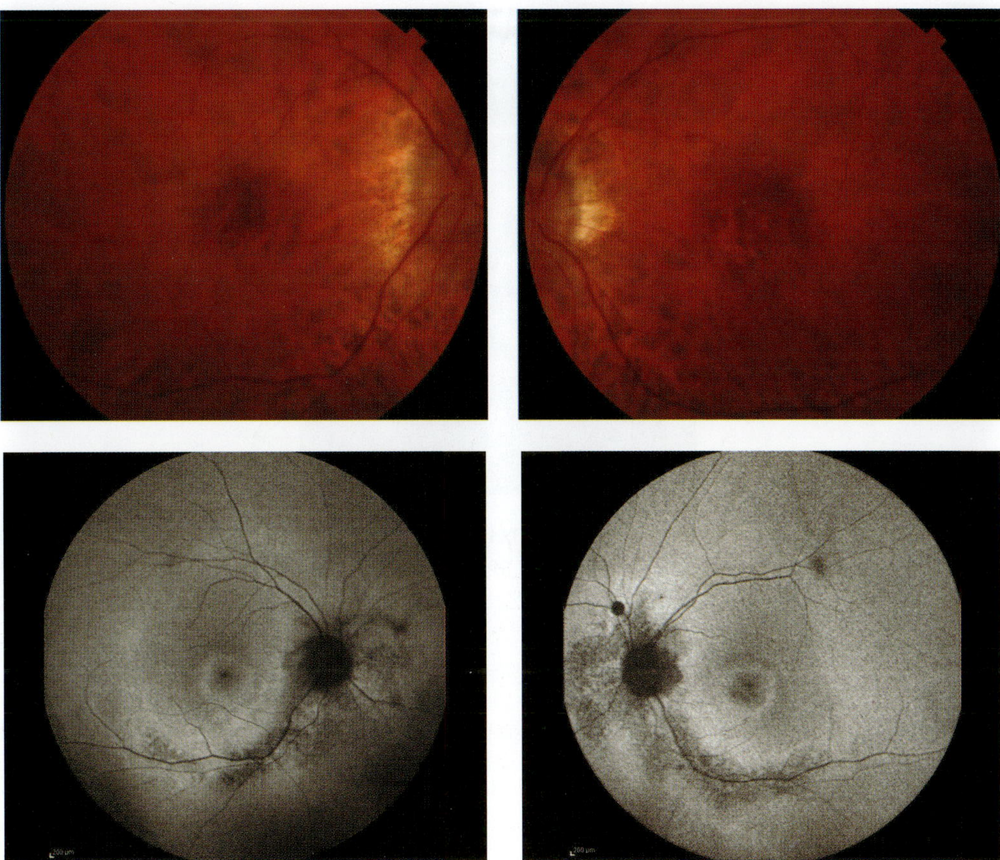

Fig. 93.1 (*Above, left*) Color fundus photograph of the right eye in a patient with cone–rod dystrophy, showing macular depigmentation and peripapillary chorioretinal atrophy. (*Above, right*) Color fundus photograph of left eye with similar findings. (*Below, left*) Fundus autofluorescence of the right eye showing a perifoveal ring of hypoautofluorescence (bull's eye maculopathy), which was not clearly evident on the fundus photo, and decreased autofluorescence of the peripapillary and inferotemporal regions. (*Below, right*) Fundus autofluorescence of the left eye showing a similar decreased autofluoresce pattern.

hypoautofluorescence around the fovea that revealed the bull's eye pattern that was not evident on the fundus photos, and hypoautofluorescence in the peripapillary region and along the inferior temporal arcade (Fig. 93.1). SD-OCT showed atrophy of photoreceptor and RPE layers in the parafoveal regions in both eyes (Fig. 93.2).

Full-field ERG showed decreased scotopic and photopic responses, and an absent flicker response (Fig. 93.3). The multifocal electroretinography (mfERG) only showed noise (Fig. 93.3). Visual fields demonstrated nasal, superior, and superonasal field defects, corresponding to the retinal and RPE atrophy seen on FA and autofluorescence (Fig. 93.3). The above clinical and diagnostic findings were consistent with cone–rod degeneration.

CONCLUSION

Ophthalmoscopic examination and ERG are currently the gold standards in diagnosing cone–rod dystrophies. In the past several years, SD-OCT has become a useful adjunct in diagnosing and monitoring this condition in particular, to monitor in vivo photoreceptor appearance. The specific findings vary depending on the stage of the

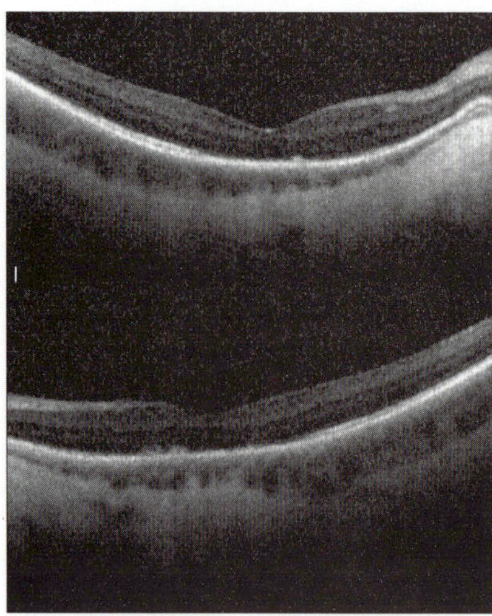

Fig. 93.2 Spectral-domain optical coherence tomography (SD-OCT) (SPECTRALIS™ OCT, Heidelberg Engineering) of the right eye (*above*) and left eye (*below*), showing loss of perifoveal photoreceptor and retinal pigment epithelial (RPE) structures.

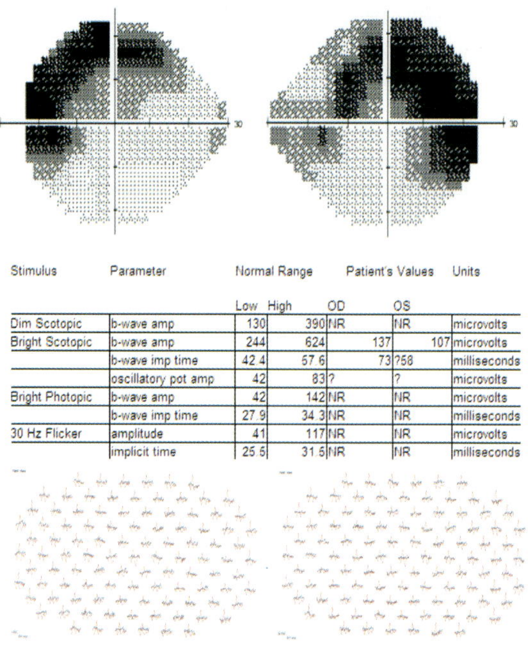

Stimulus	Parameter	Normal Range		Patient's Values		Units
		Low	High	OD	OS	
Dim Scotopic	b-wave amp	130	390	NR	NR	microvolts
Bright Scotopic	b-wave amp	244	624	137	107	microvolts
	b-wave imp time	42.4	57.6	73	?58	milliseconds
	oscillatory pot amp	42	83	?	?	microvolts
Bright Photopic	b-wave amp	42	142	NR	NR	microvolts
	b-wave imp time	27.9	34.3	NR	NR	milliseconds
30 Hz Flicker	amplitude	41	117	NR	NR	microvolts
	implicit time	25.5	31.5	NR	NR	milliseconds

Fig. 93.3 (*Above*) 24-2 Humphrey visual fields showing nasal, superior, and superonasal visual field deficits in both eyes, with relative sparing of central vision. (*Middle*) Full-field ERG results showing diminished scotopic, photopic, and flicker responses. (*Below, left*) A multifocal electroretinography (mfERG) of the right eye showing only noise and absent waveforms. (*Below, right*) An mfERG of the left eye, also with only noise and absent waveforms.

dystrophy. Future studies will provide a better understanding of the role of SD-OCT in disease management of the cone–rod dystrophies.

FURTHER READING

1. Albert D, Miller J, Azar D, Blodi B, eds.: *Albert & Jakobiec's Principles and Practice of Ophthalmology*. 3rd ed. Philadelphia: Saunders, 2253–2260, 2008.
2. Thiadens AA, Phan TM, Zekveld-Vroon RC, et al.: Clinical course, genetic etiology, and visual outcome in cone and cone-rod dystrophy. *Ophthalmology* 119:819–826, 2012.
3. Lim JI, Tan O, Fawzi AA, et al.: A pilot study of Fourier-domain optical coherence tomography of retinal dystrophy patients. *Am J Ophthalmol* 146:417–426, 2008.
4. Sergouniotis PI, Holder GE, Robson AG, et al.: High-resolution optical coherence tomography imaging in KCNV2 retinopathy. *Br J Ophthalmol* 2011, doi:10.1136/bjo.
5. Kim BJ, Ibrahim MA, Goldberg MF.: Use of spectral domain OCT to visualize photoreceptor abnormalities in cone/rod dystrophy-6. *Retin Cases Brief Rep* 5:56–61, 2011.
6. Vingolo EM, Salvatore S, Grenga PL, et al.: High-resolution spectral domain optical coherence tomography images of alstrom syndrome. *J Pediatr Ophthalmol Strabismus* 47 Online:e1–3, 2010, doi:10.3928/01913913-20100507-05.

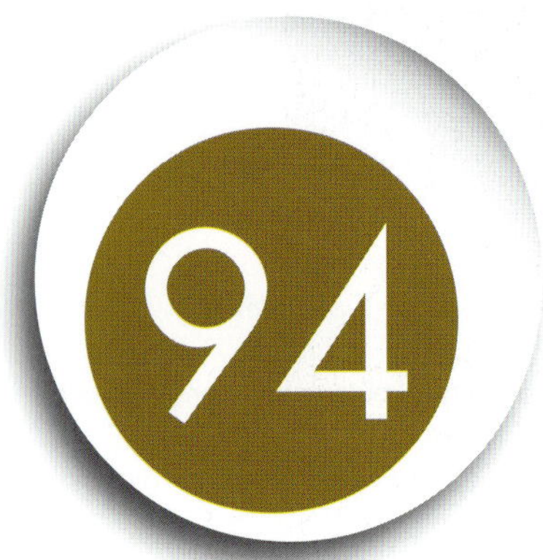

Leber's Congenital Amaurosis

Anand Vinekar

Leber's congenital amaurosis (LCA) is a group of hereditary retinal dystrophies characterized by severe loss of visual function early in life.

Clinical features usually include abnormal electroretinogram (ERG) findings, which can vary from markedly reduced to complete absence of scotopic and photopic waveforms. Others include nystagmus, roving eye movements, and eye poking, often referred to as oculodigital sign. The fundus appearance varies from near normal (Fig. 94.1) to salt-and-pepper pigmented changes.

There is a considerable genetic heterogeneity that results in variable expression of onset and progression of disease. Inheritance of LCA is most often autosomal recessive; although autosomal dominant inheritance has also been reported.

Recently, gene replacement therapy in LCA following discovery of disease coding gene mutations such as *RPE65* (retinal pigment epithelium-specific 65 kDa protein) have caused considerable excitement in the management of this disease.

The following spectral-domain optical coherence tomography (SD-OCT) images are of children who have been clinically diagnosed with LCA, with characteristic ERG changes. *RPE65* mutation was negative in all these cases.

The predominant finding on the SD-OCT is thinning of outer nuclear layer (ONL) (Fig. 94.2). The inner retinal layers (IRLs) previously described in this text are also poorly differentiated (Figs 94.2 and 94.3). In more advanced cases, there is an overall thinning of the layers at the foveal center (Fig. 94.2) and in the perifoveal

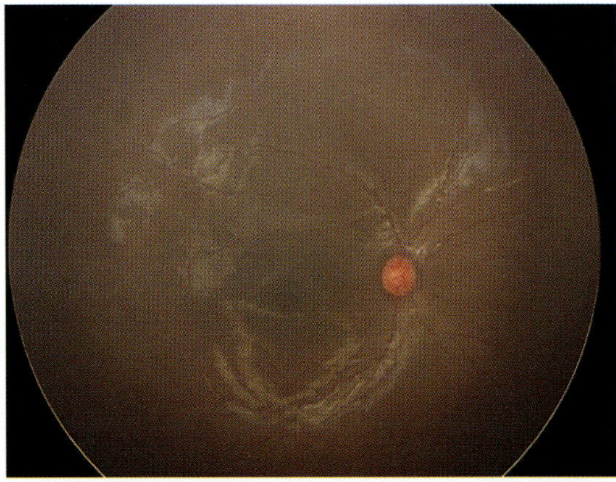

Fig. 94.1 Retcam™ (Clarity MSI, USA) image of the right eye of an infant with LCA, showing a predominantly normal appearance.

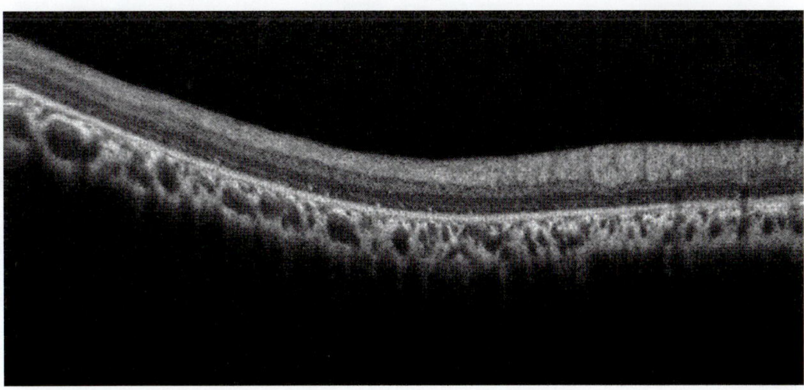

Fig. 94.2 Bioptigen image of the macular center showing persistence of the IRL, attentuation of layers and absence of foveal pit.

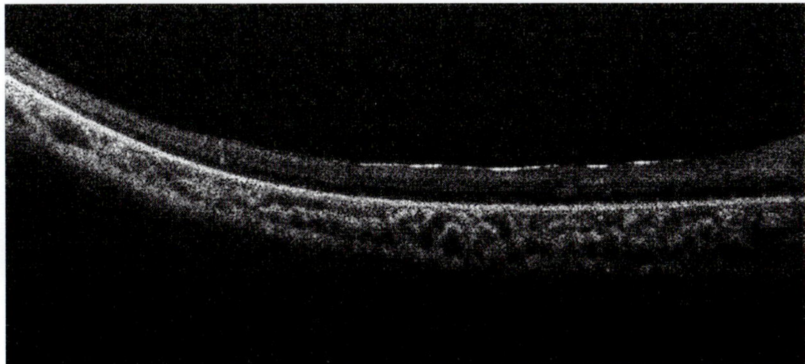

Fig. 94.3 Bioptigen scan of the peripheral retina showing gross IRL attenuation and prominence of choroidal layers.

zone (Fig. 94.3). Owing to reduced reflectance of thinned-out layers, the choroidal layers seem to be more prominent, causing a reversal of ratio between neurosensory retinal layer and choroidal complex (Fig. 94.3). However, this is not pathognomic of LCA and may be seen in any advanced retinal degeneration with loss of neurosensory retinal layers.

Photoreceptor topography in *RPE*65 mutation-positive patients aged 6–17 years have been reported with ONL foveal thinning with greater loss inferiorly compared to superiorly in the perifoveal region, possibly owing to greater density of the photoreceptors superiorly.

It is possible that optical coherence tomography (OCT) imaging of subcellular layers in the retina may be used quantitatively in the near future, especially to monitor therapeutic intervention.

FURTHER READING

Jacobson SG, Cideciyan AV, Aleman TS, et al.: Photoreceptor layer topography in children with Leber's congenital amaurosis caused by RPE65 mutations. *Invest Ophthalmol Vis Sci* 49(10):4573–4577, 2008.

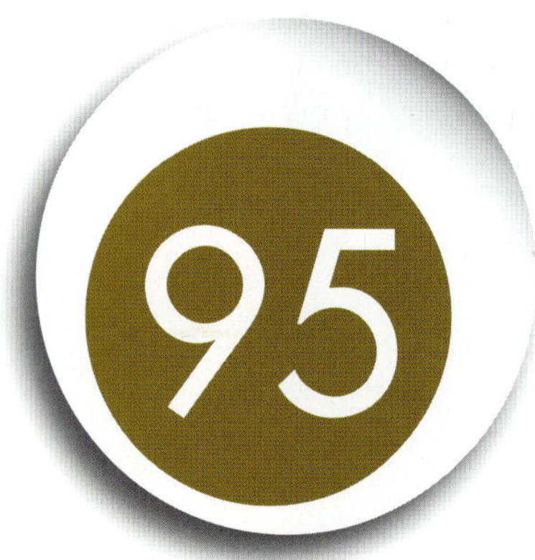

Retinoblastoma

Ashwin Mallipatna and Vandhana Suren

Retinoblastoma is a rare and unique eye cancer that mostly affects children, sometimes before they are born. It is a complicated disease triggered by genetic mutations in the cells of the retina. Incidence of retinoblastoma is 1 in 20,000 live births. If left untreated, retinoblastoma is fatal. With timely screening, diagnosis, referral, treatment, and follow-up delivered in a systematic way by a multidisciplinary team, more than 98% of children with retinoblastoma can be cured, many with useful vision.

CASE STUDY

A 3-month-old boy presented with leukocoria of the right eye noticed by parents for a month (Fig. 95.1). There was no family history of retinoblastoma. The leukocoria was evident on examination, seeming to originate from behind the lens. A dilated fundus examination of the left eye revealed presence of multiple smaller tumors.

Ocular B-mode ultrasonography was performed, which displayed the presence of an intraocular lesion filling the vitreous cavity of the right globe, with multiple highly reflective intralesional echoes with shadowing, which is suggestive of calcification. Although a CT scan would display calcification in the tumor, which will assist in the

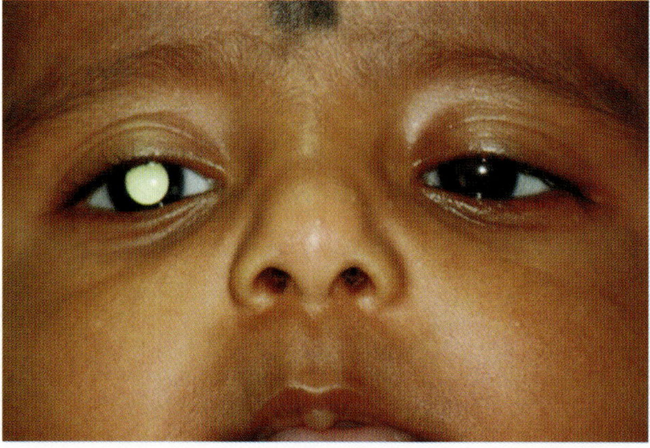

Fig. 95.1 Leukocoria of right eye caused from retinoblastoma. Notice how left eye, having small tumors, does not display the same.

diagnosis of retinoblastoma, most lesions are diagnosed clinically by an experienced ocular oncologist. A magnetic resonance image of the orbits and the brain could further stage the disease by observing for an extraocular extension and obvious optic nerve involvement. The MRI in this child showed no signs suggestive of retrolaminar optic nerve involvement or extraocular extension.

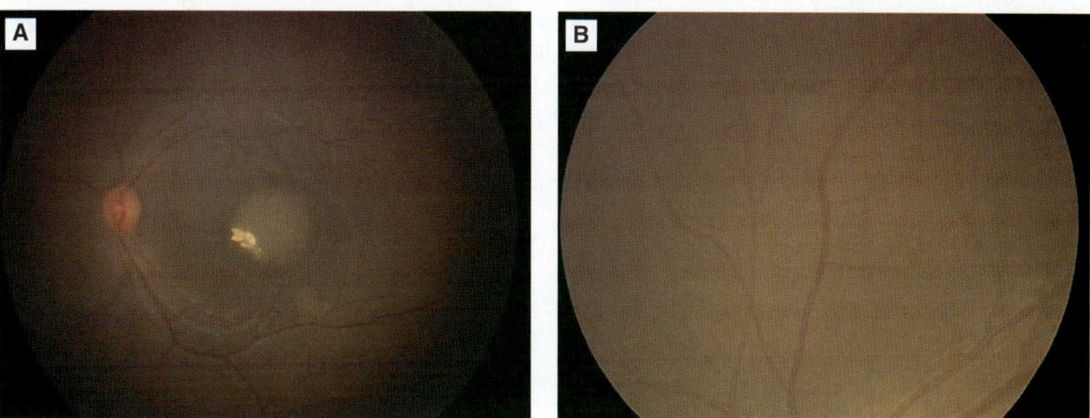

Fig. 95.2 Retcam™ (Clarity MSI, USA) images showing tumors in the left eye. Picture A shows two tumors in the posterior pole; and picture B shows one in periphery.

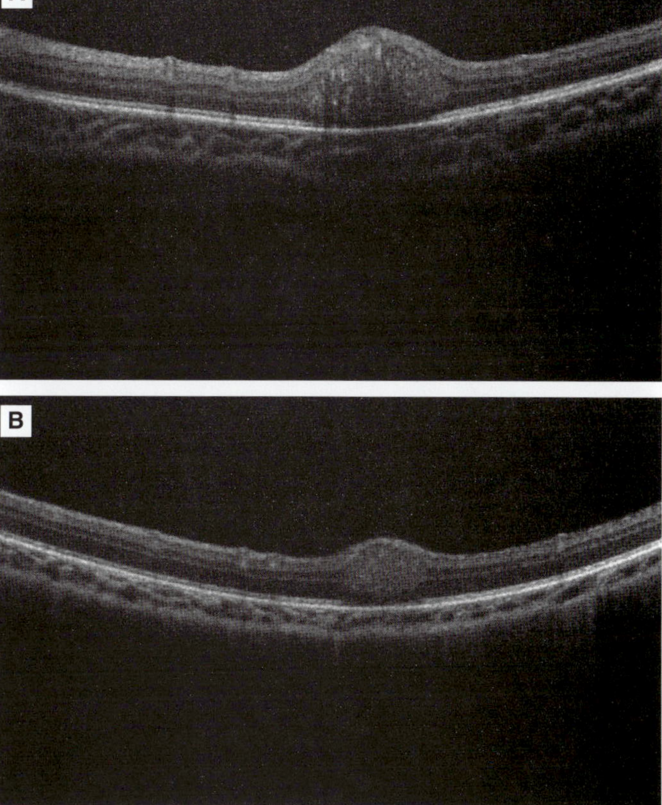

Fig. 95.3 Bioptigen (NC, USA) SD-OCT images of the small peripheral tumor. Picture A was obtained before chemotherapy was given and picture B was obtained after four cycles of chemotherapy.

The child was scheduled for an examination under anesthesia. A detailed fundus examination confirmed the diagnosis, and the right eye was found to have an intraocular pressure of 50 mmHg (Group E). The right eye was enucleated. The left eye had three tumors—two in the posterior pole and one smaller one in the periphery (Group B; Fig. 95.2). The child was staged as having T3b, N0, M0 disease. Bone marrow aspiration and lumbar puncture at diagnosis showed no evidence of metastasis. Histopathology of the right eye revealed a well-differentiated retinoblastoma with no uveal or optic nerve involvement (pT1, N0, M0). The child underwent treatment with chemotherapy and focal laser therapy. The tumor response is being closely followed-up with serial fundus images using the Retcam™.

Optical coherence tomography (OCT) was made possible during examinations under anesthesia using portable hand-held spectral domain optical coherence tomography (SD-OCT) system (Bioptigen™). Early tumors can be seen arising from the inner retinal nuclear layer (Fig. 95.3). Untreated tumors show speckled hyperintense dots from within the tumor. Once the tumors are treated with chemotherapy, the consistency of the reflectivity becomes more homogenous.

The left eye tumors were monitored using serial SD-OCT images, and areas of suspicious tumor activity were identified with the SD-OCT and treated with laser.

FURTHER READING

1. Gallie B, Erraguntla V, Heon E, et al.: Retinoblastoma. In: Taylor D, Hoyt C, eds. *Pediatric Ophthalmology and Strabismus*, ed 3, London, UK: Elsevier, 2004.
2. Murphree A: Intraocular retinoblastoma: the case for a new group classification. In: Singh A, ed: *Ophthalmic Oncology*, Ophthalmology Clinics of North America (18). Philadelphia: Elsevier Saunders, 2005.
3. Finger PT, Harbour JW, Murphree AL, et al.: Retinoblastoma. In: Edge SB, Byrd DR, Compton CC, et al., editors. *AJCC Cancer Staging Manual*, ed 7, New York, NY: Springer, 2009.

Retinopathy of Prematurity—Macular Changes

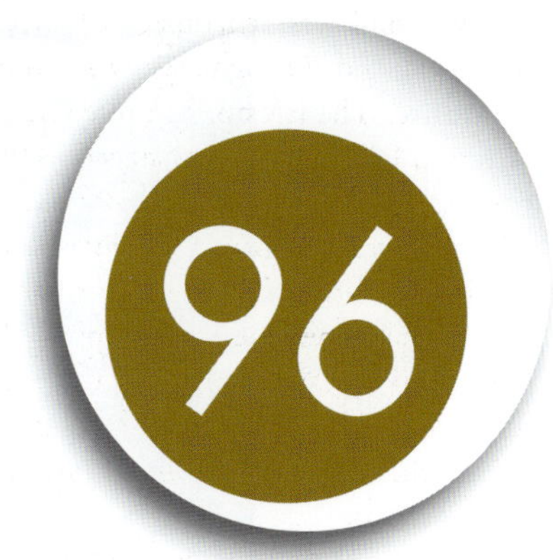

Anand Vinekar and Kavitha Avadhani

Central foveal changes in a proportion of acute Type 2 (not requiring treatment) retinopathy of prematurity (ROP) imaged on spectral-domain optical coherence tomography (SD-OCT) have been recently reported. The foveal change resembles macular edema of adults. These foveal disruptive changes on SD-OCT seem to be subclinical as these eyes appear "normal" on clinical exam. These findings are summarized in this chapter.

In a cohort of Asian Indian infants with ROP, these central foveal changes were observed in approximately 29% of clinically "normal-looking" foveae in infants with stage 2 ROP that did not warrant treatment. These changes were not seen in stage 1 ROP nor in normal premature infants without any ROP.

The foveal changes were divided into two categories based on their appearance. Pattern A: This type of central foveal change had a dome-shaped elevation resembling cystoid macular edema of the adult. Intraretinal cystoid spaces had highly reflective intervening vertical septae between the roof and the floor of the dome with complete disruption of foveal depression in all cases and were accompanied by a marked increase in central foveal thickness (**Fig. 96.1**).

Pattern B: This type of central foveal change had features of multiple, confluent, or near-confluent, vacuolated, optically empty hyporeflective spaces within the layers of the retina with a smaller number or absent septae. There was a preservation of foveal depression and a moderate increase in the central foveal thickness. (**Fig. 96.2**)

The mean central foveal thickness of eyes with and without edema was approximately 315 microns versus 159 microns, respectively. These foveal changes were seen in approximately 29% of infants with stage 2 ROP at a mean postmenstrual age of 37.18 weeks. This group did not differ in birth weight or gestational age from groups with no foveal change.

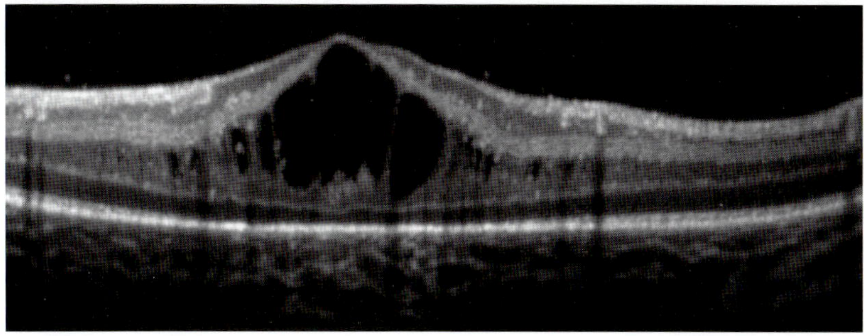

Fig. 96.1 Pattern A.

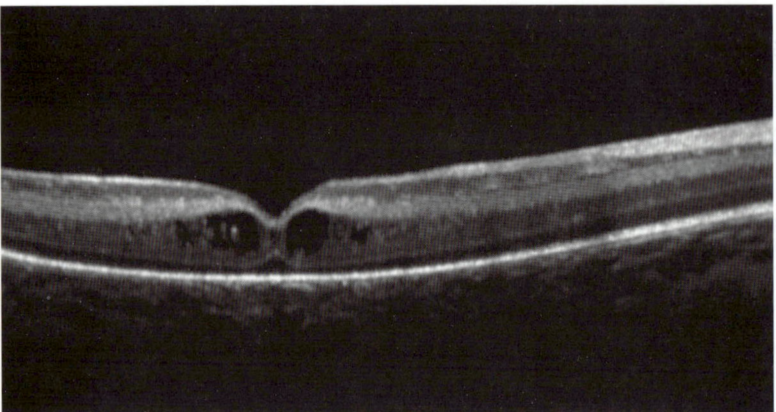

Fig. 96.2 Pattern B.

The distributions of the patterns were 52% versus 48% of A and B, respectively. What is interesting about these foveal disruptive changes, is the fact that they completely resolved within 52 weeks postmenstrual age (PMA), irrespective of the pattern they belonged to.

The etiology of this edema is currently not well established. Theories include increased vascular endothelial growth factor (VEGF) and a mechanical theory. Clinical and visual significance of these apparently transient foveal changes are also unknown at this time.

In another study, 58% of premature infants of Caucasian origin were observed to have similar macular edema in a cohort between 32 and 43 weeks PMA. In this study too, morphology of the edema varied from a single rounded hyporeflective lesion to a more extensive edema, which thickened the inner layers and disturbed the foveal contour. Although not a longitudinal study, they found the resolution of this edema between 42 and 65 weeks.

Currently, our knowledge of the long-term effect of this edema is unknown, but throws an interesting aspect of SD-OCT imaging in its ability to detect clinically undetected changes in ROP.

FURTHER READING

1. Vinekar A, Avadhani K, Munusamy S, et al.: Understanding clinically undetected macular changes in early retinopathy of prematurity on spectral domain optical coherence tomography. *Invest Ophthalmol Vis Sci* 52(8):5183–5188, 2011.
2. Maldonado RS, O'Connell RV, Sarin N, et al.: Dynamics of human foveal development after premature birth. *Ophthalmology* 118(12):2315–2325, 2011.

Retinopathy of Prematurity— Neovascularization

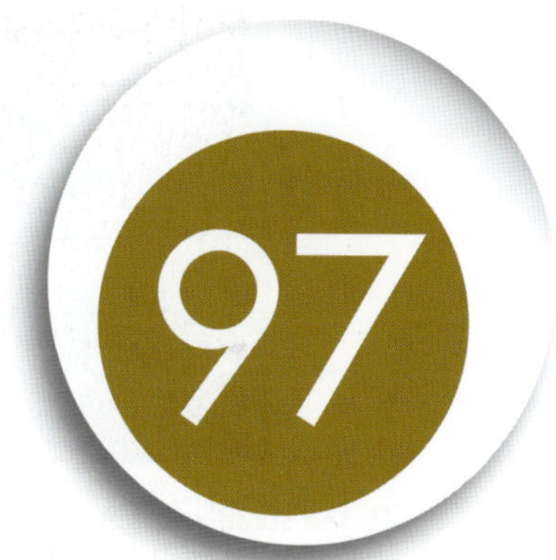

Anand Vinekar, Harsha Pai, and Hemanth Anaspure

Abnormal vascularization or neovascularization is a common feature of ischemic retinal diseases in retinal conditions. However, this is not a pathognomic finding. Although best reported in retinopathy of prematurity (ROP), it may occur in familial exudative vitreoretinopathy, incontinentia pigmenti, Norrie's disease, Coats' disease, and tumors such as retinoblastoma.

We had previously reported the ability of the spectral-domain optical coherence tomography (SD-OCT) (SPECTRALIS™, Heidelberg, Germany) to image flat neovascularization (FNV) in cases of aggressive posterior ROP (APROP). This was particularly useful when media haze after recent laser had precluded accurate localization of residual FNV (Fig. 97.1).

This led to selective ablation of persistent FNV, which was observed to disappear on subsequent OCT imaging (Fig. 97.2).

Although imaging is possible by our technique of dismantling table-top device (see Chapter 88), it must be kept in mind that images would be laterally inverted.

Incontinentia pigmenti (IP) is another condition that is much rarer than retinopathy of prematurity that can present with neovascularization. Using the hand-held Bioptigen (NC, USA), we were able to image subtle neovascularization that was clinically suspected in one eye (Fig. 97.3).

Fluorescein angiogram performed at the same sitting also confirmed an ischemic periphery and leakage of dye from the neovascularized fronds in that eye. Following laser photoablation, regression of the neovascularization was also demonstrated on the Bioptigen.

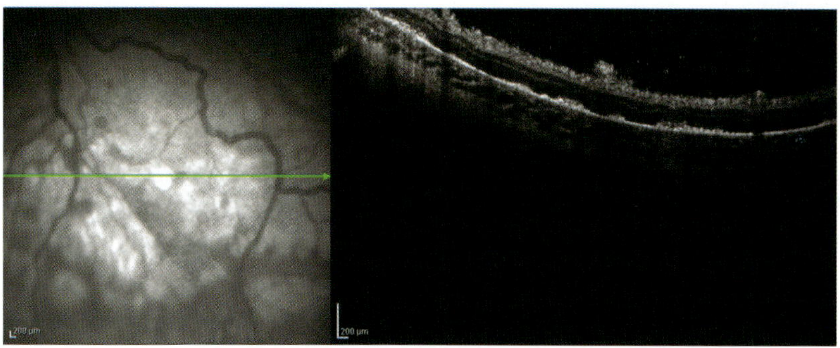

Fig. 97.1 (*Right panel*) This shows an irregular, raised, frond of neovascularization protruding from the retinal surface. Adjoining infrared (IR) image (*left panel*) helps localization of the lesion. It is possible to capture these images despite a hazy media following extensive laser for aggressive posterior retinopathy of prematurity (APROP).

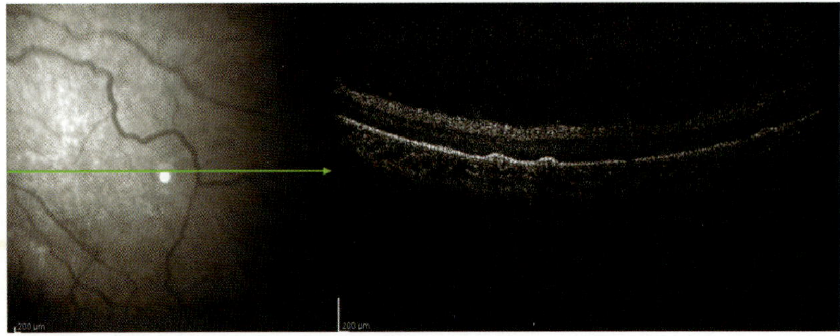

Fig. 97.2 The same location as in Figure 97.1 has been imaged a week following supplement laser performed over the FNV image, confirming resolution of fronds. OCT-guided selective laser ablation of neovascularization results in high accuracy and rapid resolution.

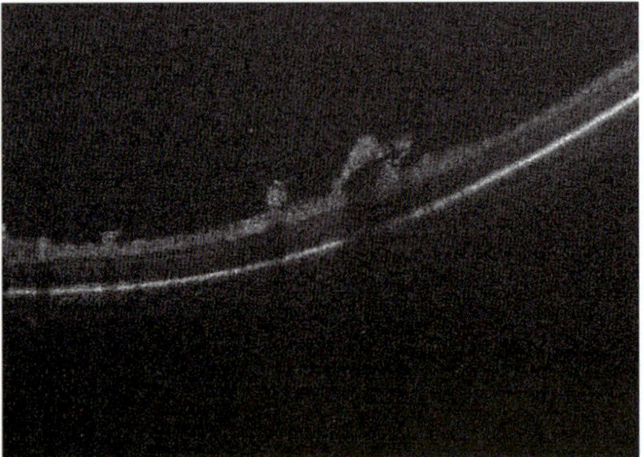

Fig. 97.3 The SD-OCT image of the right eye of a 34-day-old male infant, who was referred with classical skin lesions of IP and suspected neovascularization in one eye, shows irregular, multiple, fronds protruding from the retinal surface. These are often not easily discernible on routine fundus examination.

Hence, with SD-OCT confirmation of neovascularization in clinically difficult situations or even as a substitute for angiography is possible.

FURTHER READING

Vinekar A, Sivakumar M, Shetty R, et al. A novel technique using spectral-domain optical coherence tomography (Spectralis™, SD-OCT + HRA) to image supine non-anaesthetized infants: utility demonstrated in aggressive posterior retinopathy of prematurity. *Eye* (Lond) 24(2):379–382, 2010.

Retinopathy of Prematurity—Postvitrectomy

Anand Vinekar and Naresh Kumar Yadav

Retinal detachment in retinopathy of prematurity (ROP) is staged as 4A or 4B if it is subtotal and is either macula on or macula off, respectively. Considerable success has been reported following lens-sparing surgery in these cases, if the timing and technique is appropriate. Lens sparing vitrectomy (LSV) has been reported to result in visual acuities between 20/200 and 20/40 postoperatively. Despite the macula being "on" in 4A or being reattached in 4B cases, vision does not always improve despite anatomical improvement.

Optical coherence tomography (OCT) has been used to explain this variability in visual outcome after LSV in stage 4A cases. Time-domain optical coherence tomography (TD-OCT) has been previously reported to detect macular involvement in over 15% of eyes selected for LSV, with preoperative diffuse intraretinal posterior pole changes not apparent ophthalmoscopically. Postoperatively, these eyes did not do well visually and demonstrated an absent foveal avascular zone on angiography as well as abnormal architecture on TD-OCT.

In this chapter, preoperative changes in the macula in an eye undergoing LSV and its subsequent improvement on spectral-domain optical coherence tomography (SD-OCT) postoperatively with a positive correlation with the visual acuity have been described.

CASE STUDY

An Asian Indian infant weighing 1400 gm at birth with a gestational age of 34 weeks presented with stage 4 ROP with no previous history of ROP screening or laser treatment. Preoperative Retcam™ (Clarity MSI, USA) images show peripheral raised tractional retinal detachment (**Fig. 98.1A**) with an attached macula (**Fig. 98.1B**). However, the SD-OCT imaging performed preoperatively (Bioptigen, NC, USA) showed foveal involvement. The SD-OCT image showed a disruptive inner retina with poor differentiation of inner retinal layers (**Fig. 98.2**), and extension of intraretinal hyporeflective areas from the location of detached retina peripherally to the center of the fovea. It has been argued that involvement of the macula on the OCT could possibly reclassify the stage as 4B.

The eye underwent 23-gauge LSV and showed successive improvement structurally. Peripheral traction settled down with an improvement of the macular contour ophthalmoscopically. There was residual narrowing of the arcade (**Fig. 98.3A**). The SD-OCT images showed an improvement in the inner retinal architecture and more details of photoreceptor layers were visible 8 weeks following surgery. The optically hollow spaces had reduced and there was

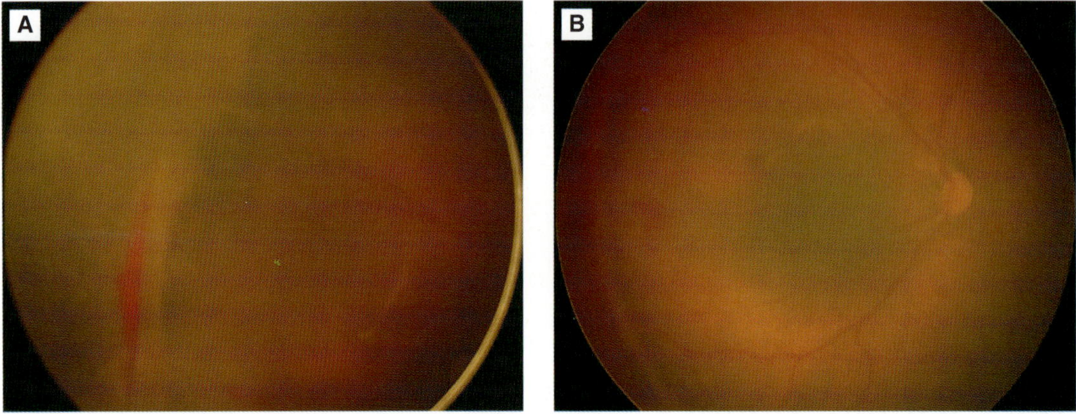

Fig. 98.1 **(A)** Right eye temporal periphery imaged on the Retcam™ (Clarity MSI, USA), showing tractional retinal detachment. **(B)** The posterior pole of the right eye of the same eye in A was attached ophthalmoscopically.

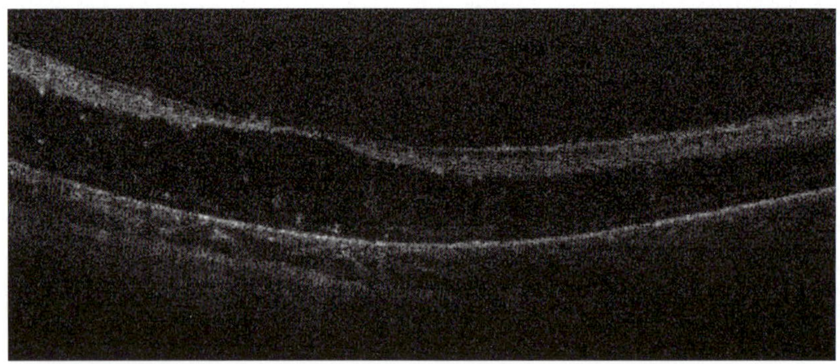

Fig. 98.2 SD-OCT image (Bioptigen™) of the foveal center shows inner retinal layer disruption with extensive hyporeflective areas.

less distortion at the foveal center (Fig. 98.3B). The visual acuity had improved from <20/2000 on Teller Acuity Charts to 20/540 in this eye.

Hence, SD-OCT imaging of the ROP detachments performed pre-, intra-, and postoperatively may not only help to plan the modality of surgery better, but also help us to understand why certain cases do and do not improve following apparently "successful" surgeries. This would help prognosticate outcome to parents before surgery.

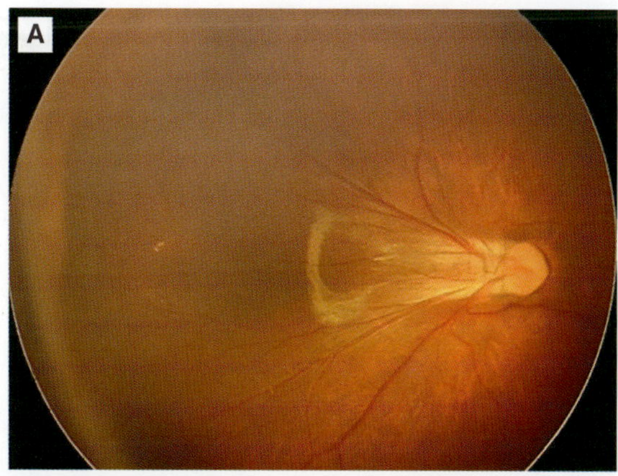

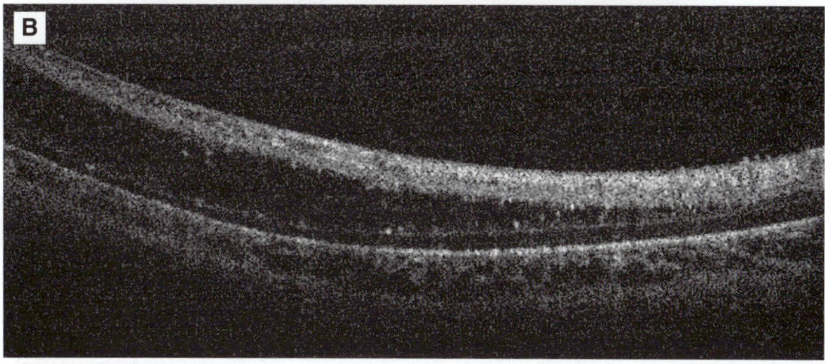

Fig. 98.3 (A) Retcam™ image obtained after 8 weeks of lens sparing vitrectomy (LSV) showing anatomical improvement. The macula is on and the traction has reduced in height. (B) The SD-OCT image shows an improved contour of the inner retinal layers centrally. The peripheral hyporeflective disruption is consistent with the stable traction in the periphery.

FURTHER READING

1. Joshi MM, Trese MT, Capone A Jr.: Optical coherence tomography findings in stage 4A retinopathy of prematurity: a theory for visual variability. *Ophthalmology* 113(4):657–660, Apr 2006.
2. Capone A Jr, Trese MT: Lens-sparing vitreous surgery for tractional stage 4A retinopathy of prematurity retinal detachments. *Ophthalmology* 108(11):2068–2070, Nov 2001.
3. El Rayes EN, Vinekar A, Capone A Jr.: Three-year anatomic and visual outcomes after vitrectomy for stage 4B retinopathy of prematurity. *Retina* 28(4):568–572, Apr 2008.

Rubella Retinopathy

Jyoti Matalia and Anand Vinekar

Congenital rubella syndrome is the classic triad of ocular abnormalities, heart disease, and deafness. Among ocular findings, cataract is the most common and is believed to account for 25% of the congenital cataracts in India.

Rubella retinopathy is reported to occur from 13.3% to 61% of the affected population, and is reported as a fine pigmentary mottling of the retina with tiny flecks of dark pigment mixed with fine areas of whitish depigmentation giving it the classical description of "salt-and-pepper" retinopathy.

CASE STUDY

A 4-month-old Asian Indian boy with bilateral microphthalmos and cataracts presented with a previous diagnosis of congenital heart disease with the echocardiographic evidence of a patent ductus arteriosis (PDA) with a left-to-right shunt—along with left ventricular hypertrophy, coarctation of aorta, and bicuspid aortic valves with mild aortic stenosis. The TORCH (toxoplasmosis, rubella, cytomegalovirus, herpes simplex, and herpes zoster) screening done within 1 month of birth had showed positive titres for rubella IgG and IgM. The child had delay in development. He was subsequently found to have severe otological abnormalities. A diagnosis of congenital rubella syndrome was made.

The child underwent bilateral extracapsular cataract extraction and was rehabilitated with aphakic contact lenses. The vision gradually improved to 20/360 @ 38 cms measured using Teller Acuity Cards in both eyes with 80% reliability after 6 months of contact lens use.

Retinal examination revealed the classical "salt-and-pepper" appearance owing to the distribution of areas of increased and decreased pigmentation (Fig. 99.1). Bioptigen spectral-domain optical coherence tomography (SD-OCT)

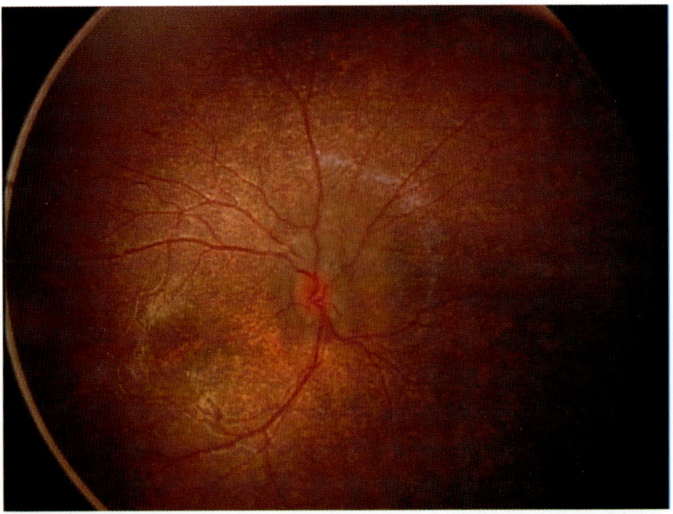

Fig. 99.1 Retcam™ image of the right eye following cataract surgery reveals the classical "salt-and-pepper" appearance.

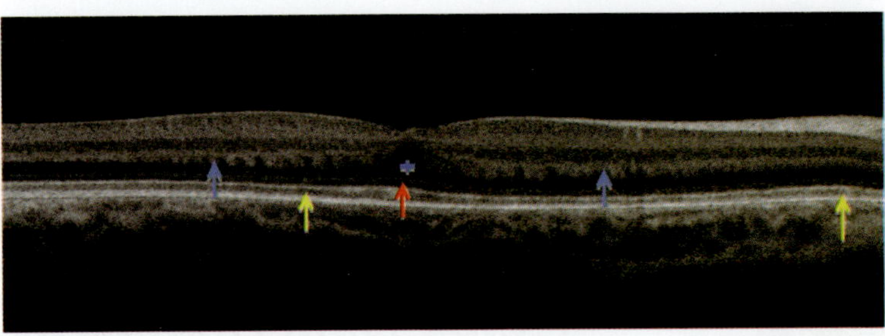

Fig. 99.2 Bioptigen SD-OCT image of the foveal center showing irregular, jagged edges of the outer plexiform layer (*blue arrows*), a thin outer nuclear layer (ONL) (*blue cross*), an attenuated inner segment–outer segment (IS–OS) layer with absent foveal tent (*red arrow*), and diffuse irregularities in the RPE (*yellow arrows*).

of the retina showed four features (Fig. 99.2): (a) irregular and jagged outer plexiform layer – "scalloped sign"; (b) an attenuated outer nuclear layer; (c) attenuated inner segment–outer segment (IS–OS) with absent foveal tent; and (d) diffuse irregularites in the retinal pigment epithelium (RPE).

Histological studies suggest that there is a diffuse damage of the RPE with mild-to-variable effect on vision. Neural retinal or choroidal changes are less well described.

It is noteworthy that none of these optical coherence tomography (OCT) findings are pathognomic of rubella retinopathy. In the absence of evidence in literature of OCT characterization of retinal changes caused due to rubella, we must await larger, multicentric studies to evaluate the different changes and correlate these to the stage of the disease and to visual acuity to appreciate the true clinical potential of these findings in the management of these cases.

FURTHER READING

1. Vijayalakshmi P, Kakkar G, Samprathi A, et al.: Ocular manifestations of congenital rubella syndrome. *Ind J Ophthalmol* 50:307–311, 2002.
2. Mark EO: Pigmentary abnormalities in children congenitally deaf following maternal German measles. *Br J Ophthalmol* 31:119, 1947.
3. Krill AE: The retinal disease of rubella. *Arch Ophthalmol* 77(4):445–449, 1967.

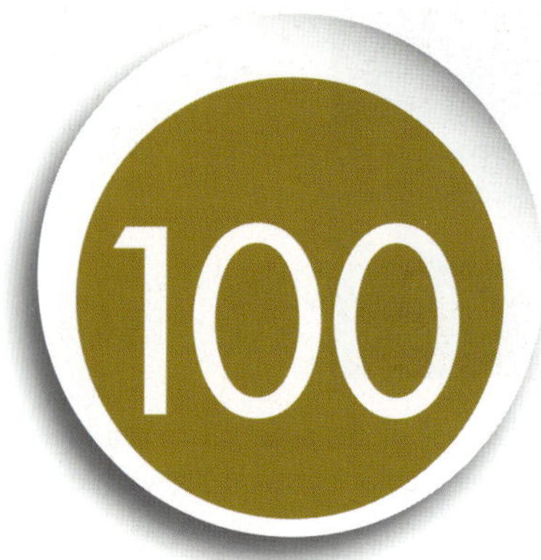

Shaken Baby Syndrome

Vishak John, Audina Berrocal, and Ditte Hess

Shaken baby syndrome (SBS) or nonaccidental trauma (NAT) is the leading cause of infant death from injury around the world. This condition is associated with various ophthalmic findings, including blood in all three layers of the retina, retinal detachments, perimacular folds, traumatic retinoschisis, and macular holes. In fact, when SBS or NAT is suspected, ophthalmologists are often asked to examine the retina because a vast majority of babies (83%) will have retinal hemorrhages.

The exact mechanism of retinal hemorrhages in SBS remains controversial. Some theorize that bleeding is secondary to raised retinal venous pressures from increased intracranial and intrathoracic pressures. While others postulate that the hemorrhage is a direct product of significant vitreoretinal traction from repeated mechanical shaking. The advent of new imaging, especially spectral-domain optical coherence tomography (SD-OCT) has shed important light in this matter. Specifically for imaging infants with suspected SBS, the hand-held SD-OCT Bioptigen and Retcam™ has been invaluable. SD-OCT has demonstrated, in multiple studies, the presence of focal posterior vitreous separation, multilayered tractional schisis, disinsertion of the internal limiting membrane, and preretinal hemorrhages. These studies essentially confirmed that retinal hemorrhages in SBS are mainly due to shaking, which induces shearing forces at the vitreoretinal interface. In addition, 360° peripheral nonperfusion in both eyes after nonaccidental trauma has also been recently reported.

Significance of correctly diagnosing SBS/NAT cannot be overstated. Clinical suspicion needs to be high in the setting of bilateral retinal hemorrhages, retinal folds, and/or traumatic retinoschisis in a young, nonverbal child.

CASE STUDY

A 7-month-old boy was referred to pediatric ophthalmology service at Bascom Palmer with suspicion of nonaccidental trauma. Examination in the clinic revealed possible submacular demarcation lines in both eyes suspicious for prior trauma and preretinal hemorrhages over the macula (**Fig. 100.1**). The child underwent exam under anesthesia, and Retcam™ photography and Bioptigen, hand-held SD-OCT (HH-SD-OCT) documented the findings (**Figs 100.2 and 100.3**). Peripheral retinal exam revealed significant retinal ischemia as well, for which the child underwent diode laser ablation.

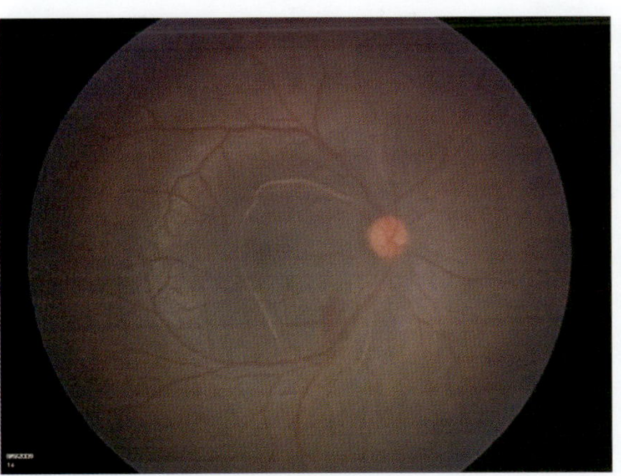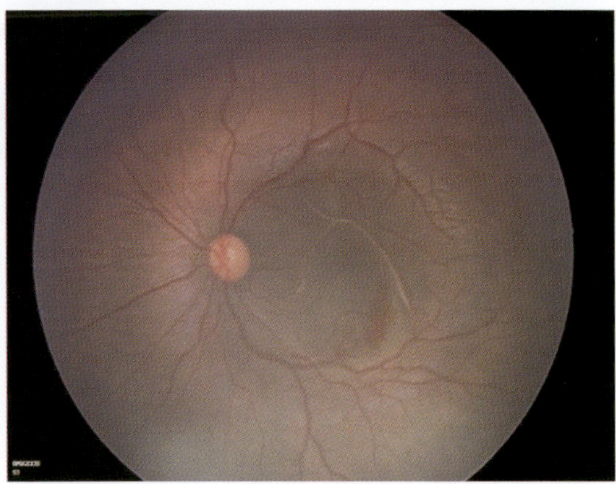

Fig. 100.1 Retcam™ photos demonstrating preretinal hemorrhages and submacular demarcation lines suggestive of recent and prior trauma.

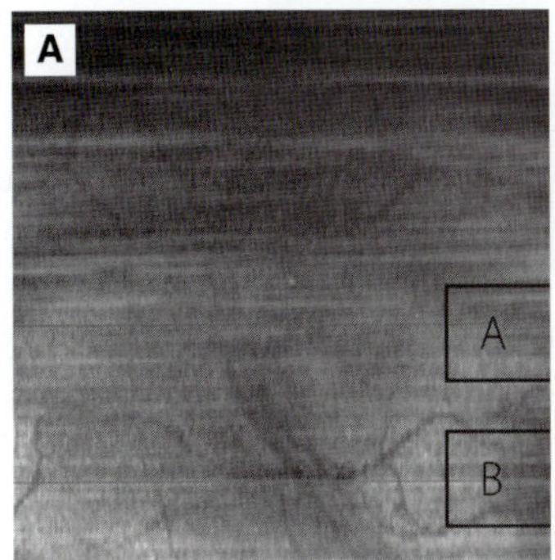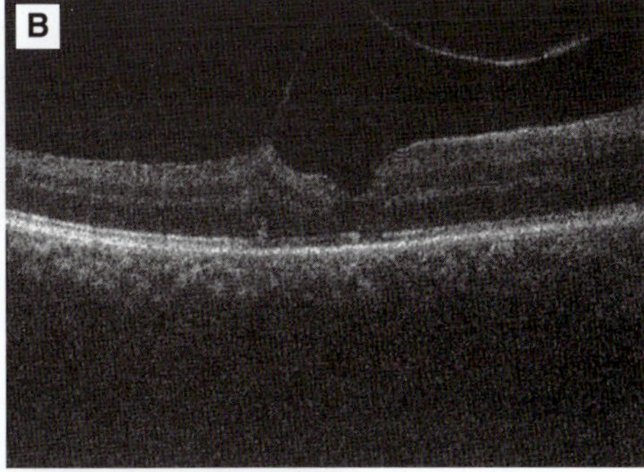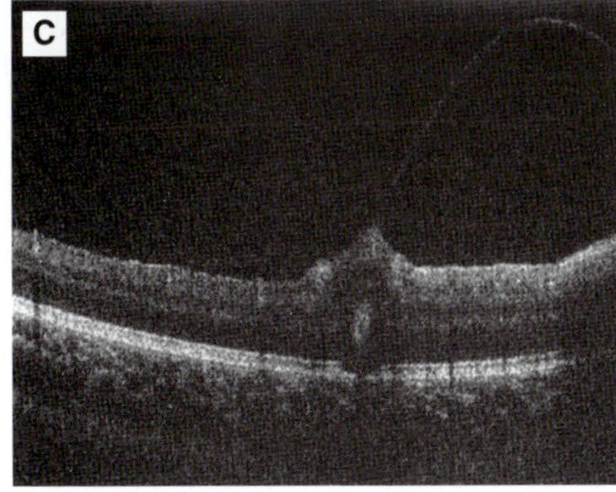

Fig. 100.2 SD-OCT scans of the right macula demonstrating focal vitreous traction and separation.

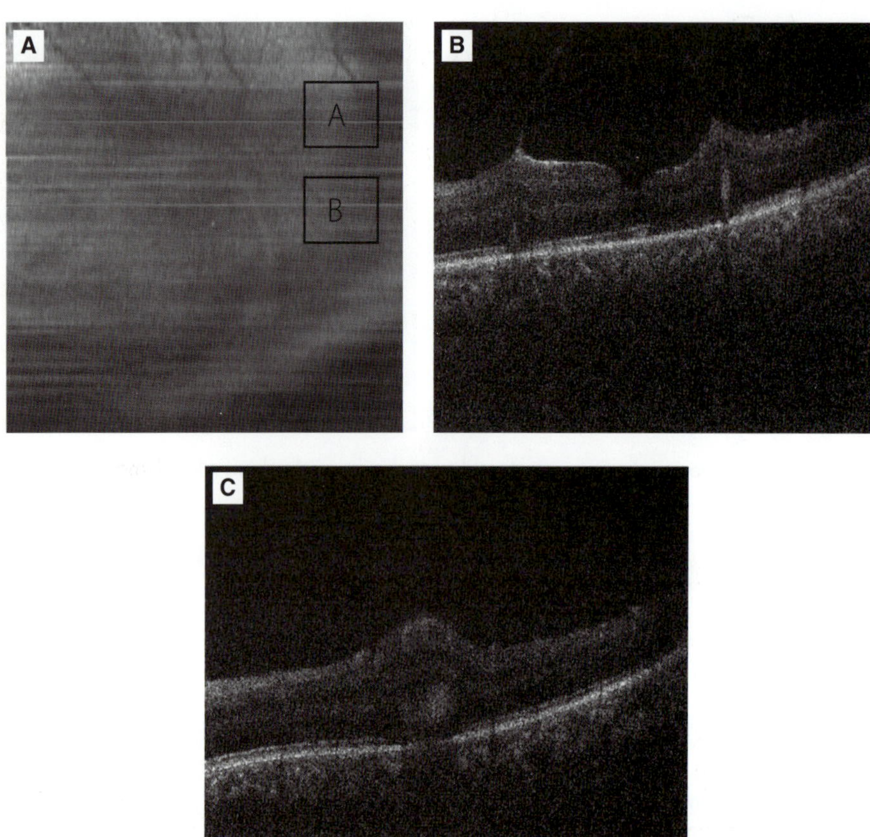

Fig. 100.3 SD-OCT scans of the left macula demonstrating focal vitreous traction, and areas of retinal elevation corresponding to retinal folds.

Shaken baby syndrome (SBS) is a leading cause of infant death from injuries. Ophthalmologists play a key role in diagnosis of this condition. Characteristic retinal findings of SBS include multilayered hemorrhages, retinal detachments, perimacular folds, retinoschisis, and macular holes. Bilateral flame hemorrhages in a nonverbal child is highly suspicious and specific for SBS. With the advent of SD-OCT, pathophysiologic mechanism of SBS is better understood as being due to mechanical shearing.

FURTHER READING

1. Sturm V, Landau K, Menke MN: Optical coherence tomography findings in shaken baby syndrome. *Am J Ophthalmol* 146:363–368, 2008.
2. Muni RH, Kohly RP, Sohn EH, et al.: Hand-held spectral domain optical coherence tomography finding in shaken baby syndrome. *Retina* 30(4 suppl):S45–S50, 2010.
3. Gardner H. Letter to the Editor. OCT Findings in Shaken Baby Syndrome: Forbes Editorial. *Am J Ophthalmol* 146:559, 2008.
4. Bielory BP, Dubovy SR, Olmos LC, et al.: Fluorescein angiographic and histopathologic findings of bilateral peripheral retinal nonperfusion in nonaccidental injury: a case series. *Arch Ophthalmol* 130(3):383–387, 2012, doi:10.1001/archopthalmol. 2011.1674.

X-linked Retinoschisis

Vishak John, Audina Berrocal, and Ditte Hess

X-linked retinoschisis (XLRS) is a bilateral vitreoretinal degenerative condition affecting males, which was first described by Haas in 1898. This has a worldwide prevalence of 1 in 5000 to 1 in 25,000, with highest incidence in Finland. Foveal stellate cysts are seen in almost all patients, and peripheral retinoschisis can be found in about 50% of the individuals. Vision loss from XLRS is mainly due to maculopathy, and manifests usually between ages 5 and 10 as reading difficulties in school. Other common complications of this condition include vitreous hemorrhage and retinal detachment in patients developing inner and outer retinal holes.

*XLRS*1, the disease-causing gene, codes for retinoschisin—a protein expressed on photoreceptor cells and bipolar cells, which is involved in cellular adhesion and cell–cell interaction. Although previous histopathologic studies reported split in the retina at the level of nerve fiber layer (NFL), newer imaging modalities including time-domain and spectral-domain optical coherence tomography (TD-OCT and SD-OCT) demonstrate that the schisis can occur at multiple levels of the retina, including the inner nuclear layer (INL) and outer plexiform layer (OPL).

CASE STUDY 1

A 3-month-old boy was referred to the pediatric retina service after his mother noticed eccentric gaze with decreased visual function for 1 month prior to presentation. The child was born at 37 weeks gestational age via spontaneous vaginal delivery without any peripartum complications. On exam, the child grimaced to light in both eyes, had symmetric pupils with no relative afferent pupillary defect (RAPD), and both eyes were soft to palpation. On dilated fundus examination, prominent schisis cavities were noted temporally in the right eye and superiorly in the left eye (Fig. 101.1). Under anesthesia, optical coherence tomography (OCT) images of his eyes were obtained and demonstrated retinal schisis in the macula, without any evidence of retinal detachment (Fig. 101.2).

On follow-up examination under anesthesia in 3 months, the patient was noted to have a retinal detachment involving the macula in the right eye, and underwent scleral buckle, pars plana vitrectomy with silicone oil (Fig. 101.3).

CASE STUDY 2

A 45-year-old male presented for evaluation of macular edema in both eyes. He reported poor vision since the age of 10, and had a best-corrected visual acuity (BCVA) of 20/40 in the right eye and 20/50 in the left eye. Fundus examination demonstrated foveal cysts and vitreous veils in both eyes consistent with XLRS (Fig. 101.4) and classical OCT features (Fig. 101.5).

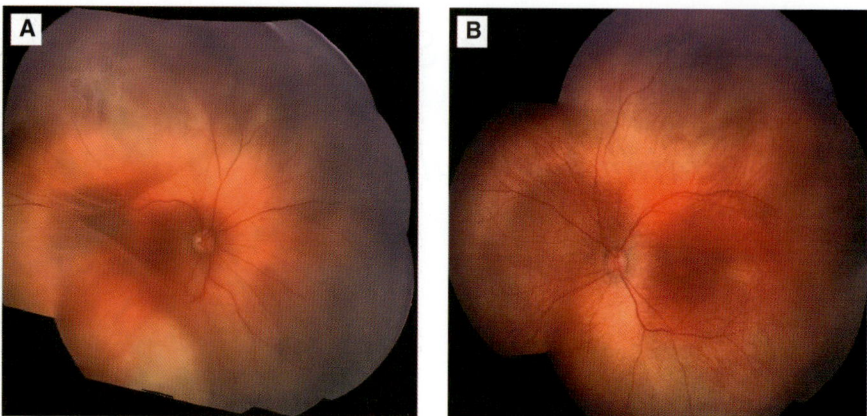

Fig. 101.1 Retcam™ fundus photos of the right and left eyes showing peripheral schisis cavities.

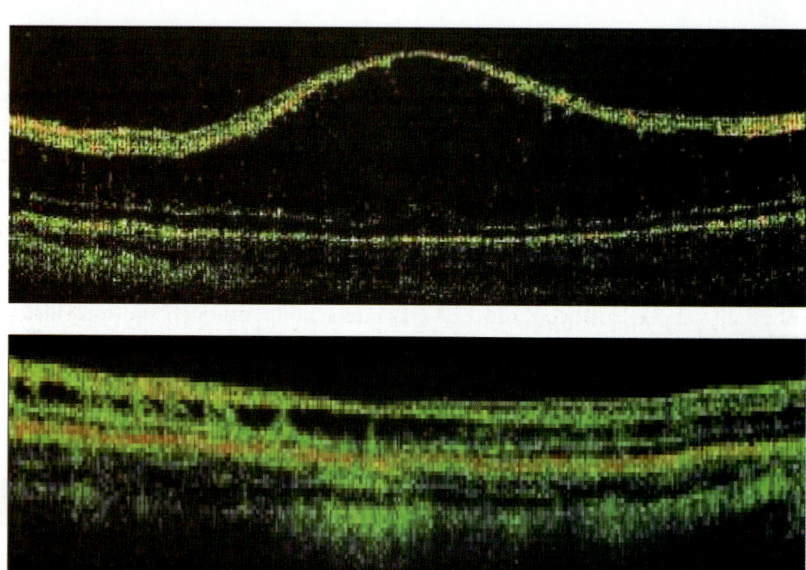

Fig. 101.2 Stratus OCT demonstrating inner retinal schisis cavity, right eye (*top*), left eye (*below*).

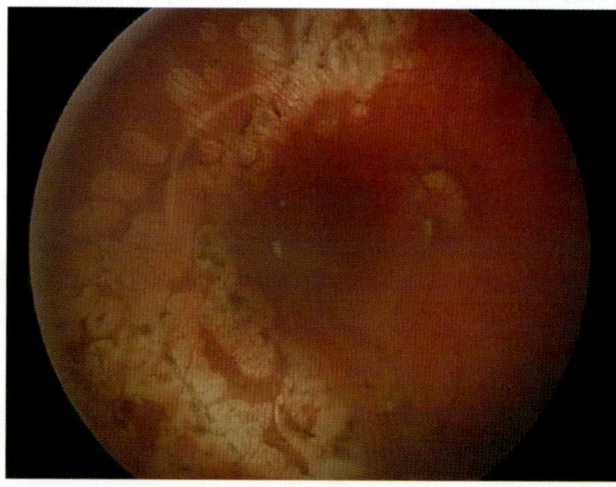

Fig. 101.3 Retcam™ photo after patient underwent retinal reattachment surgery in the right eye.

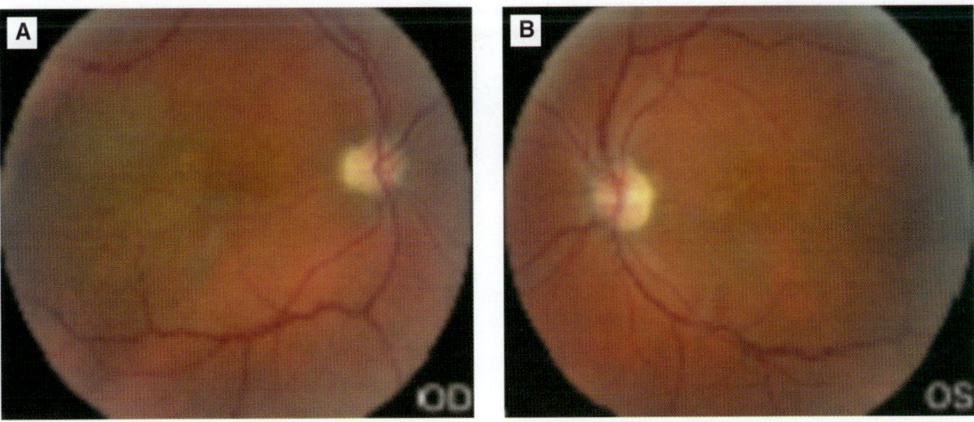

Fig. 101.4 Fundus photographs of the right **(A)** and left eye **(B)** at the time of referral for evaluation of macular edema.

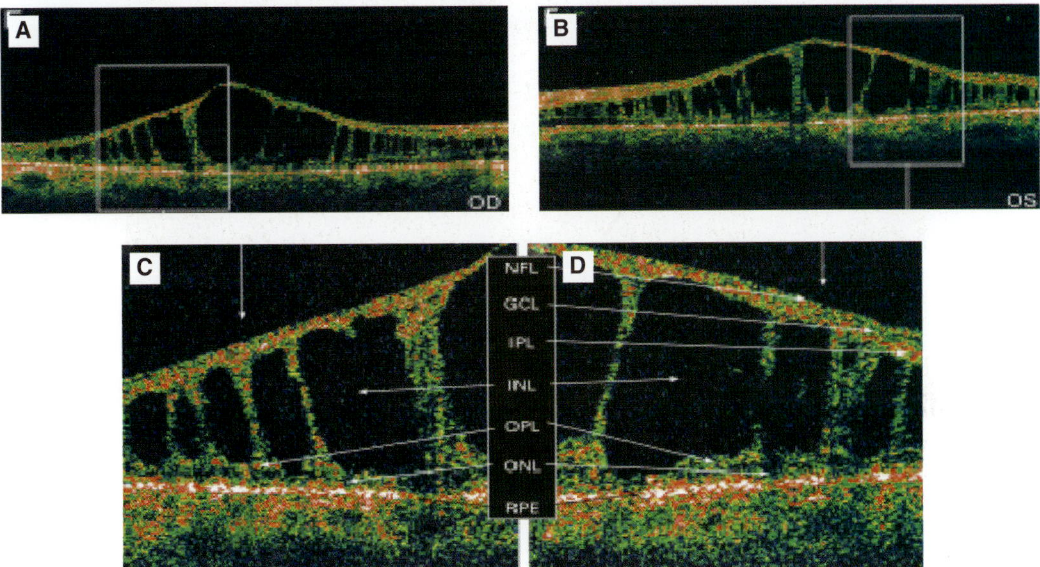

Fig. 101.5 Spectral-domain optical coherence tomography (SD-OCT) showed splitting of inner nuclear layer and abnormally thin outer plexiform layer.

FURTHER READING

1. Yanoff and Duker. X-Linked Retinoschisis. Ophthalmology, Third edition 580–581, 2009.
2. Tantri A, Vrabec TR, Cu-Unjieng A, et al.: X-linked retinoschisis. A clinical and molecular genetic review. *Surv Ophthalmol* 49(2):214–230, 2004.
3. Gregori NZ, Berrocal AM, Gregory G, et al.: Macular spectral-domain optical coherence tomography in patients with X linked retinoschisis. *Br J Ophthalmol* 93:373–378, 2009.

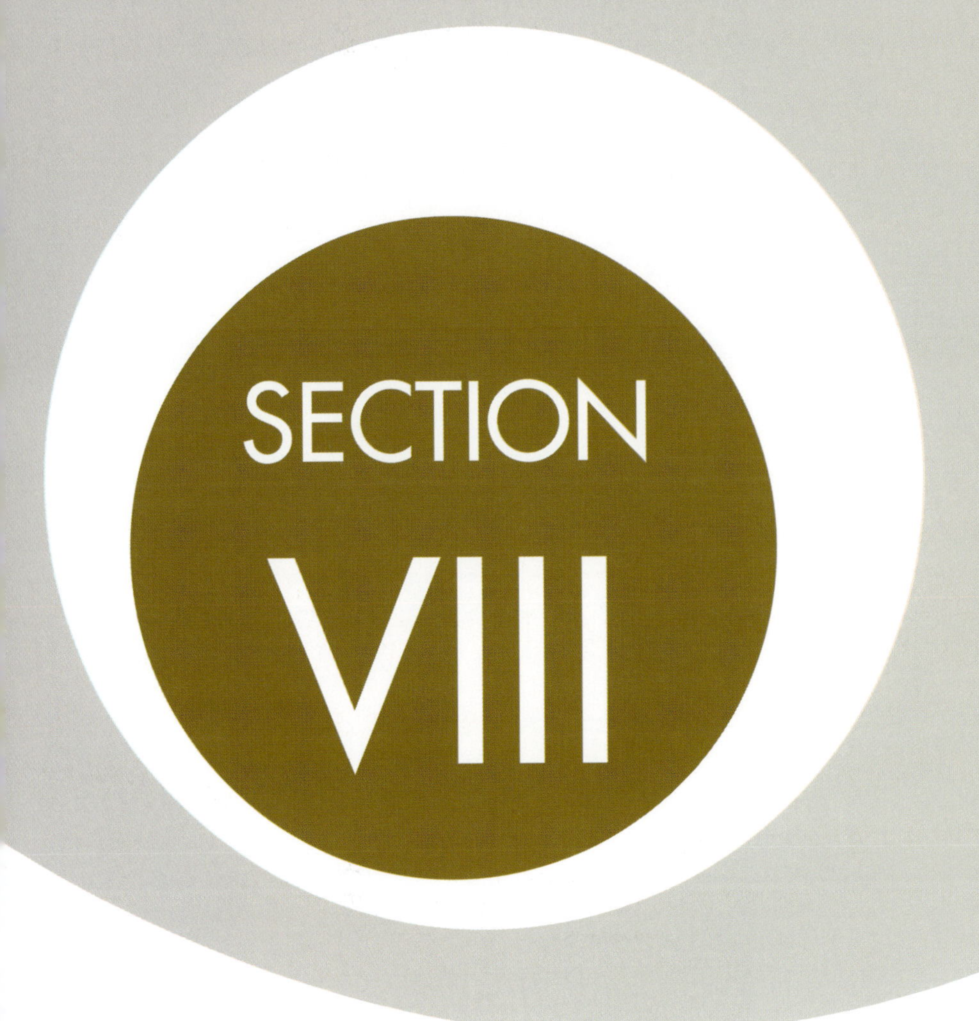

Uvea

Acute Retinal Necrosis

Kavitha Avadhani and Padmamalini Mahendradas

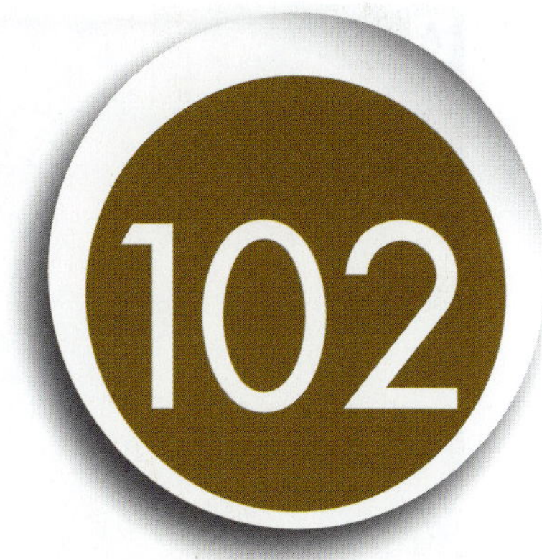

Acute retinal necrosis (ARN) is a form of retinitis that occurs in healthy, immunocompetent individuals, and is believed to be caused by the herpes group of viruses. Classical features of ARN include intense vitritis, multiple patchy yellow–white areas in the retinal midperiphery that coalesce over time, retinal vasculitis, and sometimes optic neuropathy. Treatment of ARN is done with a course of systemic acyclovir (intravenous followed by oral medications). Visual loss often occurs secondary to retinal detachment or optic neuropathy.

CASE STUDY

A 24-year-old female presented with complaints of redness, pain, and blurred vision in the left eye for a week. Vision in the right eye was poor since childhood (anisometropic amblyopia). Best-corrected visual acuity in the left eye was 20/80. Anterior segment examination was normal in the right eye, while the left eye showed fine keratic precipitates and an anterior chamber reaction of 2+ cells. Fundus examination of the right eye showed a tessellated myopic fundus. The left eye fundus evaluation revealed vitritis 3+, hyperemic disc (**Fig. 102.1A**), and multiple (often coalescent) yellowish, ill-defined areas of retinitis in the midperiphery (**Fig. 102.1B**) all around. Retinal vessels adjacent to the areas of retinitis showed sheathing suggesting active vasculitis. A spectral-domain optical coherence tomography (SD-OCT) scan through the retinal lesions showed a clear demarcation between normal and affected retina (**Fig. 102.1C**). Diseased retina showed hyperreflectivity of inner retinal layers along with fluid accumulation in the outer retina (**Fig. 102.1D**). The intense vitritis was clearly seen on the SD-OCT as multiple hyperreflective spots anterior to the retina.

A diagnosis of left eye ARN was made and the patient was started on intravenous acyclovir. A week later her best-corrected visual acuity had improved to 20/40 in the left eye. The vitritis had reduced and the retinal lesions were now showing signs of healing (**Fig. 102.2A**). The SD-OCT at this visit showed absence of posterior vitreous cells and complete disruption of normal retinal anatomy, with only a thinned-out hyperreflective layer seen now in place of the retina (**Fig. 102.2B**).

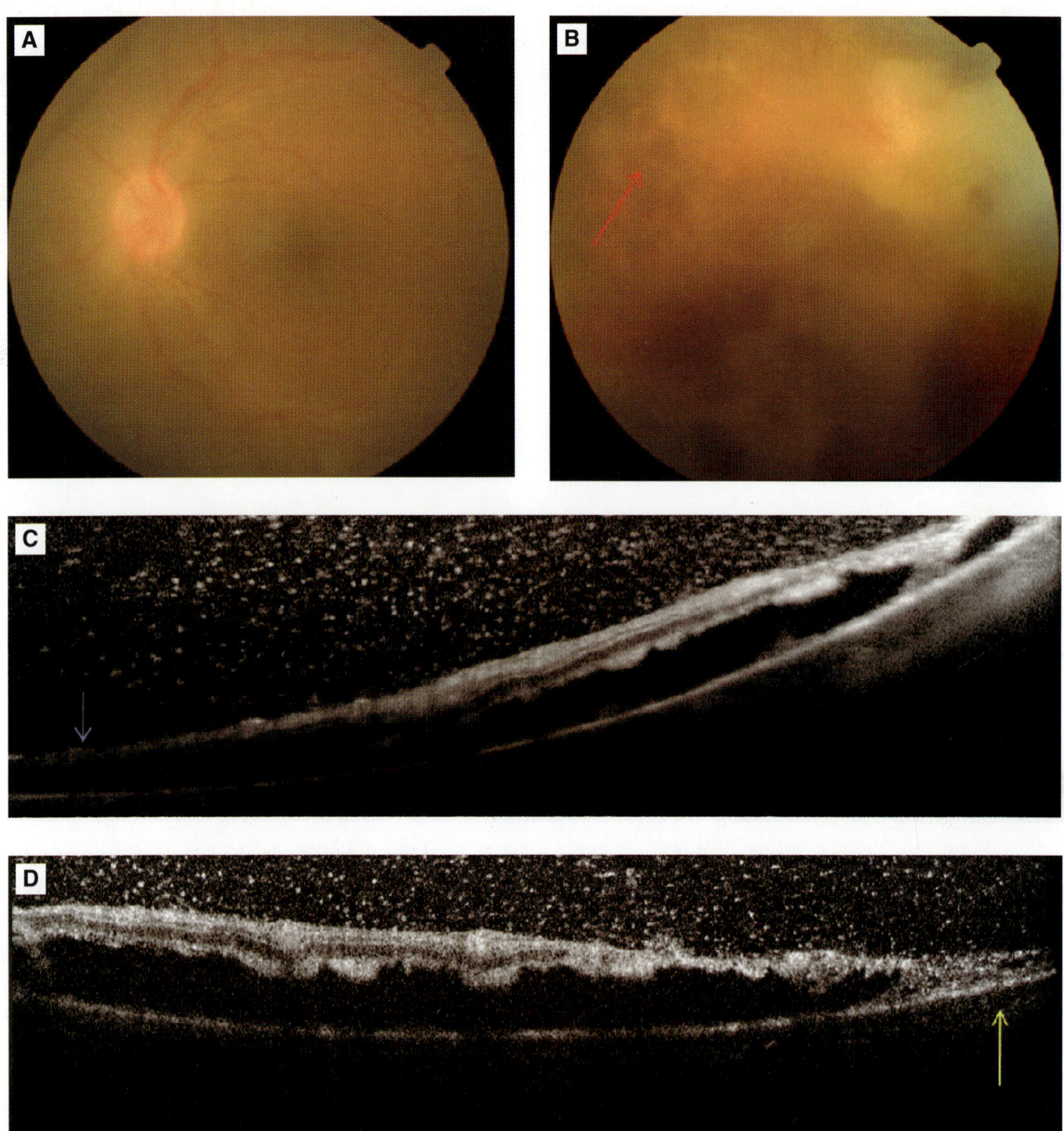

Fig. 102.1 **(A)** Fundus photograph of the posterior pole of left eye of the patient showing a hyperemic disc and a hazy media secondary to vitritis. **(B)** Fundus photo of the inferotemporal midperiphery of left eye showing large coalescent yellow lesions on the retina. Adjacent retinal vessels show sheathing (*red arrow*) suggestive of active inflammation of retinal vessels in acute retinal necrosis. **(C)** SD-OCT done in the same area as in "B" showing normal/uninvolved retina (*blue arrow*) and adjacent diseased retina. There is hyperreflectivity of inner retinal layers with accumulation of fluid in outer retinal layers seen as a hyporeflectivity on OCT. Small mounds of hyperreflectivity in the outer retinal layers probably correspond to RPE hypertrophy caused due to a perturbation of the RPE. Plenty of posterior vitreous cells are also clearly visible. **(D)** A scan taken slightly more anterior to the previous one shows similar findings. In addition, on the right hand side of the scan a portion of the retina (*yellow arrow*) where there is complete disruption of all retinal layers and absence of retinal fluid is also seen, suggesting that the lesion here has probably healed, leaving behind atrophic retina.

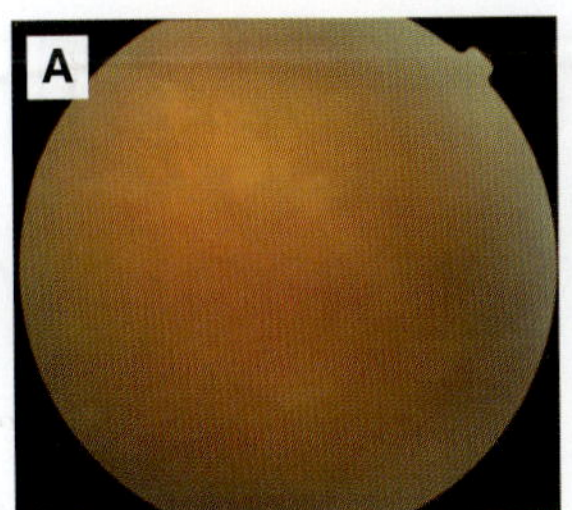 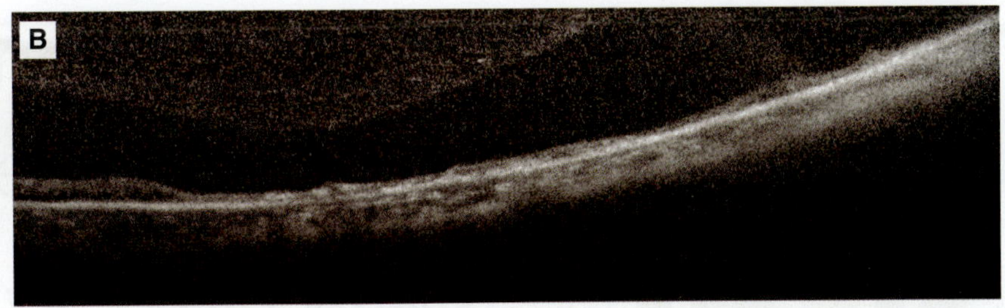

Fig. 102.2 **(A)** Fundus photograph of the same area seen in Figure 102.1B showing disappearance of yellow retinal lesions following 1 week of treatment with intravenous acyclovir. The retina now appears pale and atrophic. **(B)** SD-OCT through this area shows absence of all retinal layers (atrophic retina) and disappearance of posterior vitreous cells seen in the scan at presentation.

FURTHER READING

1. Suzuki J, Goto H, Minoda H, et al.: Analysis of retinal findings of acute retinal necrosis using optical coherence tomography. *Ocul Immunol Inflamm* 14(3):165–170, 2006.
2. Fisher JP, Lewis ML, Blumenkranz M, et al.: The acute retinal necrosis syndrome. Part 1: Clinical manifestations. *Ophthalmology* 89(12):1309–1316, 1982.
3. Culbertson WW, Blumenkranz MS, Haines H, et al.: The acute retinal necrosis syndrome. Part 2: Histopathology and etiology. *Ophthalmology* 89(12):1317–1325, 1982.
4. Gorman BD, Nadel AJ, Coles RS: Acute retinal necrosis. *Ophthalmology* 89(7):809–814, 1982.

Acute Zonal Occult Outer Retinopathy

Sumeer Thinda and Anita Agarwal

Acute zonal occult outer retinopathy (AZOOR) is a disease characterized by damage to broad zones of outer retina. Patients tend to be young women who present with acute visual field loss and photopsias. Examination typically reveals a normal-appearing fundus early in the disease process with vitreous cells occasionally. The electroretinography (ERG) is abnormal and can show either or both rod and cone dysfunction. Vision loss tends to be stabilized by 6 months. The disease can be unilateral or bilateral with occasional recurrences. Late fundus findings that correlate with areas of visual field loss include atrophy and migration of retinal pigment epithelium and attenuation of arterioles. The etiology of AZOOR is unknown but possible models of pathogenesis include a primary viral infection of photoreceptors that alters its antigenicity, or an autoimmune mechanism.

CASE STUDY

A 39-year-old female with a history of panuveitis of the right eye previously treated with acyclovir and steroids presented with new-onset photopsias and a scotoma in her left eye. Her symptoms began in the right eye several years prior with constant photopsias and progressive vision loss. She now presented with a temporal visual field defect in the left eye associated with photopsias projected to the zone of field loss. Examination revealed vision of hand motions in the right eye and 20/20 in the left eye. Amsler grid (**Fig. 103.1**), Goldmann visual fields (**Fig. 103.2**),

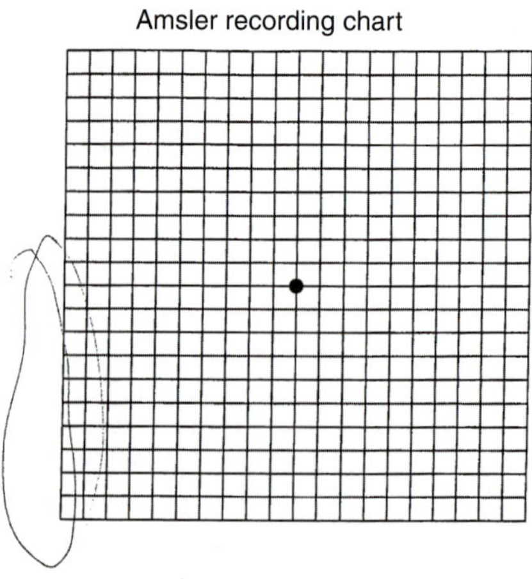

Fig. 103.1 Amsler grid of the left eye showed a temporal scotoma.

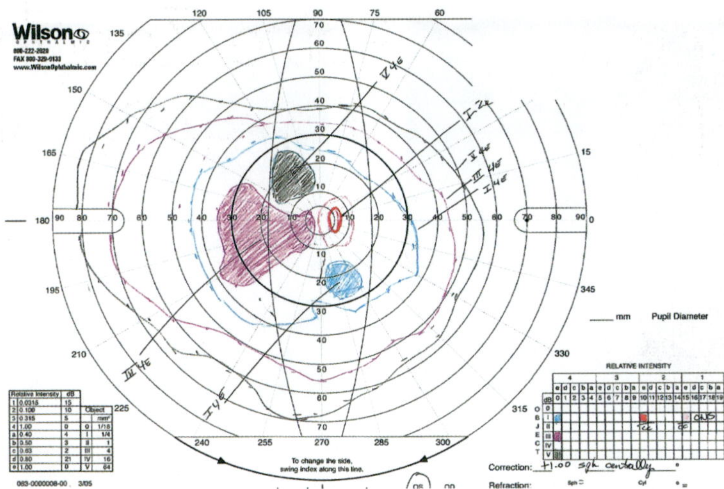

Fig. 103.2 Goldmann visual field of the left eye showed a temporal field defect and two paracentral defects—one superior and one inferior to fixation.

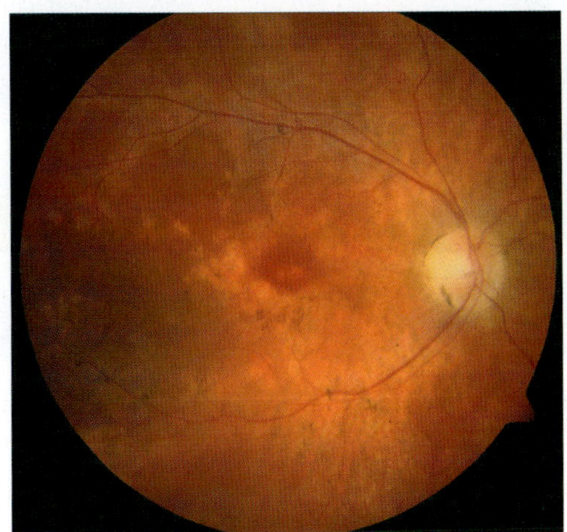

Fig. 103.3 Fundus photograph of the right eye showed optic nerve pallor, narrowed retinal vessels, retinal pigment epithelium disturbance, and retinal pigment epithelium migration throughout the fundus.

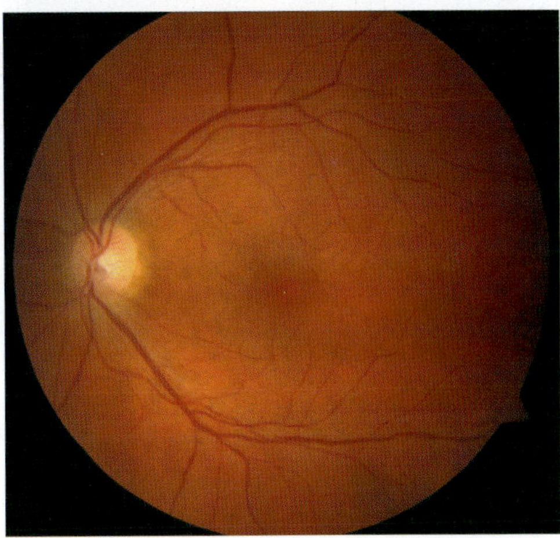

Fig. 103.4 Fundus photograph of the left eye showed mild retinal arteriolar narrowing.

fundus photographs (**Figs 103.3 and 103.4**), fundus autofluorescence (**Figs 103.5 and 103.6**), optical coherence tomography (OCT) images (**Figs 103.7–103.9**) and ERG findings (**Fig. 103.10**) are shown below.

This case shows chronic changes from prior AZOOR in the right eye and new-onset AZOOR in the left eye. The patient was initially tried on oral prednisone and acyclovir with continued progression of visual field defect in the left eye. She was then switched to methotrexate with later addition of mycophenolate mofetil. She is currently stable on aforementioned immunosuppressive therapy.

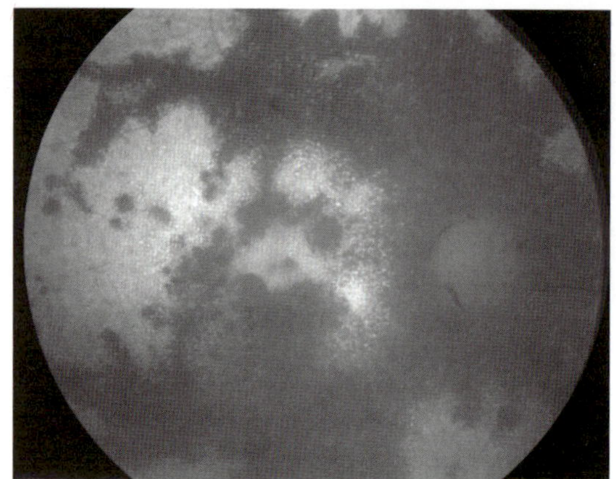

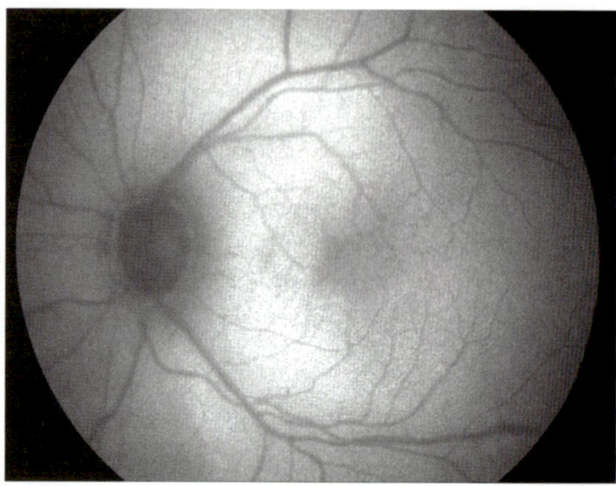

Fig. 103.5 Fundus autofluorescence of the right eye showed decreased autofluorescence, especially along retinal veins corresponding to zones of retinal pigment epithelial loss.

Fig. 103.6 Fundus autofluorescence of the left eye was normal.

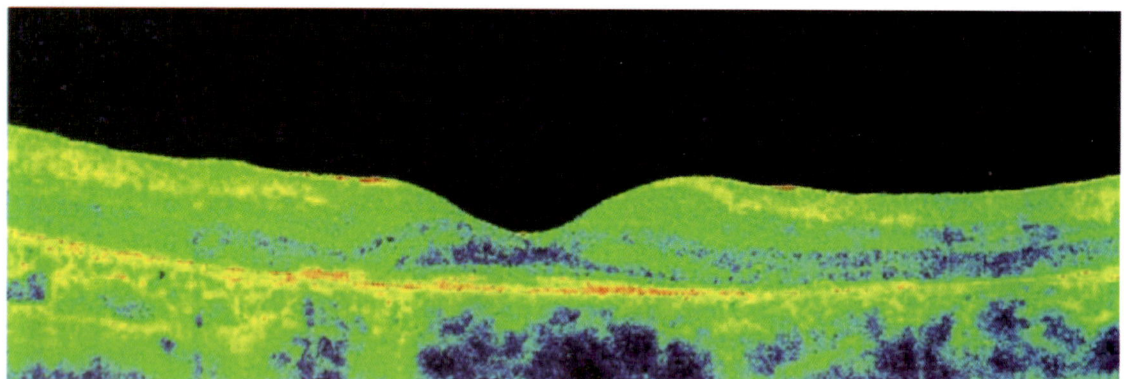

Fig. 103.7 Spectral-domain Cirrus HD OCT of the right eye showed diffuse loss of photoreceptor layer throughout the macular and peripapillary area in the right eye.

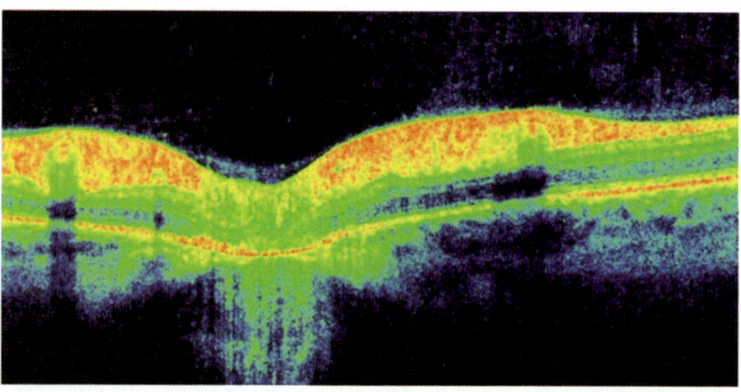

Fig. 103.8 Spectral-domain Cirrus HD OCT of the left eye showed loss of photoreceptors in the juxtapapillary area.

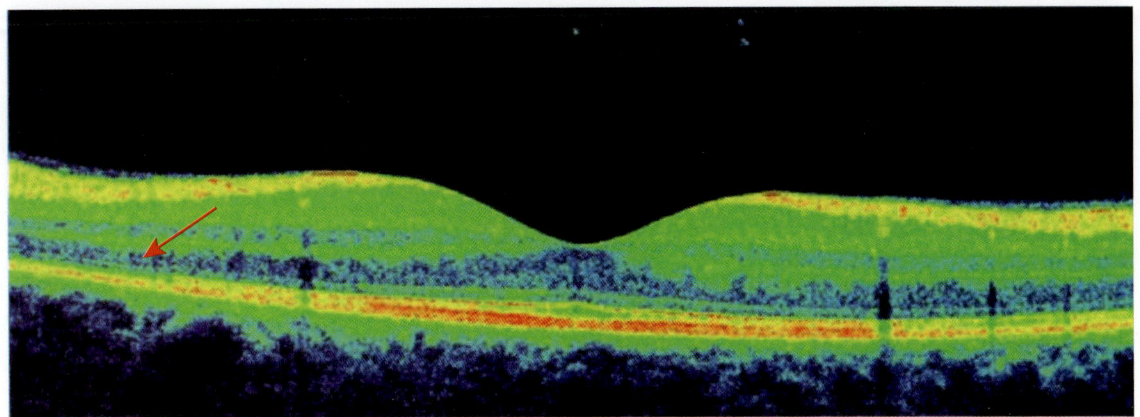

Fig. 103.9 Spectral-domain Cirrus HD OCT of the left eye showed a normal foveal center, but loss of photoreceptors in temporal peripapillary area (*arrow*).

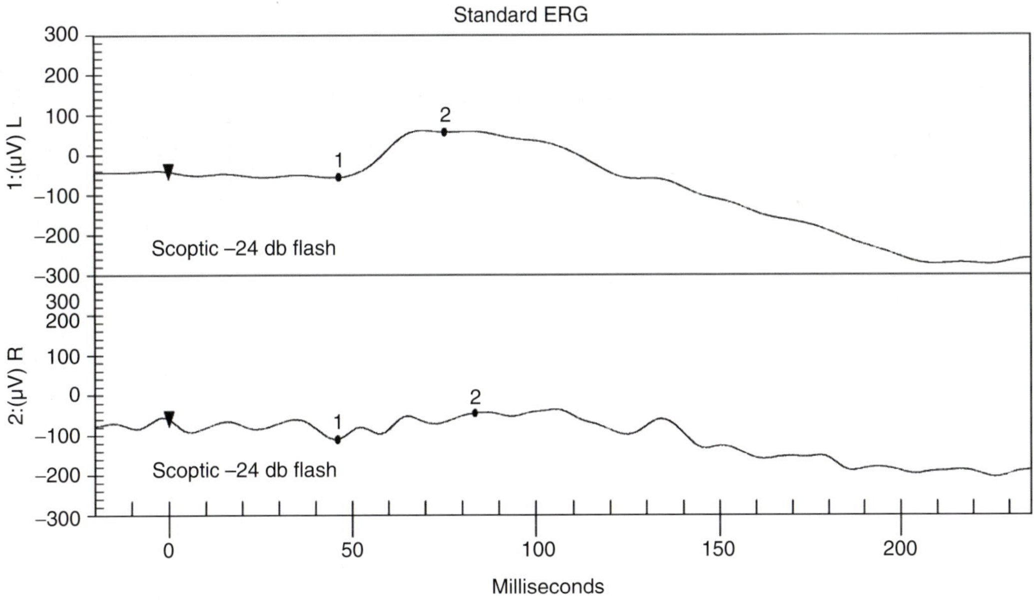

Fig. 103.10 *(Continued)*

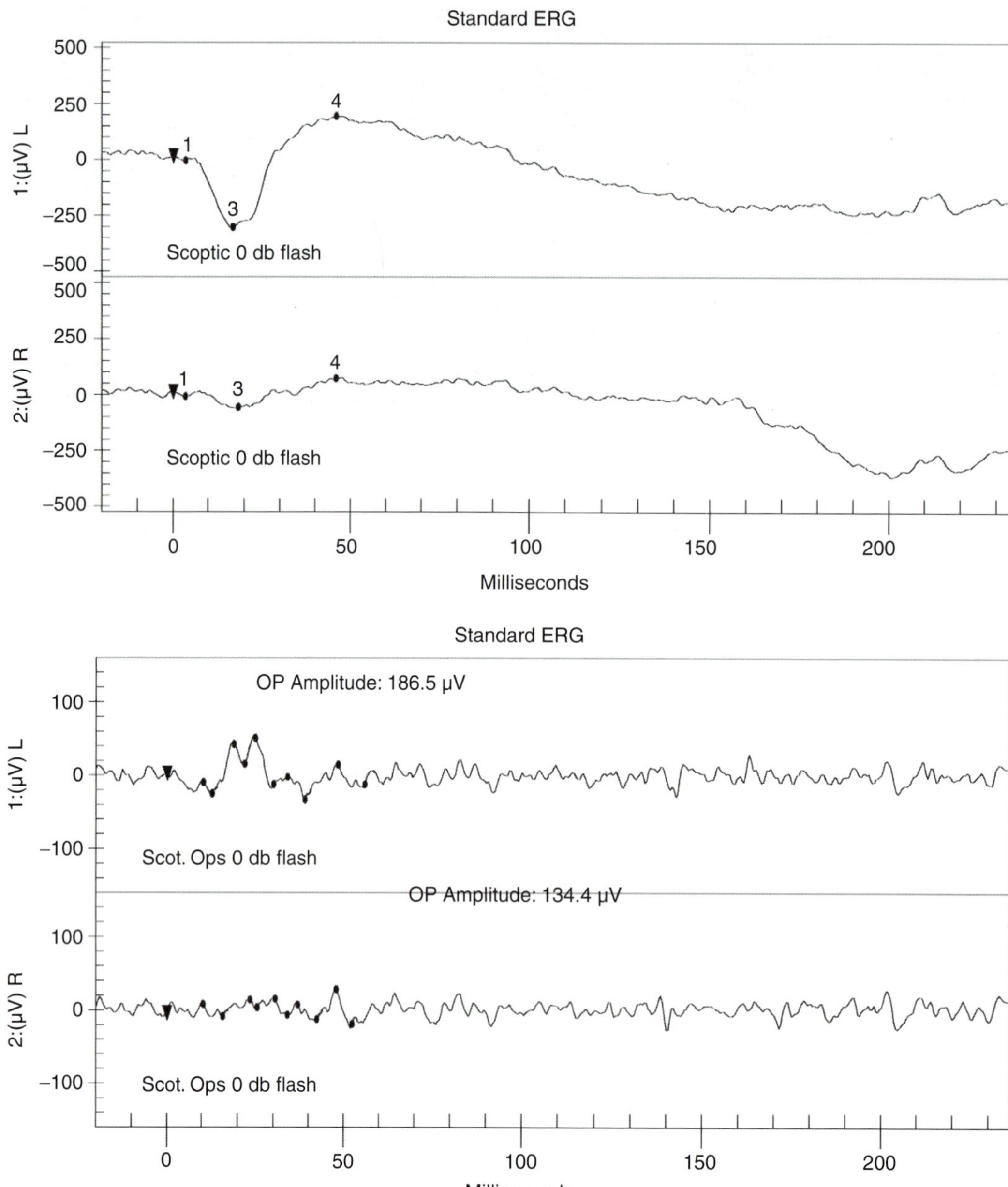

Fig. 103.10 *(Continued)*

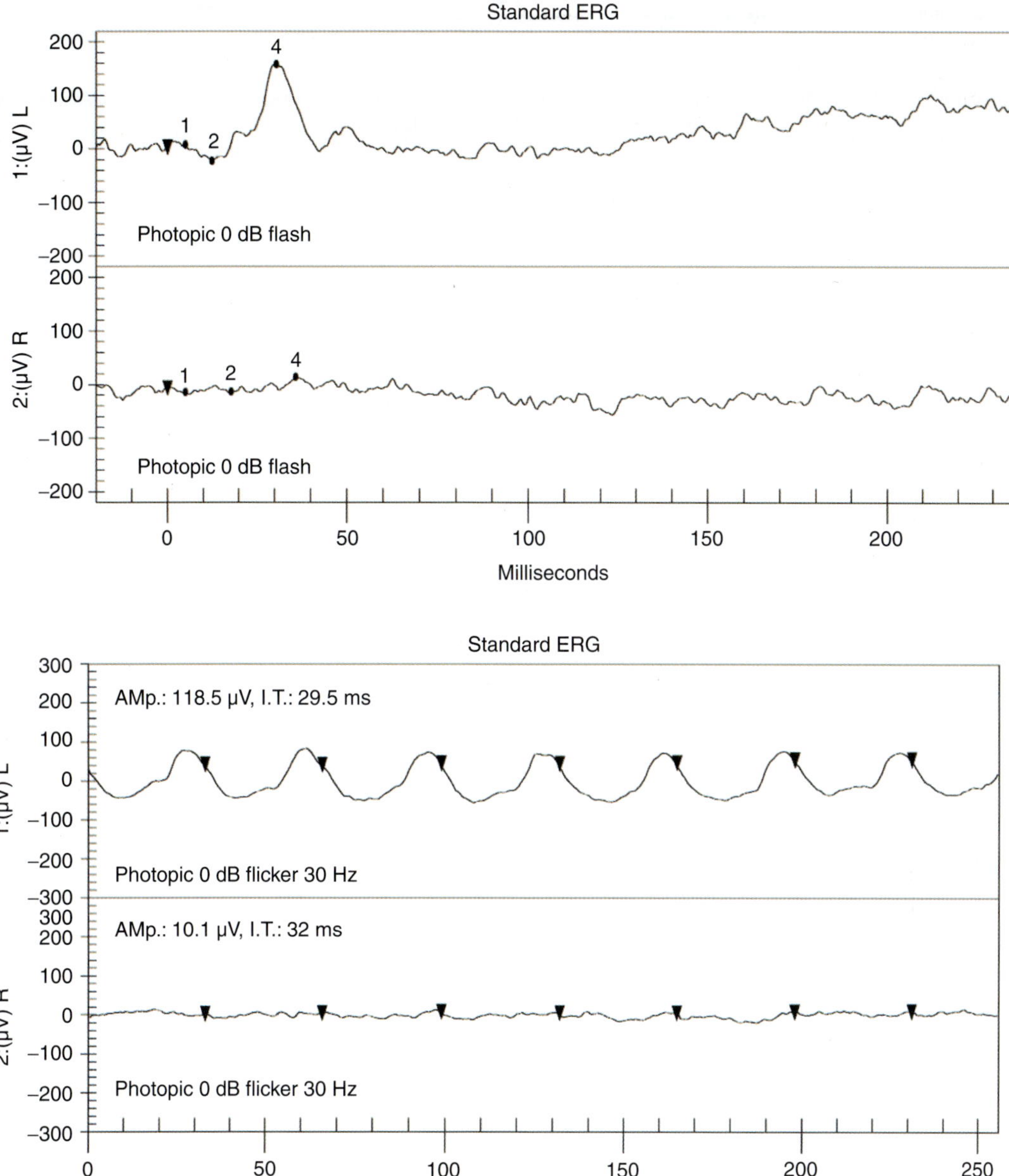

Fig. 103.10 Electroretinogram showed decreased scotopic and photopic amplitudes—which were markedly worse in the right eye compared to the left eye.

FURTHER READING

1. Gass JD. Acute zonal occult outer retinopathy. Donders Lecture: The Netherlands Ophthalmological Society, Maastricht, Holland, June 19, 1992. *J Clin Neuroophthalmol* 13:79–97, 1993.
2. Gass JD, Agarwal A, Scott IU. Acute zonal occult outer retinopathy: Along-term follow-up study. *Am J Ophthalmol* 134:329–339, 2002.
3. Gass JD. Are acute zonal occult outer retinopathy and the white spot syndromes (AZOOR complex) specific autoimmune diseases? *Am J Ophthalmol* 135:380–381, 2003.

4. Fujiwara T, Imamura Y, Giovinazzo VJ, et al.: Fundus autofluorescence and optical coherence tomographic findings in acute zonal occult outer retinopathy. *Retina* 30:1206–1216, 2010.

5. Monson DM, Smith JR. Acute zonal occult outer retinopathy. *Surv Ophthalmol* 56:23–35, 2011.

6. Mkrtchyan M, Lujan BJ, Merino D, et al.: Outer retinal structure in patients with acute zonal occult outer retinopathy. *Am J Ophthalmol* 153(4):757–768, Apr 2012; 768.e1. Epub 20 Nov 2011.

Acute Macular Neuroretinopathy

Maziar Lalezary and Anita Agarwal

Acute macular neuroretinopathy (AMN) was first described by Bos and Deutman as peculiar, reddish, wedge-shaped lesions that develop in the macula of young patients who complain of paracentral vision loss following a flu-like syndrome. Since this description, numerous other etiologic associations have been reported including use of sympathomimetics, hypotensive shock, oral contraceptives, and trauma. The scotoma(s) occurs suddenly, affecting one or both eyes with mildly decreased visual acuity. Biomicroscopically lesions are typically multiple, well-defined flat lesions that are wedge shaped and arranged in a petalloid fashion around the macula. The lesions may vary in color from reddish to purple or brown, depending on fundal pigmentation. The lesions correspond to shape and location of the scotomas. Fluorescein angiography is typically, but not always, normal. Optical coherence tomography (OCT) localizes pathology within these lesions to outer retina. While the outer retina and photo receptors are damaged, the OCT imaging of the lesions in very-early phases have recently been reported to show thickening of outer plexiform layer (OPL). Symptoms may be self-limiting or persistent, as fundus lesions usually fade with time. There is no treatment known to affect the course of this condition.

CASE STUDY

A 23-year-old healthy female noted a sudden-onset scotoma in the right eye upon waking in the morning. Her only medication included oral contraceptives. Visual acuity measured 20/20 in both eyes. She described missing lines superotemporal to fixation on Amsler grid testing. Fundus examination was normal at presentation (Fig. 104.1); however, fluorescein angiography revealed early choroidal hypoperfusion (Fig. 104.2). At this time, oral contraceptives were stopped. The patient's symptoms were unchanged when re-examined at 6 weeks. Fundus examination revealed a faint, solitary, petal-shaped area of reddish-bronze coloration in the juxtafoveal area in the right eye (Fig. 104.3). Infrared imaging better highlighted the lesion (Fig. 104.4). The OCT through the lesion showed disruption of the inner segment–outer segment (IS–OS) junction (Figs 104.5 and 104.6). At this time, a diagnosis of AMN was clinched.

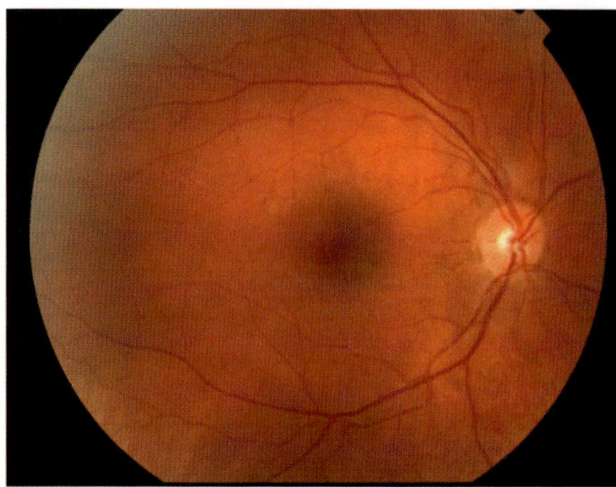

Fig. 104.1 Normal fundus appearance of a 23-year-old female who presented with acute-onset scotoma in the right eye. (Photo courtesy: Gass Atlas of Macular Diseases by Anita Agarwal, 5th edition, Vol. II, Fig. 11.25 (A), p. 997, Elsevier, 2012.)

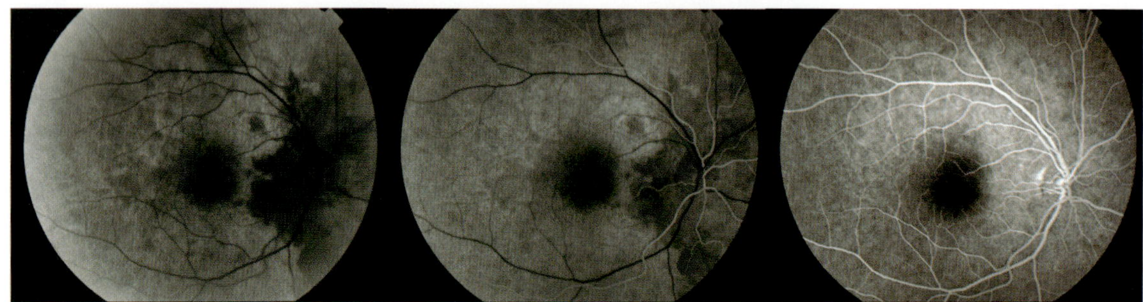

Fig. 104.2 Fluorescein angiogram (three frames shown in temporal sequence) of the described patient shows delayed choroidal filling. (Photo courtesy: (Photo courtesy: Gass Atlas of Macular Diseases by Anita Agarwal, 5th edition, Vol. II, Figs 11.25 (B), (C), and (E), p. 997, Elsevier, 2012.)

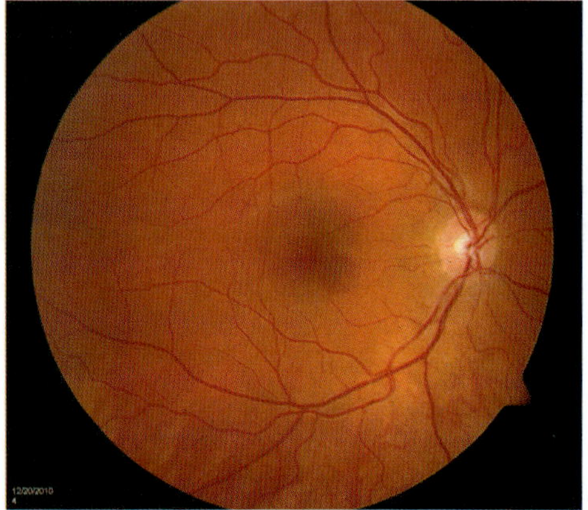

Fig. 104.3 Fundus photograph of the right eye 6 weeks after presentation showed a faint reddish-bronze discoloration of juxta foveal region typical for acute macular neuroretinopathy (AMN). (Photo courtesy: Gass Atlas of Macular Diseases by Anita Agarwal, 5th edition, Vol. II, Fig. 11.25 (F), p. 997, Elsevier, 2012.)

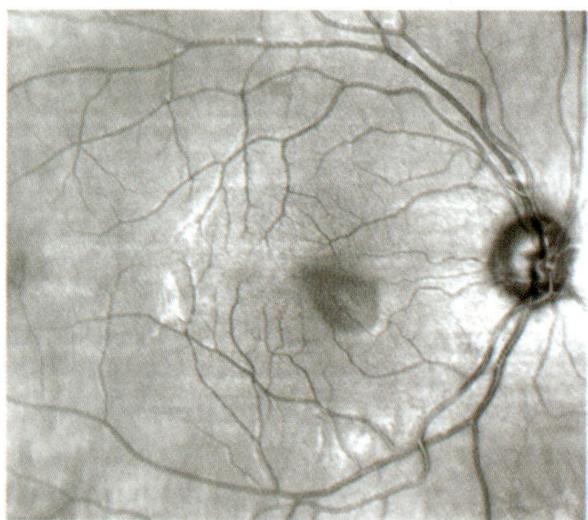

Fig. 104.4 Infrared image of the right eye highlighted a distinct petal-shaped darkened lesion in the inferonasal foveal region. (Photo courtesy: Gass Atlas of Macular Diseases by Anita Agarwal, 5th edition, Vol. II, Fig. 11.25 (H), p. 997, Elsevier, 2012.)

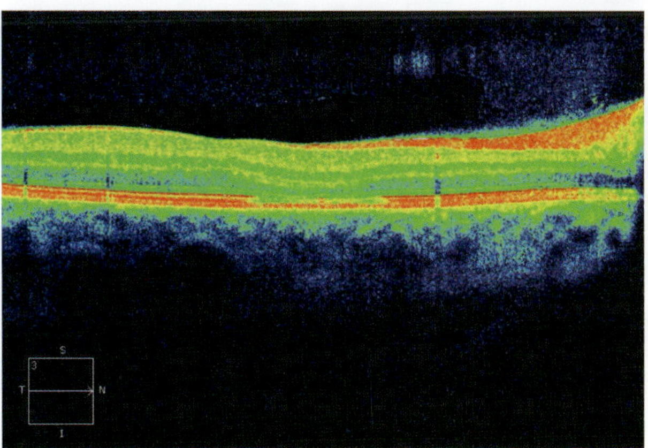

Fig. 104.5 Spectral-domain OCT image (Cirrus) through lesion of the right eye revealed disruption of inner segment–outer segment (IS–OS) junction. Subtle stretching of outer plexiform layer (OPL) was also noted. (Photo courtesy: Gass Atlas of Macular Diseases by Anita Agarwal, 5th edition, Vol. II, Fig. 11.25 (I), p. 997, Elsevier, 2012.)

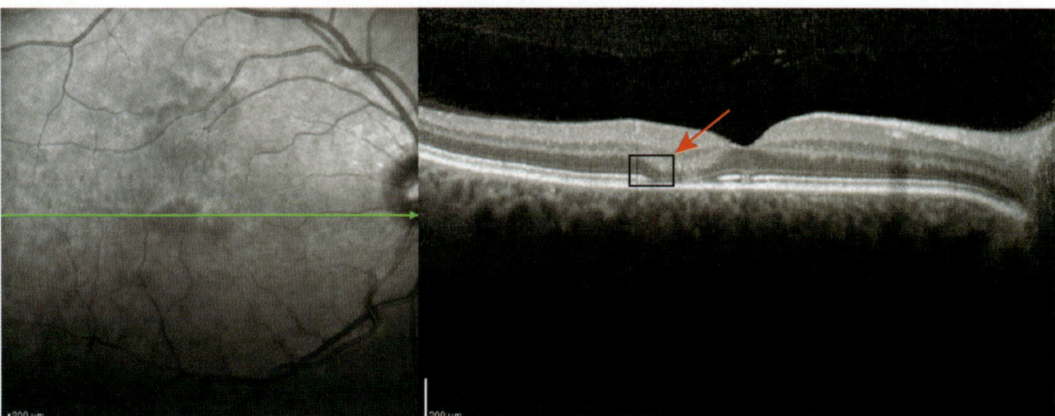

Fig. 104.6 Infrared and spectral-domain optical coherence tomography (SD-OCT) images (SPECTRALIS™) of a lesion from a different patient with AMN. The infrared image on left highlights lesions with a green line corresponding to location of OCT scan on right. OPL was thickened (*red arrow*) and outer retina was thinned. (Submitted to journal *Cases and Brief reports*, Walters Kluver, 2012.)

FURTHER READING

1. Bos PJ, Deutman AF. Acute macular neuroretinopathy. *Am J Ophthalmol* 80:573–584, 1975.
2. Agarwal A. Gass' Atlas of Macular Diseases. Philadelphia: Elsevier Saunders, Fifth Edition, Vol 2, 994–997.
3. O'Brien DM, Farmer SG, Kalina RE, et al.: Acute macular neuroretinopathy following intravenous sympathomimetics. *Retina* 9:281–286, 1989.
4. Leys M, Van Slycken S, Koller J, et al.: Acute macular neuroretinopathy after shock. *Bull Soc Belge Ophtalmol* 241: 95–104, 1991.
5. Gillies M, Sarks J, Dunlop C, et al.: Traumatic retinopathy resembling acute macular neuroretinopathy. *Aust NZ J Ophthalmol* 25:207–210, 1997.
6. Baumüller S, Holz FG. Early spectral-domain optical coherence tomography findings in acute macular neuroretinopathy. *Retina* 32(2):409–410, 2012.

Acute Posterior Multifocal Placoid Pigment Epitheliopathy

Scott Schoenberger and Anita Agarwal

Acute posterior multifocal placoid pigment epitheliopathy (APMPPE) is an acute inflammatory condition that usually occurs in young adults following a viral prodrome. Patients may have one eye involved at onset of disease, but contralateral eye becomes involved within days to weeks in most cases. It is characterized by creamy colored, multifocal, flat placoid lesions at the level of retinal pigment epithelium (RPE) in the posterior pole. Vision loss may be significant. Over ensuing weeks, the vision improves as the lesions heal, leaving permanent retinal pigment epithelial alterations.

CASE STUDY

A 19-year-old male presented with severe decreased vision oculus dexter (OD) for 1 week and oculus sinister (OS) for 2 days. He had a recent illness with fever and headache. He had no past ocular history or other systemic symptoms. His visual acuity was counting fingers oculi uterque (OU). There were no signs of intraocular inflammation. Dilated ophthalmic examination and fluorescein angiography were consistent with a diagnosis of APMPPE. Because of severe vision loss in OU, the patient was treated with systemic corticosteroids. Over the ensuing few weeks, he noted a dramatic improvement in the vision.

Fundus photography of both the eyes (Figs. 105.1A–D) shows creamy-yellow placoid lesions in the macula at the level of retinal pigment epithelium. The lesions are multifocal and involve the fovea OU. There is no peripapillary involvement. Both eyes show midperipheral small-to-medium-sized areas of chorioretinal atrophy, consistent with a more subacute or chronic component to his disease. Fundus Fluorescein angiography of both eyes (Fig. 105.2) showed early hypofluorescence and late hyperfluorescence with diffuse staining of the lesions.

Infrared imaging and spectral-domain optical coherence tomography of right eye (Fig. 105.3A) and left eye (Fig. 105.3B) are included. Lesions are visible on infrared imaging, but are less vivid than on color photographs and fluorescein angiogram. In the region of placoid lesions, optical coherence tomography (OCT) shows hyperreflectivity of outer nuclear layer and disruption of external limiting membrane (ELM), inner segment–outer segment (IS–OS) junction, and outer segments. Also present in the left eye (Fig. 105.3B) is outer retinal fluid superficial to the outer segments.

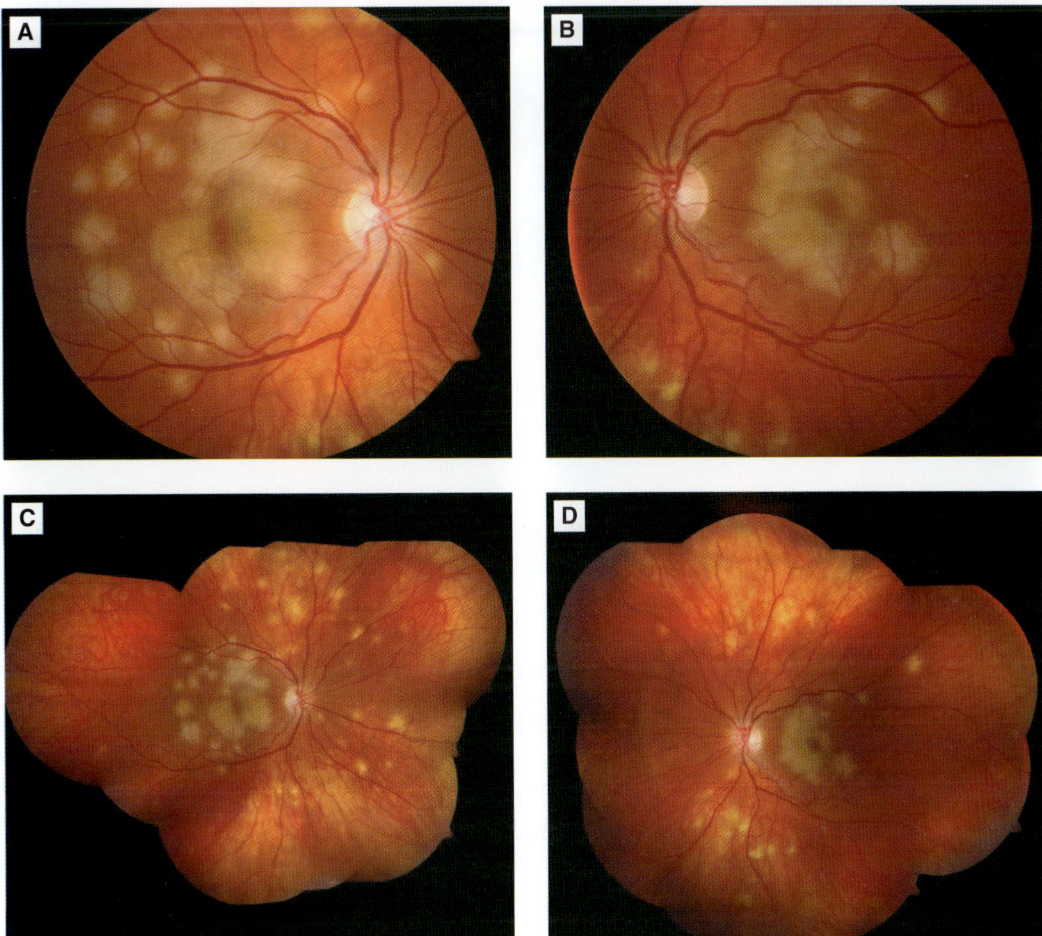

Fig 105.1 (A) and (B) Fundus photograph of the right (A) and left (B) eyes showing multifocal creamy yellow placoid lesions involving the fovea. (C) and (D) Montage fundus photographs of the right (C) and left (D) eyes showing mid-peripheral areas of chorioretinal atrophy in addition to the acute yellow placoid lesions.

APMPPE is an inflammatory disorder affecting the outer retina and retinal pigment epithelium (RPE). Its pathogenesis is most consistent with inflammation within the RPE and contiguous structures. Evidence for choroidal ischemia as a cause is lacking, given the diffuse late hyperfluorescence of the lesions. If there is an occlusion of the precapillary choroidal arteriole, the lesions should show a gradually increasing hyperfluorescence from the periphery. The condition primarily affects healthy young adults, and a viral prodrome is common. The patients usually develop rapid vision loss in one or both the eyes, and may experience scotomas. The patients with unilateral disease frequently develop contralateral eye involvement within days or weeks. Macular lesions as in the above case are highly characteristic of this disorder. A mild amount of vitreous cells are seen in one-half of the cases. As seen above, fluorescein angiogram shows early blockage and late even staining of the lesions. The OCT typically shows disruption of the RPE and outer retinal structures, including the photoreceptors, IS–OS junction, and ELM. The presence of subretinal

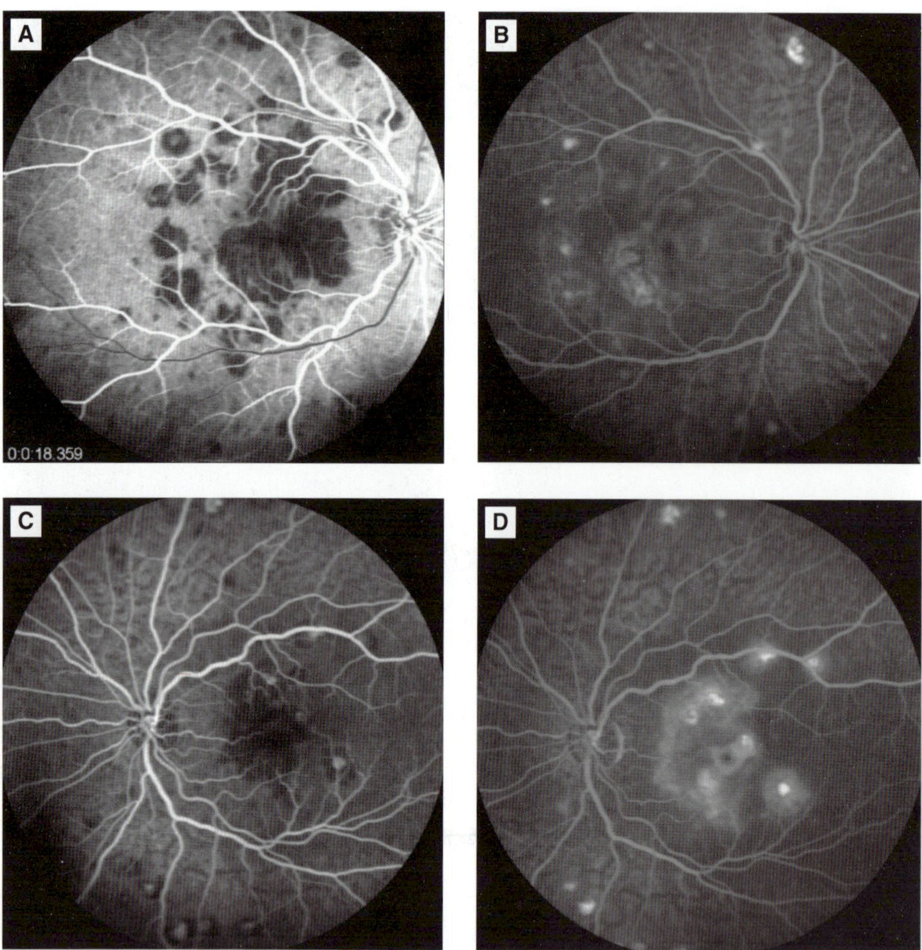

Fig. 105.2 Fluorescein angiography of the right **(A, B)** and left **(C, D)** eyes at presentation. In early phase of the right eye **(A)**, the lesions block choroidal fluorescence. In late phase of the right eye **(B)**, the lesions show staining. In the left eye, most lesions are still hypofluorescent except partially healed lesions that show transmission hyperfluorescence **(C)** in the midphase of the angiogram. The late phase reveals diffuse staining of the lesions **(D)**.

fluid on OCT is an uncommon feature that has been previously reported. There is an association between APMPPE and central nervous system (CNS) vasculitis. Other organ systems are less commonly involved and include urinary casts, hepatitis, erythema nodosum, and episcleritis.

Differential diagnosis of placoid chorioretinal lesions includes syphilis, sarcoidosis, tuberculosis, serpiginous choroiditis, persistent placoid maculopathy, and relentless placoid choroidopathy. The treatment of APMPPE is controversial. Most patients exhibit a spontaneous improvement of vision to normal or near-normal levels. Corticosteroids are sometimes offered in patients with severe loss, and are used in the patients with CNS vasculitis. Within weeks, the lesions turn inactive and are replaced by areas of RPE depigmentation and significant pigment clumping.

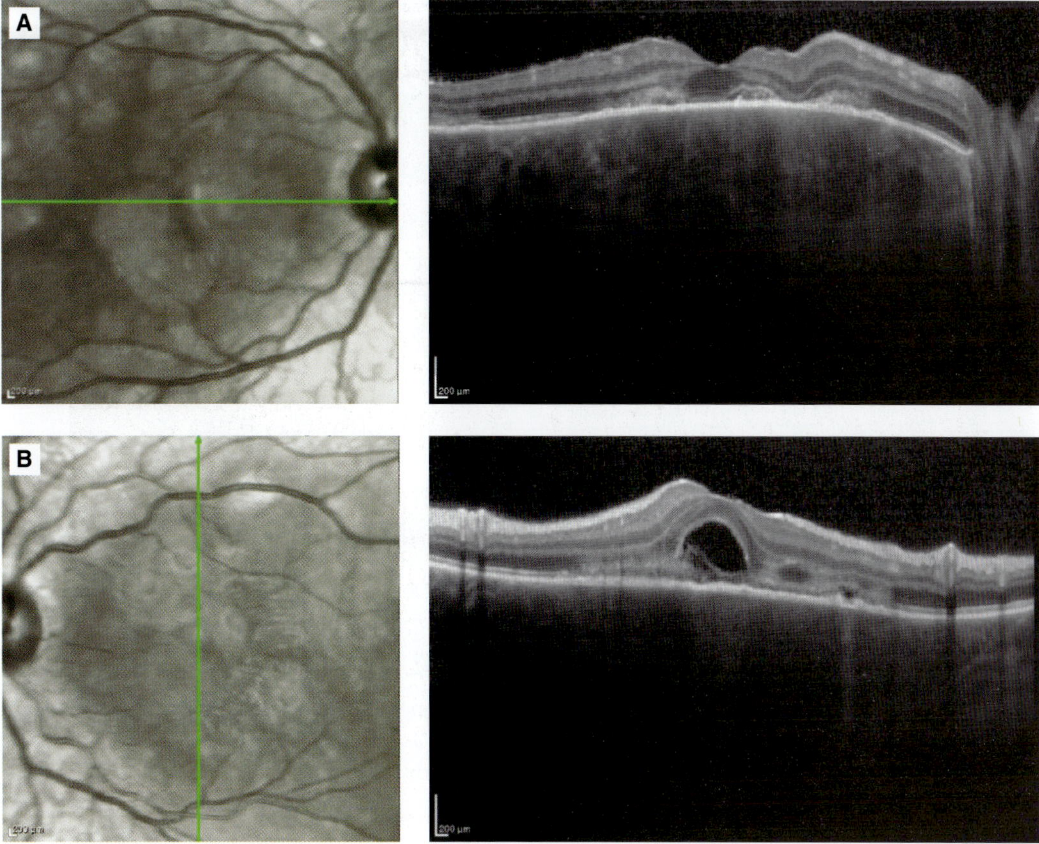

Fig 105.3 **(A)** and **(B)** Spectral-domain optical coherence tomography of the right **(A)** and left **(B)** eyes showing hyperreflectivity of outer nuclear layer and disruption of external limiting membrane, inner segment–outer segment junction and outer segments. **Figure 105.3 (B)** also shows the presence of outer retinal fluid.

FURTHER READING

1. Gass JDM. Acute posterior multifocal placoid pigment epitheliopathy. *Arch Ophthalmol* 80:177–185, 1968.
2. Deutman AF, Lion F. Choriocapillaris nonperfusion in acute multifocal placoid pigment epitheliopathy. *Am J Ophthalmol* 84:652–657, 1977.
3. Sigelman J, Behrens M, Hilal S. Acute posterior multifocal placoid pigment epitheliopathy associated with cerebral vasculitis and homonymous hemianopia. *Am J Ophthalmol* 88:919–924, 1979.
4. Birnbaum AD, Blair MP, Tessler HH, et al.: Subretinal fluid in acute posterior multifocal placoid pigment epitheliopathy. *Retina* 30:810–814, 2010.
5. Hsu CT, Harlan JB, Goldberg MF, et al.: Acute posterior multifocal placoid pigment epitheliopathy associated with a systemic necrotizing vasculitis. *Retina* 23:64–68, 2003.

Cat Scratch Disease

Anita Agarwal

Cat scratch disease (CSD) is the commonest cause of neuroretinitis in young and middle-aged people. It is caused by a pleomorphic gram-negative bacillus, *Bartonella,* previously termed *Rochalimaea.* This zoonotic disease is worldwide in distribution, the cat flea *Ctenocephalides felis* is the transmitting vector between cats. *Bartonella henselae, B. quintana, B. elizabethae, and B. grahamii* cause ocular lesions.

CASE STUDY

A 25-year-old nursing mother noted a sudden decrease in vision that began 2 weeks prior following fever and a presumed viral illness. She owned two cats, but did not recall being scratched or licked by them. Her visual acuity was 20/200 in the right eye and 20/20 in the left eye. The right fundus revealed swelling and dilated vessels of the inferior-half of the optic disc along with a macular star (Fig. 106.1). She also had two areas of white retinitis in the superonasal retina (Fig. 106.2). The left fundus was normal (Fig. 106.3). A fluorescein angiogram revealed dilated vessels on the disc that leaked late (Fig. 106.4). Optical coherence tomography showed subfoveal fluid and intraretinal lipid in the outer plexiform layer (Fig. 106.5). She was treated with oral azithromycin for 10 days. The disc swelling and prominent vessels gradually improved with complete resolution and visual recovery to 20/20 over 4 months (Fig. 106.6).

Cat scratch disease presents as a neuroretinitis with a macular star and a swollen optic nerve. Focal white retinal lesions of CSD may occur anywhere in the fundus, but show some predilection for occurring adjacent to, and obstructing major retinal arteries and less often veins. These retinal lesions, as well as similar lesions involving the optic nerve head, may be associated with an angioma-like proliferation of capillaries. White lesions typically involve the inner-half of the retina and may or may not be associated with overlying vitreous cells. These may resemble cotton-wool spots, but are not distributed along a first-order arteriole, as is the case with cotton-wool spots. Occasionally, severe occlusive vasculitis with involvement of both arteries and veins can be seen. The focal white retinal and optic disc lesions, swelling of the optic disc, and macular star figure typically clear spontaneously within several weeks or months (Figs 106.1, 106.2, and 106.6); and the visual acuity usually returns to normal or near normal. Most of the retinal lesions resolve without causing RPE damage. Detection of antibodies to cat scratch bacillus is helpful

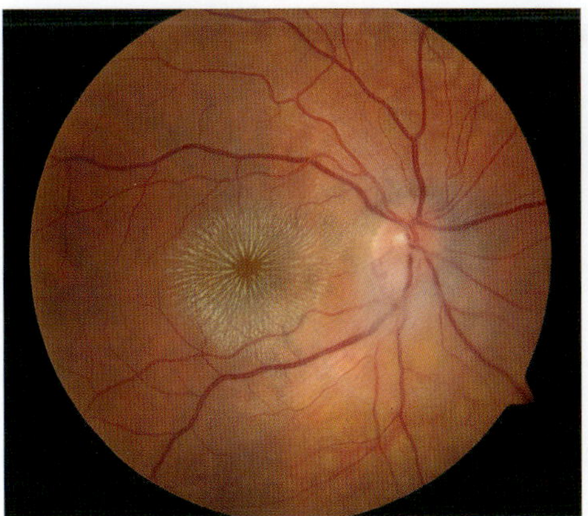

Fig. 106.1 Right eye has swelling of the inferior half of the optic disc with dilated vessels on its surface. The macula shows lipid exudates arranged in a "star".

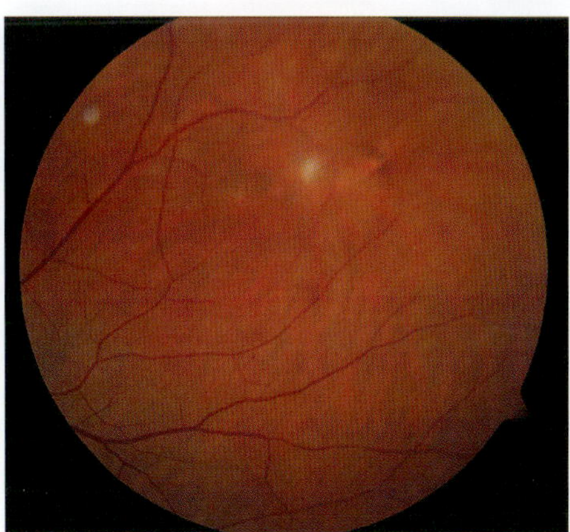

Fig. 106.2 Focal white infiltrates are seen in the inner retina in the upper nasal quadrant.

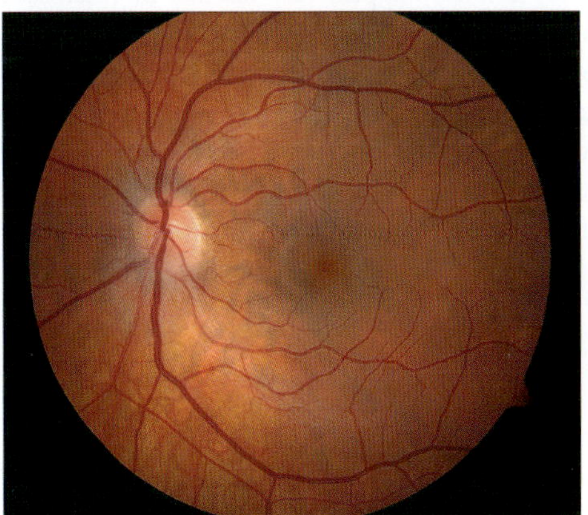

Fig. 106.3 The left optic disc, blood vessels and macula are unaffected.

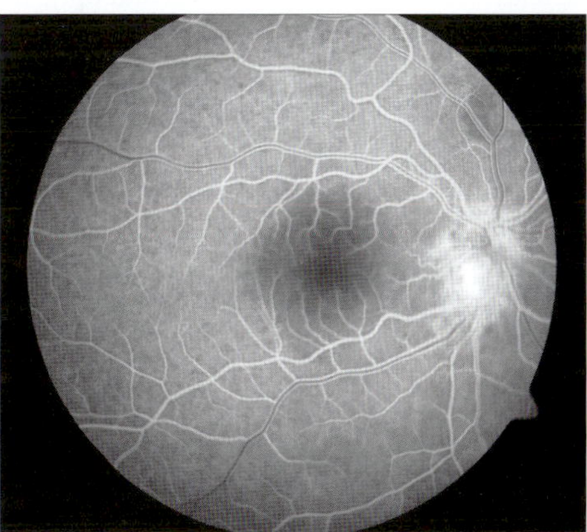

Fig. 106.4 The dilated optic disc vessels are visible on the angiogram in the right eye.

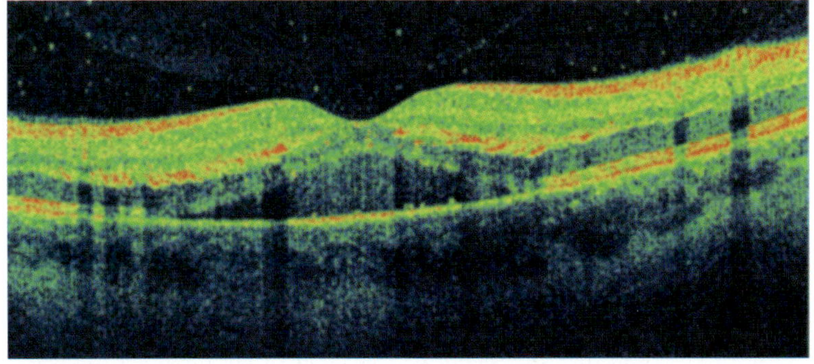

Fig. 106.5 SD-OCT of the macula demonstrates subretinal fluid and lipid exudates in the outer plexiform layer.

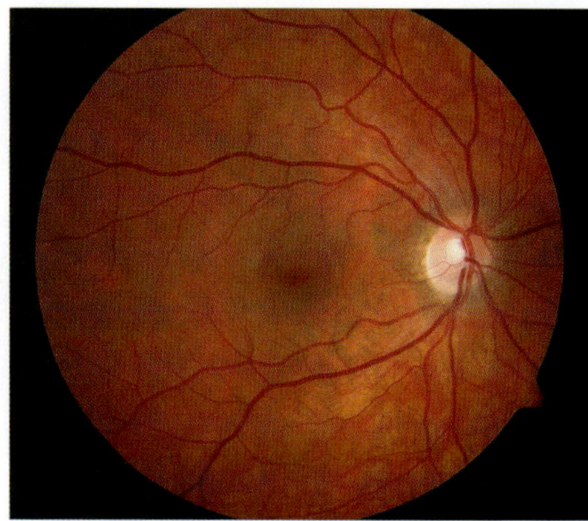

Fig. 106.6 The right eye 4 months after onset is back to a normal appearance with resolution of the optic disc edema and macular exudates.

in diagnosis. Indirect fluorescent antibody assay for *B. henselae* and *B. quintana,* available through the Centers for Disease Control and Prevention in Atlanta, is sensitive for diagnosis of CSD.

The tendency for some of the retinal and optic nerve inflammatory lesions to appear very vascular biomicroscopically and angiographically may be an important feature of cat scratch infection. Angioma-like masses referred to as epithelioid angiomatosis and caused by cat scratch bacillus have occurred on skin and mucous membranes of the patients with AIDS. In these patients, the lesions may resemble Kaposi's sarcoma clinically. In the eye, the lesions may simulate capillary angiomas or astrocytic hamartomas of the retina. The treatment is indicated only for those with significant loss of vision or when associated with immunocompromised state, as in the patients with AIDS. The organism is susceptible to several antibiotics, including trimethoprim and sulfamethaxazole, rifampicin, azithromycin, doxycycline, ciprofloxacin, and others.

FURTHER READING

1. Dalton MJ, Robinson LE, et al.: Use of Bartonella antigens for serologic diagnosis of cat-scratch disease at a national referral center. *Arch Intern Med* 155(15):1670–1676, 1995.
2. Gass JDM (1997). Stereoscopic atlas of macular diseases: Diagnosis and treatment. St. Louis, CV Mosby: 604–606.
3. Agarwal A. Gass' Atlas of Macular Diseases. 812–815, 2012.
4. Stoler MH, Bonfiglio TA, Steigbigel RT et al.: An atypical subcutaneous infection associated with acquired immune deficiency syndrome. *Am J Clin Pathol* 80:714–718, 1983.

Chikungunya Retinitis

Padmamalini Mahendradas and Kavitha Avadhani

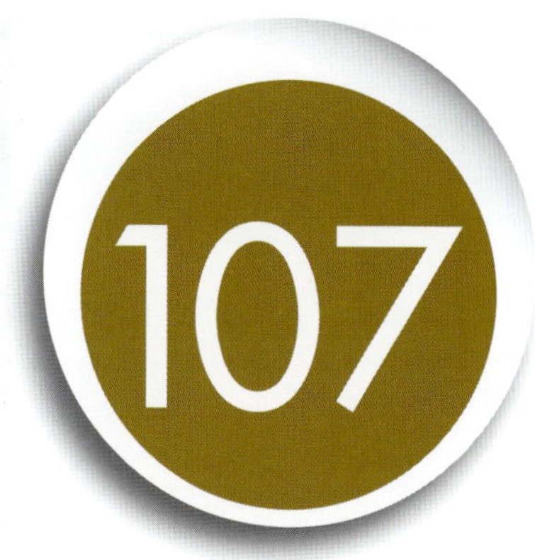

INTRODUCTION

Chikungunya retinitis is caused by the chikungunya virus, which is a single-stranded RNA virus of genus *Alphavirus* in family Togaviridae. It occurs following the bite of infected mosquitoes, primarily *Aedes aegypti* and sometimes by *A. albopictus*. Systemic features of chikungunya infection include sudden onset of fever with chills, headache, malaise, arthralgia or arthritis, myalgia, vomiting, and skin rash. It is a self-limiting illness. Many patients experience persistent joint symptoms for longer duration.

Chikungunya retinitis can present at the time of fever or can manifest after many weeks or months. Clinical features include vitritis, hyperemic disc, multifocal retinitis, retinal hemorrhages, neuroretinitis, and optic neuritis. Diagnosis is done by demonstration of chikungunya IgM antibody in the serum and also by reverse transcriptase–polymerase chain reaction (RT-PCR) analysis from ocular fluids and serum. Management is done by symptomatic treatment with topical and systemic steroids to control inflammation. Prevention of the disease is done by using protective measures against the mosquito bite.

CASE STUDY

A 38-year-old male presented with complaints of decreased vision in the left eye since 1 week. He also gave a history of fever 15 days back, which was associated with vomiting and skin rashes. On examination, right eye was normal. The left eye revealed best-corrected visual acuity (BCVA) of 6/36, N36. Intraocular pressure (IOP) was normal. The slit lamp biomicroscopic examination revealed fine diffuse keratic precipitates, flare++, cells++, and anterior vitreous cells++ in the left eye. Fundus examination revealed vitreous haze++, mild hyperemic disc, area of retinitis associated with retinal hemorrhage, and macular star (**Fig. 107.1**).

On investigation, enzyme-linked immunosorbent assay (ELISA) for IgM antibody for chikungunya was positive. Other investigations including platelet count, peripheral smear, total count, differential count, *Treponema pallidum* hemagglutination assay (TPHA), and HIV-1 and HIV-2 were negative. Spectral-domain optical coherence tomography (SD-OCT) revealed the presence of posterior vitreous cells and hyperreflective area in the inner retina with after shadowing corresponding to the area of retinitis (**Fig. 107.2**).

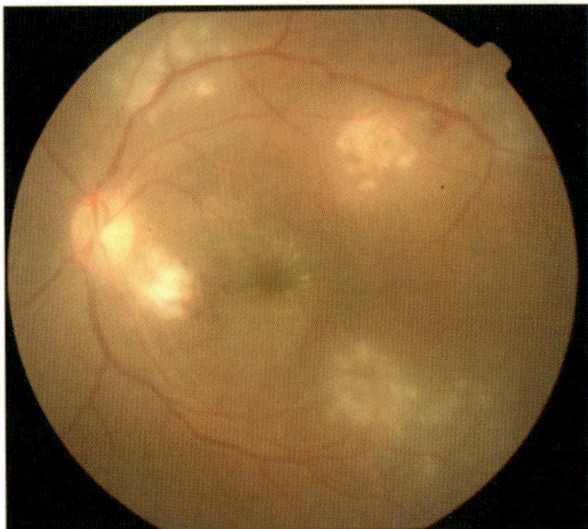

Fig. 107.1 Color fundus photograph of the left eye showing hyperemic disc, area of retinitis inferotemporal to the disc with confluent areas of whitening, especially along arcades associated with superficial hemorrhage and macular star.

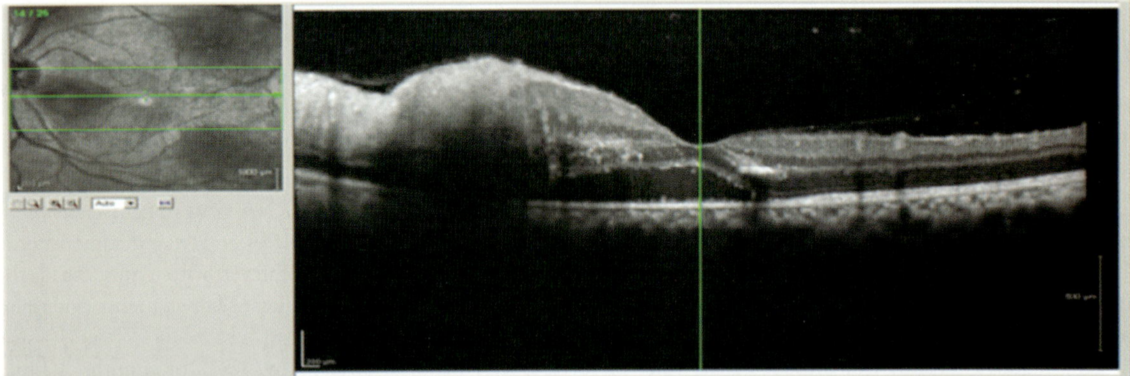

Fig. 107.2 SD-OCT (*horizontal line scan*) revealed presence of posterior vitreous cells, hyperreflective area in the inner retina with aftershadowing corresponding to area of retinitis, hyperreflective dots suggestive of hard exudates with fluid-filled spaces in the outer retina.

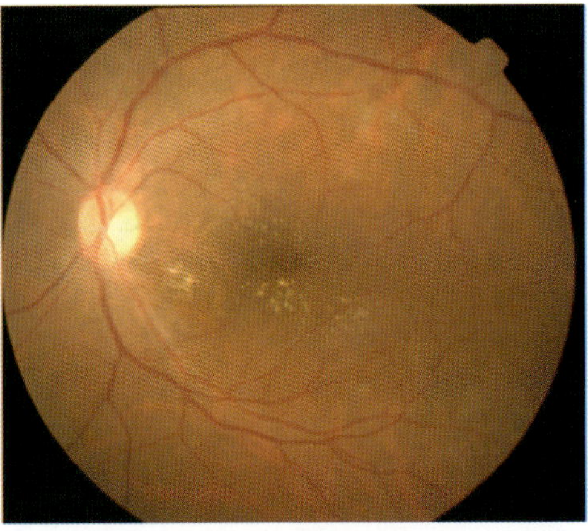

Fig. 107.3 Follow-up color fundus photograph showing resolved retinitis with resolving macular star in the left eye.

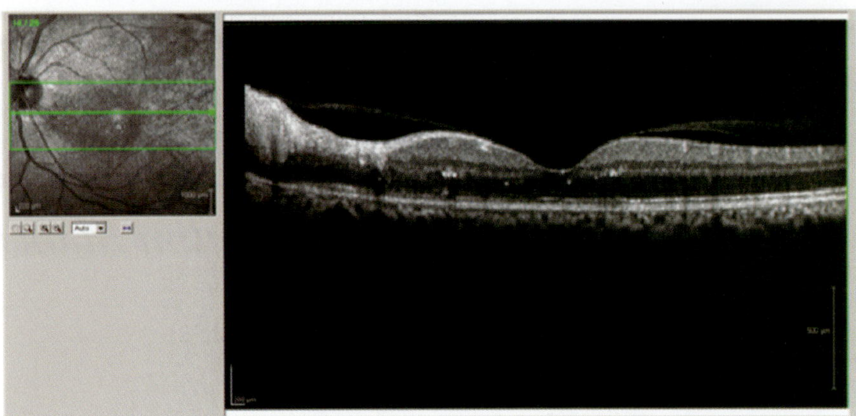

Fig. 107.4 SD-OCT follow-up scan revealed partial posterior vitreous detachment and healed retinitis with few hyper-reflective echoes in retina suggestive of resolving macular star.

Patient was treated with topical prednisolone acetate, homatropine, and oral prednisolone acetate 40 mg/day; and it was tapered over a period of 6 weeks along with oral calcium supplements and tablet ranitidine.

Follow-up after 6 weeks revealed BCVA of 6/6, N6 in the left eye. Anterior segment was quiet. The fundus examination revealed occasional vitreous cells with resolved retinitis, sclerosis of the retinal vessel along with the resolving macular star (**Fig. 107.3**).

The SD-OCT follow-up scan revealed partial posterior vitreous detachment, healed retinitis with a few hyper-reflective echoes in the inner plexiform layer suggestive of resolving macular star (**Fig. 107.4**).

FURTHER READING

1. Mahendradas P, Ranganna SK, Shetty R, et al.: Ocular manifestations associated with chikungunya. *Ophthalmology* 115(2): 287–291, 2008.
2. Mittal A, Mittal S, Bharati MJ, et al.: Optic neuritis associated with chikungunya virus infection in South India. *Arch Ophthalmol* 125(10):1381–1386, 2007.
3. Lalitha P, Rathinam S, Banushree K, et al.: Ocular involvement associated with an epidemic outbreak of chikungunya virus infection. *Am J Ophthalmol* 144(4):552–556, 2007.
4. Murthy KR, Venkataraman N, Satish V, et al.: Bilateral retinitis following chikungunya fever. *Indian J Ophthalmol* 56(4): 329–331, 2008.
5. Mahesh G, Giridhar A, Shedbele A, et al.: A case of bilateral presumed chikungunya neuroretinitis. *Indian J Ophthalmol* 57(2):148–150, 2009.
6. Khairallah M, Chee SP, Rathinam SR, et al.: Novel infectious agents causing uveitis. *Int Ophthalmol* 30(5):465–483, 2010.

Chorioretinal Folds

Kavitha Avadhani and Padmamalini Mahendradas

Chorioretinal folds or folds in the inner choroid, Bruch's membrane, retinal pigment epithelium (RPE), and retina are produced due to compression of the sclera. These may be idiopathic (often bilateral and symmetric) or may be secondary to inflammation, hypotony, tumors, papilledema, etc. Retinal folds (without any choroidal involvement) maybe seen in epiretinal membranes, optic disc edema (Paton's lines), etc. These folds (except idiopathic ones) resolve with treatment of the underlying disease.

CASE STUDY 1

A 26-year-old Asian Indian female presented with complaints of metamorphopsia and pain in both eyes. Best-corrected visual acuity was 20/30 in both the eyes. Anterior segment examination of the right eye was normal, while left eye showed fine keratic precipitates, cells 1+, and flare 1+. Fundus examination showed vitritis+ with disc edema and subtle retinal folds in both the eyes (Fig. 108.1A). Fluorescein angiography (FA) only showed disc hyperfluorescence (Fig. 108.1B). The folds did not appear on angiogram.

Spectral-domain optical coherence tomography (SD-OCT) clearly demonstrated the inner retina that was thrown into folds (Fig. 108.1C), in fact showing more folds than were even visible clinically. (*These multiple folds were secondary to the disc edema and most probably accounted for the metamorphopsia the patient was experiencing.*) The patient was treated with systemic steroids after baseline investigations. The disc edema and associated retinal folds resolved (Fig. 108.1D) with the treatment.

CASE STUDY 2

A 52-year-old patient was seen in the outpatient department, where she presented for a routine eye examination. The patient had no systemic illness. Her best-corrected visual activity was 20/20, N6 in both the eyes. Intraocular pressure was 12 mmHg in both the eyes. Anterior segment examination was normal in both the eyes. Fundus examination showed multiple choroidal folds (Fig. 108.2A) in both the eyes. There was no evidence of active ocular inflammation. She was diagnosed to have idiopathic choroidal folds in both the eyes. The SD-OCT showed the folds clearly without any subretinal/intraretinal fluid and a normal choroidal thickness (Fig. 108.2B).

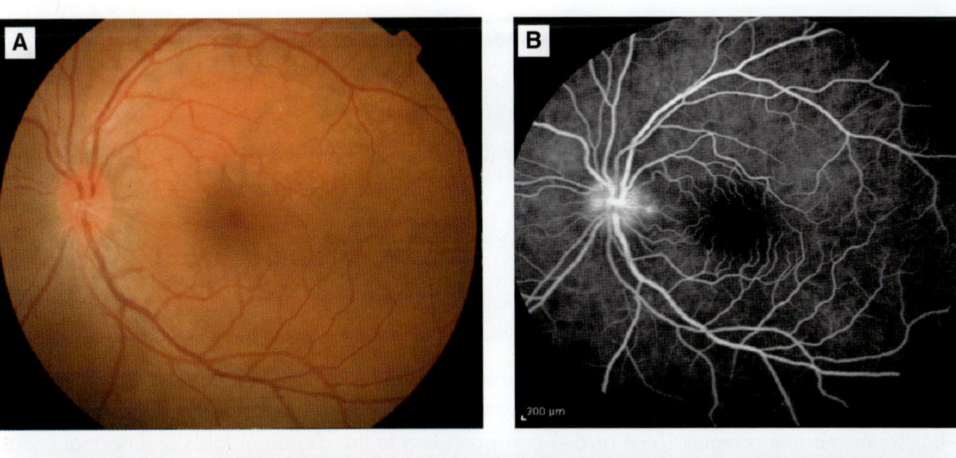

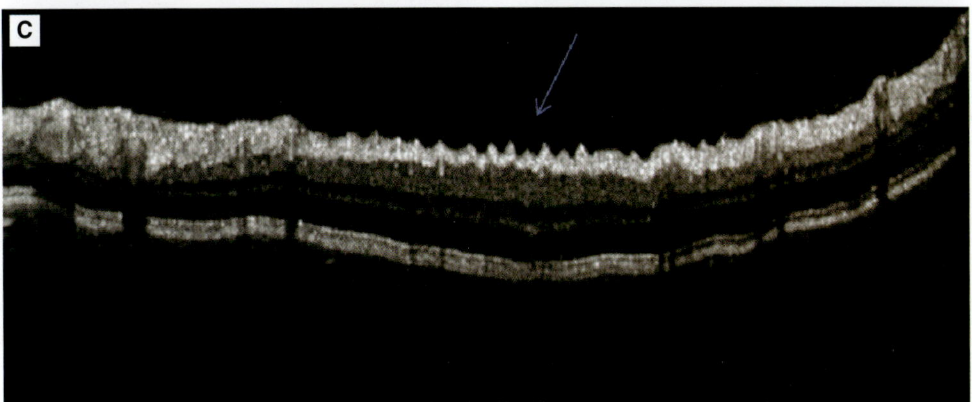

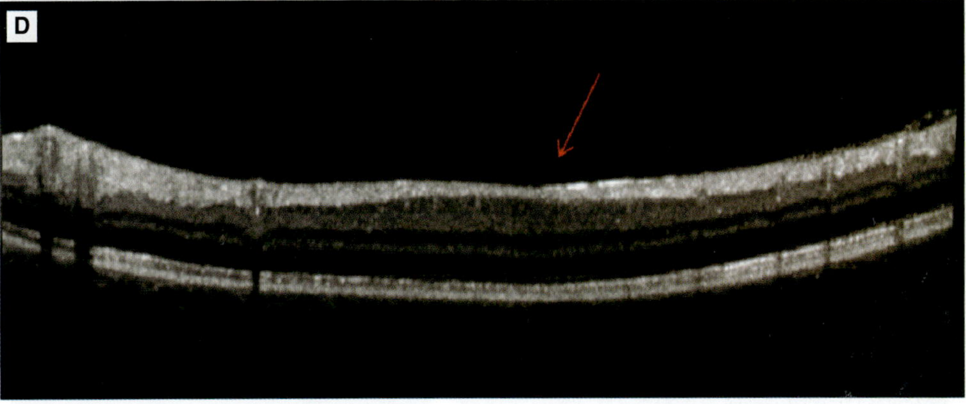

Fig. 108.1 **(A)** The left eye fundus photograph of a 26-year-old female showing blurring of disc margins with subtle retinal folds. **(B)** Fluorescein angiogram of the left eye demonstrating hyperfluorescence of optic disc in the left eye. **(C)** SD-OCT of the left eye (*vertical scan*) shows inner retina thrown into multiple folds (*blue arrow*). Other retinal layers and choroid appear normal. **(D)** The SD-OCT scan of the same area as in **(C)** following treatment shows resolution of these folds (*red arrow*).

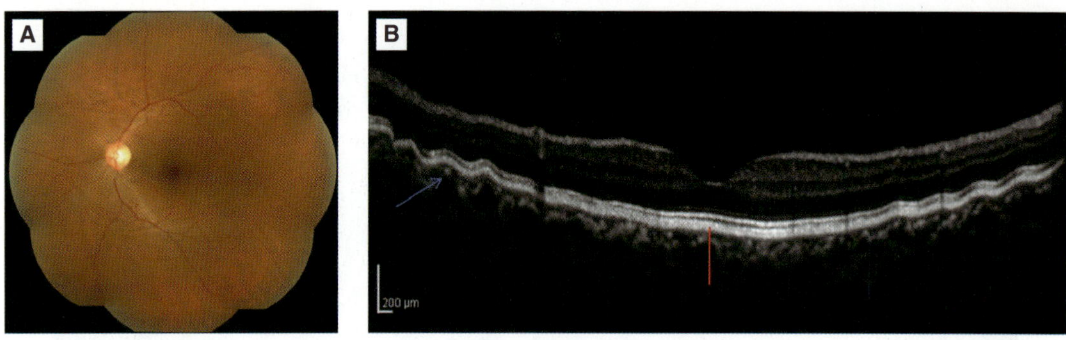

Fig. 108.2 (A) The left eye montage fundus photograph of a 52-year-old female showing multiple dark lines suggestive of choroidal folds. **(B)** SD-OCT of the left eye (*vertical scan*) shows multiple undulations in the retinal pigment epithelium–Bruch's membrane complex (*blue arrow*) corresponding to the choroidal folds and normal choroidal thickness (*red line*).

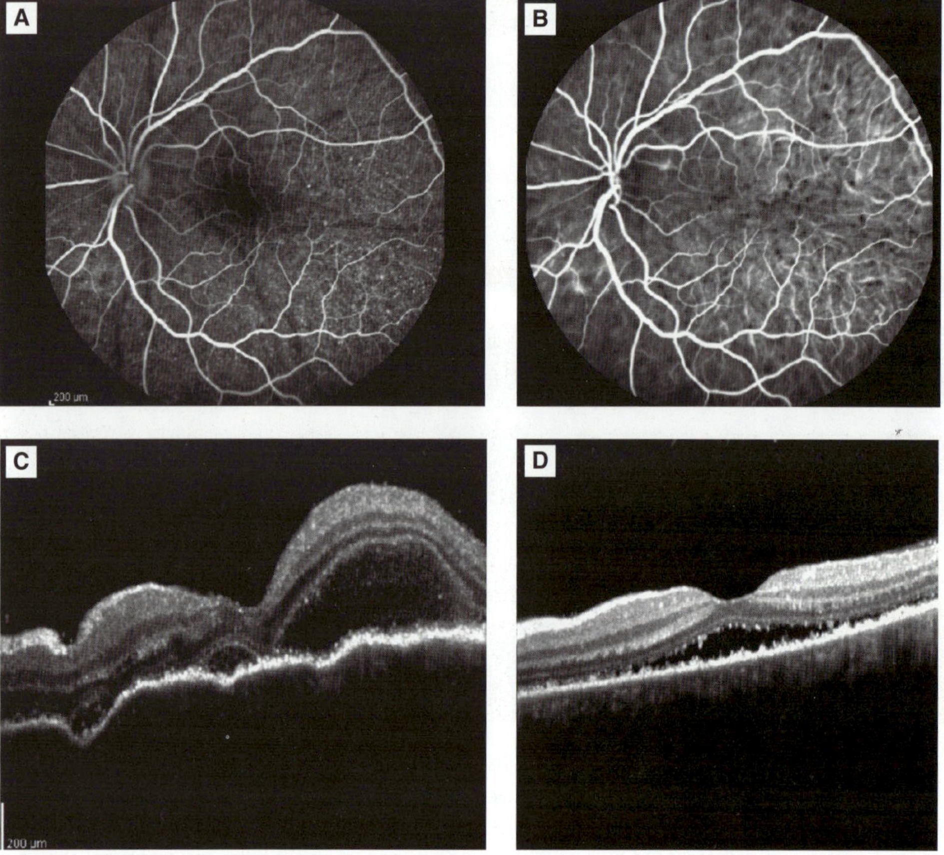

Fig. 108.3 (A) The left eye fluorescein angiogram (*early phase*) of a 45-year-old female showing dark lines radiating outwards from the disc suggestive of choroidal folds. **(B)** Indocyanine green angiogram of the left eye demonstrating multiple hypofluorescent areas corresponding to areas of active choroidal inflammation. The folds are only seen as faint dark lines. **(C)** SD-OCT of the left eye (vertical scan) shows retinal edema and subretinal fluid accumulation along with undulations in the RPE–Bruch's membrane complex (*choroidal folds*). **(D)** Repeat SD-OCT after systemic steroid therapy shows complete resolution of the choroidal folds and resolving subretinal fluid.

CASE STUDY 3

A 45-year-old Asian Indian female presented with complaints of headache and bilateral decrease in vision (counting fingers in right eye and 20/200 in left eye). The fundus examination showed vitritis++, exudative retinal detachment, and multiple alternating light and dark bands suggestive of chorioretinal folds in both the eyes. On FA (**Fig. 108.3A**), the folds were seen as alternating bands of hyper- (at peaks of the folds) and hypofluorescence (in troughs of the folds). In addition to this, pinpoint hyperfluorescence with late leakage of dye was seen suggestive of Vogt–Koyanagi–Harada (VKH) disease. On the indocyanine green angiography (**Fig. 108.3B**), multiple hypofluorescent areas were seen while the folds were not as clearly visible as seen on FA.

The SD-OCT (**Figs 108.3C and D**) showed both hollows and bulges of the folds very clearly *(These are particularly clear when scans are performed perpendicular to the folds.).* Other changes seen in active VKH such as subretinal fluid, as well as retinal and choroidal thickening were also observed on optical coherence tomography (OCT).

In some very early cases of VKH (**Fig. 108.4A**), chorioretinal folds may be the only clinical sign of VKH without any other classical signs such as exudative detachments, disc edema, etc. The SD-OCT in these cases demonstrates the folds very clearly (**Fig. 108.4B**) and also shows increased choroidal thickness noted in the patients with VKH disease. These signs resolve well with systemic steroid therapy (**Figs 108.4C and D**).

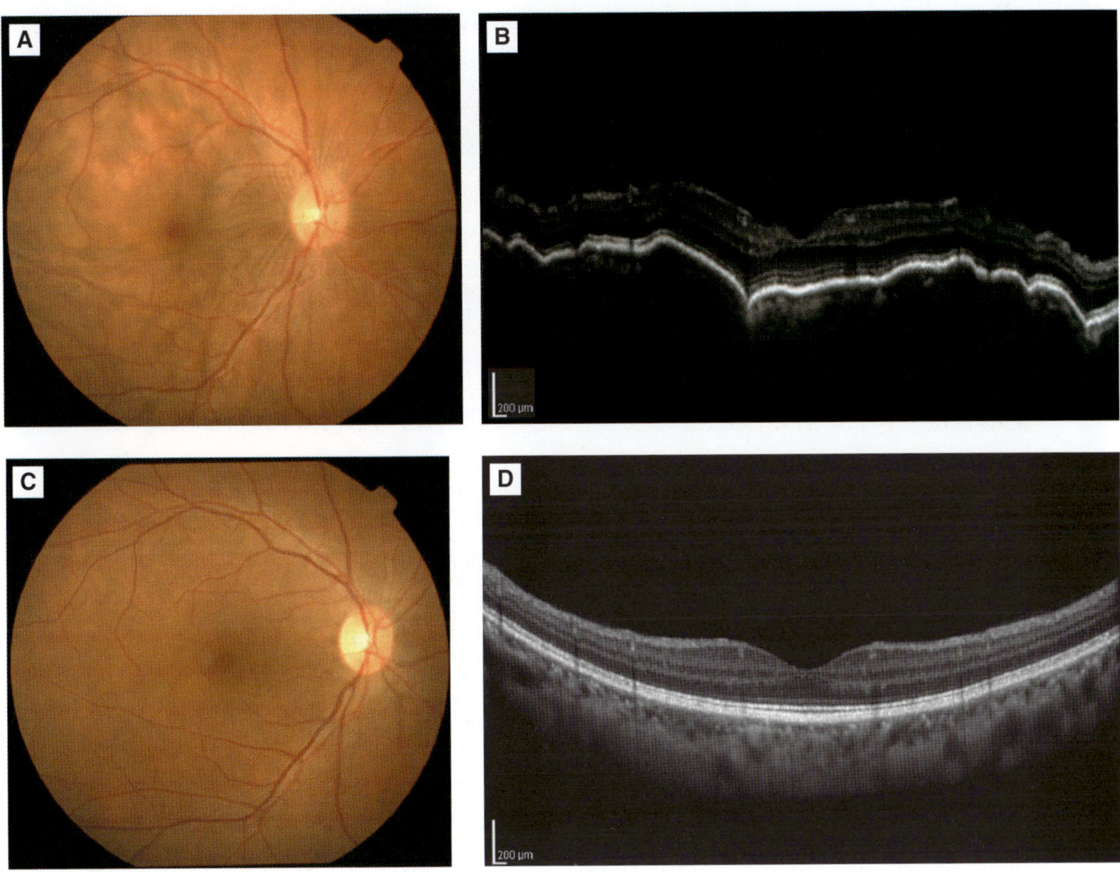

Fig. 108.4 A 40-year-old female with headache and blurred vision was diagnosed with bilateral panuveitis (VKH). **(A)** The right eye fundus photograph showing multiple chorioretinal folds. **(B)** SD-OCT of the right eye showed multiple undulations of both retina and the RPE–Bruch's membrane complex suggestive of chorioretinal folds. Increased choroidal thickness was also observed on OCT. **(C)** Fundus photograph of the right eye showing complete resolution of the folds after systemic steroid therapy. **(D)** Repeat SD-OCT following treatment through the same area showing normal retinal and choroidal architecture.

FURTHER READING

1. Wu W, Wen F, Huang S, et al.: Choroidal folds in Vogt-Koyanagi-Harada disease. *Am J Ophthalmol* 143(5):900–901, 2007.
2. Giuffrè G, Distefano MG: Optical coherence tomography of chorioretinal and choroidal folds. *Acta Ophthalmol Scand* 85(3):333–336, 2007.
3. Fine HF, Cunningham ET, Kim E, et al.: Autofluorescence imaging findings in long-standing chorioretinal folds. *Retin Cases Brief Rep* 3(2):137–139, 2009.
4. Zhao C, Zhang M, Wen X, et al.: Choroidal folds in acute Vogt-Koyanagi-Harada disease. *Ocul Immunol Inflamm* 17(4):282–288, 2009.

Choroidal Granuloma

Padmamalini Mahendradas and Kavitha Avadhani

Choroidal granulomas can occur in various granulomatous inflammations of the eye, which are seen as elevated yellowish-white subretinal masses with fuzzy, ill-defined margins. A choroidal granuloma may be suspected to be inflammatory, infective, or neoplastic.

CASE STUDY 1

A 34-year-old male presented with complaints of blurring of vision in left eye. He gave history of abdominal Koch's on treatment with antituberculosis treatment (ATT). He was also diagnosed to have multifocal choroiditis on treatment with systemic steroids in addition to the ATT.

On examination his best-corrected visual acuity (BCVA) was 6/6, N6 in the right eye, 6/9, N6 in the left eye. The examination of the right eye was normal. Examination of the left eye revealed traces of anterior vitreous cells, healing multifocal choroiditis lesions with a hypopigmented subretinal yellowish lesion inferotemporal to macula, suggestive of the choroidal granuloma (Fig. 109.1 A–F).

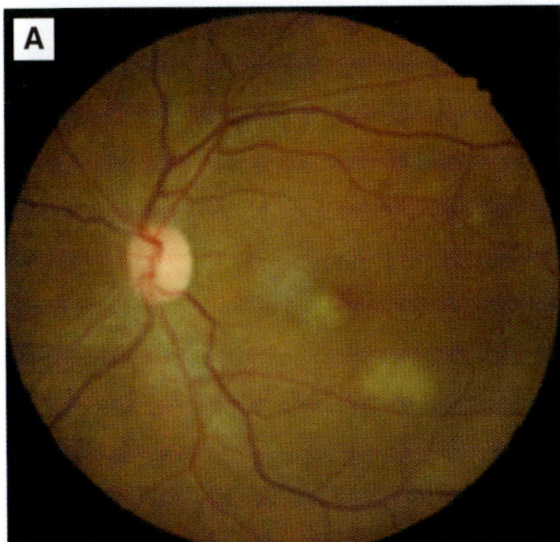
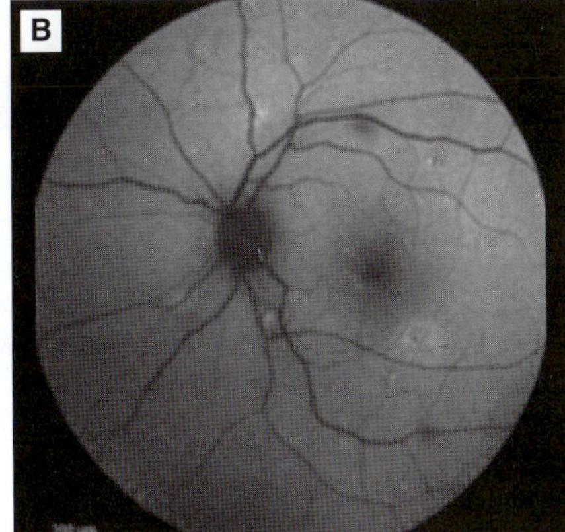

Fig. 109.1 (A) A color fundus photograph reveals multiple healing choroiditis lesions with a well-defined yellowish-white subretinal lesion inferotemporal to macula, suggestive of choroidal granuloma. **(B)** Autofluorescence imaging shows area of mottled hypo- with hyperautofluorescence in the area of the choroidal granuloma.

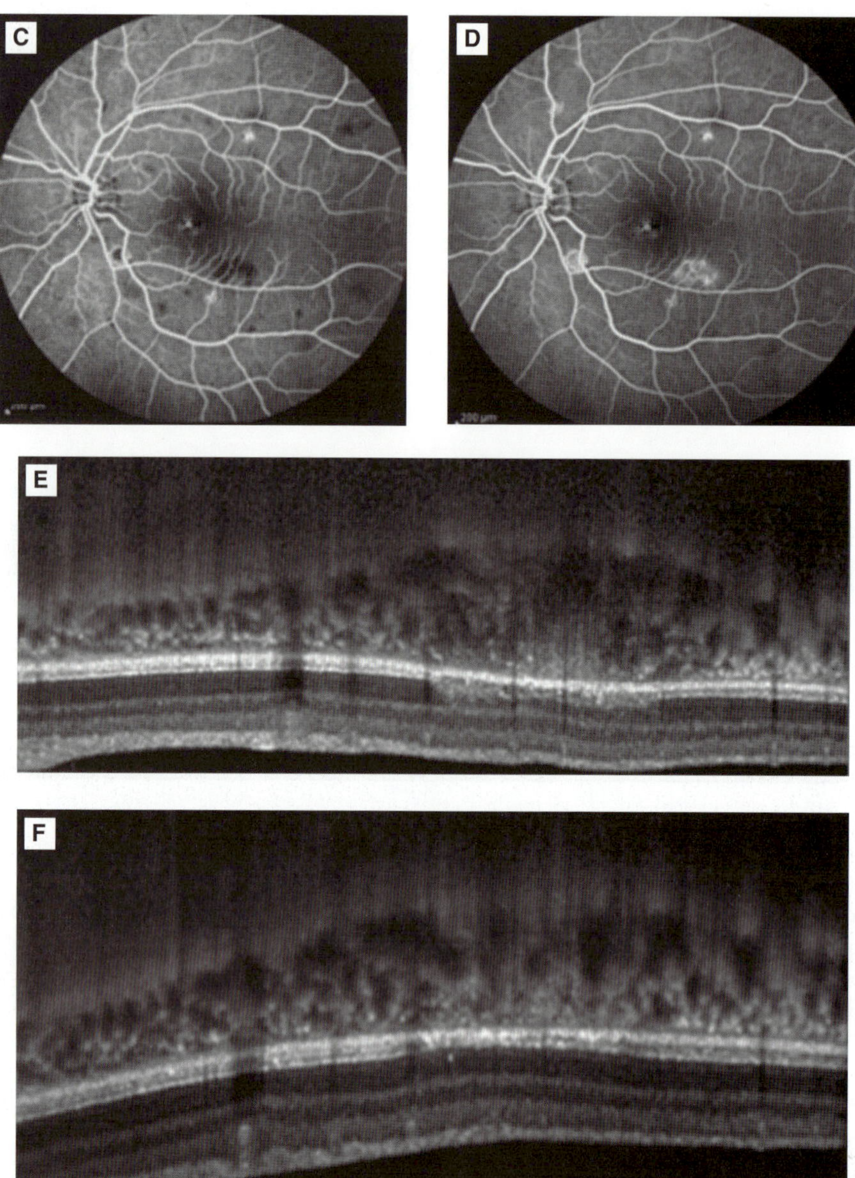

Fig. 109.1 (C) Fundus fluorescein angiography reveals early hypofluorescence with late hyperfluorescence **(D)** of choroidal granuloma in the left eye. **(E)** Spectral-domain optical coherence tomography (SD-OCT)–enhanced depth imaging (EDI) of the choroid revealed hyporeflective choroidal lesion with increased choroidal thickness associated with destruction of IS–OS junction with infiltrates in the outer retina and choroid. **(F)** Repeat SD-OCT with ATT and systemic steroid therapy shows that there is a decrease in size of the hyporeflective lesion with decrease in choroidal thickness.

CASE STUDY 2

A 58-year-old female presented with decreased vision in the left eye. She was diagnosed to have retinochoroiditis (**Fig. 109.2 A–G**) with inferior snowball opacities in the eye, suggestive of posterior uveitis. On investigation, Mantoux was 14 mm, and Toxoplasma IgG +ve. Anterior chamber paracentesis was done. Polymerase chain reaction

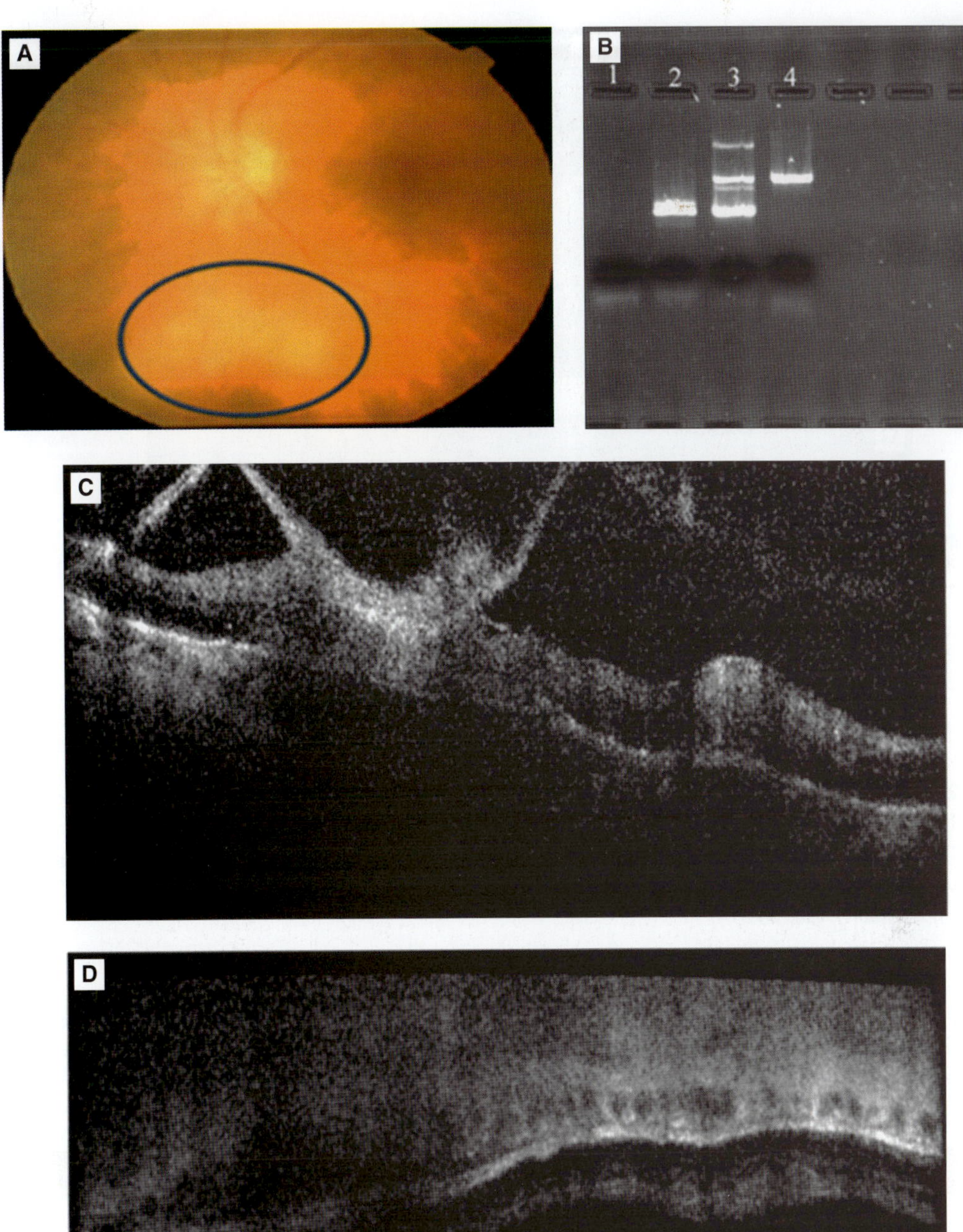

Fig. 109.2 **(A)** The left eye color fundus photograph shows grade 2 media haze, hyperemic disc, yellowish-white, ill-defined retinochoroiditis lesion. **(B)** PCR for panfungal genome was positive from aqueous humor. (Lane 1: Negative control, Lane 2: Patient J, Lane 3: Second round positive control, Lane 4: First round positive control.) **(C)** SD-OCT shows presence of vitreous membranes, hyperreflective retinal lesion with ill-defined hyporeflective choroidal lesion. **(D)** SD-OCT-EDI (enhanced depth imaging) scan shows the presence of a well-delineated hyporeflective lesion suggestive of choroidal granuloma.

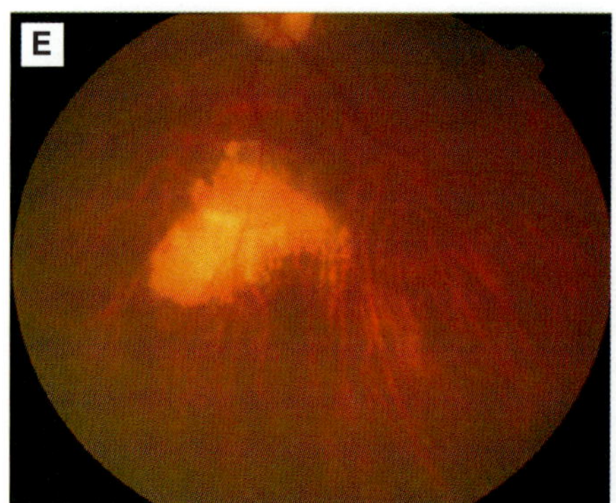

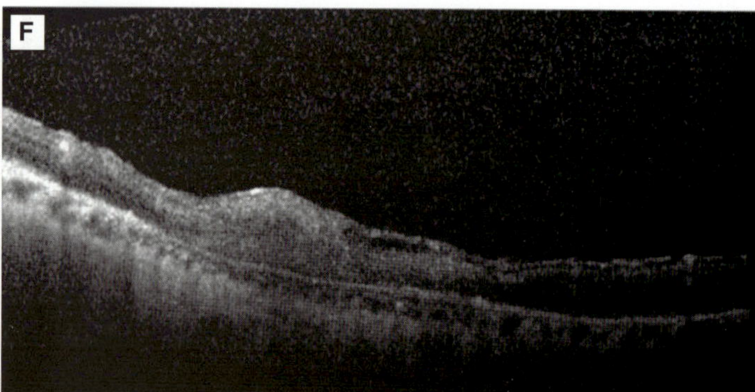

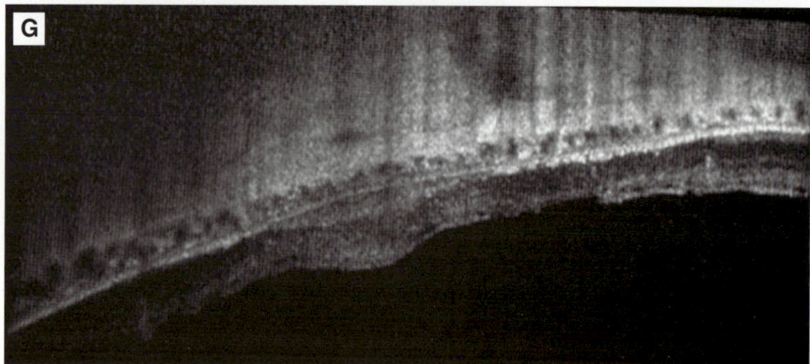

Fig. 109.2 (E) The left eye color fundus photograph shows healed choroidal granuloma. **(F)** SD-OCT shows presence of epiretinal membrane with hyperreflective echoes in the retina and choroid, suggestive of healed retinochoroiditis. **(G)** SD-OCT–EDI post-treatment scan shows hyperreflectivity in the retina and choroid with disappearance of the hyporeflective lesion in the choroid seen in Figure 109.2D suggestive of a healed lesion (Photo courtesy: *Ocul Immunol Inflamm* 18(5):408–410, Oct 2010.)

(PCR) for *Mycobacterium tuberculosis* was negative while that for panfungal genome was positive. She was treated with systemic antifungal oral fluconazole and intravitreal voriconazole injections. Follow-up after 2 weeks showed resolution of inflammation in the left eye.

CASE STUDY 3

A 56-year-old female presented with discomfort in both the eyes. On examination, her best-corrected visual acuity (BCVA) was 6/9. Slit lamp biomicroscopic examination revealed the presence of mutton fat keratic precipitates in both the eyes with multiple hypopigmented ill-defined lesions in the choroid suggestive of choroidal granuloma. On investigation, the Mantoux test was negative, chest X-ray revealed bilateral hilar lymph adenopathy, serum ACE level was 65 U/L. Clinically, the patient was diagnosed to have bilateral granulomatous panuveitis due to sarcoidosis. She was started on oral prednisolone acetate 40 mg/day, topical prednisolone, homatropine, along with immunosuppressive therapy (tab. methotrexate). Follow-up examination after 6 weeks revealed, BCVA of 6/5 in both the eyes, normal intraocular pressure, with resolution of anterior segment inflammation and resolving choroidal granuloma in both the eyes (**Fig. 109.3 A–T**).

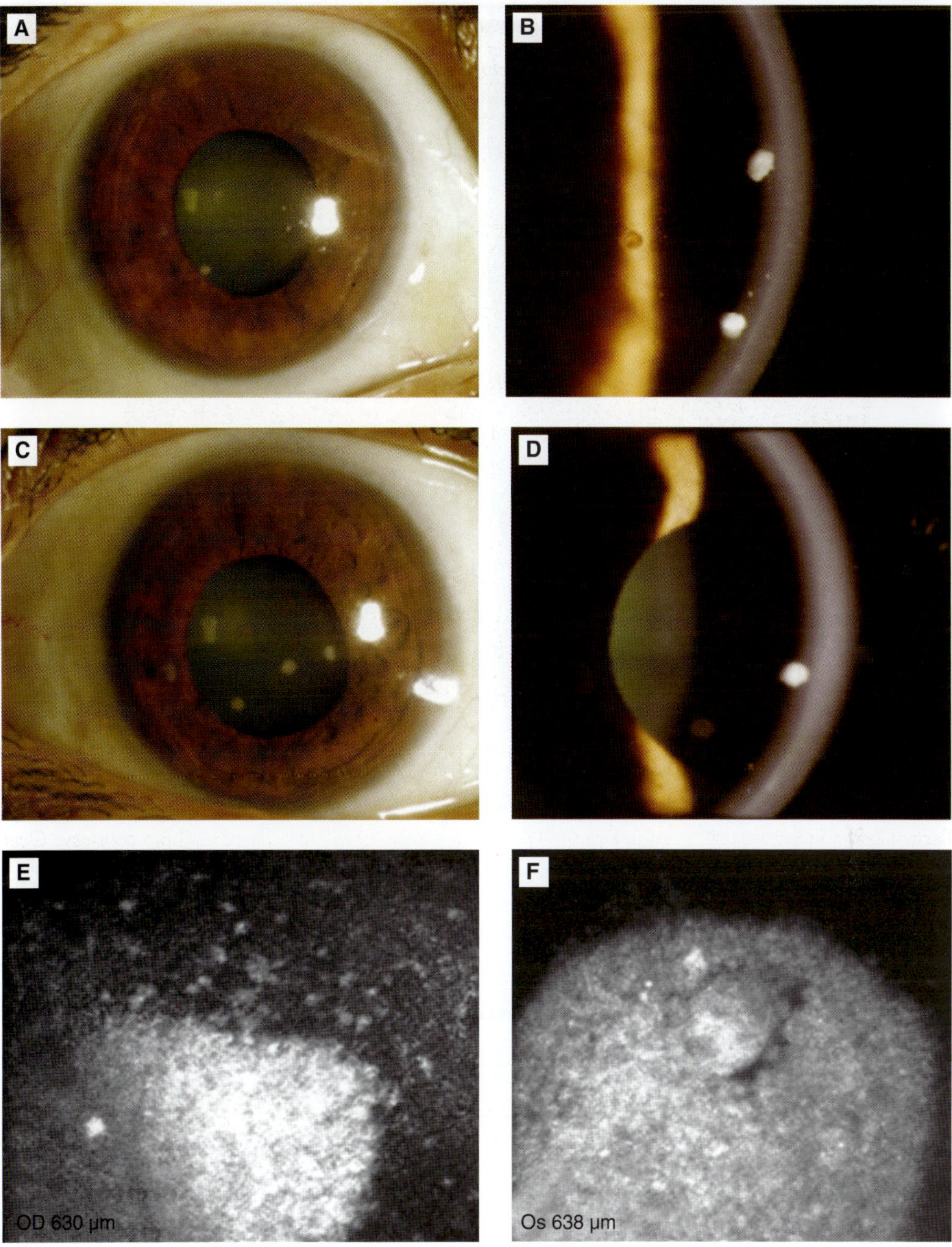

Fig. 109.3 Slit lamp anterior segment photograph shows the presence of mutton-fat keratic precipitates in the right **(A and B)** and left eye **(C and D)**. Confocal microscopy reveals globular pattern of keratic precipitate on endothelium in the right **(E)** and left eyes **(F)**.

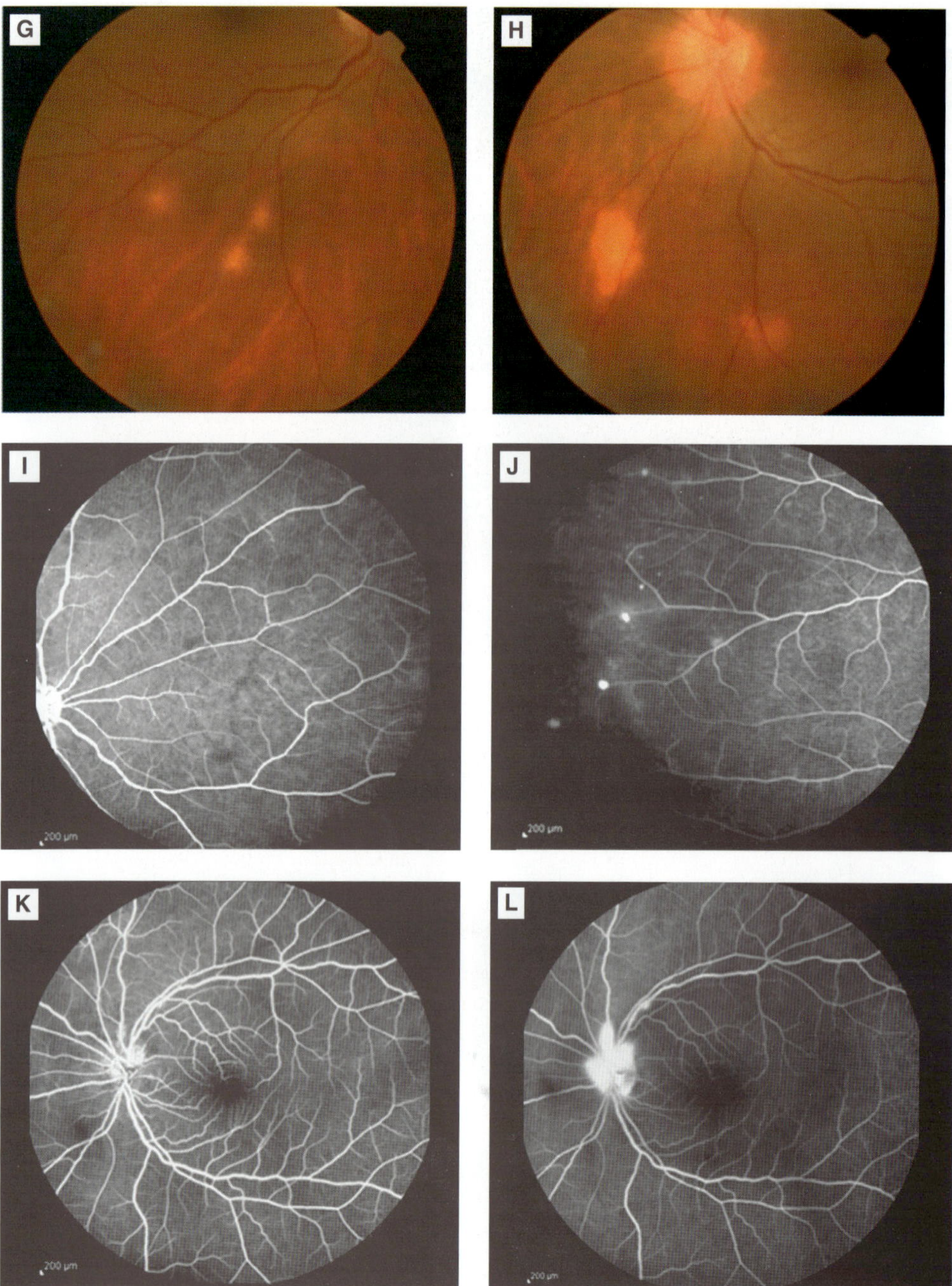

Fig. 109.3 Color fundus photographs show the presence of hypopigmented multiple choroidal granuloma in both the eyes **(G and H)**. Fundus fluorescein angiography shows early hypofluorescence **(I)** suggestive of choroidal granuloma, with staining and leakage from temporal retinal peripheral vessels with capillary nonperfusion areas **(J)** in the right eye. The left eye FFA shows early hypofluorescence **(K)**, which changes into isofluorescence in late phase with disc leak and staining of vessels **(L)**.

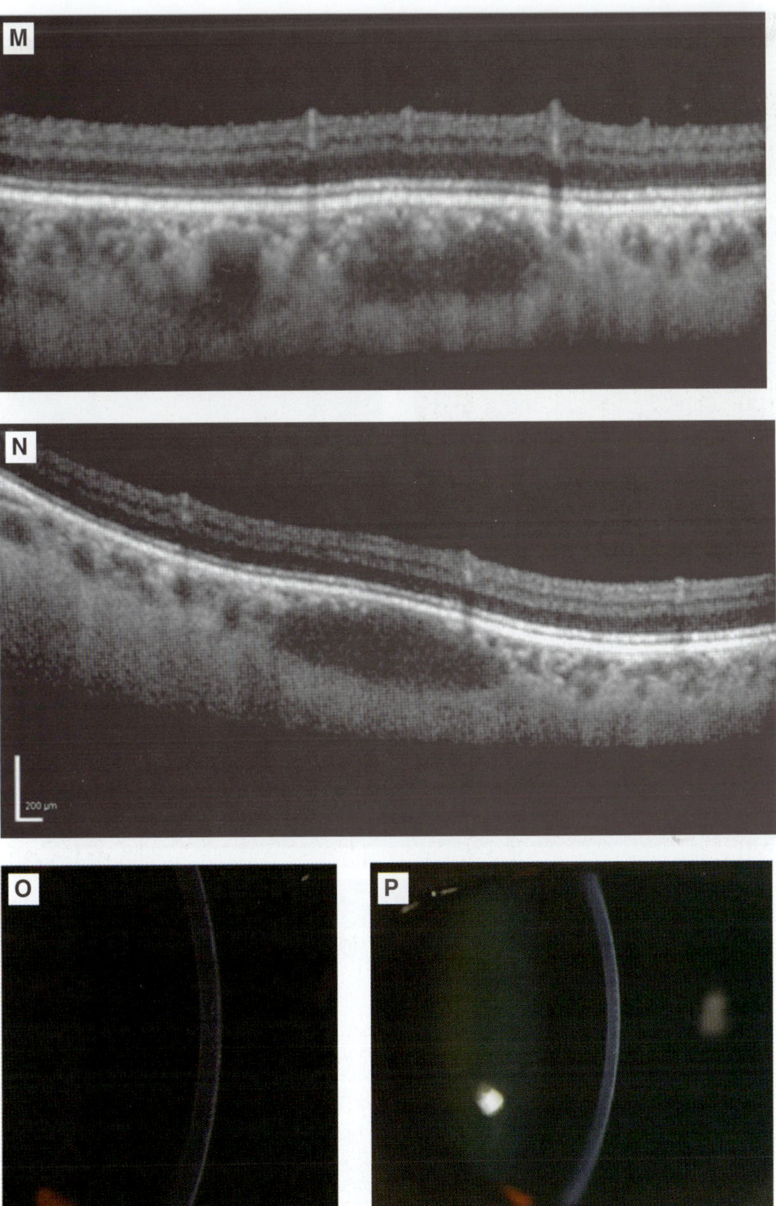

Fig. 109.3 SD-OCT–EDI scan shows the presence of hyporeflective lesion in the choroid suggestive of choroidal granuloma. **(M)** in the right eye and **(N)** in the left eye. Following treatment with topical and systemic steroids and immunosuppressive therapy with oral methotrexate resolution of anterior segment inflammation is seen **(O and P)**.

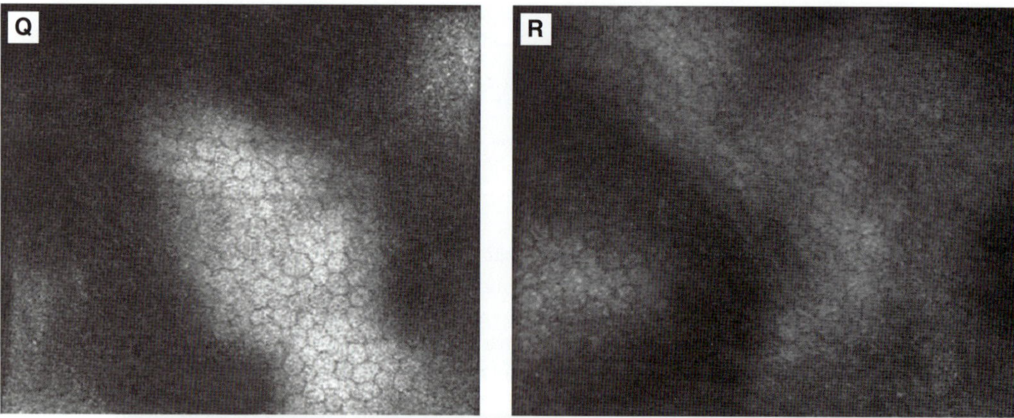

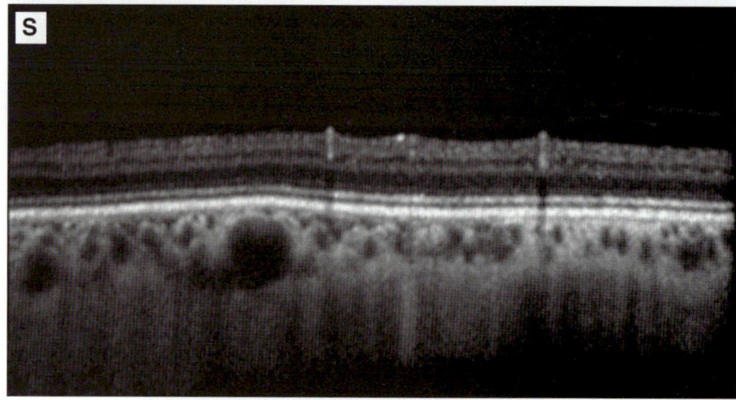

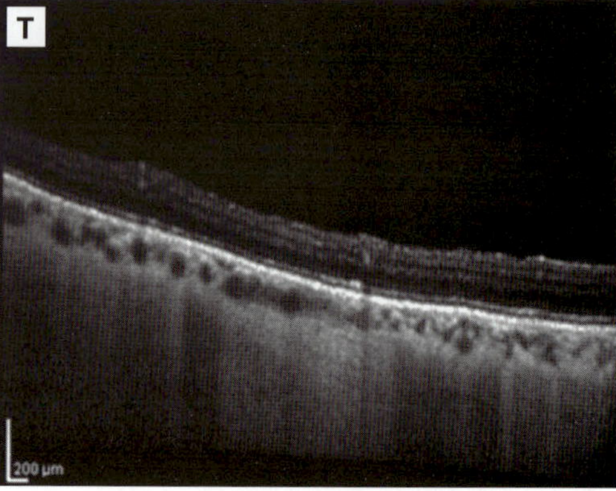

Fig. 109.3 Confocal microscopy showed normal endothelium following treatment. **(Q and R)** SD-OCT EDI also showed healing choroidal granuloma **(S)** in the right eye and **(T)** in the left eye.

FURTHER READING

1. Desai UR, Tawansy KA, Joondeph BC, et al.: Choroidal granulomas in systemic sarcoidosis. *Retina* 21:40–47, 2001.
2. Yanoff M, Sassani JW: Granulomatous inflammation. In: Ocular Pathology, ed 6, Mosby Elsevier, China, 73–103, 2009.
3. Mahendradas P, Avadhani K, Yadav NK, et al.: Role of Spectralis HRA + OCT spectral domain optical coherence tomography in the diagnosis and management of fungal choroidal granuloma. *Ocul Immunol Inflamm* 18(5):408–410, 2010.
4. Salman A, Parmar P, Rajamohan M, et al.: Optical coherence tomography in choroidal tuberculosis. *Am J Ophthalmol* 142(1):170–172, 2006.
5. Marcus DF, Bovino JA, Burton TC: Sarcoid granuloma of the choroid. *Ophthalmology* 89(12):1326–1330, 1982.
6. van der Vaart R, Greven C, Manning R, et al.: Unilateral solitary choroidal granuloma as presenting sign of secondary syphilis. *Graefes Arch Clin Exp Ophthalmol* 249(10):1575–1577, 2011.

Cytomegalovirus Retinitis

Kavitha Avadhani and Padmamalini Mahendradas

Cytomegalovirus (CMV) infection of the retina or CMV retinitis is seen primarily as an opportunistic infection in immunosuppressed persons (either in those who are on lifelong immunosuppression following transplant or in those with HIV infection). The risk of infection increases significantly once the CD4 count drops to below 50 cells/µl. Two clinical presentations are commonly encountered: the classical "Pizza Pie" retinitis with white fluffy retinal lesions associated with hemorrhages and "granular" form with fewer hemorrhages. Vision is affected only in cases affecting the disc or macula and in those who develop rhegmatogenous retinal detachment as a consequence of retinitis. Treatment consists of antiretroviral therapy (ART) combined with systemic and/or intravitreal ganciclovir.

CASE STUDY 1

A 38-year-old male, a known case of the HIV infection and not on ART, presented with blurring of vision in the right eye for past 2 days. His recent CD4 counts were173 cells/µl. His best-corrected visual acuity was 20/80 in the right eye. On examination, anterior segment in both the eyes was normal. Fundus examination of the right eye showed a deep yellowish-white granular lesion between the optic disc and macula (**Fig. 110.1A**). The left eye was normal. A diagnosis of granular CMV retinitis of the right eye was made.

Spectral-domain optical coherence tomography (SD-OCT) through the lesion revealed hyperreflectivity of inner retinal layers along with multiple cystic spaces, and disruption and loss of outer retinal layers (**Fig. 110.1B**).

CASE STUDY 2

A 65-year-old patient, a known case of HIV infection and on the ART, presented with some visual disturbance for the past 2 weeks. His best-corrected visual acuity was 20/20 in the both eyes. On examination, anterior segment was normal in both the eyes. The fundus examination of both the eyes showed perivascular fluffy yellow-white lesions along with associated hemorrhages in midperiphery (**Fig. 110.2A**). A diagnosis of bilateral CMV retinitis was made. The patient was started on systemic and intravitreal ganciclovir in addition to the ART. Most of the lesions appeared healed 6 weeks after the therapy (**Fig. 110.2B**).

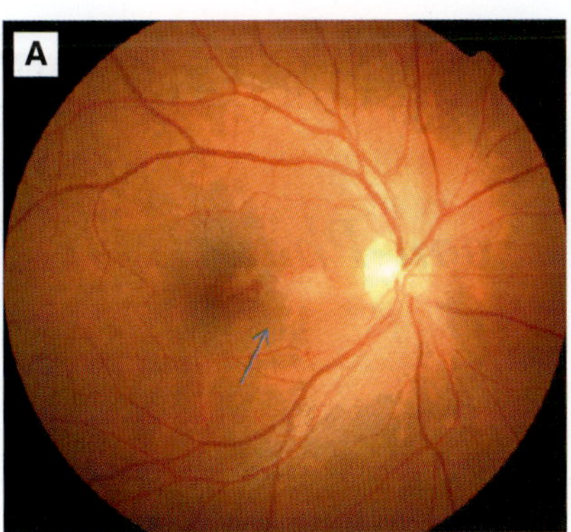 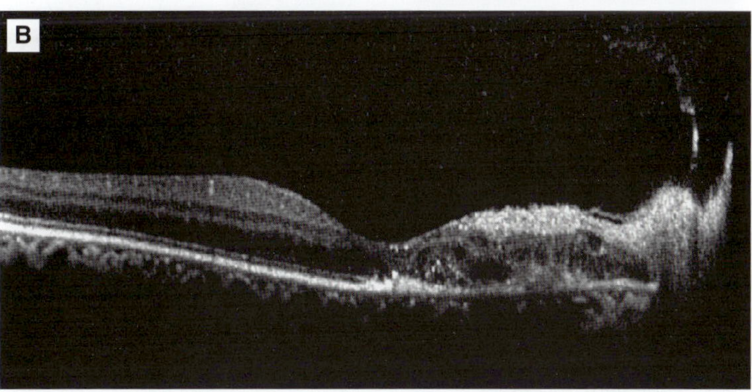

Fig. 110.1 (A) Fundus photograph of right eye of the patient in Case study 1 showing a granular-appearing yellow lesion (*blue arrow*) in the posterior pole. **(B)** SD-OCT through the same lesion showing hyperreflectivity in inner retinal layers, retinal edema with cystic spaces, and loss/disruption of outer retinal layers. A few posterior vitreous cells are also seen.

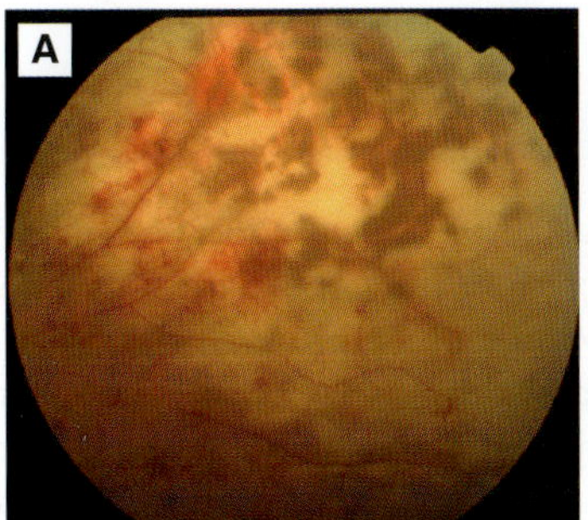 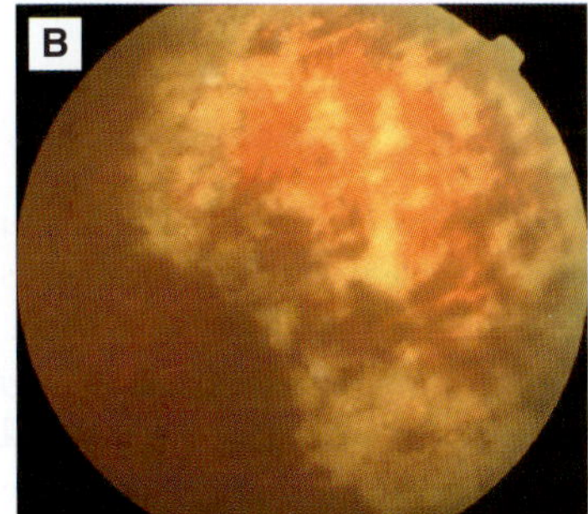 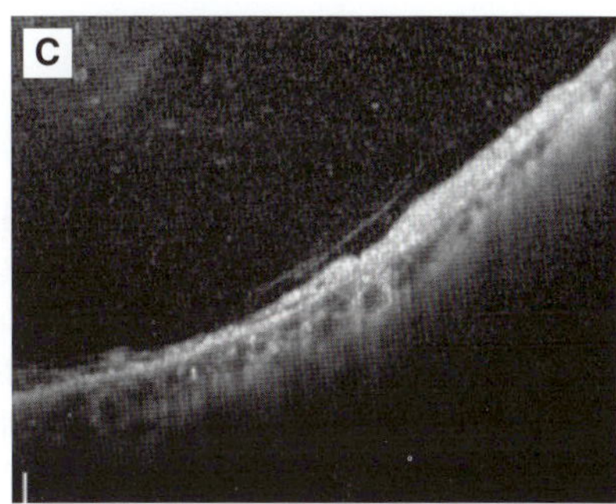

Fig. 110.2 (A) Fundus photograph of superotemporal midperiphery of the right eye of patient in Case study 2 at presentation showing multiple yellow-white lesions with associated hemorrhages. **(B)** Fundus photograph of same quadrant as in A, 6 weeks after treatment showing healed lesions and absence of hemorrhages. **(C)** SD-OCT of same area done after 6 weeks of treatment showing a few posterior vitreous cells, complete loss of retinal architecture, and a hyperreflective band of tissue corresponding to atrophic retina.

The SD-OCT done at this time showed complete destruction of all the retinal layers, with only a hyperreflective band remaining in its place representing atrophic retina (**Fig. 110.2C**) left behind after active retinitis had healed.

FURTHER READING

1. Friedman AH, Orellana J, Freeman WR, et al.: Cytomegalovirus retinitis: a manifestation of the acquired immune deficiency syndrome (AIDS). *Br J Ophthalmol* 67(6):372–380, 1983.
2. Murray HW: CMV retinitis. *Br Med J* 2(6043):1071, 1976.
3. Astle JN, Ellis PP: Ocular complications in renal transplant patients. *Ann Ophthalmol* 6(12):1269–1274, 1974.
4. Egbert PR, Pollard RB, Gallagher JG, et al.: Cytomegalovirus retinitis in immunosuppressed hosts. II. Ocular manifestations. *Ann Intern Med* 93:664–670, 1980.

Dengue Maculopathy

Aliza JAP and Soon-Phaik CHEE

Dengue fever, a mosquito-borne infection caused by *Flavivirus* family, is endemic in most continents with 2.5 billion people being at risk and up to 50 million people developing an infection every year. Its presentation includes subclinical infection, dengue fever, dengue hemorrhagic fever, or dengue shock syndrome.

Ocular complications of dengue fever involve primarily the posterior segment and include cotton-wool spots, foveolitis, retinal hemorrhages, retinal edema, vitritis, vasculitis, choriocapillaris and choroidal involvement, and optic neuropathy. Prevalence of dengue maculopathy varies with the prevalent serotype, ranging from no cases to 10%. The average interval from onset of fever to onset of ocular symptoms is 1 week (range 0–30 days). Management of patients with dengue maculopathy has been empirical, with corticosteroids being used on the presumption that it is secondary to an immune-mediated inflammation. The majority of patients regain good visual acuity (VA); however, permanent visual loss may occur in those who had severe occlusive disease.

ROLE OF IMAGING STUDIES IN DIAGNOSIS OF DENGUE MACULOPATHY

The diagnosis of the dengue maculopathy is based on the presence of clinical features of dengue fever, including a positive dengue IgM and the presence of fundus lesions that are not attributable to other conditions such as diabetes mellitus, occurring within 1 month of the onset of dengue fever.

Not a single imaging modality is superior to the others in the diagnosis of the dengue maculopathy. For example, optical coherence tomography (OCT) may be normal in symptomatic patients who have normal-appearing fundus; yet they have abnormalities on electroretinography. Furthermore, the OCT changes seen in the dengue maculopathy are variable, ranging from an increase in retinal thickness without apparent fluid accumulation to a collection of fluid (or as in Case study 2, of perhaps exudative material as well) in subretinal and/or deep retinal layers. Even in the eyes with similar clinical features, as in Case studies 2 and 3, who both had foveolitis, there may be some differences in the OCT. In Case study 2, in addition to the localized subretinal fluid, there was also surrounding deep intraretinal fluid.

Except for Case study 1, who had fairly large amount of fluid on the OCT, the fluorescein angiography (FA) in other cases was unremarkable, except for some small patches of hypoperfusion and mild leakage. Indocyanine green angiography (ICGA) was also unremarkable, except for diffuse choroidal leak in Case Study 5. Hence, although current imaging techniques such as the OCT have contributed to understanding of pathogenesis of the dengue maculopathy, there is still much that remains unknown and further research is required.

The diagnosis of the dengue fever in these patients was made based on typical clinical features and a positive dengue IgM. All the patients were Chinese and were females, except for Case study 3. The interval between the onset of the fever and the onset of the ocular symptoms ranged from 4–8 days.

CASE STUDY 1

A 32-year-old woman had bilateral central scotoma, causing a reduction of her VA to 6/120 in both eyes. Fundal examination (Fig. 111.1) showed bilateral macula edema with sheathing of vessels and small dot hemorrhages. She was treated with intravenous hydrocortisone for 1 week, followed by a tapering dose of oral prednisolone. Retinal changes resolved with mild retinal pigment epithelial changes with her VA returning back to 6/6 by 2 months.

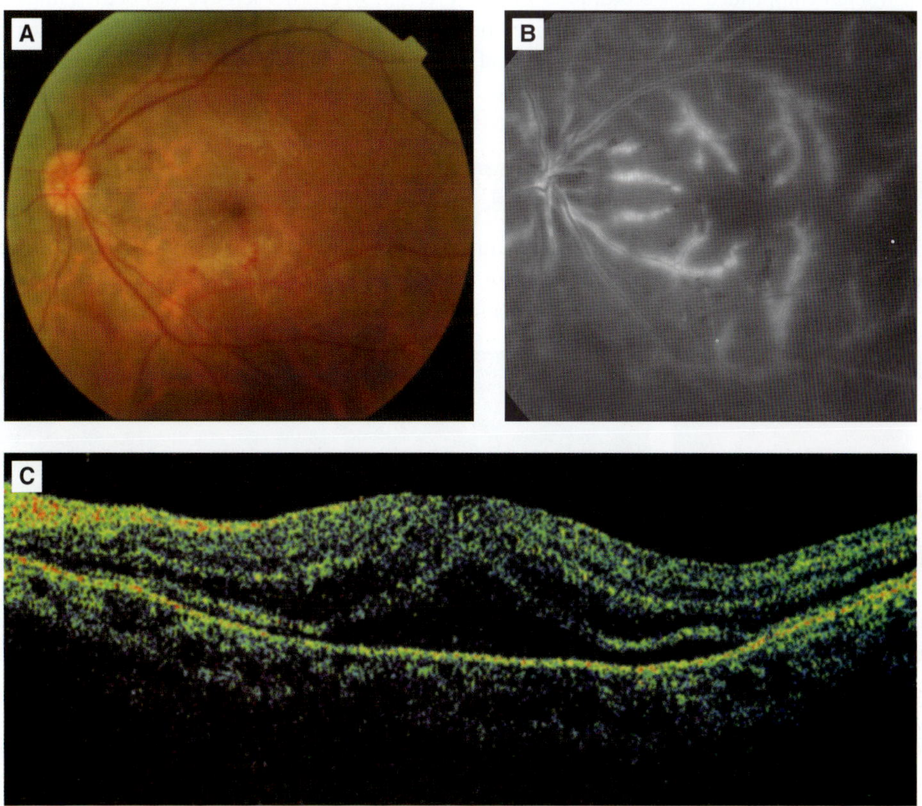

Fig. 111.1 Images of the left fundus obtained at onset of symptoms. **(A)** Color photograph showing macular edema with vasculitis and dot hemorrhages. **(B)** Fluorescein angiography at 3 minutes showing staining and mild leakage with areas of masking by retinal hemorrhages. **(C)** Optical coherence tomography showing localized subretinal and adjacent deep intraretinal fluid.

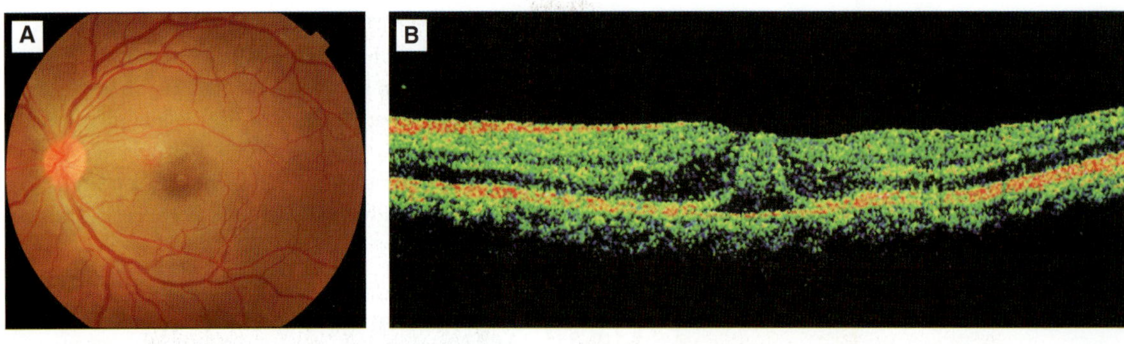

Fig. 111.2 Images of the left fundus obtained at onset of symptoms. **(A)** Color photograph showing a well-circumscribed round orange-yellow lesion at fovea (foveolitis) with flame-shaped hemorrhages and cotton-wool spots. **(B)** Optical coherence tomography showing disruption of photoreceptor layer at fovea with surrounding deep intraretinal edema. In addition to fluid, there is also a solid plaque-like lesion in subretinal space.

CASE STUDY 2

A 26-year-old woman complained of a scotoma in her left eye. The VA in her left eye was 6/21. Fundal examination (Fig. 111.2) of the left eye showed a small, well-defined orange-yellow lesion at fovea with retinal dot hemorrhages and cotton-wool spots. The FA shows scattered tiny areas of hypofluorescence around macula. The ICGA showed mild hypofluorescence.

CASE STUDY 3 (FIG. 111.3)

A 34-year-old patient had bilateral scotoma with counting fingers VA in both eyes. The FA and ICGA were unremarkable.

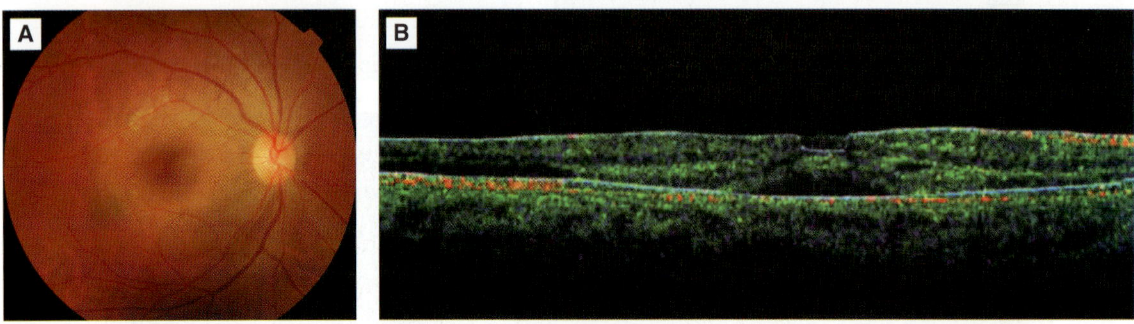

Fig. 111.3 Images of the right eye obtained 4 days after onset of symptoms. **(A)** Color photograph showing foveolitis. **(B)** Optical coherence tomography showing localized subretinal fluid.

CASE STUDY 4

A 25-year-old man noticed a scotoma in his left eye. Left VA was counting fingers at 0.5 meter and right VA was 6/12. There were 2+ cells in anterior chamber (AC) of both the eyes. Fundal examination (Fig. 111.4) showed bilateral vitritis, macula edema, and retinal hemorrhages. He was treated with intravenous methylprednisolone and oral prednisolone along with periocular steroids. His VA improved to 6/6 in both the eyes, with resolution of all the cellular activity and retinal signs.

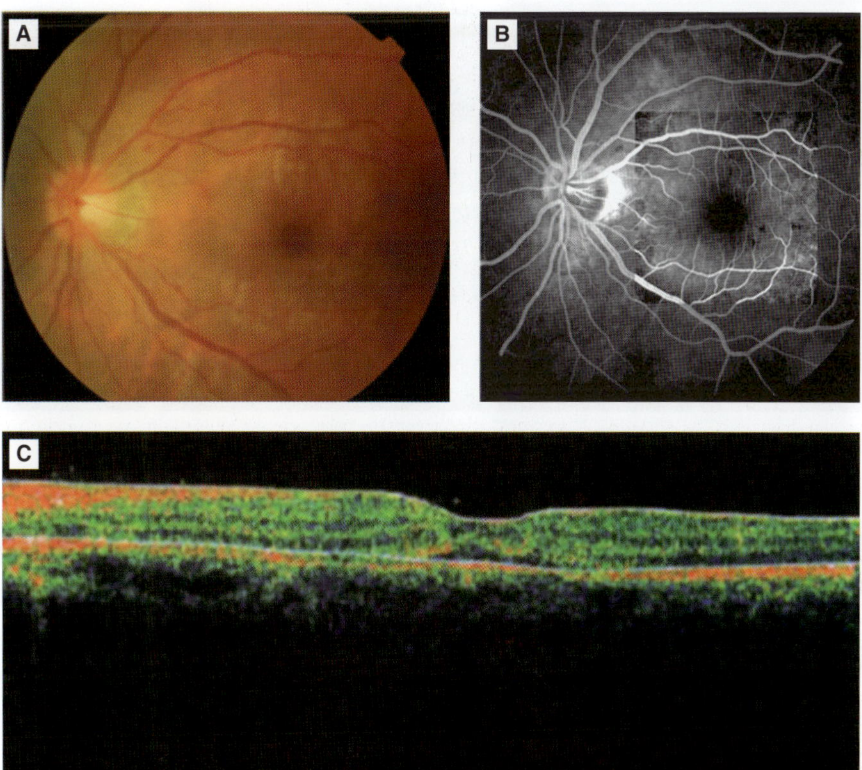

Fig. 111.4 Images of left fundus obtained 2 days after onset of symptoms. **(A)** Color photograph showing macular edema and one flame-shaped retinal hemorrhage. **(B)** Fluorescein angiography showing scattered tiny patches of hypoperfusion at macula with mild leakage. **(C)** Optical coherence tomography showing diffuse macular thickening.

CASE STUDY 5

A 20-year-old female complained of scotoma in both the eyes with her VA being 6/9 in the right eye and 6/45 in the left eye. Fundal examination (**Fig. 111.5**) showed macular edema with cotton-wool spots and perivascular cuffing in

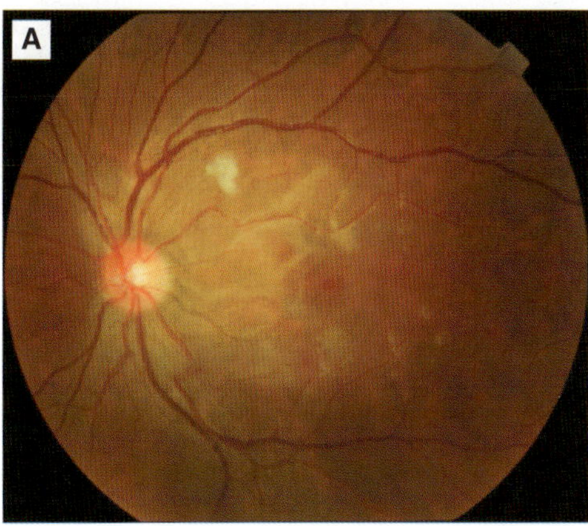
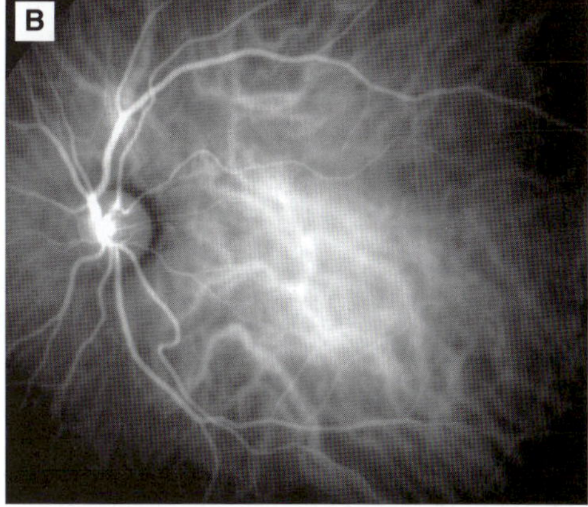

Fig. 111.5 Images of left fundus obtained at 4 days after onset of symptoms. **(A)** Color photograph showing macular edema, perivascular sheathing, and cotton-wool spots. **(B)** Indocyanine green angiography showing diffuse choroidal leakage over macula area.

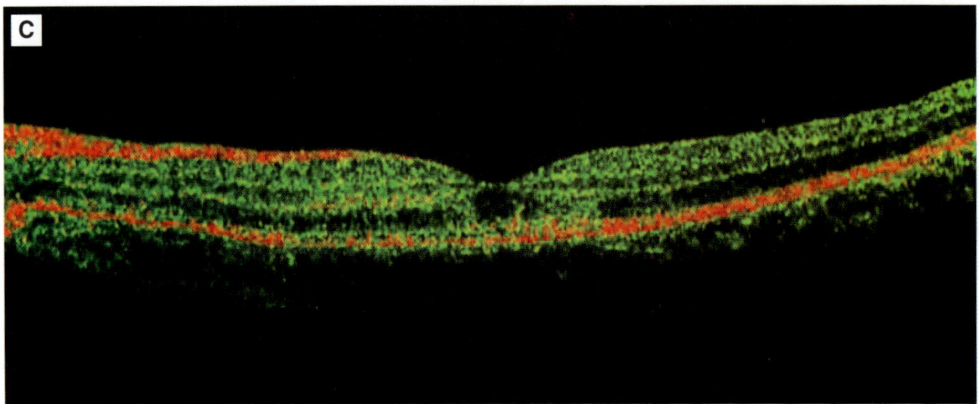

Fig. 111.5 (C) Optical coherence tomography showing diffuse subretinal fluid.

both the eyes. The FA was within normal limits. She was also treated with systemic corticosteroids; her VA recovered to 6/6 in both the eyes with resolution of the edema, but the left eye had residual retinal pigment epithelial mottling.

FURTHER READING

1. Lim WK, Mathur R, Koh A, et al.: Ocular manifestations of dengue fever. *Ophthalmology* 111:2057–2064, 2004.
2. Bacsal KE, Chee SP, Cheng CL, et al.: Dengue-associated maculopathy. *Arch Ophthalmol* 125:501–510, 2007.
3. Chia A, Luu CD, Mathur R, et al.: Electrophysiological findings in patients with dengue-related maculopathy. *Arch Ophthalmol* 124:1421–1426.
4. Su DH, Bacsal K, Chee SP, et al.: Dengue Maculopathy Study Group. Prevalence of dengue maculopathy in patients hospitalized for dengue fever. *Ophthalmology* 114:1743–1747, 2007.
5. Chee E, Sims JL, Jap A, et al.: Comparison of prevalence of dengue maculopathy during two epidemics with differing predominant serotypes. *Am J Ophthalmol* 148:910–913, 2009.
6. Teoh SC, Chee CK, Laude A, et al.: Eye Institute Dengue-related Ophthalmic Complications Workgroup. Optical coherence tomography patterns as predictors of visual outcome in dengue-related maculopathy. *Retina* 30:390–398, 2010.

Fuchs' Uveitis

Carl P Herbort and Nadia Bouchenaki

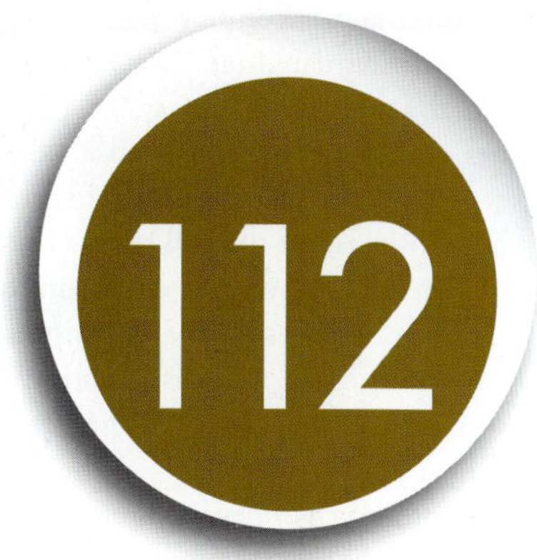

Fuchs' uveitis (FU), formerly called Fuchs' heterochromic iridocyclitis, is an intraocular inflammatory condition, unilateral in about 90% of cases, involving vitreous humor, lens, optic disc, and anterior segment. It is a universally occurring condition at similar frequencies all over the world. Vitritis, one of the most frequent findings, present in over 95% of cases, is associated anteriorly with a typical anterior uveitis and presence of posterior polar opacification of crystalline lens or a frank, sometimes white cataract (50%–90% of cases depending on when the diagnosis is made). The main characteristics of the FU granulomatous anterior uveitis are: (1) stellate fine granulomatous keratic precipitates (KPs) randomly distributed all over endothelium, including the area above midline (over 90% of cases), (2) atrophic changes in iris structure of the affected eye (over 95%), (3) presence of Koeppe's nodules at iris–pupillary rim in 40%–50% of cases, (4) abnormal vessels in iridocorneal angle (20%–30%), and (5) absence of iridolenticular synechiae in quasi 100% of cases. Posterior findings include a hyperfluorescent disc on fluorescein angiography (FA) in diseased eye in almost all cases, and, as long as no intraocular surgery has been performed, there is absence of inflammatory macular edema in all cases, how-so-ever pronounced the vitritis is, representing a strong diagnostic criterion. Heterochromia, which should no longer be considered as a disease-defining sign, is only present in 30%–50% of Caucasian populations and absent in brown irises. Hence, the eponym "Fuchs' heterochromic iridocyclitis" should not be used any more, as heterochromia is not present in major part of the world population having brown irises and the disease is characterized not only by an iridocyclitis but also by a vitritis and a papillitis. Trigger of the disease is most probably caused by rubella virus, as almost all cases aqueous humor show an increase of antirubella antibodies as compared to serum (Goldman–Witmer coefficient). Diagnosis of FU is often missed or delayed substantially because of failure of the clinician to associate vitritis and disc hyperfluorescence with FU and because the diagnosis is not thought of in the absence of heterochromia, which sometimes leads to the administration of deleterious systemic inflammation suppressive therapy.

CASE STUDY

A 24-year-old Caucasian woman treated for 12 months with systemic steroids (20 mg of prednisone tapered down from an initial dose of 60 mg) and systemic cyclosporine (4 mg/kg) for a "unilateral panuveitis" consulted for a second opinion as the treatment had brought no improvement and caused substantial discomfort, including a gain of weight of 9.6 kg, hirsutism, and hypertrophy of gums. It was the mother of the patient coming from a

Mediterranean country who took the appointment, as she was very concerned by the weight gain of her not-yet-married daughter. The history revealed that the patient had consulted to adjust her spectacles. Best-corrected visual acuity (BCVA) was 0.8 oculus dexter (OD) and 0.9 oculus sinister (OS). During ophthalmic examination, her eye doctor had detected a substantial vitreous infiltration in her right eye and referred the patient to a uveitis center. In the specialized uveitis referral center, the diagnosis of right "panuveitis" was made after FA had shown a hyperfluorescent disc OD (Fig. 112.1).

The patient was put on prednisone (60 mg) for 1 month, and then was tapered slowly to 40 mg after 3 months. As there was absolutely no improvement, cyclosporine (5 mg/kg tapered after 3 months to 4 mg/kg) was given and, as after 12 months situation was identical, the patient sought a second opinion. At presentation, the BCVA was 0.8 OD and 0.9 OS. The left eye showed fine, granulomatous KPs distributed all over the corneal endothelium (Fig. 112.2).

Anterior chamber inflammation measured by laser flare photometry (using a Kowa FM-500 laser flare photometer) was 9.8 photons per millisecond (ph/ms) OD, whereas value was normal OS (3.8 ph/ms). Intraocular pressure was 9 mmHg in right Fuchs' eye and 14 mmHg in left normal eye. The brown irises were isochromic; however, the iris structure appeared slightly atrophic in OD (Fig. 112.3).

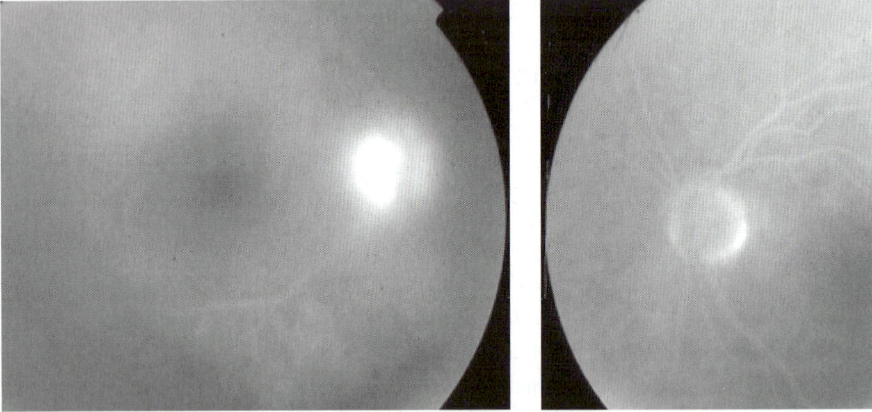

Fig. 112.1 Fluorescein angiography showing disc hyperfluorescence in affected Fuchs' eye (*right eye, left image*); note blurred image due to vitritis.

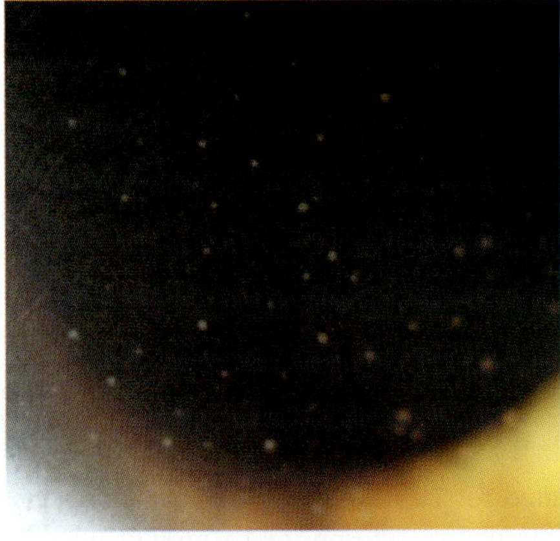

Fig. 112.2 Fine, granulomatous, stellate KPs randomly distributed all over the endothelium including corneal area above midline.

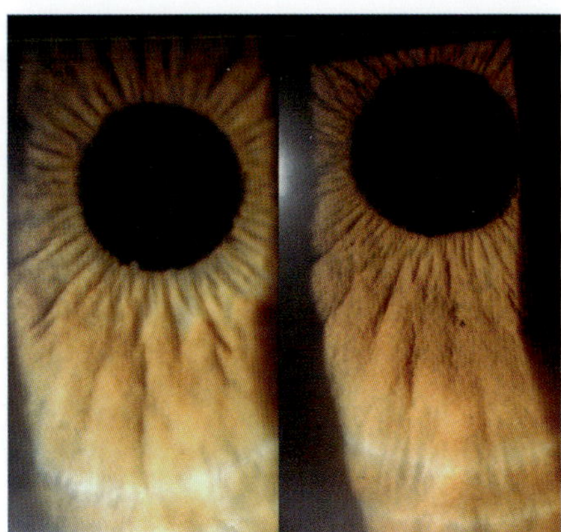

Fig. 112.3 Iris structure atrophic changes in Fuchs' eye (*right eye, left picture*), especially around pupillary margin, as compared to normal left eye (*right picture*).

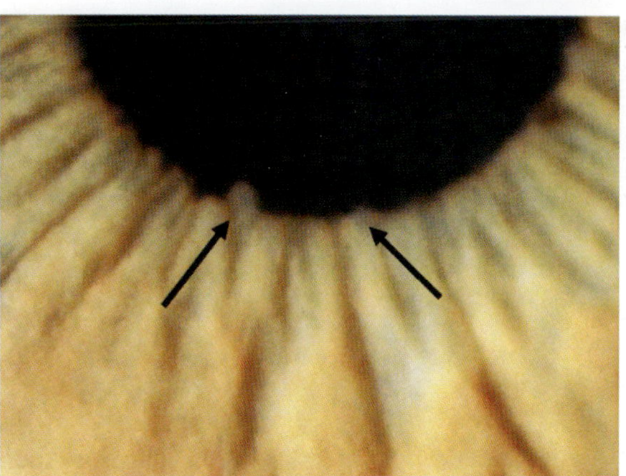

Fig. 112.4 Koeppe's nodules on pupillary margin (*arrows*).

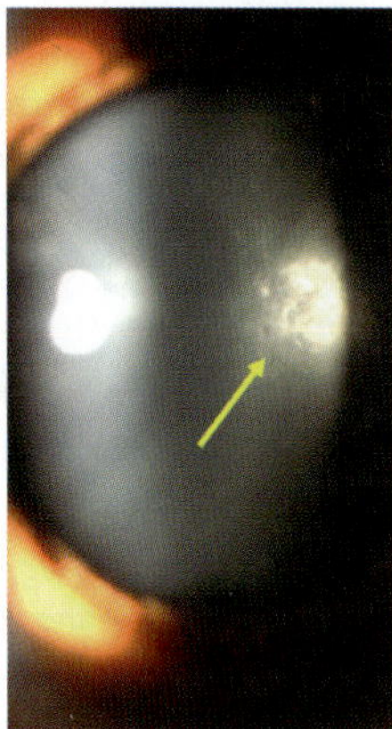

Fig. 112.5 Central polar capsular opacification of lens capsule (*arrow*).

And on the pupillary margin there were a few Koeppe's nodules OD (**Fig. 112.4**).

On dilatation, in the right eye, there was a slight opacification of posterior lenticular capsule probably explaining the slightly lower visual acuity OD (**Fig. 112.5**).

Spectral-domain optical coherence tomography (SD-OCT) showed hyperreflective dots in vitreous humor and on retinal surface as well as an incipient epiretinal membrane (**Fig. 112.6**).

The diagnosis of the FU was made, the treatment of cyclosporine was discontinued at once, and prednisone was tapered over a period of 2 months when patient was seen again with same findings. Laser flare photometry measurement of inflammation OD was stable with a slightly lower value of 8.4 ph/ms. Check-up every 6–12 months was recommended to patient in order to check intraocular pressure, as a glaucomatous evolution is always possible and to check evolution of cataract.

This case illustrates well the fact that vitreous infiltration is not recognized as being a classical feature of FU, having lead the clinician, in the absence of heterochromia, towards an erroneous diagnosis of "panuveitis" that was even confirmed by the presence of disc hyperfluorescence on the FA. In our series of patients, most of whom were referred, the proportion of nondiagnosed patients was 77.1% and mean diagnostic delay was 3.04 years, with

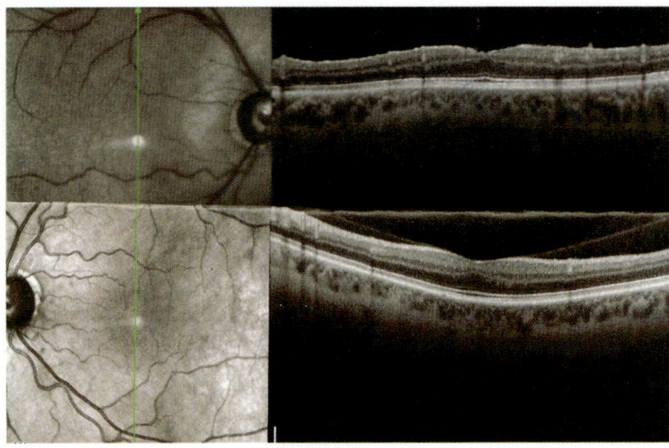

Fig. 112.6 Spectral-domain optical coherence tomography (SD–OCT) shows hyperreflective dots in vitreous humor and on retinal surface and incipient epiretinal membrane in right Fuchs' eye (*top picture*). Normal left eye is shown in bottom picture.

the proportion of patients having received systemic corticosteroids and/or immunosuppressive drugs being 38.7%. Spectral-domain optical coherence tomography (SD-OCT) shows that vitreoretinal modifications are seen in 90% of the FU patients, including hyperreflective dots in the vitreous humor and on the surface of the retina (45%), thickening of posterior hyaloid (38.7%), posterior vitreous detachment (32.3%), vitreoretinal traction (29%), and epiretinal membrane (25.8%) with optical coherence tomography (OCT) examination being normal in 9.6% of cases.

FURTHER READING

1. Fuchs E: Ueber Komplikationen der Heterochromie. *Zeitschrift für Augenheilkunde* 15:191–212, 1906.
2. Herbort CP, Khairallah M: Fuchs' uveitis: from imperial Vienna to global appraisal (editorial). *Int Ophthalmol* 30:449–452, 2010.
3. Bouchenaki N, Herbort CP: Fuchs' uveitis: failure to associate vitritis and disc hyperfluorescence with the disease is the major factor for misdiagnosis and diagnostic delay. *Middle East Afr J Ophthalmol* 16:239–244, 2009.
4. Tugal-Tutkun I, Guney-Tefekli E, Kamaci-Duman F, et al.: A cross-sectional and longitudinal study of Fuchs uveitis syndrome in Turkey. *Am J Ophthalmol* 148:510–515, 2009.
5. Bouchenaki N, Herbort CP: Fluorescein angiographic findings and clinical features in Fuchs' uveitis. *Int Ophthalmol* 30:511–519, 2010.
6. Quentin C, Reiber H: Fuchs' heterochromic cyclitis: rubella virus antibodies and genome in acqueous humor. *Am J Ophthalmol* 138:46–54, 2004.

Intermediate Uveitis

Padmamalini Mahendradas and
Kavitha Avadhani

Intermediate uveitis has been defined as an inflammatory syndrome, mainly involving the anterior vitreous, peripheral retina, and ciliary body. Optical coherence tomography (OCT) has become a standard diagnostic tool in intermediate uveitis patients for the diagnosis of cystoid macular edema, vitreoretinal interface abnormalities, measuring retinal thickness, and monitoring response to treatment.

Gupta et al. demonstrated the advantage of spectral-domain optical coherence tomography (SD-OCT) over time-domain optical coherence tomography (TD-OCT) in detecting macular abnormalities like posterior vitreous detachment, cystoid retinal spaces, etc., in eyes with intermediate uveitis.

CASE STUDY 1

A 53-year-old female presented with complaints of blurred vision and pain in both the eyes. She also gave a history of dry cough. On examination, her best-corrected visual acuity (BCVA) was 6/18, N10 in right eye, and 6/18, N6 in left eye. Intraocular pressure was normal in both the eyes. Slit lamp biomicroscopic examination revealed 2+ anterior vitreous cells in both the eyes. Fundus examination (**Figs 113.1–113.3**) revealed grade 2 media haze, macular edema with inferior multiple snowball opacities in both the eyes. On investigation, Schirmer's test was 7 mm in the right eye and 8 mm in the left eye. Mantoux test was negative. Chest X-ray revealed bilateral hilar lymphadenopathy, which was also confirmed by CT scan of the thorax. Serum angiotensin-converting enzyme was 68.8 IU/L. Clinical diagnosis of bilateral intermediate uveitis with dry eyes due to sarcoidosis was made. Patient was treated with oral prednisolone along with topical steroids and lubricants with good response to treatment (**Figs 113.4 and 113.5**). After 4 weeks, immunosuppressive therapy with methotrexate was started in addition to tapering dose of systemic steroids.

CASE STUDY 2

A 40-year-old male presented with complaints of decreased vision in both the eyes since 2 weeks. On examination, his BCVA was 6/9, N8 in right eye and 6/9, N10 in left eye. Intraocular pressure was normal. Anterior segment examination was normal. Fundus examination revealed vitreous haze++, cells++ macular edema, and inferior

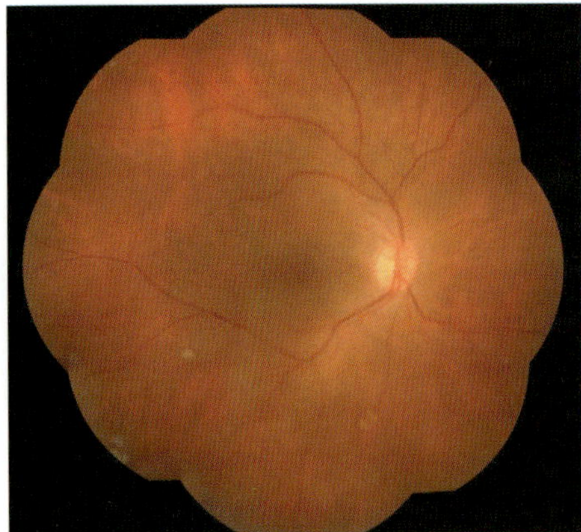

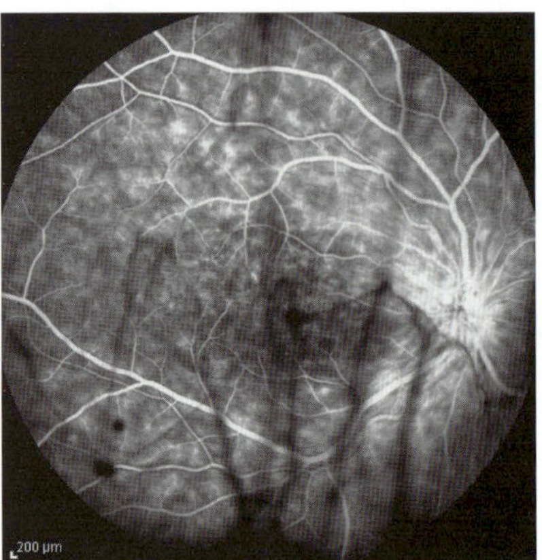

Fig. 113.1 A montage color fundus photograph of the right eye reveals macular edema with multiple inferior snowball opacities.

Fig. 113.2 Fundus fluorescein angiography reveals disc leak, diffuse perivascular leak with cystoid macular edema in the right eye.

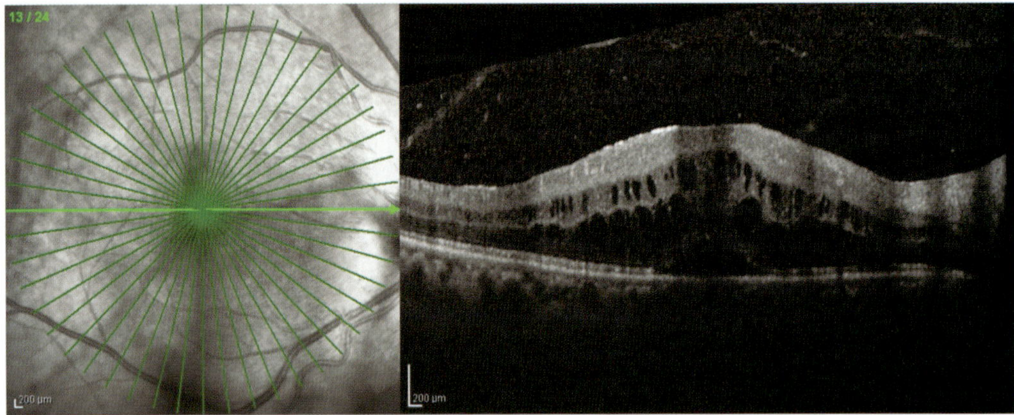

Fig. 113.3 SD-OCT reveals posterior vitreous cells, posterior vitreous detachment, loss of foveal contour, multiple hyporeflective cystic spaces with intervening high-reflective septae with subfoveal serous retinal detachment with central retinal thickness of 543 microns in the right eye.

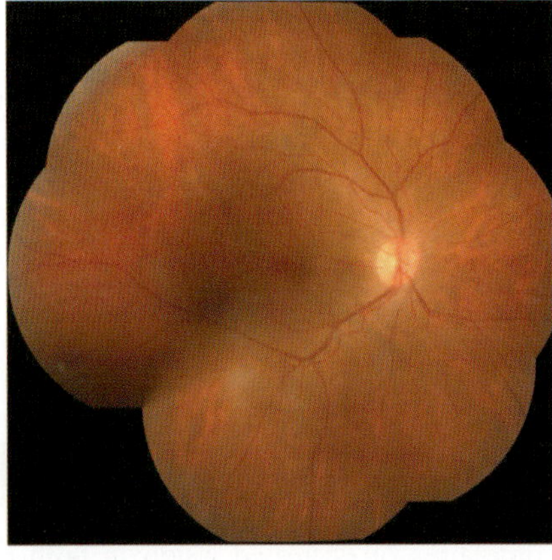

Fig. 113.4 Montage color fundus photograph shows resolved macular edema with disappearance of snowball opacities in the right eye.

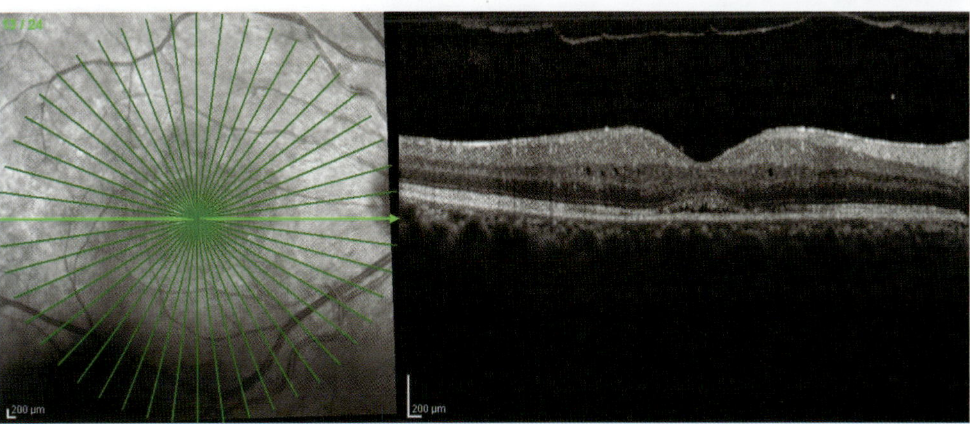

Fig. 113.5 Follow-up SD-OCT scan reveals disappearance of posterior vitreous cells, posterior vitreous detachment, normal foveal contour, with few tiny cystic spaces along with resolving subfoveal serous retinal detachment in the right eye.

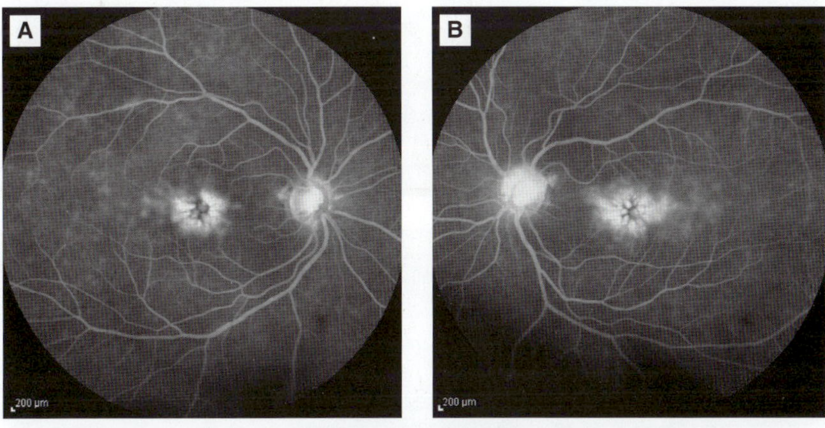

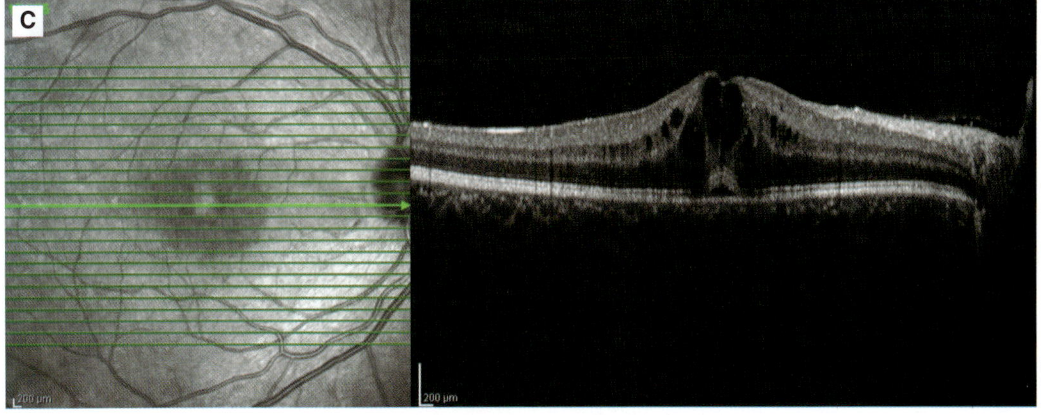

Fig. 113.6 **(A)** Fundus fluorescein angiography (FFA) of the right eye reveals disc staining, staining of retinal veins with diffuse perivascular leak along with classical flower petal pattern in macula suggestive of cystoid macular edema. **(B)** FFA of the left eye reveals disc leak, diffuse perivascular leak with cystoid macular edema.

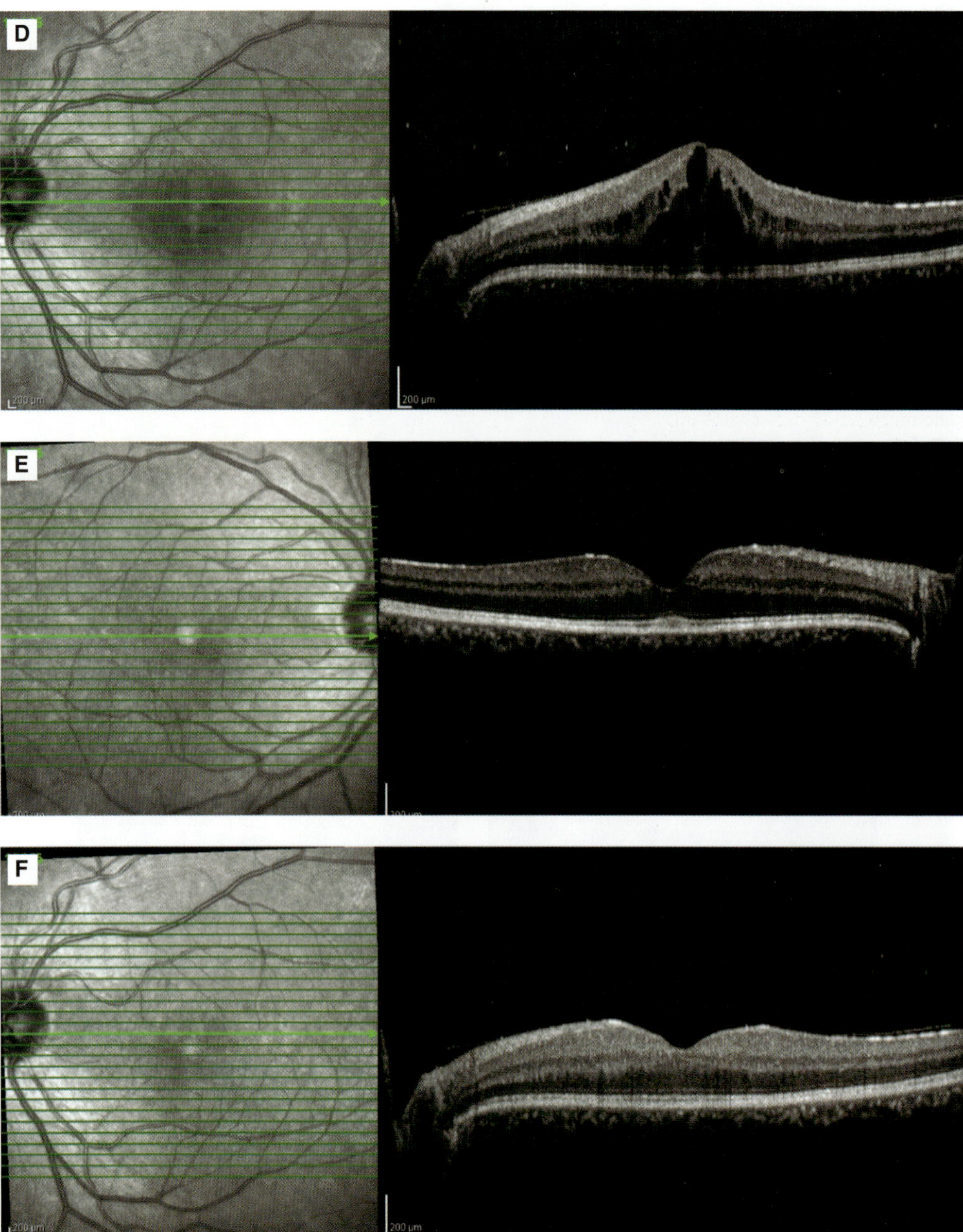

Fig. 113.6 (*Continued*) **(C, D)** SD-OCT scan reveals posterior vitreous cells, loss of foveal contour with hyporeflective cystic spaces with intervening high-reflective septae with subfoveal serous retinal detachment with central retinal thickness of 513 microns in the right eye and 639 microns in the left eye. **(E)** and **(F)** On follow-up after 4 weeks, following treatment with ATT and systemic steroids, there was resolution of inflammation in both the eyes. SD-OCT scan reveals normal foveal contour with resolution of cystoid macular edema in both the eyes.

snowball opacities and snow banking in both the eyes. Fundus fluorescein angiogram showed disc leak, perivascular leak along with petaloid pattern of hyperfluorescence in the fovea suggestive of cystoid macular edema (**Figs 113.6A and 113.6B**) On investigation, Mantoux test was 16 mm, and QuantiFERON®-TB Gold test was positive. Clinical diagnosis of bilateral intermediate uveitis due to presumed ocular tuberculosis was made and patient was started on antituberculous treatment and systemic steroid therapy. Follow-up after 4 weeks revealed decreased inflammation with disappearance of macular edema in both the eyes (**Figs 113.6C–F**).

FURTHER READING

1. Markomichelakis NN, Halkiadakis I, Pantelia E, et al.: Patterns of macular edema in patients with uveitis: Qualitative and quantitative assessment using optical coherence tomography. *Ophthalmology* 111(5):946–953, 2004.
2. Reinthal EK, Völker M, Freudenthaler N, et al.: Optical coherence tomography in the diagnosis and follow-up of patients with uveitic macular edema. *Ophthalmologe* 101(12):1181–1188, 2004.
3. Holland GN: The enigma of pars planitis. Revised. *Am J Ophthalmol* 141:729–730, 2006.
4. Venkatesh P, Abhas Z, Garg S, et al.: Prospective optical coherence tomographic evaluation of the efficacy of oral and posterior subtenon corticosteroids in patients with intermediate uveitis. *Graefes Arch Clin Exp Ophthalmol* 245(1):59–67, 2007.
5. Gupta V, Gupta P, Singh R, et al.: Spectral-domain Cirrus high-definition optical coherence tomography is better than time-domain stratus optical coherence tomography for evaluation of macular pathologic features in uveitis. *Am J Ophthalmol* 145:1018–1022, 2008.
6. Payne JF, Bruce BB, Lee LB, et al.: Logarithmic transformation of spectral-domain optical coherence tomography data in uveitis-associated macular edema. *Invest Ophthalmol Vis Sci* 52(12):8939–8943, 2011.

Multiple Evanescent White Dot Syndrome

114

Kavitha Avadhani and Padmamalini Mahendradas

Multiple evanescent white dot syndrome (MEWDS) is an inflammatory choriocapillaropathy of unknown origin that was first described in 1984 by Jampol et al. It predominantly affects young females and a flu-like illness may precede the disease in some cases. Patients of MEWDS typically present with complaints of scotoma and decreased vision, but most of them recover fully without any treatment in 1–2 months.

CASE STUDY

A 42-year-old Asian Indian female presented with complaints of sudden painless blurring of vision associated with flashes in her left eye for the past 4 days. Visual acuity at presentation was 20/20 in both the eyes. She had no other systemic illness or preceding flu-like illness. Ophthalmoscopic examination revealed multiple 100–200 micron yellowish-white dots deep in the retina in both the posterior pole and up to midperiphery in the left eye along with foveal granularity (Fig. 114.1).

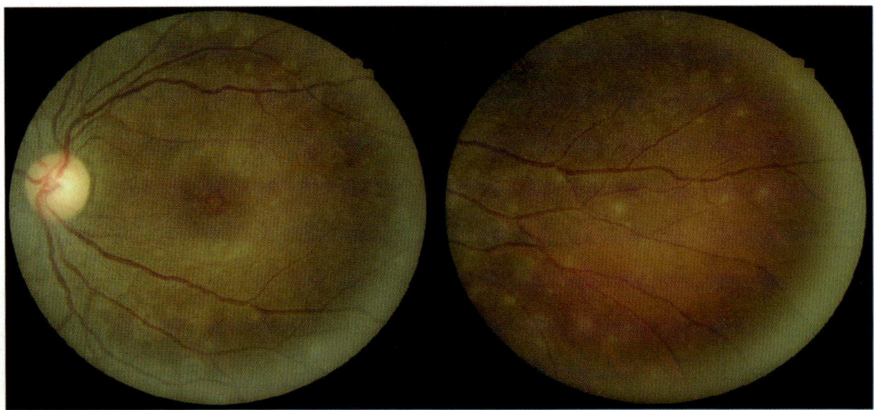

Fig. 114.1 Fundus photograph of the left eye showing multiple yellowish-white lesions in the posterior pole (*left*) and midperiphery (*right*).

On autofluorescence, many more lesions were visible than seen clinically as hyperfluorescent areas. Fluorescein angiography showed stippled hyperfluorescence corresponding to yellow-white lesions [*indocyanine green angiography (ICGA) has been reported to show multiple hypofluorescent areas. Hypofluorescence on ICGA suggests that MEWDS involves outer retina (blocked fluorescence) and/or inner choroid (nonperfusion)*]. Visual field of the left eye showed an enlarged blind spot (**Fig. 114.2**).

Spectral-domain optical coherence tomography (SD-OCT) through lesions showed a disruption in inner segment-outer segment (IS–OS) junction along with focal hyperreflectivity along with posterior vitreous cells (**Fig. 114.3**). These findings indicate that photoreceptor is involved in the disease. (*This corroborates well with electrophysiology findings seen in MEWDS, which suggest that the disease process occurs in outer retina and/or retinal pigment epithelium.*)

The patient was followed-up at weekly intervals. Nearly all lesions seen clinically had disappeared, 5 weeks after initial presentation. Visual field in the left eye showed disappearance of the scotoma (**Fig. 114.4**).

The SD-OCT through same areas imaged at presentation showed complete restoration of the IS–OS junction with disappearance of the focal lesions (**Fig. 114.5**).

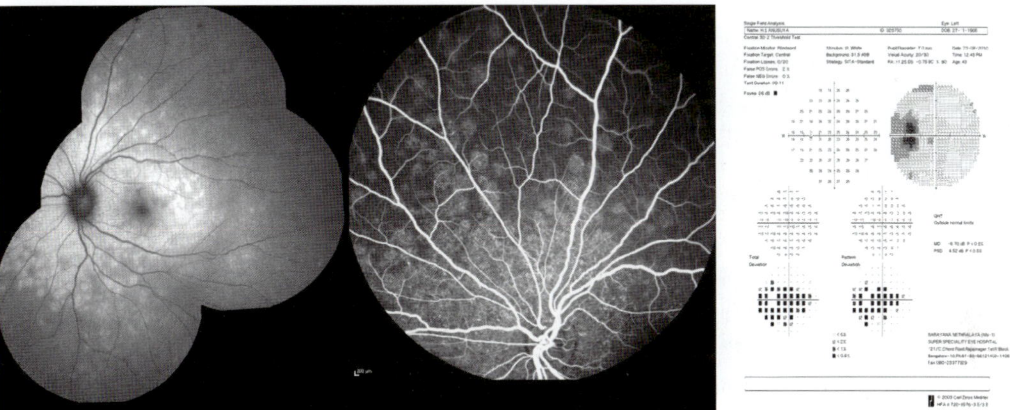

Fig. 114.2 Autofluorescence (*left*) image showing hyperfluorescence of the active lesions. Fundus Fluorescein angiography (*middle*) showing stippled hyperfluorescence in the area corresponding to the lesions. Visual field (*right*) showed an enlargement of the blind spot.

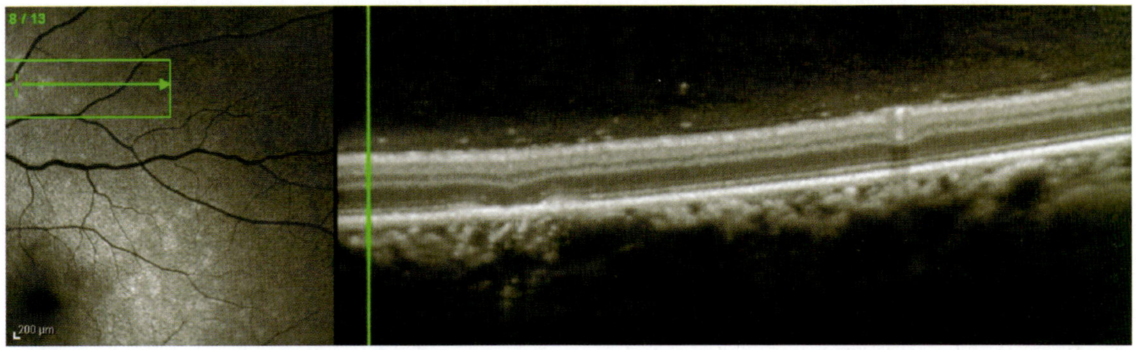

Fig. 114.3 SD-OCT through the active lesion showed disruption of the IS–OS junction along with a focal hyperreflectivity.

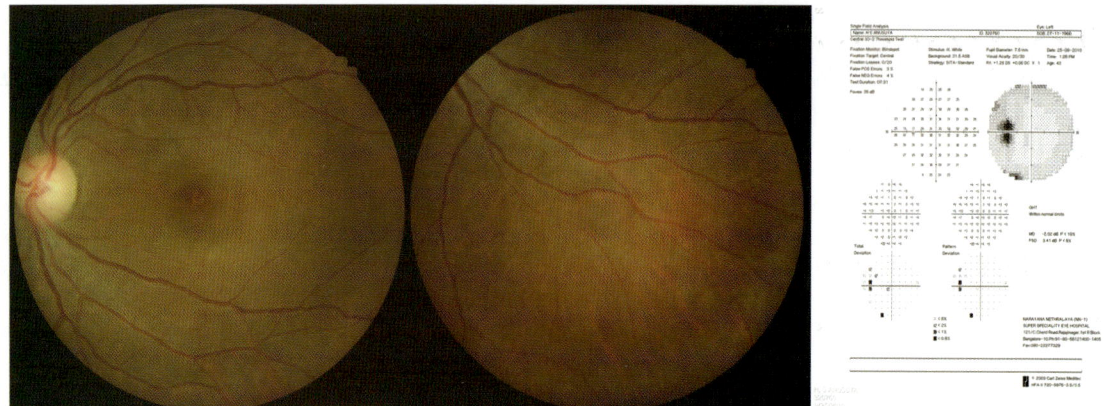

Fig. 114.4 Fundus photograph of the posterior pole (*left*) and midperiphery (*middle*) of the left eye showing disappearance of the lesions 5 weeks after initial presentation. Visual field (*right*) also showed the disappearance of the scotoma.

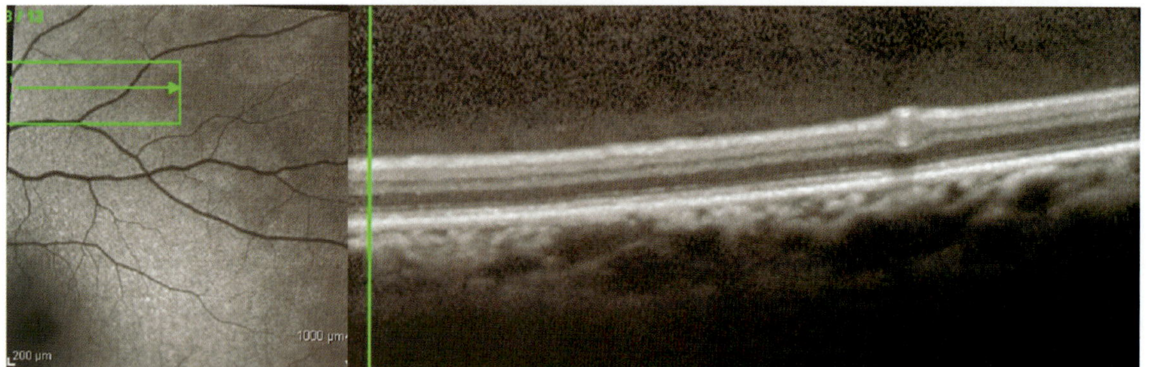

Fig. 114.5 SD-OCT 5 weeks after initial presentation through the same area as seen in Figure 111.3 shows disappearance of the focal abnormalities with restoration of normal IS–OS junction.

FURTHER READING

1. Nguyen MH, Witkin AJ, Reichel E, et al.: Microstructural abnormalities in MEWDS demonstrated by ultrahigh resolution optical coherence tomography. *Retina* 27(4):414–418, 2007.
2. Sikorski BL, Wojtkowski M, Kaluzny JJ, et al.: Correlation of spectral optical coherence tomography with fluorescein and indocyanine green angiography in multiple evanescent white dot syndrome. *Br J Ophthalmol* 92(11):1552–1557, 2008.
3. Gass JD: Acute zonal occult outer retinopathy. Donders Lecture: The Netherlands Ophthalmological Society, Maastricht, Holland, June 19, 1992. *J Clin Neuroophthalmol* 13(2):79–97, 1993.
4. Spaide RF, Koizumi H, Freund KB: Photoreceptor outer segment abnormalities as a cause of blind spot enlargement in acute zonal occult outer retinopathy-complex diseases. *Am J Ophthalmol* 146(1):111–120. Epub 2008 Apr 24. Erratum in: *Am J Ophthalmol* 2008, 2008.

Progressive Outer Retinal Necrosis

Kavitha Avadhani and Padmamalini Mahendradas

Progressive outer retinal necrosis (PORN) is a necrotizing viral retinitis caused most often by varicella zoster virus (VZV) or herpes simplex virus in an immunocompromised host. It is characterized by minimal vitritis and multifocal yellowish retinal lesions that progress rapidly and relentlessly leave behind a completely atrophic retina and pale optic disc. It is very resistant to treatment and is associated with very poor prognosis.

CASE STUDY

A 33-year-old Asian Indian male, a known case of HIV infection with a CD4 count of 50, presented with blurring of vision in both eyes. He was on treatment with highly active antiretroviral therapy (HAART). His best-corrected visual acuity in both the eyes was 20/30. Fundus examination revealed minimal vitritis with fuzzy yellowish lesions suggestive of retinitis in the posterior pole of both the eyes (**Fig. 115.1A**). Anterior chamber paracentesis was performed and subjected to polymerase chain reaction (PCR) for identification of possible etiological agent. The PCR for VZV was positive. A diagnosis of PORN due to VZV was made. The patient was treated with intravenous acyclovir and intravitreal ganciclovir. The lesions, despite treatment, continued to progress in size and number (**Fig. 115.1B**).These then went on to become confluent, involving the entire retina (**Fig. 115.1C**). Visual acuity deteriorated to light perception in both the eyes over a period of 3 weeks.

Spectral-domain optical coherence tomography (SD-OCT) was performed serially and showed diffuse retinal thickening (specially seen in the inner retinal layers) in the acute phase (**Fig. 115.2A**). The optical coherence tomography (OCT) showed progressive disorganization of all the retinal layers with the disease progression (**Figs 115.2B and C**). By 3 weeks, despite treatment, the retina turned completely atrophic with significant tissue loss (involving full thickness of the retina) that was clearly visible on the OCT (**Fig. 115.2D**).

Sequential OCT is very useful and clearly documents progression of the disease in PORN. In the acute phase, the lesions are seen as inner retinal edema and opacification. Continued tissue breakdown involving all the retinal layers (outer more than inner) is clearly seen on the OCT. The retina in late phases of the disease appears completely attenuated on the OCT.

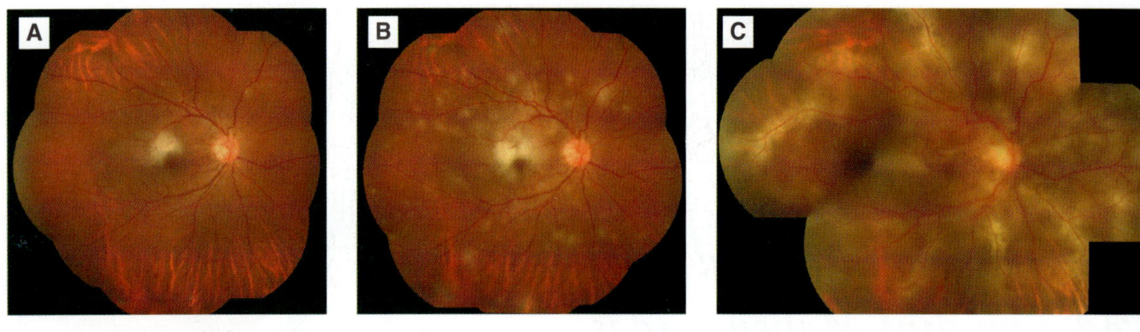

Fig. 115.1 **(A)** Fundus photograph of the right eye at presentation showing deep yellowish-white retinal lesions involving the posterior pole with a couple of subtle lesions beyond the vascular arcade. **(B)** Fundus photograph of the right eye 1 week since presentation showing the appearance of several new retinal lesions all over the fundus. **(C)** Fundus photograph of the right eye 3 weeks from the time of presentation showing further progression with confluence of the retinal lesions. The retina, especially in the posterior pole, appears atrophic and disc appears pale.

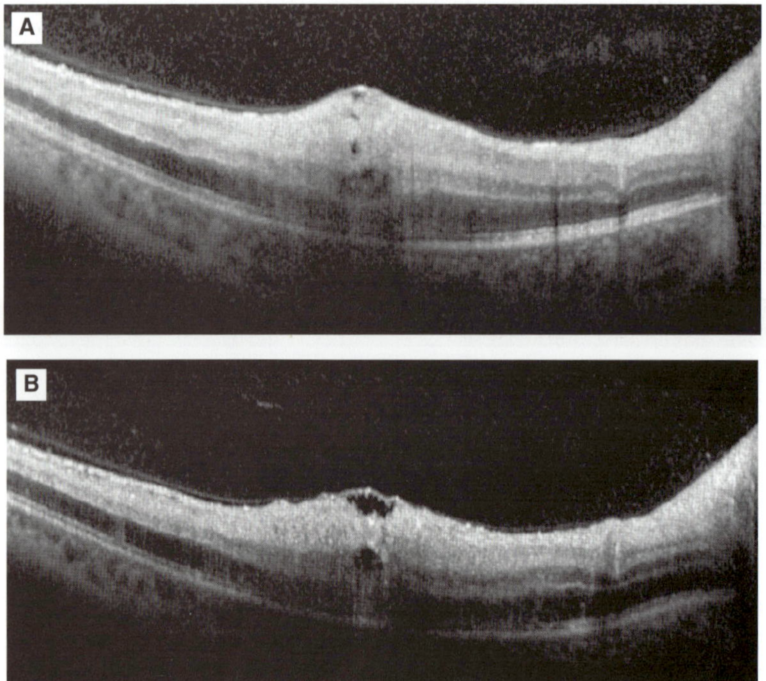

Fig. 115.2 **(A)** SD-OCT at presentation showing hyperreflectivity of the inner retinal layers along with retinal thickening and outer retinal edema. **(B)** OCT scan through same area 1 week after presentation showing persistence of the inner retinal hyperreflectivity along with hyporeflective areas in the outer retina, suggesting a breakdown of the outer retinal layers.

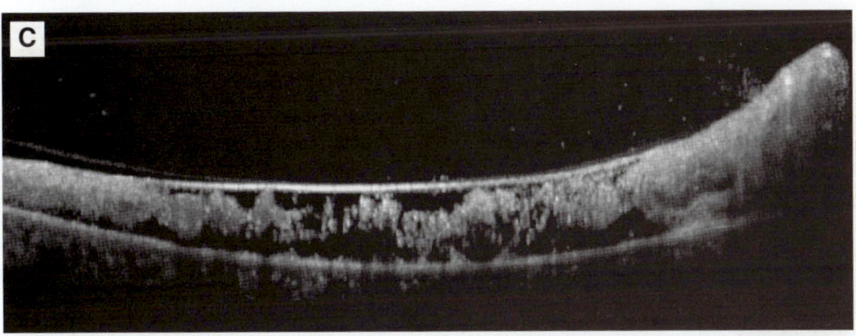

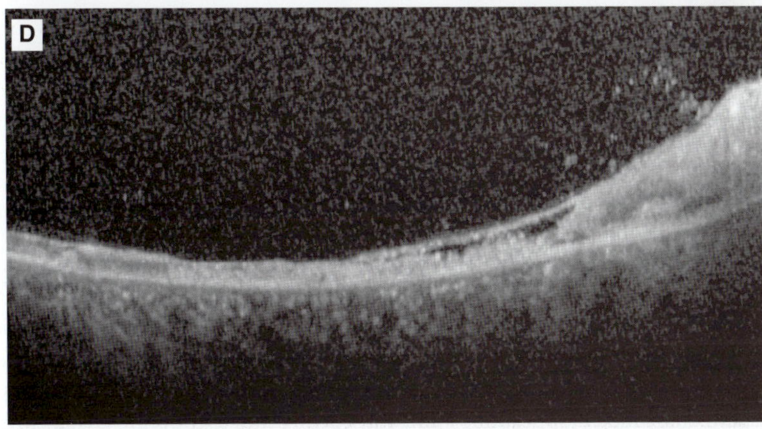

Fig. 115.2 **(C)** OCT scan done at 2 weeks from the time of presentation showing complete disruption of all the retinal layers and a total loss of retinal architecture. **(D)** At 3 weeks from the time of presentation, only a thin hyperreflective layer persists, representing a completely atrophic retina. Underlying choroid also appears to have thinned out with each progressive scan.

FURTHER READING

1. Forster DJ, Dugel PU, Frangieh GT, et al.: Rapidly progressive outer retinal necrosis in the acquired immunodeficiency syndrome. *Am J Ophthalmol* 110:341–348, 1990.
2. Yeh S, Wong WT, Weichel ED, et al.: Fundus autofluorescence and OCT in the management of progressive outer retinal necrosis. *Ophthalmic Surg Lasers Imaging* 1–4, 2010.
3. Engstrom RE Jr, Holland GN, Margolis TP, et al.: The progressive outer retinal necrosis syndrome. A variant of necrotizing herpetic retinopathy in patients with AIDS. *Ophthalmology* 101(9):1488–1502, 1994.
4. Greven CM, Ford J, Stanton C, et al.: Progressive outer retinal necrosis secondary to varicella zoster virus in acquired immune deficiency syndrome. *Retina* 15(1):14–20, 1995.
5. Pavesio CE, Mitchell SM, Barton K, et al.: Progressive outer retinal necrosis (PORN) in AIDS patients: a different appearance of varicella-zoster retinitis. *Eye (Lond)* 9 (Pt 3):271–276, 1995.
6. Blair MP, Goldstein DA, Shapiro MJ: Optical coherence tomography of progressive outer retinal necrosis. *Retina* 27(9): 1313–1314, 2007.

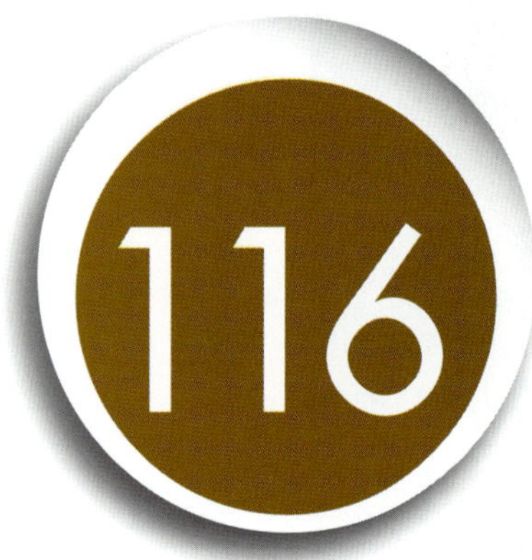

Rickettsial Retinitis

*Moncef Khairallah, Sonia Attia,
Rim Kahloun, and Sonia Zaouali*

Rickettsioses are worldwide distributed zoonotic diseases caused by obligate intracellular small gram-negative bacteria. Human infection results from the bite of contaminated arthropods, mainly ticks. The rickettsial agents include three categories: spotted fever group, typhus group, and scrub typhus group. A rickettsial disease should be kept in mind in the presence of high fever, headache, general malaise, and skin rash, during warm seasons, in a patient living in or traveling back from a region endemic for the rickettsial infection. Systemic rickettsioses usually have a good prognosis; however, severe systemic complications and subsequent death can occur. Ocular involvement associated with rickettsial infection is more common than previously thought, and can be asymptomatic or less frequently symptomatic.

CASE STUDY

A 20-year-old man with a 3-week's history of fever and skin rash complained of acute visual loss in the left eye since last 5 days. Visual acuity was 20/20 in the right eye and 20/200 in the left eye. Results of fundus examination of the right eye were unremarkable. There were 2+ vitreous cells in the left eye. The fundus examination of the left eye showed a focus of retinitis along the superior temporal arcade, retinal hemorrhages, serous retinal detachment (SRD), hard exudates, and optic disc edema (**Fig. 116.1**). The patient underwent color fundus photography (**Fig. 116.1**), fluorescein angiography (FA), and optical coherence tomography (OCT).

Fluorescein angiography (FA) at presentation showed early hypofluorescence (**Fig. 116.2A**) and late staining (**Fig. 116.2B**) of the white retinal lesion seen clinically, blockage effect by retinal hemorrhages, retinal vascular leakage, and optic disc hyperfluorescence.

Oblique optical coherence tomography (OCT) section scan over the lesion showed increased internal reflectivity with posterior shadowing due to the retinitis, retinal thickening, SRD, and thickened posterior hyaloid (**Fig. 116.3**).

Initial work-up for common infectious and noninfectious causes of retinitis was negative. The indirect immunofluorescence test was positive for *Rickettsia conorii* (causative agent of Mediterranean spotted fever) with a titer of 1:320 (normal < 1:80). The patient was treated with doxycycline 200 mg/day and prednisone 60 mg/day, with gradual tapering for 4 weeks.

Fundus photograph of the left eye taken 3 months after initial examination showed complete resolution of the white retinal lesion as well as all associated findings without residual retinal pigment epithelial changes (**Fig. 116.4**). The visual acuity had improved to 20/25.

Ocular involvement, usually asymptomatic and self-limiting, is very common in patients with rickettsioses. However, it may be associated with ocular symptoms including decreased visual acuity, redness, floaters, and scotoma. Retinitis is the most common clinical finding in the rickettsioses and presents as white lesions infiltrating

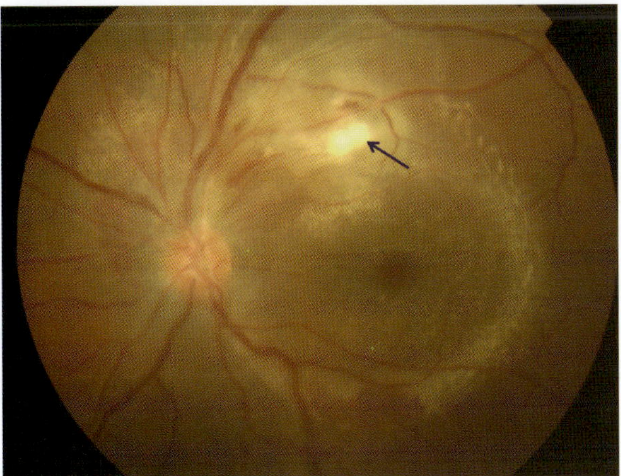

Fig. 116.1 Fundus photograph of the left eye of a patient with rickettsioses shows a white retinal lesion adjacent to superotemporal vascular arcade (*arrow*) with associated serous retinal detachment, retinal hard exudates with macular star, and superficial and deep retinal hemorrhages.

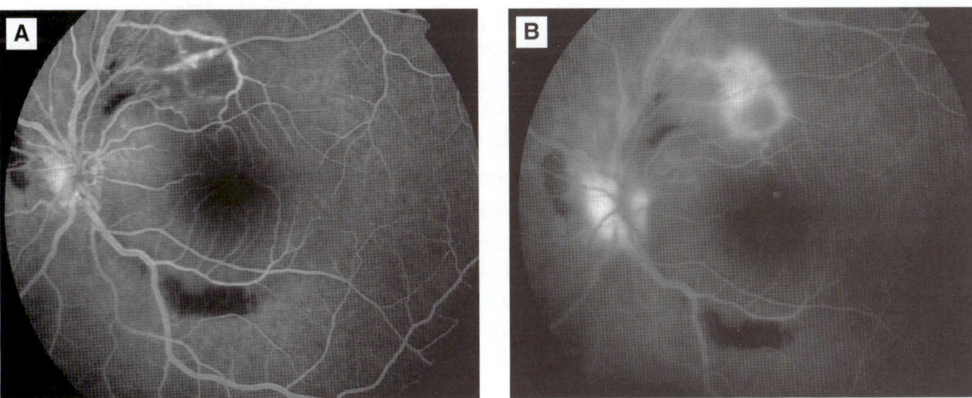

Fig. 116.2 (A) Early-phase fluorescein angiogram shows early hypofluorescence of the focus of retinitis. **(B)** Late-phase fluorescein angiogram shows staining of retinal lesion, blockage effect by retinal hemorrhages, retinal vascular leakage, and optic disc hyperfluorescence.

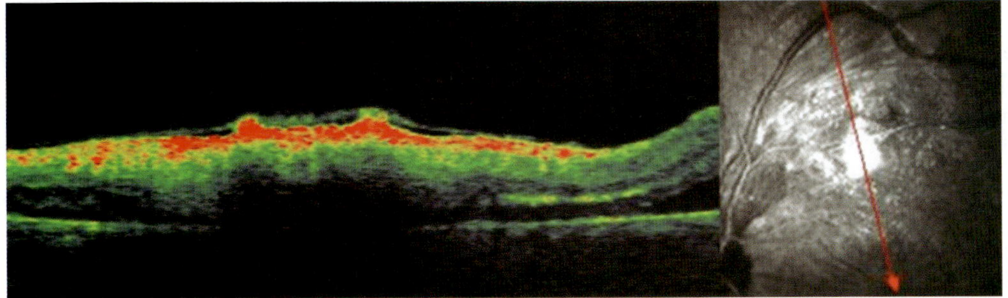

Fig. 116.3 Optical coherence tomography shows increased internal reflectivity with posterior shadowing due to retinitis, retinal thickening, serous retinal detachment, and thickened posterior hyaloid.

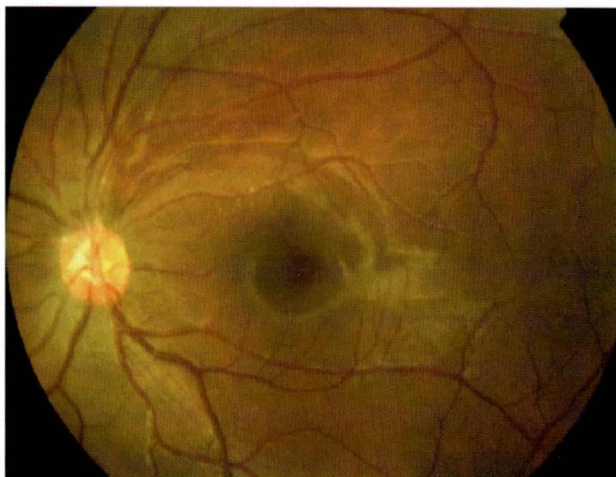

Fig. 116.4 Fundus photograph of the left eye 3 months after initial examination shows complete resolution of the white retinal lesion and associated findings without residual retinal pigment epithelial changes.

primarily the inner retina with or without associated mild vitritis. The retinal lesions are variable in number, size, and topography, and are typically adjacent to retinal vessels. On FA, large retinal lesions show early hypofluorescence and late staining, though small retinal lesions are slightly hypofluorescent or isofluorescent. The OCT, showing internal hyperreflective lesion, reveals that the inner retinal layers are the primary location of rickettsial retinitis. OCT is also useful in detecting retinal edema and SRD that frequently accompany large retinitis foci.

Other common ocular manifestations of rickettsial disease that may be asymptomatic or symptomatic include nonocclusive or occlusive retinal vasculitis and optic nerve involvement.

This case demonstrates that rickettsial infection should be considered in the differential diagnosis of retinitis, retinal vasculitis, and optic nerve involvement in any patient with a history of fever and/or skin rash living in or returning from a specific endemic area, especially during warm seasons. FA and OCT are useful tools in evaluation of rickettsial retinitis and detecting associated retinal and optic disc changes.

A systematic ophthalmic examination, revealing frequently abnormal, fairly typical findings, mainly retinitis, can help establish an early clinical diagnosis of systemic rickettsial disease while the serologic testing is pending.

FURTHER READING

1. Parola P, Raould D: Rickettsioses éruptives. EMC (Elsevier Paris) Maladies infectieuses, 8-137-I-20, 1998.
2. Mc Dade JE. Rickettsial diseases In: Hausler WJ, Sussman M, editors. *Topley and Wilson's Microbiology and Microbial Infections*, ed 9, London: Arnold, 3:995–1011, 1998.
3. Khairallah M, Ladjimi A, Chakroun M, et al.: Posterior segment manifestations of *Rickettsia conorii* infection. *Ophthalmology* 111:529–534, 2004.
4. Khairallah M, Ben Yahia S, Toumi A, et al.: Ocular manifestations associated with murine typhus. *Br J Opthalmol* 93(7):938–942, Epub 2009 May 3.
5. Khairallah M, Chee SP, Rathinam SR, et al.: Novel infectious agents causing uveitis. *Int Ophthalmol* 30:465–483, 2010.
6. Khairallah M, Ben Yahia S, Zaouali S: Rickettsial Diseases. In: Gupta A, Gupta V, Herbort CP, Khairallah M, editors: *Uveitis text and imaging*. India: Jaypee Brothers Medical Publishers. pp 687–693, 2009.
7. Alio J, Ruiz-Beltran R, Herrero-Herrero JI, et al.: Retinal manifestations of Mediterranean spotted fever. *Ophthalmologica* 195:31–37, 1987.
8. Khairallah M, Zaouali S, Ben Yahia S, et al.: Anterior ischemic optic neuropathy associated with *Rickettsia conorii* infection. *J Neuroophthalmol* 25:212–214.
9. Khairallah M, Yahia SB, Jelliti B, et al.: Diagnostic value of ocular examination in Mediterranean spotted fever. *Clin Microbiol Infect* 15 Suppl 2:273–274, 2009.

Serpiginous Choroiditis

Vishali Gupta and Amod Gupta

Serpiginous choroiditis (SC) is a bilateral, chronic, progressive, recurrent inflammation of choriocapillaris, choroid, and retinal pigment epithelium (RPE). This disease is primarily believed to be autoimmune. However, tuberculosis can present as serpiginous-like choroiditis and should be ruled out especially in a population endemic for tuberculosis. The patients with tubercular serpiginous-like choroiditis have younger age of onset, greater incidence of unilaterality, and may have associated anterior segment and vitreous inflammation, perivascular choroiditis patches, and vasculitis that provide a possible clue towards possible tubercular etiology. Clinical presentations include: (1) multifocal progressive choroiditis initially presenting as few discrete areas of choroiditis that show a wave-like progression to confluent, diffuse choroiditis, eventually resembling SC; (2) diffuse choroiditis presenting as confluent, plaque-like choroiditis with amoeboid pattern suggestive of SC at initial presentation; and (3) a mixed variety in which opposite eyes have different features. These patients have systemic evidence of active or latent tuberculosis, and show repeated recurrences when treated alone with corticosteroid therapy. Diagnosis is based on classic clinical picture in addition to a positive Mantoux test, a chest radiograph suggestive of tuberculosis, or a positive polymerase chain reaction (PCR) result from aqueous or vitreous humor for *Mycobacterium tuberculosis*. The treatment regimen consists of a prolonged course of four-drug antituberculosis treatment (ATT) in addition to oral corticosteroids. Prognosis is favorable with significant visual recovery in nearly all eyes, with only occasional episodes of recurrence.

CASE STUDY

A 28-year-old man was seen with macular SC in his left eye (**Fig. 117.1**). Fundus fluorescein angiogram shows early hypofluorescence (**Fig. 117.2**) with late hyperfluorescence and leak of dye along superior temporal active edge (**Fig. 117.3**).

Autofluorescence image of the active lesion showed an area of increased autofluorescence. A fuzzy area of hyperreflectivity in the outer retinal layers (including RPE, external limiting membrane (ELM), photoreceptor outer segment tips (POST), photoreceptor inner segment–outer segment (IS–OS) junction, and outer nuclear layer [ONL]) was seen on OCT. Mild distortion of inner retinal layers with absence of any backscattering from inner choroid was also noted (**Fig. 117.4**).

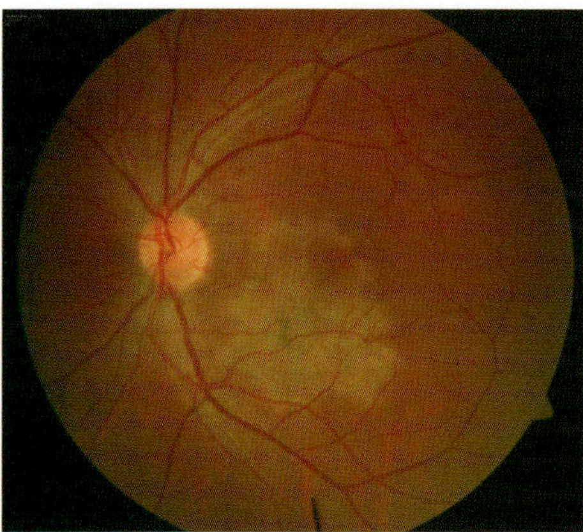

Fig. 117.1 Fundus photograph of the left eye showing a yellowish area of choroiditis involving macula. Lesion is active along an edge that appears to be progressing temporal to fovea.

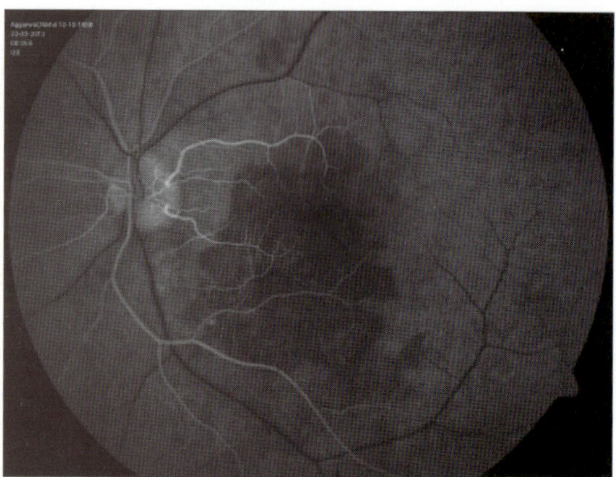

Fig. 117.2 Early phase fundus fluorescein angiogram of the left eye of same patient as in Figure 117.1 showing hypofluorescence corresponding to area of choroiditis.

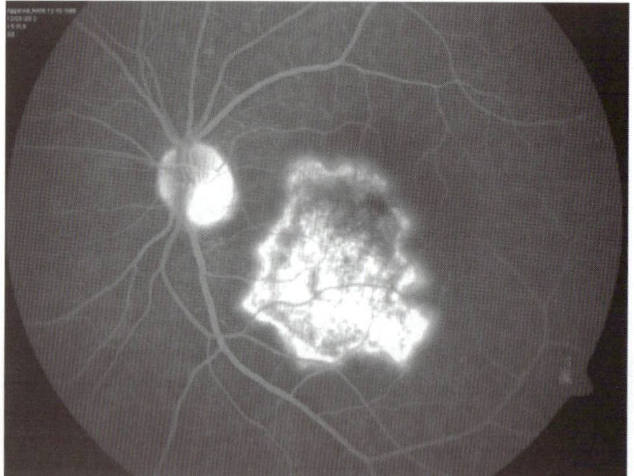

Fig. 117.3 Late phase angiogram of the same eye as in Figure 117.1 showing hyperfluorescence and leakage of dye along temporal active edge.

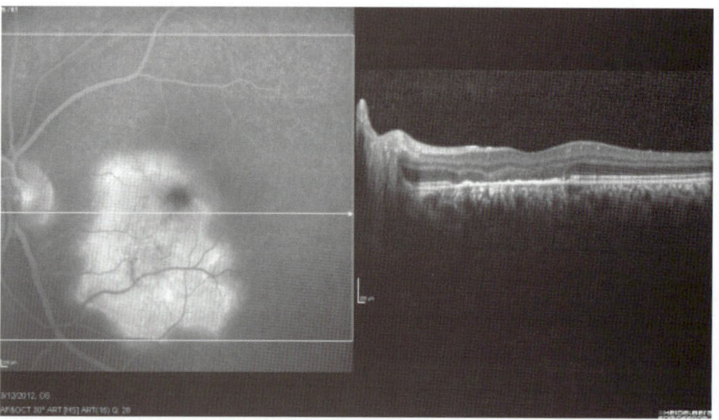

Fig. 117.4 Spectral-domain optical coherence tomography (*right panel*) showing fuzzy hyperreflectivity involving outer retinal layers in the area corresponding to the area of choroiditis.

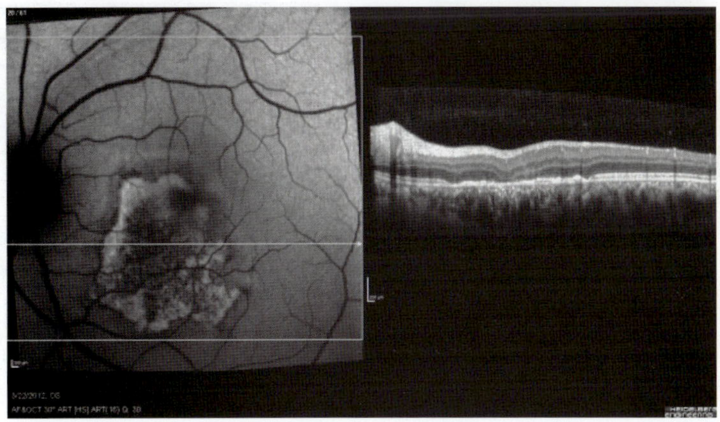

Fig. 117.5 Following treatment, autofluorescence image (*left panel*) shows hypofluorescent border with central stippling suggestive of healing. SD-OCT image (*right panel*) shows irregular knob-like elevations with indistinguishable outer retinal layers in the healing phase.

The patient had a positive QuantiFERON®-TB Gold test, positive purified protein derivative (PPD) skin test, and hilar lymphadenopathy on chest X-ray. He received antituberculosis treatment with systemic corticosteroids. As the lesions healed, they became well defined with a thin hypo-autofluorescent border and stippled central autofluorescence. The spectral-domain optical coherence tomography (SD-OCT) showed irregular knob-like elevations of the outer retinal layers. The RPE, POST, IS–OS junction, and ELM could not be distinguished and an increased reflectance was noted from choroidal layers as a result of the disappearance of the RPE–photoreceptor complex (**Fig. 117.5**).

FURTHER READING

1. Bansal R, Kulkarni P, Gupta A, et al.: High-resolution spectral-domain optical coherence tomography and fundus autofluorescence correlation in tubercular serpiginous-like choroiditis. *J Ophthalmic Inflamm Infect* 4:157–163, 2011.
2. Gupta V, Gupta A, Sachdev N. Presumed tubercular serpiginous-like choroiditis. In: Gupta A, Gupta V, Herbort CP, Khairallah M. Uveitis Text and Imaging. Jaypee Bros Medical Publishers Ltd. chap 22; 479–491, 2009.

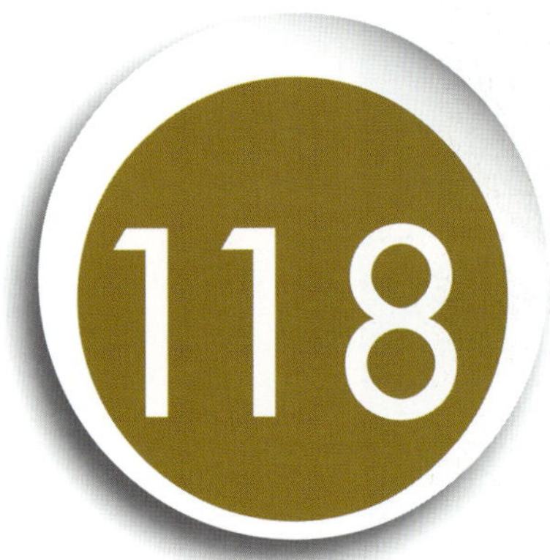

Sympathetic Ophthalmia

118

Padmamalini Mahendradas and Kavitha Avadhani

Sympathetic ophthalmia is a bilateral, diffuse, granulomatous panuveitis that occurs after trauma or surgery in one or both eyes. The eye that endures a penetrating injury or surgery and is responsible for the initiation of inflammation is known as the exciting eye, while the fellow eye with the inflammatory response is known as the sympathizing eye. The sparing of choriocapillaries is one of the classic findings in sympathetic ophthalmia. Management includes long-term corticosteroids as well as immunosuppressive agents. Visual prognosis is favorable with timely diagnosis and early initiation of immunosuppressive therapy.

CASE STUDY

A 13-year-old Indian boy with repaired open-globe injury in the right eye (Fig. 118.1) developed a granulomatous panuveitis with mutton-fat keratic precipitates (KPs), anterior chamber flare ++, cells ++ in the left eye (Fig. 118.2) 6 weeks after the ocular trauma. Fundus examination revealed vitritis ++, papillitis, extensive retinal detachment (Fig. 118.3) in the left eye. Visual acuity at presentation was no perception of light in the right eye; perception of light with accurate projection of rays in the left eye. Montage fundus fluorescein angiography (FFA) picture of the same patient showed disc leak, multiple hyperfluorescent lesions with leakage, and pooling of dye in late phase (Fig. 118.4); and indocyanine green angiography (ICGA) of the same patient showed multiple hypofluorescent lesions with staining and leakage of choroidal vessels (Fig. 118.4). Spectral-domain optical coherence tomography (SD-OCT) revealed the presence of posterior vitreous cells as well as internal limiting membrane (ILM) folds with exudative retinal detachment (Fig. 118.5) in the left eye.

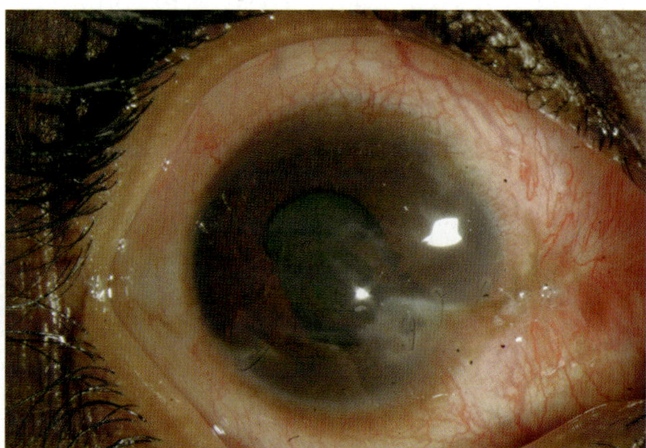

Fig. 118.1 Anterior-segment photograph of the right eye reveals sutured corneoscleral wound with complicated cataract.

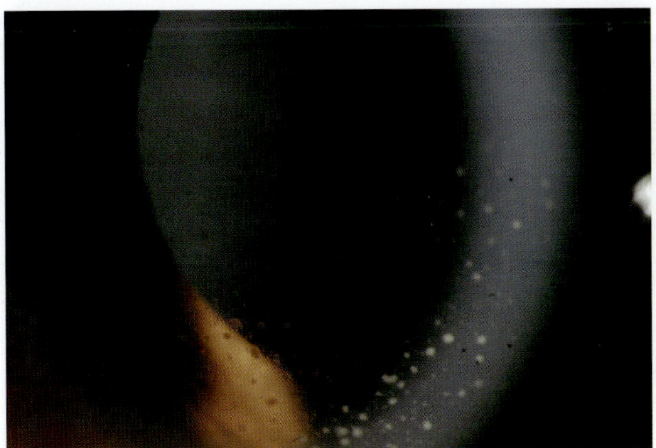

Fig. 118.2 Slit lamp microphotograph reveals the presence of medium-sized and mutton-fat keratic precipitates in the left eye.

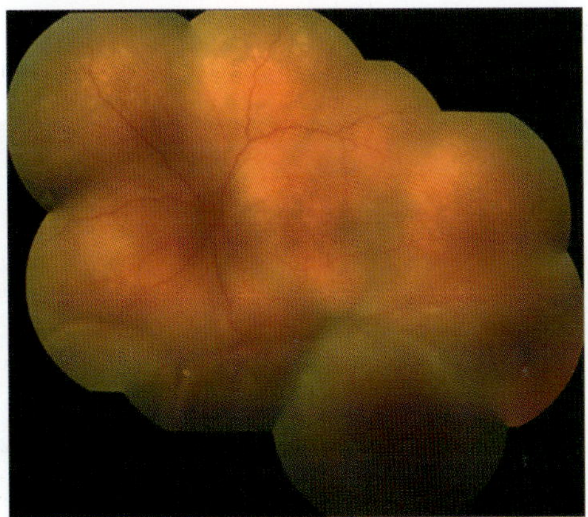

Fig. 118.3 Montage color fundus photograph of the left eye shows disc edema with exudative retinal detachment.

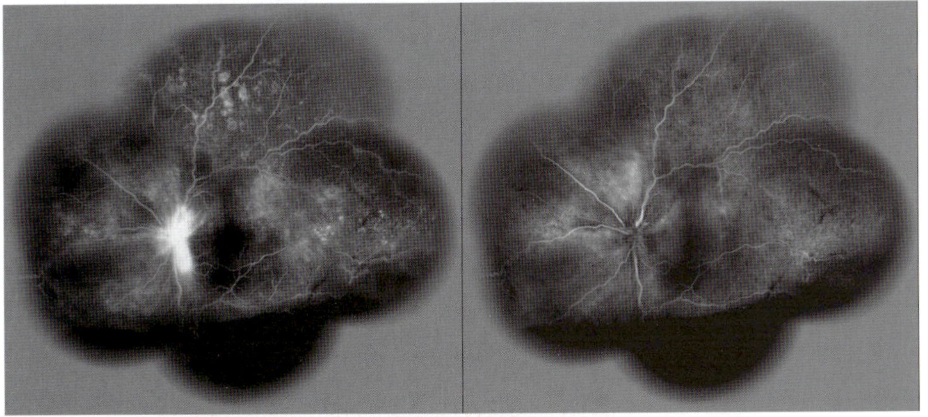

Fig. 118.4 FFA (*left panel*) reveals disc leak, multiple hyperfluorescent lesions with leakage, and pooling of the dye in late phase. Indocyanine green angiography (ICGA) (*right panel*) reveals multiple hypofluorescent lesions with staining and leakage of the choroidal vessels.

The patient was managed with topical steroids, cycloplegic agent, and intravenous methylprednisolone 1 gm/day for 3 days. Follow-up after 3 days revealed best-corrected visual acuity (BCVA) of 6/24 in the left eye with minimal inferior retinal detachment (**Fig. 118.6**). SD-OCT revealed posterior vitreous cells and ILM folds, with choroidal infiltrates (**Fig. 118.7**) in the left eye. The patient was continued on treatment with oral steroids and tablet azathioprine

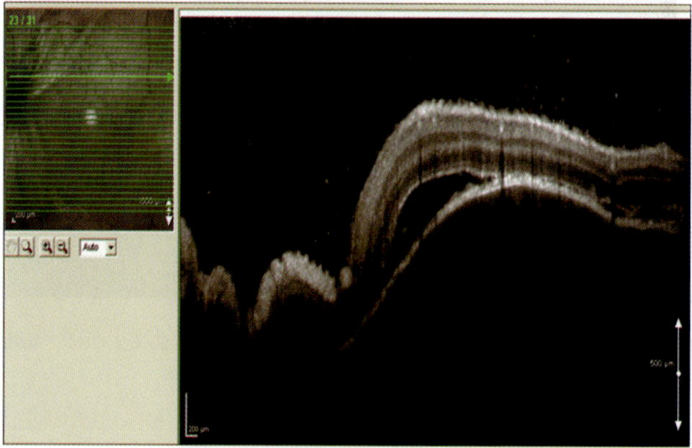

Fig. 118.5 Spectral-domain optical coherence tomography (SD-OCT) showing the presence of posterior vitreous cells, internal limiting membrane (ILM) folds along with exudative retinal detachment in the left eye.

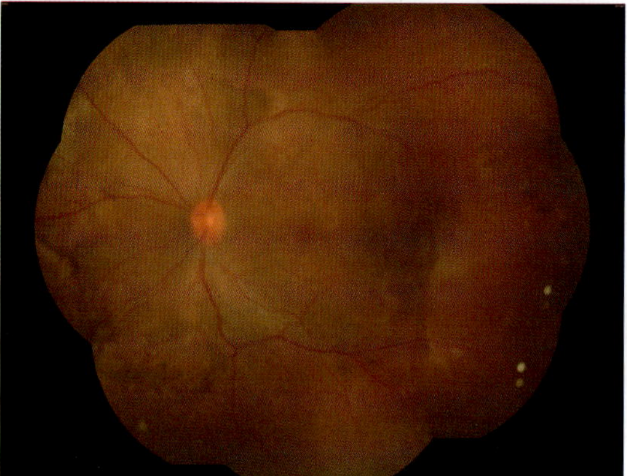

Fig. 118.6 Follow-up after 3 days of IVMP therapy shows the complete resolution of disc edema with a near total resolution of the exudative retinal detachment.

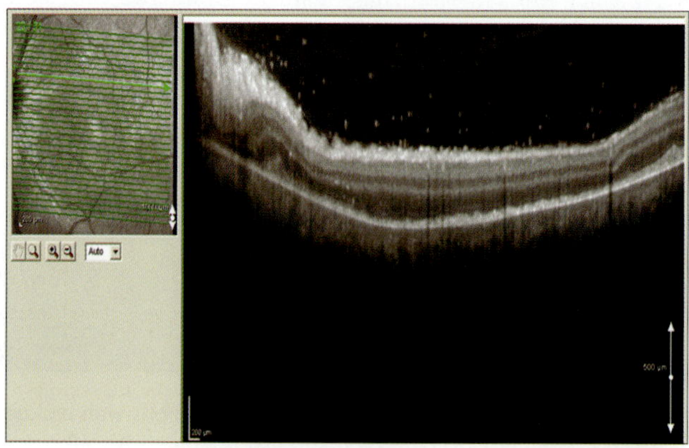

Fig. 118.7 Follow-up OCT showing the presence of posterior vitreous cells as well as ILM folds with choroidal infiltrates.

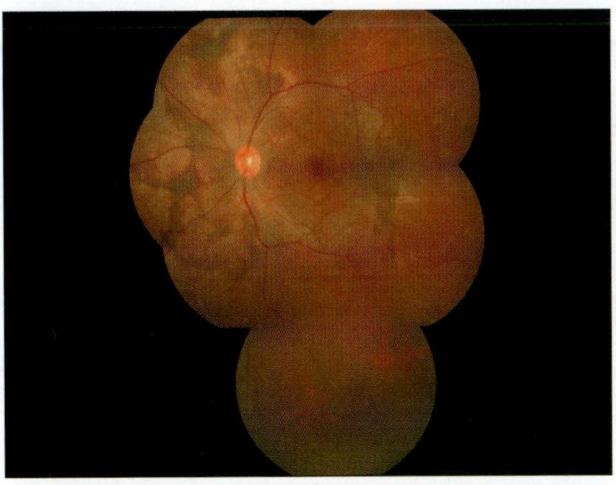

Fig. 118.8 Follow-up after 6 months showing the presence of a sunset-glow fundus with diffuse retinal pigment epithelial changes.

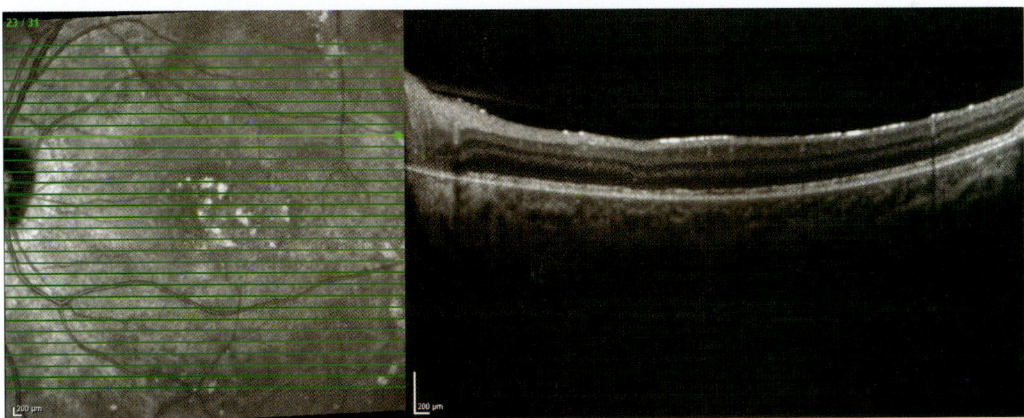

Fig. 118.9 SD-OCT at 6 months showing normal retinal thickness with the resolution of inflammation.

was added. Follow-up after 6 months revealed a sunset-glow fundus (**Fig. 118.8**) with visual acuity of 6/6 p, N6. The SD-OCT revealed altered retinal pigment epithelium (RPE) morphology with normal retinal thickness in the left eye (**Fig. 118.9**).

FURTHER READING

1. Albert DM, Diaz-Rohena R: A historical review of sympathetic ophthalmia and its epidemiology. *Surv Ophthalmol* 34:1–14, 1989.
2. Fuchs E: On sympathetic inflammation. *Graefes Arch Clin Exp Ophthalmol* 61:365–456, 1905.
3. Sharp DC, Bell RA, Patterson E, et al.: Sympathetic Ophthalmia. Histopathologic and fluorescein angiographic correlation. *Arch Ophthalmol* 102:232–235, 1984.

Toxoplasmic Retinochoroiditis

Padmamalini Mahendradas and Kavitha Avadhani

Toxoplasmic retinochoroiditis caused by *Toxoplasma gondii*, an obligate intracellular parasite, is the commonest cause of posterior uveitis in an immunocompetent patient. It can be transmitted congenitally or acquired after birth usually by ingestion of oocysts or contaminated water. Ocular toxoplasmosis generally affects younger individuals and is characterized by recurrences.

New lesions often appear adjacent to a healed chorioretinal scar and are seen as yellowish-white areas of retinitis involving the inner retinal layers often associated with intense vitritis, and adjacent choroiditis and vasculitis. Diagnosis is usually based on clinical features and serology. Polymerase chain reaction (PCR) and determination of local antibody production is useful in atypical presentations.

Antitoxoplasmic treatment along with systemic steroids is used in the management to control inflammation.

CASE STUDY 1: CONGENITAL TOXOPLASMOSIS

A 22-year-old individual, presented with a history of decreased vision in the right eye. On examination, visual acuity in the right eye was counting finger 2 meter, and in the left eye was 6/6, N6. Slit lamp biomicroscopic examination of the anterior segment revealed flare+, cells+ in anterior chamber of the right eye. Fundus examination revealed reactivated toxoplasmic retinochoroiditis (**Figs 119.1 and 119.2**) scar in the right eye. On investigation, antitoxoplasma IgG antibody was 70.21 IU/ml and IgM was negative. The patient was treated with antitoxoplasma drugs such as sulphadiazine and pyrimethamine along with systemic steroids. On follow-up, after 6 weeks, there was a healing retinochoroiditis (**Figs 119.3 and 119.4**) lesion in the right eye with visual acuity of 6/36, N18.

CASE STUDY 2: ACQUIRED TOXOPLASMOSIS

A 24-year-old female presented with a history of sudden blurring of vision in the right eye since 7 days. On examination, her best-corrected visual acuity (BCVA) was 6/12, N8 in the right eye and 6/6, N6 in the left eye. Intraocular pressure (IOP) was normal. Slit lamp biomicroscopic examination revealed medium-sized keratic precipitates flare++, cells+ and anterior vitreous cells+ in the right eye. Fundus examination (**Figs 119.5–119.7**) revealed grade 2 media haze, hyperemic disc, active focus of retinitis superotemporal to disc showing central white core representing the necrotizing

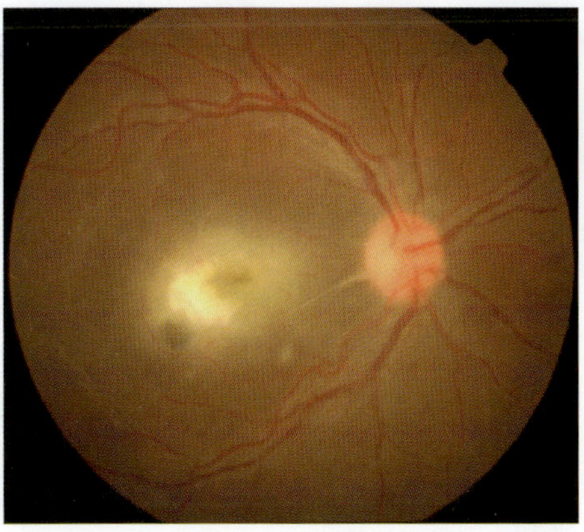

Fig. 119.1 Color fundus photograph shows hyperemic disc with active toxoplasmic retinochoroiditis lesion adjacent to a healed scar in the right eye.

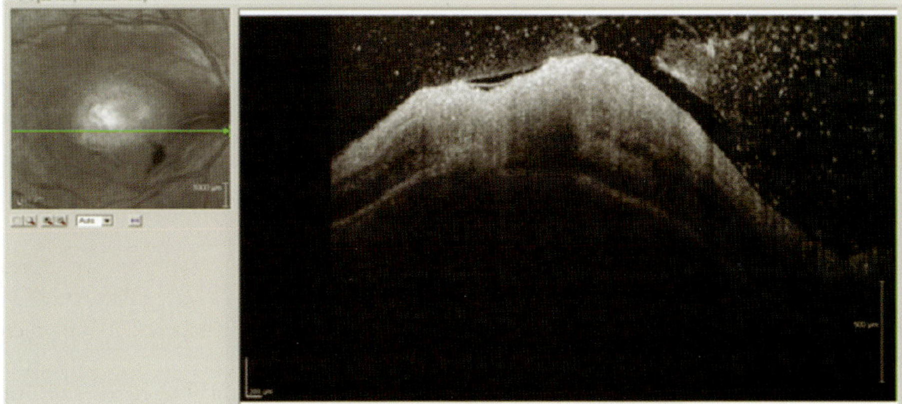

Fig. 119.2 Horizontal line scan on SD-OCT reveals the presence of posterior vitreous cells with incomplete PVD; hyperreflective lesion in the retina suggestive of active retinitis with hyporeflective lesion in the outer retina, which is suggestive of fluid-filled spaces with hyperreflective area corresponding to area of chorioretinal scar in the outer retina.

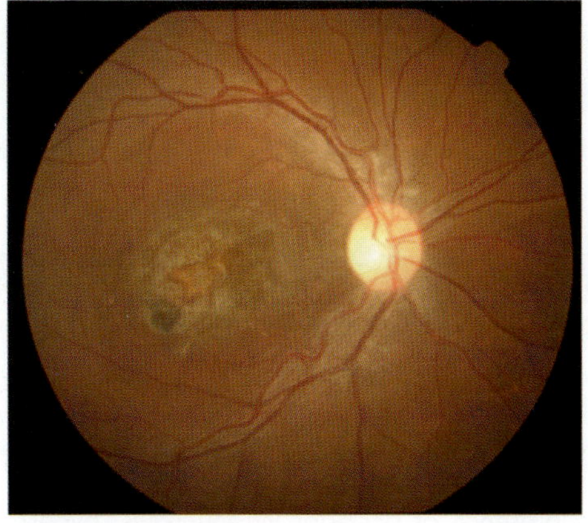

Fig. 119.3 Follow-up, color fundus photograph shows healing retinochoroiditis lesion in the right eye.

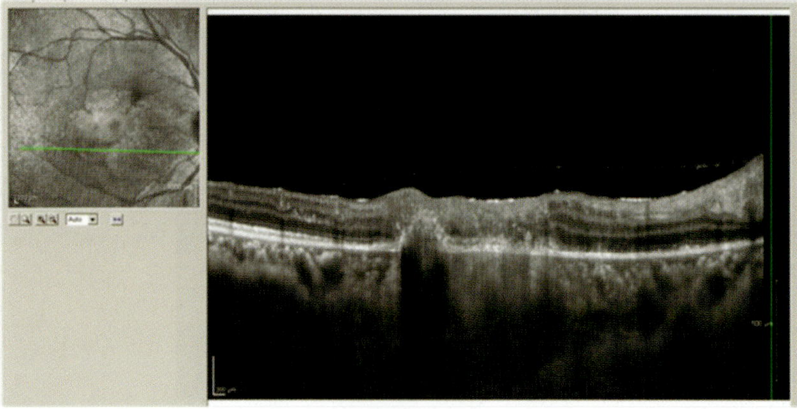

Fig. 119.4 SD-OCT horizontal line repeat scan reveals PVD, reduced posterior vitreous cells, hyperreflective disorganized retinal layers with an area of hyperreflectivity with after shadowing, suggestive of healing retinochoroiditis lesion in the right eye.

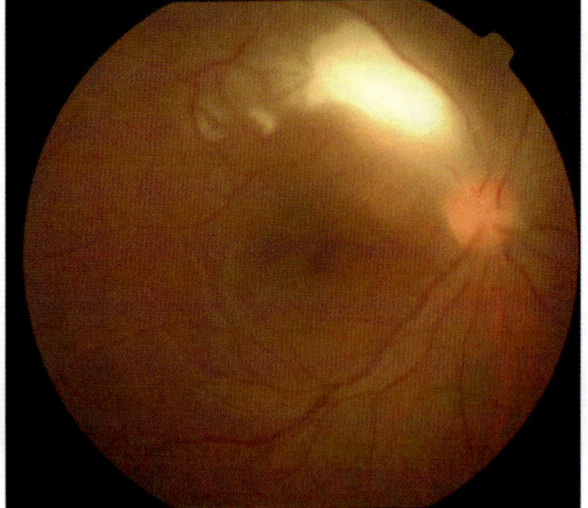

Fig. 119.5 A color fundus photograph shows hyperemic disc with active area of retinitis superotemporal to disc.

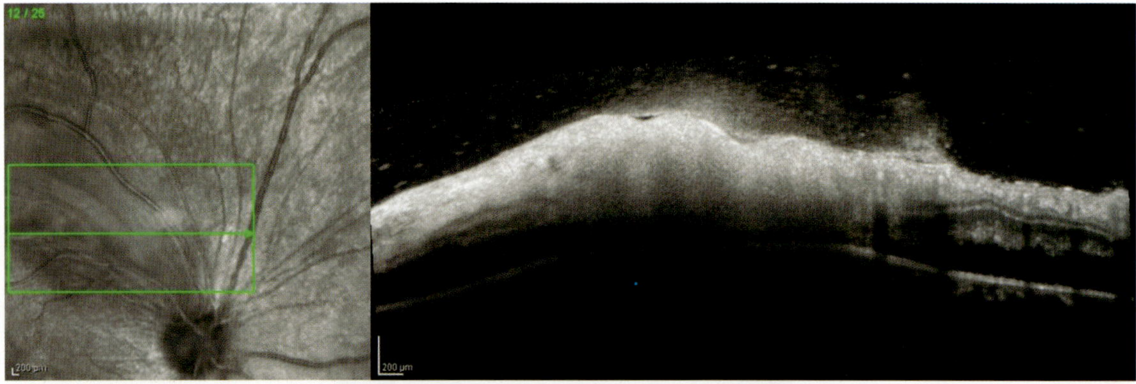

Fig. 119.6 SD-OCT showing the presence of posterior vitreous cells, hyperreflectivity in inner retinal layer with increased retinal thickness along with disorganization of retinal layers with subretinal fluid at lesion site.

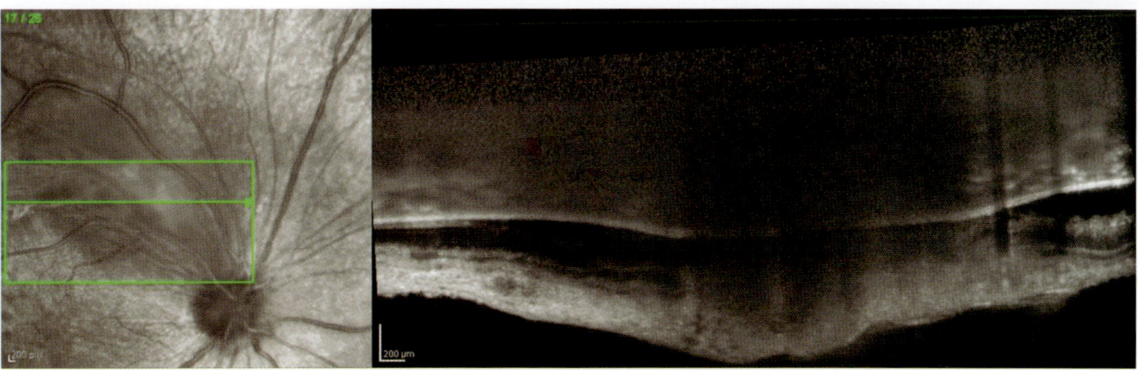

Fig. 119.7 SD-OCT EDI scan shows increased reflectivity in inner retinal layer with fluid-filled areas in outer retina with hyporeflective lesion in choroid.

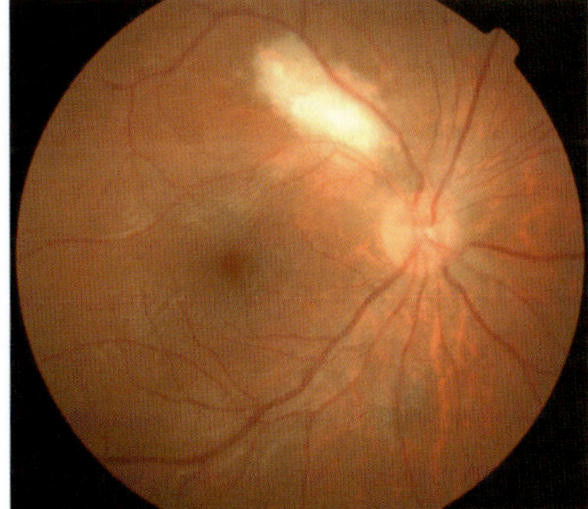

Fig. 119.8 Follow-up color fundus photograph reveals the presence of healed retinochoroiditis scar with internal limiting membrane folds in the right eye.

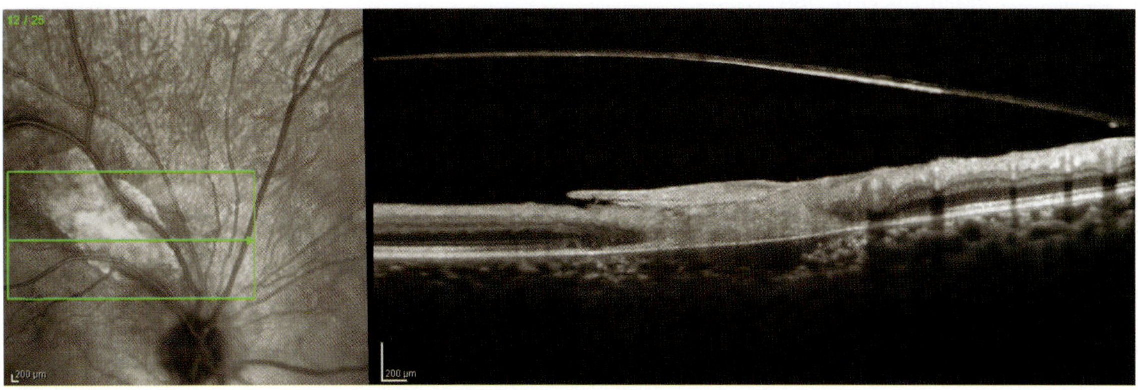

Fig. 119.9 Follow-up SD-OCT horizontal line scan shows posterior vitreous detachment, epiretinal membrane, hyperreflective disorganized retina suggestive of healed retinochoroiditis scar in the right eye.

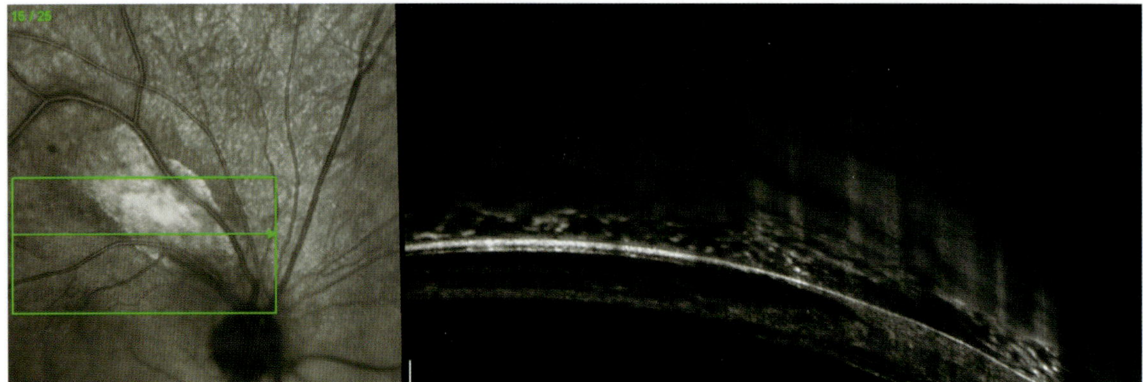

Fig. 119.10 SD-OCT–enhanced depth imaging (EDI) scan reveals epiretinal membrane (ERM), hyperreflective retinochoroidal echoes suggestive of healed chorioretinal scar.

process surrounded by retinal edema. On investigation, ELISA for antitoxo-IgM antibody was negative and IgG was 20 IU/ml (value more than 8 is considered positive). The patient gave history of allergy to sulpha drugs. She was treated with oral clindamycin, azithromycin along with systemic steroids. Following treatment her BCVA improved to 6/6, N6 with healed retinitis (**Figs 119.8–119.10**) in the right eye.

FURTHER READING

1. Cho DY, Nam W: A case of ocular toxoplasmosis imaged with spectral domain optical coherence tomography. *Korean J Ophthalmol* 26(1):58–60, 2012.
2. Diniz B, Regatieri C, Andrade R, et al.: Evaluation of spectral domain and time domain optical coherence tomography findings in toxoplasmic retinochoroiditis. *Clin Ophthalmol* 2011;5:645–650.
3. Singh M, Chee CK: Spectral domain optical coherence tomography imaging of retinal diseases in Singapore. *Ophthalmic Surg Lasers Imaging* 40(3):336–341, 2009.
4. Englander M, Young LH: Ocular toxoplasmosis: advances in detection and treatment. *Int Ophthalmol Clin* 51(4):13–23, Fall 2011.
5. Mahendradas P, Kamath G, Mahalakshmi B, et al.: Serpiginous choroiditis-like picture due to ocular toxoplasmosis. *Ocul Immunol Inflamm* 15(2):127–130, 2007.
6. Fardeau C, Romand S, Rao NA, et al.: Diagnosis of toxoplasmic retinochoroiditis with atypical clinical features. *Am J Ophthalmol* 134(2):196–203, 2002.

Vogt–Koyanagi–Harada Disease

Daniel Vitor Vasconcelos-Santos

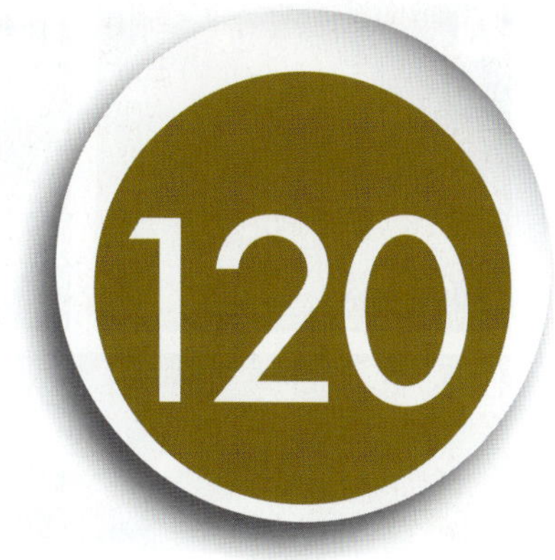

Vogt–Koyanagi–Harada disease (VKH) is a bilateral, granulomatous panuveitis associated with autoimmunity against a tyrosinase-related peptide present in melanocytes. The disease occurs especially in young women, and is more prevalent in Asian, Indian, and Hispanic ethnicities. Association of VKH with specific HLA haplotypes such as HLA-DR4/DR53, HLA-DR1, HLA-DRB1 has been consistently reported worldwide.

The disease follows two main distinct phases. The acute uveitic phase is often preceded by neurologic (headache, meningismus) and auditory (tinnitus, dysacousia) prodromes, and is characterized by diffuse granulomatous inflammation of uveal tract, resulting in bilateral exudative retinal detachments and optic disc hyperemia/edema, as along with inflammatory cells in vitreous and anterior chamber of eye.

In chronic phase, progressive depigmentation of choroid ensues, leading to typical *sunset-glow fundus* change. Extraocular depigmentation in the form of vitiligo and poliosis may also develop. Nummular atrophic scars are common in retinal periphery, in addition to variable retinal pigment epithelium (RPE) changes. Some patients evolve with relapsing intraocular inflammation (chronic recurrent stage), associated with proliferation of the RPE. Secondary glaucoma, choroidal neovascularization (CNV), and subretinal fibrosis may also complicate these cases.

Prompt and aggressive treatment is essential, using high-dose corticosteroids with very-slow tapering, in the acute phase, and a combination of corticosteroids and immunosuppressive agents, as needed, in the chronic recurrent stage.

CASE STUDY 1

A 27-year-old Brazilian female presented with suddenly decreased vision in both the eyes (hand motions), associated with headache and tinnitus. Uveitis work-up was negative, including investigations for tuberculosis and syphilis. On admission, biomicroscopy revealed small keratic precipitates (KPs), 3+ cells, and 2+ flare in anterior chamber of both the eyes. The vitreous showed 2+ cells bilaterally. Fundus examination revealed marked hyperemia and edema of optic discs along with bullous retinal detachments in both the eyes (**Figs 120.1A and D**).

Fluorescein angiography (FA) revealed multiple pinpoint leaks at level of the RPE along with progressive hyperfluorescence of the optic disc (**Figs 120.1B and C**). Echography (B-scan) disclosed bilateral diffuse choroidal thickening and spectral-domain optical coherence tomography (SD-OCT) confirmed retinal edema and serous detachment extending to macular area (**Figs 120.1E and F**).

The patient was appropriately treated with high-dose intravenous methylprednisolone followed by oral steroids, the latter with slow tapering over several months. Immunosuppressive agents were also added later. Recovery was slow, but vision eventually reached 20/20 in each eye.

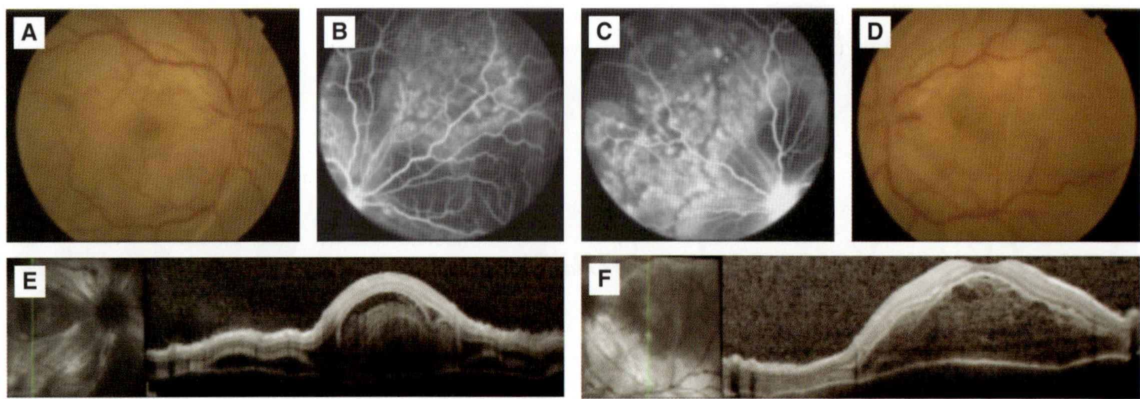

Fig. 120.1 Aspects of *Case 1*, a 27-year-old woman presenting with the acute phase of Vogt–Koyanagi–Harada disease. Fundus photographs **(A and D)** show exudative retinal detachments, and optic nerve hyperemia and edema. FA **(B and C)** reveals multiple pinpoint leaks, as well as marked disc hyperfluorescence in both the eyes. SD-OCT **(E and F)** discloses bullous retinal detachment involving maculas. The subretinal space contains partially organized hyperreflective material consistent with fibrin. Undulations in the RPE–Bruch's membrane layer support the presence of choroidal folds. Hyperreflective dots representing inflammatory cells in vitreous can also be seen close to vitreoretinal interface **(E and F)**.

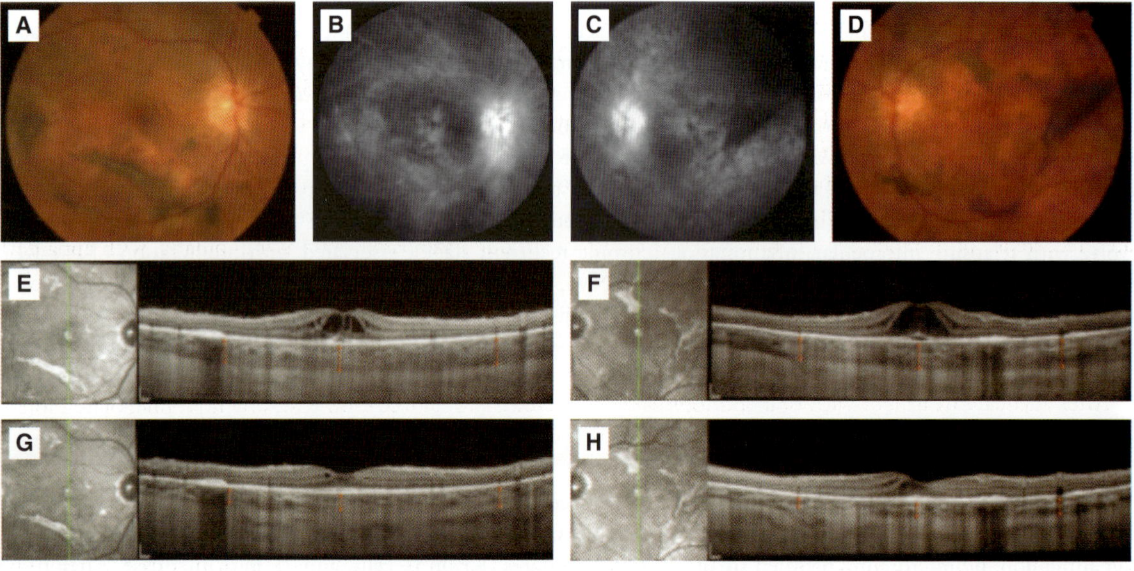

Fig. 120.2 *Case 1* in chronic phase of Vogt–Koyanagi–Harada disease after resolution of exudative retinal detachment. Fundus photographs **(A and D)** reveal reddish discoloration indicative of sunset-glow fundus change bilaterally, as well as formation of multiple irregular and sometimes curvilinear pigmented plaques (scimitar sign) associated with proliferation of RPE. Some other minor RPE changes can also be seen. FA **(B and C)** discloses perifoveal petaloid leakage consistent with cystoid macular edema in both the eyes. Optic disc hyperfluorescence as along with window defects corresponding to foci of RPE atrophy can also be observed. SD-OCT **(E and F)** delineates large cystoid spaces in central macula and even a small pocket of subfoveal fluid bilaterally. Choroidal thickening can also be appreciated on SD-OCT (*red arrows*). Foci of thickening of RPE–Bruch's membrane layer are also shown, corresponding to pigmented plaques of RPE proliferation **(E and F)**. Retinal edema almost got completely resolved and this was paralleled by a thinning of the choroids (*red arrows*) on SD-OCT **(G and H)**, 3 weeks following treatment with corticosteroids and immunosuppressants.

The patient came back complaining of decreased vision and metamorphopsia in both the eyes 3 months later, after inadvertent discontinuation of immunosuppressive therapy. Examination revealed small KPs bilaterally, 3+ cells, and 2+ flare in anterior chamber of both the eyes as well as iris nodules. There were also 2+ cells in the anterior vitreous of both the eyes. The fundus examination disclosed changes consistent with chronic VKH (**Fig. 120.2A and D**). However, FA showed bilateral perifoveal and optic disc leakage in both the eyes (**Figs 120.2B and C**). SD-OCT confirmed the presence of intraretinal cystoid spaces as well as minimal subretinal fluid bilaterally. In addition, choroidal thickening could also be appreciated on the SD-OCT (**Figs 120.2E and F**). Vision again recovered to 20/20 in each eye, with significant improvement of chorioretinal changes on the SD-OCT, 3 weeks after corticosteroid therapy, and re-initiation of azathioprine and cyclosporine (**Figs 120.2G and H**).

CASE STUDY 2

A 6-year-old Brazilian girl presented with a history of "idiopathic uveitis," previously treated with topical and oral corticosteroids. Review of systems was significant for mild poliosis of parietal region (scalp) as well as a small depigmented patch in genital area, consistent with vitiligo. Vision was 20/20 in right eye oculus dexter (OD) and 20/200 in left eye oculus sinister (OS). Anterior segment examination was normal, without any signs of intraocular inflammation in each eye.

The fundus examination of both the eyes revealed a reddish discoloration consistent with a sunset-glow fundus change. An atrophic halo could also be seen around the optic discs. Multiple RPE changes, including tiny hypopigmented and hyperpigmented spots, were also present in the fundi, as along with numerous peripheral atrophic nummular scars (**Figs 120.3A and B**). In the left eye, an elevated and partially pigmented grayish subretinal lesion consistent with the CNV could also be seen nasal to the fovea, associated with minor overlying retinal edema. Pigmented patches were also observed nasally to the left optic disc (**Fig. 120.3B**).

The right eye had a normal macular area on the SD-OCT, despite subtle RPE changes (**Fig. 120.3C**). The SD-OCT of the left eye, on the other hand, disclosed a highly reflective subretinal structure consistent with a fibrotic neovascular membrane (**Fig. 120.3D**). A small amount of overlying intraretinal fluid was also present. Outer retinal structure was clearly disrupted in the left foveal area (**Figs 120.3D and F**).

Based on clinical findings, the patient was diagnosed with chronic VKH, but no anti-inflammatory therapy was initiated at that time because of lack of signs of an active process. However, on a regular follow-up visit 2 months later, recurrence of intraocular inflammation was detected; although the patient was asymptomatic, with apparently quiet eyes and maintained visual acuity. Slit lamp biomicroscopy then showed anterior chamber cells (3+) and flare (2+), in addition to small keratic precipitates and iris nodules. Vitreous cavity had also 2+ cells. Fundus examination was stable and retinal morphology was unaltered on the SD-OCT, when compared to previous examination. The choroids, however, were significantly increased in thickness (**Figs 120.3G and F**).

After adequate treatment with oral and topical corticosteroids, in combination with oral mycophenolate mofetil, intraocular inflammation resolved and choroidal thickness decreased to baseline levels.

VKH is a potentially severe disorder, frequently diagnosed in the acute phase when exudative retinal detachments and inflammation of the optic disc result in markedly decreased vision bilaterally, as seen in first case. After ruling out infectious etiologies, as well as posterior scleritis, aggressive therapy with systemic corticosteroids should be promptly initiated and tapered over several months.

However, some patients may present in the chronic phase (with acute phase having been "overlooked") and in these individuals, the presence of the sunset-glow fundus changes (and the peripheral nummular atrophic scars) are an important clue to diagnosis, as seen in second case. In chronic phase, some individuals not only develop relapsing episodes of intraocular inflammation, with anterior chamber and vitreous inflammatory cells, but also choroidal thickening, which can be followed by the SD-OCT. Persistent intraocular inflammation may lead to proliferation and even fibrous metaplasia of the RPE, resulting in subretinal fibrosis. The CNV is also another common sight-threatening complication, in addition to glaucoma and cataract. Advanced cases may eventually develop extensive chorioretinal atrophy.

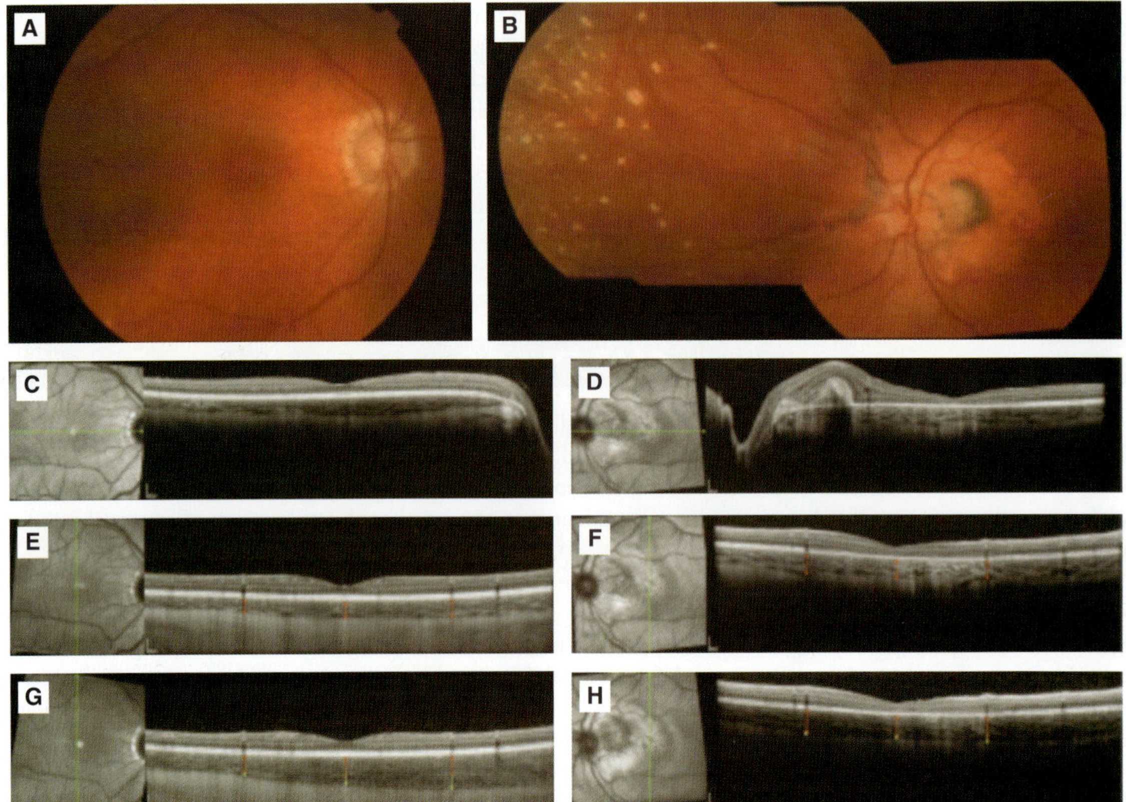

Fig. 120.3 Aspects of *Case 2*, a 6-year-old girl diagnosed in chronic phase of Vogt–Koyanagi–Harada disease. Fundus photographs **(A and B)** depict sunset-glow fundi. Peridiscal atrophic haloes along with multiple peripheral atrophic nummular scars can also be seen. The left eye also shows a pigmented curved plaque nasally (scimitar sign) and a partially pigmented gray-whitish lesion deep to maculodiscal bundle, consistent with fibrotic choroidal neovascular (CNV) membrane **(B)**. SD-OCT at baseline examination reveals normal retinochoroidal architecture in the right eye **(C and E)** and a hyperreflective subretinal lesion representing a fibrotic CNV in left eye; a small amount of overlying intraretinal fluid can also be appreciated **(D)**. At left fovea, outer retinal structure is completely disrupted, with discontinuation of bands corresponding to junction of inner and outer segments of photoreceptors (IS–OS junction), external limiting membrane, and even outer nuclear layer **(D and F)**. At that time, there was no sign of active intraocular inflammation. However, patient returned to a follow-up visit 2 months later, with inflammatory cells in anterior chamber and vitreous cavity of both the eyes. Despite relatively stable retinal profile, choroids were markedly thickened [*red arrows demarcate baseline thickness; green arrows indicate increase in thickness* **(G and H)**].

FURTHER READING

1. Fong AH, Li KK, Wong D: Choroidal evaluation using enhanced depth imaging spectral-domain optical coherence tomography in Vogt–Koyanagi–Harada disease. *Retina* 31(3):502–509, 2011.
2. Heussen FM, Vasconcelos-Santos DV, Pappuru RR, et al.: Ultra-wide-field green-light (532 nm) autofluorescence imaging in chronic Vogt–Koyanagi–Harada disease. *Ophthalmic Surg Lasers Imaging* 42(4):272–277, 2011.
3. Moorthy RS, Inomata H, Rao NA: Vogt–Koyanagi–Harada syndrome. *Surv Ophthalmol* 39(4):265–292, 1995.
4. Rao NA, Gupta A, Dustin L, et al.: Frequency of distinguishing clinical features in Vogt–Koyanagi–Harada disease. *Ophthalmology* 117(3):591–599, 9 e1, 2010.
5. Rao NA: Pathology of Vogt–Koyanagi–Harada disease. *Int Ophthalmol* 27(2–3):81–85, 2007.
6. Vasconcelos-Santos DV, Sohn EH, Sadda S, et al.: Retinal pigment epithelial changes in chronic Vogt–Koyanagi–Harada disease: fundus autofluorescence and spectral-domain optical coherence tomography findings. *Retina* 30(1):33–41, 2010.

Acknowledgments: Prof. Fernando Orefice and Centro Brasileiro de Ciências Visuais.

Index

let us be social

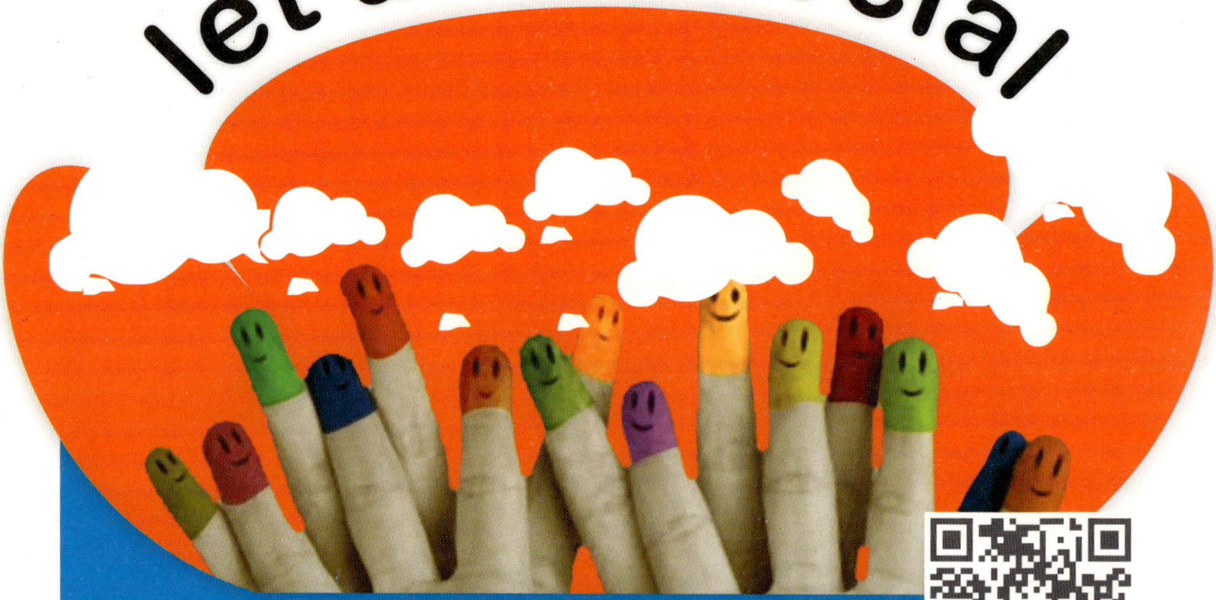

Join India's largest health professionals and students community at facebook.com/ElsevierIndia

- Latest and most relevant information
- Exciting competitions
- Invitations to author events and group discussions
- Connect with your peers and start thought provoking discussions
- Feed us back to make our products more suited to your needs

Connect with us!

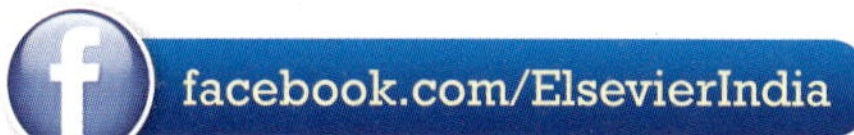

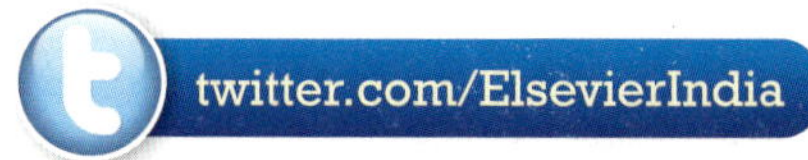

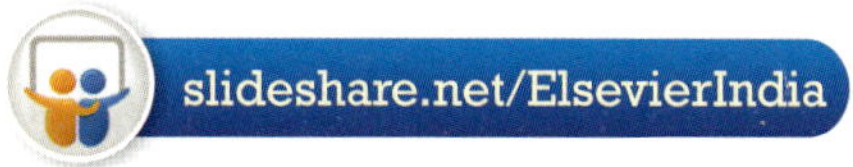

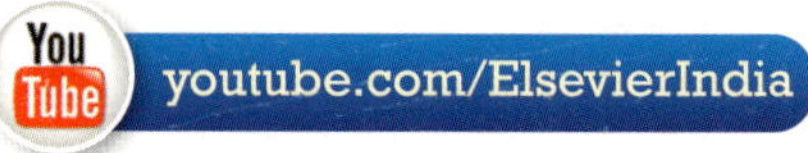

Can't find Elsevier Books? Call/SMS **+91-8527622422**

To know more, please visit **www.elsevier.co.in**

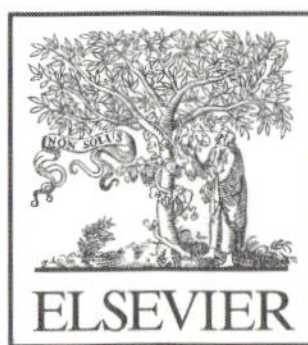